First Aid
Manual

Authorised by the

Irish   ORDER
Red Cross   OF MALTA

First Aid
Manual

Dr Andrew Kelly DCH DObs MICGP
Chief Medical Adviser, Irish Red Cross

DK

LONDON, NEW YORK, MUNICH, MELBOURNE, DELHI

St. John Ambulance, a registered charity, St. Andrew's Ambulance Association, a registered
charity in Scotland, and the British Red Cross Society, a registered charity, receive a royalty
for every copy of this book sold by Dorling Kindersley. Details of the royalties payable to
the Societies can be obtained by writing to the publishers, Dorling Kindersley Limited at
80 Strand, London WC2R 0RL. For the purposes of the Charities Act 1992 no further seller
of the Manual shall be deemed to be a commercial participator with these three Societies.

SENIOR EDITOR	Janet Mohun
EDITOR	Katie John
PROJECT ART EDITOR	Janice English
ART EDITOR	Sara Freeman
DESIGN ASSISTANT	Iona Hoyle
DTP DESIGNER	Julian Dams
CONSULTANT MANAGING EDITOR	Jemima Dunne
MANAGING ART EDITOR	Louise Dick
PRODUCTION CONTROLLER	Rita Sinha
PRODUCTION MANAGER	Michelle Thomas
ILLUSTRATOR	Richard Tibbitts
PHOTOGRAPHER	Gary Ombler

Text revised in line with the latest guidelines from the American Heart Association.
Note: The masculine pronoun "he" is used when referring to the first aider or casualty, unless the individual
shown in the photograph is female. This is for convenience and clarity and does not reflect a preference for either sex.

This Irish edition first published in Ireland in 2003 by Dorling Kindersley Limited
Eighth edition first published in Great Britain in 2002 by
Dorling Kindersley Limited, 80 Strand, London WC2R 0RL

A Penguin Company

6 8 10 9 7

Illustration copyright © 2002, 2003 Dorling Kindersley Limited, except as listed in acknowledgments, p.288
Text copyright © 2002, 2003 St. John Ambulance;
St. Andrew's Ambulance Association; The British Red Cross Society

A CIP catalogue record for this book is available from
the British Library

ISBN 0 7513 4964 X (Paperback)

Reproduced in Singapore by Colourscan
Printed and bound in Slovakia by TBB s.r.o.

See our complete catalogue at
www.dk.com

FOREWORD

With the onset of the new millennium, the value of
first aid skills as a means of personal and community
empowerment is emphasised in new ways. In Ireland
health service reforms, first responder schemes in rural
communities, public access defibrillation, and increased
emphasis on primary care combine to underscore the
importance of ensuring a wide knowledge of current
first aid actions.

This new 8th edition *First Aid Manual* is the standard
reference in the home, sports ground, workplace, and
community. It has been extensively updated with the
latest public resuscitation measures.

Given the practical nature of first aid, the skills
of emergency actions are best practised at a recognised
first aid course. For details of Irish Red Cross basic or
occupational first aid courses contact your local
Branch or National Head Office.

IRISH RED CROSS

CONTENTS

2 TECHNIQUES AND EQUIPMENT   39

3 LIFE-SAVING PROCEDURES   71

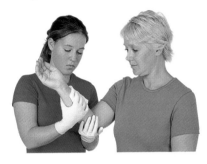

8 NERVOUS SYSTEM PROBLEMS 175

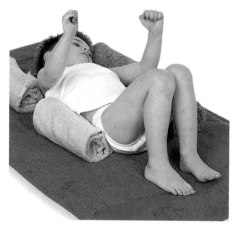

9 ENVIRONMENTAL INJURIES 189

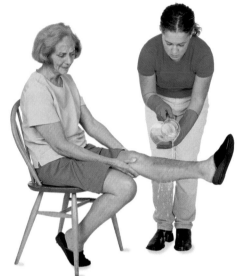

10 FOREIGN OBJECTS 209

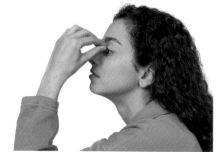

INTRODUCTION

This publication is the authorised manual of the Irish Red Cross and Order of Malta. They have endeavoured to ensure that it reflects the relevant guidance from informed authoritative sources, which is current at the time of publication. The material contained in this manual provides guidance on initial care and treatment but must not be regarded as a substitute for medical advice.

Neither the Irish Red Cross nor Order of Malta accepts responsibility for any claims arising from the use of this manual when the guidelines have not been followed. First aiders are advised to keep up to date with developments, to recognise the limits of their competence, and to obtain first-aid training from a qualified trainer.

The first part of this book enables you to look at your role as a first aider and become competent in the techniques you will need to use, including life-saving procedures for all age groups. Specific problems are described in more detail in relevant chapters.

The emergency first-aid section at the back of the book gives you at-a-glance action plans for all emergency situations. It is also provided as a separate booklet for you to keep in your first-aid kit or to carry with you at all times.

HOW TO USE THIS BOOK

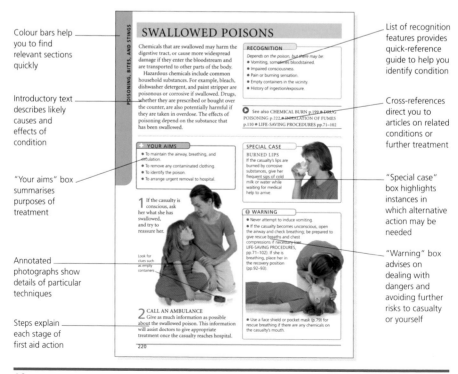

Colour bars help you to find relevant sections quickly

Introductory text describes likely causes and effects of condition

"Your aims" box summarises purposes of treatment

Annotated photographs show details of particular techniques

Steps explain each stage of first aid action

List of recognition features provides quick-reference guide to help you identify condition

Cross-references direct you to articles on related conditions or further treatment

"Special case" box highlights instances in which alternative action may be needed

"Warning" box advises on dealing with dangers and avoiding further risks to casualty or yourself

1

FIRST AID is the initial assistance or treatment given to someone who is injured or suddenly taken ill. This chapter describes the sequence of priorities for giving first aid, providing essential information on how to deal with emergencies, and how to look after yourself. It also covers the steps involved in assessing and treating a casualty.

LEARNING FIRST-AID SKILLS
By following the guidance in this book, most people can give effective first aid. However, to become a fully competent first aider you should complete a programme of study and gain an appropriate certificate. The standard first-aid certificate is awarded by the Irish Red Cross and the Order of Malta. The certificate is valid for 3 years and to maintain it you must be reassessed.

✚ FIRST-AID PRIORITIES

- Assess the situation quickly and calmly.
- Protect yourself and the casualties from danger.
- Assess the conditions of all casualties.
- Comfort and reassure the casualties.
- Deal with any life-threatening conditions.
- Obtain medical aid if necessary. Call an ambulance if you suspect a serious illness or injury.

CONTENTS

BEING A FIRST AIDER

The first aid learned from a manual or study programme is not quite like reality. Most of us feel apprehensive when dealing with "the real thing". By facing up to these feelings, we are better able to cope with the unexpected.

DOING YOUR BEST

First aid is not an exact science and is open to human error. Even with appropriate treatment, and however hard you try, a casualty may not respond as you hoped. Some conditions are inevitably fatal, even with the best medical care. If you do your best, your conscience can be clear.

ASSESSING RISKS

The golden rule is, "First do no harm", while applying the principle of "calculated risk". You should use the treatment that is most likely to be of benefit to a casualty, but do not use a treatment that you are not sure about just for the sake of doing something.

The principle of the "Good Samaritan" supports those who act in an emergency situation to provide help to others but not those who go beyond accepted boundaries. If you remain calm, and you follow the guidelines set out in this book, you need not fear any legal consequences.

Your responsibilities

The first aider's responsibilities are clearly defined. They are as follows:
- To assess a situation quickly and safely, and summon appropriate help.
- To protect casualties and others at the scene from possible danger.
- To identify, as far as possible, the injury or nature of the illness affecting a casualty.
- To give each casualty early and appropriate treatment, treating the most serious conditions first.

- To arrange for the casualty's removal to hospital, into the care of a doctor, or to his home as necessary.
- If medical aid is needed, to remain with a casualty until further care is available.
- To report your observations to those taking over care of the casualty, and to give further assistance if required.
- To prevent cross-infection between yourself and the casualty as far as possible (p.15).

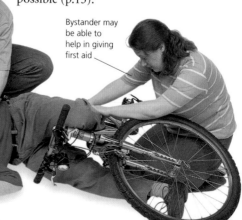

Talk to casualty to reassure him and obtain information about his condition

Bystander may be able to help in giving first aid

Treat casualty in position found

Assess the situation
Ask the casualty and any bystanders what has happened. Try to identify his injuries and treat urgent ones first. Do not move him unless it is absolutely necessary.

Giving care with confidence

Every casualty needs to feel secure and in safe hands. You can create an air of confidence and assurance by:
- Being in control both of your own reactions and of the problem.
- Acting calmly and logically.
- Being gentle, but firm.
- Speaking to the casualty kindly but in a clear and purposeful way.

BUILDING UP TRUST
While performing your examination and treatment, talk to the casualty throughout.
- Explain what you are going to do.
- Try to answer questions honestly to allay fears as best you can. If you do not know the answer, say so.
- Continue to reassure the casualty, even when the treatment is finished. In addition, find out about the next of kin, or anyone else who should be contacted about the incident. Ask if you can help to make arrangements so that any responsibilities the casualty may have, such as collecting a child from school, can be taken care of.
- Do not leave someone whom you believe to be dying, seriously ill, or badly injured. Continue to talk to the casualty, and hold his hand; never allow the person to feel alone.

TALKING TO RELATIVES
The task of informing relatives of a death is usually the job of the police or the doctor on duty. However, it may well be that you have to tell relatives or friends that someone has been injured or taken ill. Always make sure that you are speaking to the right person first. Then explain, as simply and honestly as you can, what has happened and, if appropriate, where the casualty has been taken. Do not be vague or exaggerate because this may cause unnecessary alarm. It is better to admit ignorance than to give someone misleading information about an injury or illness.

COPING WITH CHILDREN
Young children are extremely perceptive and will quickly detect any uncertainty on your part. Gain an injured or sick child's confidence by talking first to someone he trusts – a parent if possible. If the parent accepts you and believes you will help, this confidence will be conveyed to the child. Always explain simply to a child what is happening and what you intend to do; do not talk over his head. You should not separate a child from his mother, father, or other trusted person.

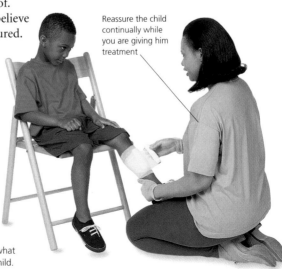

Reassure the child continually while you are giving him treatment

Giving first aid to a child
Try to make a child feel comfortable and confident with your treatment. Always explain what you are doing, no matter what the age of the child.

LOOKING AFTER YOURSELF

When carrying out first aid, it is important for you to protect yourself from injury and infection. One of the primary rules of first aid is to ensure that the situation is safe before treating a casualty. Bear in mind that infection may be a risk, even with relatively minor injuries, so you need to take steps to avoid contracting an infection from a casualty or passing on any infection that you have. In addition, you need to look after your psychological health and try to deal with stress effectively (p.16).

Personal safety

Do not attempt heroic rescues in hazardous circumstances. If you put yourself at risk, you are unlikely to be able to help casualties effectively. Always assess the situation first and make sure that the situation you are entering is safe for you (p.18).

THE "FIGHT OR FLIGHT RESPONSE"
In an emergency, your body responds by releasing certain hormones in the "fight or flight" response. When you experience this response, your heart beats faster, and your breathing is deeper and more rapid. You may also notice that you are sweating more than usual and that you are more alert.

STAYING CALM
Sometimes too great a rush of hormones may affect your ability to cope with a situation. Taking slow, deep breaths will help you to calm down, leaving you better able to remember your first-aid procedures.

Protection from infection

An important part of first aid is preventing "cross infection" (either transmitting germs to a casualty or contracting an infection yourself). This is a particular concern if you are treating open wounds.

Often, simple measures, such as washing your hands and wearing disposable gloves, will provide sufficient protection. There is a risk of infection with blood-borne viruses such as hepatitis B or C and Human Immunodeficiency Virus (HIV), but these viruses can only be transmitted by blood-to-blood contact – if an infected person's blood makes contact with yours through, for example, a cut or graze. There is no known evidence of hepatitis or HIV being transmitted during resuscitation.

IMMUNISATION
It is recommended that all first aiders are immunised against hepatitis B. Currently, there is no vaccine against hepatitis C or HIV. If you think you have been exposed to any infection after giving first aid, seek medical aid immediately.

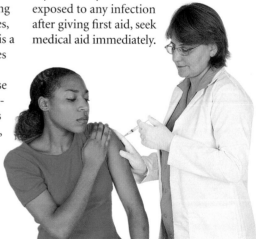

Protection from hepatitis B
All first aiders should be protected by immunisation against hepatitis B. The vaccine is given as a series of three injections in the upper arm.

Guidelines for preventing cross infection

Following good practice guidelines will help to prevent the spread of infection.

- If facilities are available, wash your hands thoroughly with soap and water before treating a casualty.
- If possible, carry protective disposable gloves with you at

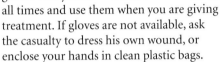

all times and use them when you are giving treatment. If gloves are not available, ask the casualty to dress his own wound, or enclose your hands in clean plastic bags.

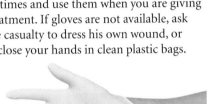

- Cover cuts and grazes on your hands with waterproof dressings.
- Wear a plastic apron when dealing with large quantities of body fluids, and wear plastic glasses to protect your eyes.
- Avoid touching a wound or touching any part of a dressing that will come into contact with a wound.
- Try not to breathe, cough, or sneeze over a wound while you are treating a casualty.
- Take care not to prick yourself with any needle found on or near a casualty or cut yourself on glass.
- If a face shield or pocket mask is available, use it when giving rescue breaths (p.79).
- Dispose of all waste safely (below).

> **⚠ WARNING**
>
> If you accidentally prick or cut your skin or splash your eyes, wash the area thoroughly and seek medical help immediately.

Dealing with waste

Once you have finished treatment, dispose of all waste material carefully to prevent the spread of infection. Place soiled items and used gloves in a plastic bag; ideally, use a special yellow bag called a biohazard bag. To dispose of sharp objects, such as needles, you should use a specially designed plastic container called a sharps container. Seal the

bag or container tightly, and label it to show that it contains clinical waste.

Biohazard bags should be destroyed by burning (incineration). If you do not have access to incineration facilities, ask your local ambulance service or local authority environmental health department how to deal with this type of waste.

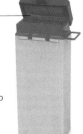

Lid can be locked or sealed after use

Sharps container
This is a plastic box designed to hold used needles and other sharp items for safe disposal. Sharps containers are usually yellow.

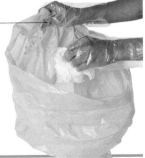

Keep gloves on until you have finished disposing of waste, then dispose of gloves

Using a biohazard bag
If you have a yellow biohazard bag available, you should use the bag to dispose safely of waste items such as soiled dressings. The bag should then be sealed and incinerated.

LOOKING AFTER YOURSELF (continued)

Dealing with stress

It is natural to feel stressed when you are called upon to administer first aid and to be very emotional once you have finished treating the casualty. Stress can interfere with a person's physical and mental well-being. Some people are more susceptible to stress than others. It is important to learn how to deal with stress to maintain your own health and effectiveness as a first aider.

FEELINGS AFTER AN INCIDENT
For all first aiders, an emergency is an emotional experience. Emotional reactions can include satisfaction or even elation, but it is more common to feel upset. After you have treated a casualty – depending on the type of incident and the outcome – you might experience:
● Satisfaction and pleasure.
● Confusion and doubt.
● Anger and sadness.
Never reproach yourself or try to hide your feelings. It is much more helpful to talk over your experience with a colleague, your line manager, your first-aid trainer, or your own doctor in the first instance. By doing so you will probably find that your feelings about the incident resolve quickly. Ideally, speak to someone else who was present at the incident because both of you may be having similar feelings.

DELAYED REACTIONS
Involvement in an incident can lead to a delayed stress reaction once you have returned to your everyday environment. The extent of the effect may depend on the level of your first-aid experience and the nature of the incident. In the longer term, stress can manifest itself in many different ways, including:
● Tremor of the hands and stomach.
● Excessive sweating.
● Flashbacks of the incident.
● Nightmares or disturbed sleep.
● Tearfulness.
● Tension and irritability.
● A feeling of withdrawal and isolation.
These symptoms should pass in time. Exercise or relaxation techniques, such as meditation or yoga, may help. In fact, doing any activity that you enjoy is a good way to relax and may help you to relieve tension.

SEVERE STRESS REACTIONS
If you have witnessed or experienced a serious threat to life, you may find yourself suffering from severe feelings of stress for some time after the incident. You might be:
● Reliving the event.
● Avoiding situations, people, and places associated with the event.
● Feeling hyperactive and restless.
If you experience intrusive or persistent symptoms associated with a stressful incident, it is important that you seek medical help from your doctor or possibly from a counsellor.

Talking to a friend
Face up to what has happened by confiding in a friend or relative. Ideally, talk to someone who also attended the incident; they may have the same feelings as you.

REGULATIONS AND LEGISLATION

First aid may be practised in any situation where accidents or illnesses have occurred. In many instances, the first person on the scene is a volunteer who wants to help, rather than someone who is medically trained. That person may or may not have knowledge of first-aid procedures and treatments. However, in some circumstances the provision of first aid, and first-aid responsibilities are defined by statutes. In the Republic of Ireland, these apply to the workplace and to mass gatherings.

First aid at work

The Safety, Health and Welfare at Work (General Application) Regulations, 1993 (S. I. No. 44 of 1993) place a general duty on employers to make first-aid provision for employees in case of injury or illness at the workplace.

Employers have a duty to provide first-aid equipment at all places of work where working conditions require it. Depending on the size and/or specific hazards of the undertaking or establishment, occupational first aiders must also be provided.

Necessary external contacts must be made as regards first-aid and emergency medical care. Information must be provided to employees and/or safety representatives as regards first-aid facilities and arrangements in place.

Occupational first-aiders are required to be trained and certified as competent at least once every three years by a recognised occupational first-aid instructor.

RECORDING FIRST-AID TREATMENT
Following an incident, the following details should be noted:
- full name and address of the casualty;
- the casualty's occupation;
- date when the entry was made;
- date and time of the incident;
- place and circumstances of the incident (describe the work process being performed by the casualty at the time);
- details concerning the injury and the treatment given;
- signature of the person making the entry.

First aid at mass gatherings

The Hamilton report was published in 1990 following the Hillsborough football ground disaster. This report made many recommendations and stated that there should be a standard approach to the provision of medical and first-aid facilities at sports stadiums and at other events where large numbers of people gather for recreational activity.

The recommendations made in the Report included:
- at least one trained first aider per 2,500 people;

- at least one approved and designated first-aid room;
- at least two doctors at any event, one of whom should be Site Medical Officer;
- one fully equipped ambulance, at any event with an expected crowd of 5,000;
- medical staff should have recognisable identification, access to public address systems, and secure communication lines.

The responsibility for providing the necessary level of first aid facilities rests with the promoter of the event.

ACTION AT AN EMERGENCY

In any emergency, you must follow a clear plan of action. This will enable you to prioritise the demands that may be made on you and help you decide on your response. The principal steps are: Assess the situation, Make the area safe, Give emergency aid, and Get help from others (below).

Before taking any action, try to control your feelings and take a moment to think. It is important to avoid placing yourself in danger, so do not rush into a potentially risky situation. Be aware of hazards such as petrol or gas. In addition, do not attempt to do too much by yourself.

FIRST-AID PRIORITIES
● Assess the situation. Quickly and calmly, observe what has happened, and look for dangers to yourself and to the casualty. Never put yourself at risk.
● Make the area safe. Protect the casualty from danger as far as you can, but be aware of your limitations.
● Give emergency aid. Assess all casualties to determine treatment priorities, and treat those with life-threatening conditions first.
● Get help from others. Quickly make sure that any necessary medical aid or other expert help has been called and is on its way.

Assess the situation

Your approach should be brisk but calm and controlled. Your priorities are to identify any risks to yourself, to the casualty, and to bystanders, then to assess the resources available to you and the kind of help you may need. When offering your help, state that you have first-aid skills. If there are no doctors, nurses, or similarly experienced people present, calmly take charge. First, ask yourself these questions:
● Is there any continuing danger?
● Is anyone's life in immediate danger?
● Are there any bystanders who can help?
● Do I need specialist help?

Make the area safe

The conditions that gave rise to the incident may still be presenting a danger. Remember that you must put your own safety first. Often, simple measures, such as turning off a switch, are enough to make the area safe. If you cannot eliminate a life-threatening hazard, you should try to put some distance between it and the casualty and minimise the danger if possible. As a last resort, you should remove the casualty from the danger (*see* CASUALTY HANDLING, pp.63–64). Usually, you will need specialist help and equipment to move a casualty.

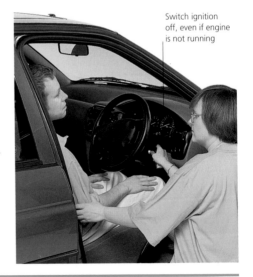

Switch ignition off, even if engine is not running

Making a vehicle safe
The first priority, when dealing with a casualty who is inside a vehicle, is to switch the ignition off. This action will reduce the risk of a spark causing a fire.

Give emergency aid

Once the area has been made safe, quickly carry out an initial assessment, or primary survey, of each casualty (p.29) so that any casualty needing emergency first aid is treated immediately. However, do not delay in summoning necessary help; if possible, ask a bystander to do this.

For each casualty, establish the following:
● Is he conscious?
● Is his airway open?
● Is he breathing?
● Does he have signs of circulation?
Your findings dictate your priorities and when and how much help is needed.

▶ **See also PRIMARY SURVEY p.29**

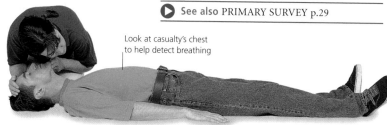

Carrying out emergency aid
As soon as it is safe to do so, carry out a primary survey: check that the casualty has an open airway, is breathing, and has signs of circulation.

Look at casualty's chest to help detect breathing

Get help from others

You may be faced with several tasks: to maintain safety, to call for help (overleaf), and to start first aid. Other people can be asked to perform the following functions:
● Make the area safe.
● Telephone for assistance.
● Fetch first-aid equipment.
● Control traffic and onlookers.
● Control bleeding or support a limb.
● Maintain the casualty's privacy.
● Transport the casualty to a safe place.

CONTROLLING BYSTANDERS
The reactions of bystanders may cause you concern or even anger. They may have had no first-aid training and may feel helpless or frightened. If they have witnessed or been involved in the incident themselves, they too may be injured and will certainly be distressed. Bear this in mind if you need to ask a bystander to help you in some way. Use a firm but gentle manner.

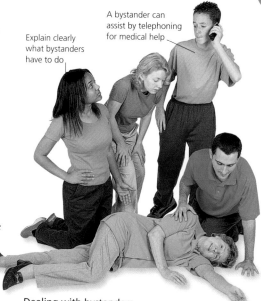

A bystander can assist by telephoning for medical help

Explain clearly what bystanders have to do

Dealing with bystanders
People at the scene of an incident may be able to help you in several ways, such as fetching equipment or controlling other onlookers. Tell them that you have first-aid training, and be clear in what you ask.

TELEPHONING FOR HELP

You can summon help by telephone from a number of sources.

- Emergency services (dial the European Union emergency number 112, or 999): Gardai, fire, and ambulance services; mine, mountain, rescue and coastguard.
- Utilities: gas, electricity, or water.
- Health services: doctor, dentist or nurse.

Emergency calls are free and can be made on any telephone, including car phones and mobile phones. On motorways, emergency telephones can be found every mile; arrows on marker posts between them indicate the direction of the nearest one. To summon help using these telephones, simply pick up the receiver and they will be answered.

If you have to leave a casualty alone in order to telephone for help, minimise the risk to the casualty by taking any vital action first (*see* PRIMARY SURVEY, p.29). Make your call short but accurate. If you ask someone else to make the call, ensure that you ask this person to come back and confirm to you that help is on the way.

Making a call

When you dial 112 or 999, you will be asked which service you require and will be put through to the correct control officer. If there are casualties, ask for the ambulance service; they will inform other services. If you are unsure of your location, do not panic – your call can be traced to any call box or motorway telephone. Stay on the telephone until the control officer clears the line. You may be asked to stay by the telephone to "lead in" the emergency services. If you delegate this task, ensure the person reports back to you.

WHAT TO TELL EMERGENCY SERVICES
State your name clearly and say that you are acting in your capacity as a first aider. The following details are essential:

- Your telephone number.
- The exact location of the incident; give a road name or number, if possible, and mention any junctions or other landmarks.
- The type and gravity of the emergency; for example, "Traffic incident, two cars, road blocked, three people are trapped".
- The number, sex, and approximate ages of the casualties, and anything you know about their condition; for example, "Man, early fifties, suspected heart attack, cardiac arrest".
- Details of any hazards such as gas, toxic substances, power-line damage, or relevant weather conditions, such as fog or ice.

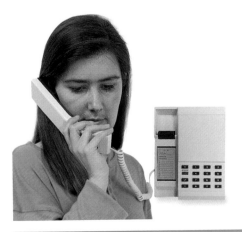

Phoning the emergency services
Try to stay calm so that you can give all the information the emergency services need. Do not hang up until the control officer has cleared the line.

MULTIPLE CASUALTIES

In situations such as major traffic incidents, you may find yourself having to deal with several casualties at the same time. You may be on your own, working with other first aiders, or assisting professionals. Whatever the situation, a systematic, calm approach is crucial in the initial chaos. Identify and attend to all unconscious casualties first, and conduct a primary survey (p.29) to find and treat any life-threatening injuries.

Dealing with the incident

Major incidents involving a large number of casualties can place overwhelming demands on rescuers. The most experienced first aider present should take charge.

The first task is to make sure that the emergency services are contacted and given accurate information about the incident. The next priority is to assess the scene and, if possible, to make it safe. Then, if it is safe to do so, start giving emergency first aid. If other first aiders come forward, give them as much information as possible.

When the emergency services arrive, the senior officer will take control of the situation. In a major incident, the police will set up rendezvous points and nominate officers to whom all rescuers will report. It is essential not to disturb any evidence at the site of the incident because there may be a legal inquiry later.

THE ROLE OF THE FIRST AIDER

At major public events, especially when there is a doctor on your team, the first aiders constitute the on-site medical team until ambulance and other services arrive. When they do arrive, your role in dealing with the incident will diminish.

At any major incident, you must leave the scene if you are asked to do so by a member of the emergency services. However, you may be asked to assist the medical team by performing simple tasks – for example, holding drips or supporting injured limbs. Always do as you are asked; your help will be greatly appreciated.

HOW YOU CAN HELP

● Identify the serious casualties and mark them for immediate treatment. Move all casualties with minor injuries quickly from the site to allow access to serious cases; minor injuries can be treated when time allows. This process is called triage.
● Leave any casualties who are obviously dead so that you can give effective help to those who need it.
● Label all casualties, and write down their names and the details about their condition, to provide accurate records for medical personnel.
● Alert workers or residents near the site of a disaster to any further hazards.

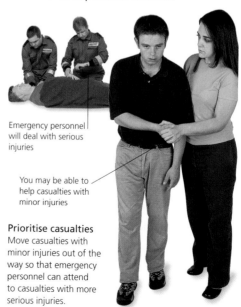

Emergency personnel will deal with serious injuries

You may be able to help casualties with minor injuries

Prioritise casualties
Move casualties with minor injuries out of the way so that emergency personnel can attend to casualties with more serious injuries.

TRAFFIC INCIDENTS

The severity of traffic incidents can range from a fall from a bicycle to a major vehicle crash that involves many casualties. Often, the incident site will present serious risks to safety, largely because of passing traffic.

It is essential to make the incident area safe before attending to any casualties. This measure enables you to protect yourself, the casualty, and other road users. Once the area is safe, quickly assess the casualties and prioritise treatment. Help those who need emergency aid before treating anyone else.

▶ **See also** ● CRUSH INJURY p.133 ● PRIMARY SURVEY p.29 ● SPINAL INJURY pp.165–167

Make the area safe

First, ensure your own safety and do not do anything that might put you in danger.
● Park safely, well clear of the incident site, and set your hazard lights flashing.
● Do not run across a busy motorway.
● At night, wear or carry something light or reflective, and use a torch.
Then take these general precautions:
● Send bystanders to warn other drivers to slow down.
● Set up warning triangles or lights at least 45 m (49 yds) from the site in each direction.
● Switch off the ignition of any damaged vehicle and, if you can, disconnect the battery. Switch off the fuel supply on diesel vehicles and motorcycles if possible.
● Stabilise vehicles. If a vehicle is upright, apply the handbrake and put it in gear, or place blocks just in front of the wheels. If a vehicle is on its side, do not attempt to right it, but try to prevent it from rolling over.
● Look out for physical dangers. Make sure that no-one smokes. Alert the emergency services to damaged power lines, spilt fuel, or any vehicles with Hazchem symbols.

HAZARDOUS SUBSTANCES
Incidents may be complicated by spillages of dangerous substances or the escape of toxic vapours. Keep bystanders away from the scene and stand upwind of it. Note any Hazchem placards on vehicles and inform the emergency services. If in doubt about your safety or the meaning of a symbol, keep your distance; take particular care if there is any spillage, or if the top left panel of a placard contains the letter "E", which indicates a public safety hazard.

Hazchem symbols
A Hazchem placard (below) indicates that a vehicle is carrying a potentially hazardous substance. A symbol indicates the nature of the potential danger (right). The information will be understood by emergency services.

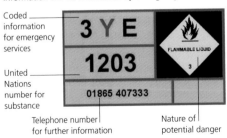

Coded information for emergency services

United Nations number for substance

Telephone number for further information

Nature of potential danger

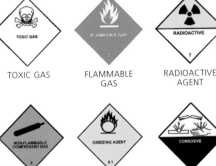

TOXIC GAS

FLAMMABLE GAS

RADIOACTIVE AGENT

COMPRESSED GAS

OXIDISING AGENT

CORROSIVE AGENT

Check the casualties

Quickly assess all casualties. If there is more than one casualty, deal first with those who may have life-threatening injuries, such as severe wounds or burns. If possible, treat casualties in the position in which you find them; move them only if they are in danger or to provide life-saving treatment.

Search the area thoroughly, so that you do not overlook any casualty who has been thrown clear or who has wandered away from the site while confused.

If a casualty is trapped inside or under a vehicle, you will need the help of the fire and rescue services, so call them at once.

When dealing with a casualty, first carry out a primary survey (p.29) and deal with any life-threatening injuries if possible. Always assume that there is a neck (spinal) injury in any casualty who has been injured in a traffic incident, and support the head with your hands until help arrives.

While waiting for specialist help, monitor and record the casualty's vital signs – level of response, pulse, and breathing (pp.42–43).

Ask helper to hold casualty's head still in case of neck injury

Get as close as possible to casualty

Dealing with casualties in the vehicle
Bystanders can help by supporting the casualty's head while you check her for any injuries that may be potentially life-threatening.

Dealing with casualties on the road
Once you are sure that the situation is safe, check the casualty for life-threatening injuries. Move the casualty only if absolutely necessary.

> **⊘ WARNING**
>
> ● Do not move the casualty unless it is absolutely necessary.
>
> ● If it is essential to move the casualty, the method you use will depend on the casualty's condition and whether help is available (*see* CASUALTY HANDLING, pp.63–64).
>
> ● Ask a bystander to mark the position of the vehicle and the casualty to provide information for the police.

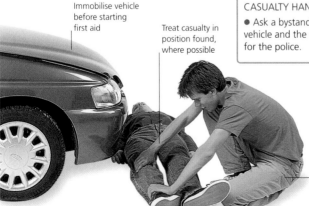

Immobilise vehicle before starting first aid

Treat casualty in position found, where possible

Place warning triangles at least 45 m (49 yds) away to alert other road users before they reach incident site

Make sure that you are not in danger

FIRES

Rapid, clear thinking at a fire is vital. Fire spreads very quickly, so your first priority is to warn any people at risk. If in a building, activate the nearest fire alarm. You should also alert the emergency services at once, but do not put your safety at risk if this action will delay your escape from the area.

Panic spreads fast among people trapped in a fire. As a first aider, you may be able to reduce panic by trying to calm anyone whose behaviour is likely to increase alarm in others. Encourage and assist people to evacuate the area. Do not delay or re-enter a burning building to collect personal possessions. Do not return to a building until cleared to do so by a fire officer.

> **⚠ WARNING**
> ● Do not use lifts under any circumstances.
> ● When arriving at an incident involving fire or burns, stop, observe, think, and do not rush into the area. There may be flammable or explosive substances, such as gas or toxic fumes, or a risk of electrocution. A minor fire can escalate in minutes to a serious blaze. If there is a risk to you, wait for the emergency services.
> ● Do not attempt to fight a fire unless you have called the emergency services and made sure that you are not putting your own safety at risk.

▶ **See also** BURNS TO THE AIRWAY p.197
● INHALATION OF FUMES pp.110–111
● SEVERE BURNS AND SCALDS pp.194–195

Dealing with fire

A fire needs three components to start and maintain it: ignition (an electric spark or naked flame); a source of fuel (petrol, wood, or fabric); and oxygen (air). Remove any one of these to break this "triangle of fire". For example:
● Switch off a car's ignition, or pull the fuel cut-off on a large diesel vehicle.

● Remove from the path of a fire any combustible materials, such as paper or cardboard, that may fuel the flames.
● Shut a door on a fire in order to cut off its oxygen supply.
● Smother flames with a fire blanket or other impervious substance to prevent oxygen from reaching them.

Leaving a burning building

If you see or suspect a fire in a building, activate the first fire alarm you see. Try to help people out of the building without putting yourself at risk. Close doors behind you to help prevent the fire from spreading. Look for fire exits and assembly points.

You should already know the evacuation procedure at your workplace. If you are visiting other premises, follow the signs for escape routes and obey any instructions.

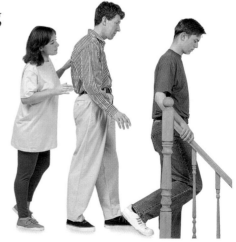

Helping escape from a burning building
Encourage people to leave the building calmly but quickly by the nearest safe exit. If you need to use stairs, make sure that people do not rush and risk falling.

Clothing on fire

Always follow this procedure: Stop, Drop, and Roll. If possible, wrap the casualty in heavy fabric before rolling him.

- Stop the casualty panicking, running around, or going outside; any movement or breeze will fan the flames.
- Drop the casualty to the ground.
- If possible, wrap the casualty tightly in a coat, curtain, blanket (not a nylon or cellular type), rug, or other heavy fabric.
- Roll the casualty along the ground until the flames have been smothered.
- If water or another non-flammable liquid is readily available, lay the casualty down with the burning side uppermost and cool the burn with the liquid.

> **⊘ WARNING**
>
> - Do not attempt to use flammable materials to smother flames.
> - If your own clothes catch fire and help is not available, extinguish the flames by wrapping yourself up tightly in suitable material and rolling along the ground.

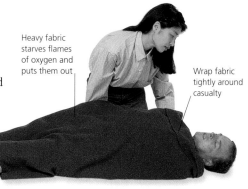

Heavy fabric starves flames of oxygen and puts them out

Wrap fabric tightly around casualty

Smoke and fumes

Any fire in a confined space creates a highly dangerous atmosphere that is low in oxygen and may be polluted by carbon monoxide and toxic fumes. Never enter a burning or fume-filled building or open a door leading to a fire. Let the emergency services do this.

WHAT YOU CAN DO

- If trapped in a burning building, go into a room with a window and shut the door. If you have to cross a smoke-filled room, stay low: air is clearest at floor level.
- If you have to escape through a window, go out feet first; lower yourself to the full length of your arms before dropping down.

Avoiding smoke and fumes

Take measures to avoid inhaling harmful smoke and fumes if you are in a burning building. Block any gaps under the door, and stay down close to the floor where you are less likely to encounter smoke.

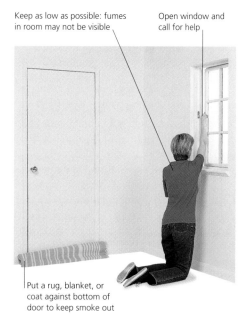

Keep as low as possible: fumes in room may not be visible

Open window and call for help

Put a rug, blanket, or coat against bottom of door to keep smoke out

25

ELECTRICAL INJURIES

When a person is electrocuted, the passage of electrical current through the body may stun him, causing his breathing and even his heartbeat to stop. The electrical current may cause burns both where it enters the body and where it exits the body to go to "earth". In some cases, the current also causes muscular spasms that may prevent a casualty from breaking contact with it, so the person may still be electrically charged ("live") when you come on the scene.

Electrical injuries usually occur in the home or workplace, due to contact with sources of low-voltage current (opposite). They may also result from contact with sources of high-voltage current (below), such as fallen power lines. People who are electrocuted by a high-voltage current rarely survive.

▶ **See also** ELECTRICAL BURN p.198
● LIFE-SAVING PROCEDURES pp.71–102

Lightning

A natural burst of electricity discharged from the atmosphere, lightning forms an intense trail of light and heat. The lightning seeks contact with the ground through the nearest tall feature in the landscape and, possibly, through anyone standing nearby. A lightning strike may set clothing on fire, knock the casualty down, or even cause instant death. Clear everyone from the site of a lightning strike as soon as possible.

High-voltage current

Contact with high-voltage current, found in power lines and overhead high-tension (HT) cables, is usually immediately fatal. Anyone who survives will have severe burns. In addition, the shock produces a muscular spasm that may propel the casualty some distance, causing injuries such as fractures.

High-voltage electricity may jump ("arc") up to 18 m (20 yds). Materials such as dry wood or clothing will not protect you. The power must be cut off and isolated before you approach the casualty; this is crucial if railway overhead power lines are damaged.

The casualty is likely to be unconscious. Once it is safe to do so, open the airway and check breathing; be ready to begin rescue breaths and chest compressions if necessary (*see* LIFE-SAVING PROCEDURES, pp.71–102). If the casualty is breathing, place him in the recovery position. Regularly monitor and record vital signs – level of response, pulse, and breathing (pp.42–43).

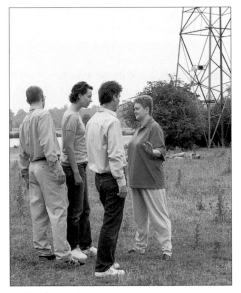

High voltage electricity
Keep any bystanders away from any incident involving high-voltage current. A safe distance is more than 18 m (20 yds) from the source of the electricity.

Low-voltage current

Domestic current, as used in homes and workplaces, can cause serious injury or even death. Incidents are usually due to faulty switches, frayed flex, or defective appliances. Young children are particularly at risk – they are naturally curious and may put fingers or other objects into electrical wall sockets.

Water, which is a dangerously efficient conductor of electricity, presents additional risks. Handling an otherwise safe electrical appliance with wet hands, or when standing on a wet floor, greatly increases the risk of an electric shock.

WHAT YOU CAN DO

Break the contact between the casualty and the electrical supply by switching off the current at the mains or meter point if it can be reached easily. Otherwise, remove the plug or wrench the cable free.

If you cannot reach the cable, socket, or mains, do the following:

● To protect yourself, stand on some dry insulating material such as a wooden box, a plastic mat, or a telephone directory.

● Using something made of wood (such as a broom), push the casualty's limbs away from the electrical source or push the source away from the casualty.

Removing the source of electricity

If you cannot switch off the electric current, stand on dry insulating material, such as a telephone directory, and use a broom handle to move the electrical source away from the casualty. Do not touch the casualty directly.

> **⚠ WARNING**
>
> ● Do not touch the casualty if he is in contact with the electrical current; he will be "live" and you risk electrocution.
>
> ● Do not use anything metallic to break the electrical contact. Stand on some dry insulating material and use a wooden object.
>
> ● If the casualty stops breathing, be prepared to give rescue breaths and chest compressions (see LIFE-SAVING PROCEDURES, pp.71–102) until emergency help arrives.

● If it is not possible to break the contact with a wooden object, loop a length of rope around the casualty's ankles or under the arms, taking great care not to touch him, and pull away from the source of the electrical current.

● If absolutely necessary, pull the casualty free by pulling at any articles of loose, dry clothing. Do this only as a last resort because the casualty may still be "live".

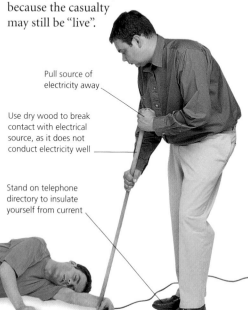

Pull source of electricity away

Use dry wood to break contact with electrical source, as it does not conduct electricity well

Stand on telephone directory to insulate yourself from current

Casualty may still be "live"

WATER RESCUE

Incidents around water may involve people of any age. Young children are at risk around even very shallow water. However, most cases of drowning involve people who have been swimming in strong currents or very cold water, or who have been swimming or boating after drinking alcohol.

DANGERS OF COLD WATER

Open water in and around Great Britain and Ireland is cold, even in summer. Sea temperatures range from 5°C (41°F) to 15°C (59°F); inland waters may be even colder.

Cold water increases the dangers to both the casualty and the rescuer because it may cause the following:

- Uncontrollable gasping when the person enters the water, with the consequent risk of water inhalation.
- A sudden rise in blood pressure, which can precipitate a heart attack.
- Sudden inability to swim.
- Hypothermia if the person is immersed in the water for a prolonged period or is exposed to the wind.

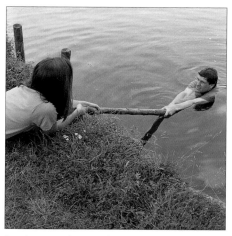

Reach out to the casualty
If possible, avoid entering the water yourself to rescue a casualty. Instead, hold out a long object such as a stick for the casualty to grasp, then pull him towards land.

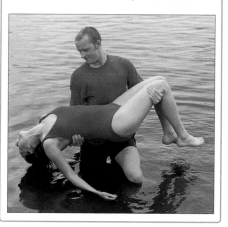

> **⚠ CAUTION**
>
> If the casualty is unconscious, lift her clear of the water, and carry her with her head lower than her chest to protect the airway if she vomits.

WHAT YOU CAN DO

Your first priority is to get the casualty on to dry land with the minimum of danger to yourself. The safest way to rescue a casualty is to stay on land and pull him from the water with your hand, a stick, a branch, or a rope; alternatively, throw him a float. If you are a trained life-saver, or if the casualty is unconscious, you may have to wade or swim to the casualty and tow him to dry land. It is safer to wade than to swim.

Once the casualty is out of the water, shield him from the wind, if possible, to prevent his body from being chilled any further, then treat him for drowning (p.109) and the effects of severe cold (*see* HYPOTHERMIA, pp.206–208).

Arrange to take or send the casualty to hospital, even if he seems to have recovered well. If necessary, or if you are at all concerned, call an ambulance.

 See also DROWNING p.109
- HYPOTHERMIA pp.206–208

ASSESSING A CASUALTY

Your first duty when attending a casualty is to assess him for life-threatening conditions that need emergency first aid. This initial assessment is called the primary survey.

Once the casualty is out of immediate danger, you should carry out a secondary survey (pp.30–31). For information on when to call an ambulance, see p.74.

PRIMARY SURVEY

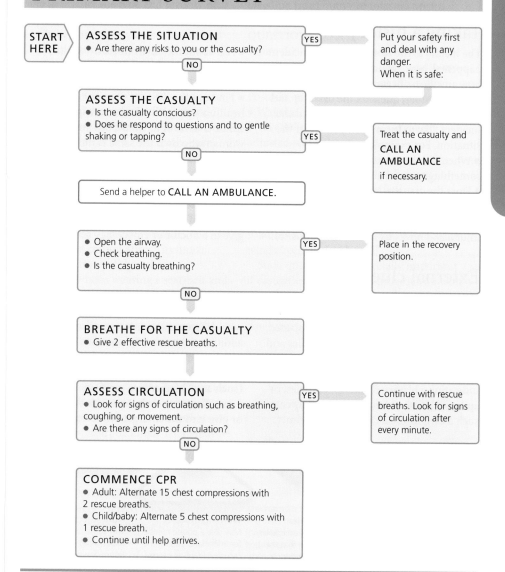

START HERE

ASSESS THE SITUATION
- Are there any risks to you or the casualty?

YES → Put your safety first and deal with any danger. When it is safe:

NO ↓

ASSESS THE CASUALTY
- Is the casualty conscious?
- Does he respond to questions and to gentle shaking or tapping?

YES → Treat the casualty and **CALL AN AMBULANCE** if necessary.

NO ↓

Send a helper to **CALL AN AMBULANCE.**

- Open the airway.
- Check breathing.
- Is the casualty breathing?

YES → Place in the recovery position.

NO ↓

BREATHE FOR THE CASUALTY
- Give 2 effective rescue breaths.

ASSESS CIRCULATION
- Look for signs of circulation such as breathing, coughing, or movement.
- Are there any signs of circulation?

YES → Continue with rescue breaths. Look for signs of circulation after every minute.

NO ↓

COMMENCE CPR
- Adult: Alternate 15 chest compressions with 2 rescue breaths.
- Child/baby: Alternate 5 chest compressions with 1 rescue breath.
- Continue until help arrives.

SYMPTOMS AND SIGNS

Injuries and illnesses usually manifest themselves as groups of distinctive features. There are two types of feature: symptoms (below), which the casualty may report, and signs (opposite), which you may detect. Some features will be obvious, but others may be missed unless you examine the casualty thoroughly (pp.34–35).

Wherever possible, examine a conscious casualty in the position in which he is found, and with any obvious injury supported.

If the casualty is unconscious, the airway must first be cleared and kept open. Do not remove items of clothing unnecessarily, and do not leave the casualty exposed to cold any longer than required. Use your senses – look, listen, feel, and smell.

Be quick and alert but thorough, and do not make unjustified assumptions. You should handle the casualty gently, but your touch must be sufficiently firm for you to detect any swelling, irregularity, or tender spot. If he is conscious, ask him to describe any sensations that your touch causes.

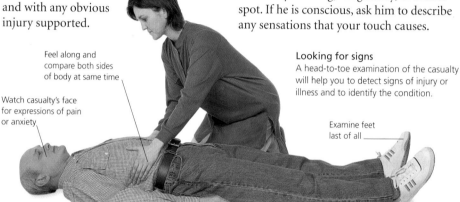

Feel along and compare both sides of body at same time

Watch casualty's face for expressions of pain or anxiety

Looking for signs
A head-to-toe examination of the casualty will help you to detect signs of injury or illness and to identify the condition.

Examine feet last of all

Assessing symptoms

Symptoms are sensations that the casualty experiences and may be able to describe. Ask if she has had any abnormal sensations. If there is pain, ask where she feels it, what type of pain it is, what makes it better or worse, and how it is affected by movement and breathing. If the pain did not follow an injury, ask how and where it began. Ask if there are other symptoms, such as nausea, giddiness, heat, cold, weakness, or thirst. If appropriate, confirm the symptoms by an examination for signs of injury or illness.

Asking about symptoms
A casualty may be able to tell you about any symptoms that she is experiencing. These details may help you to determine the nature of the injury or illness.

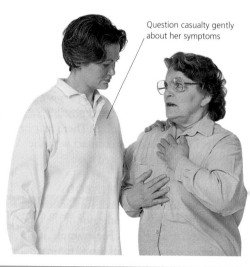

Question casualty gently about her symptoms

Looking for signs

Signs are details of a casualty's condition that you can see, feel, hear, or smell. Many are obvious, but others may be discovered only by means of a thorough examination (pp.34–35). Assess the casualty's level of response (p.42). If she is unconscious or unable to speak clearly, you may have to make a diagnosis purely on the history of the incident, information obtained from any onlookers, and the signs that you find.

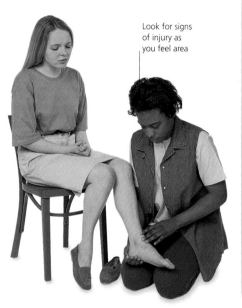

Look for signs of injury as you feel area

APPLY YOUR SENSES

Look for features such as swelling, bleeding, discoloration, or deformity. Feel the rhythm and strength of the pulse (p.42). Listen to breathing, and check for any abnormal sounds, such as crackling due to air trapped in skin tissues. Gently feel areas that are painful; note any tenderness over bones and changes in alignment. Check if the casualty is unable to perform normal functions, such as moving the limbs. Use your sense of smell to search for further clues.

Feeling for signs of injury
When examining an injured part of the body, feel for tenderness, and look for deformity or colour changes around the site of the injury. Keep the part well supported while you examine it.

SYMPTOMS AND SIGNS OF ILLNESS OR INJURY

Method of identification	Symptoms or signs
The casualty may tell you of these symptoms	Pain ● Anxiety ● Heat ● Cold ● Loss of sensation ● Abnormal sensation ● Thirst ● Nausea ● Tingling ● Pain on touch or pressure ● Faintness ● Stiffness ● Momentary unconsciousness ● Weakness ● Memory loss ● Dizziness ● Sensation of broken bone ● Sense of impending doom
You may see these signs	Anxiety and painful expression ● Unusual chest movement ● Burns ● Sweating ● Wounds ● Bleeding from orifices ● Response to touch ● Response to speech ● Bruising ● Abnormal skin colour ● Muscle spasm ● Swelling ● Deformity ● Foreign bodies ● Needle marks ● Vomit ● Incontinence ● Loss of normal movement ● Containers and other circumstantial evidence
You may feel these signs	Dampness ● Abnormal body temperature ● Swelling ● Deformity ● Irregularity ● Grating bone ends
You may hear these signs	Noisy or distressed breathing ● Groaning ● Sucking sounds (chest injury) ● Response to touch ● Response to speech ● Grating bone (crepitus)
You may smell these signs	Acetone ● Alcohol ● Burning ● Gas or fumes ● Solvents or glue ● Urine ● Faeces ● Cannabis

EXAMINING A CASUALTY

Once you have taken the history (p.30) and asked about any symptoms that the casualty has (p.32), you should carry out a detailed examination of the person. During this procedure you may have to move or remove clothing (pp.40–41), but ensure that you do not move the casualty more than is strictly necessary. Always start at the head and work down; this "head-to-toe" routine is both easily remembered and thorough.

Head-to-toe survey

1 Run your hands carefully over the scalp to feel for bleeding, swelling or depression, which may indicate a possible fracture. Be careful not to move the casualty if you suspect that she may have injured her neck.

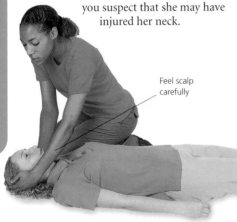

Feel scalp carefully

2 Speak clearly to the casualty in both ears to find out if she responds or if she can hear. Look for blood or clear fluid (or both) coming from either ear. These discharges may be signs of damage inside the skull.

3 Examine both eyes. Note whether the eyes are open. Check the size of the pupils, whether the pupils are equal in size (as they should be), and whether they react to light (the pupils should shrink when light falls on them). Look for any foreign object, blood, or bruising in the whites of the eyes.

4 Check the nose for discharges as you did for the ears. Look for blood or clear fluid (or a mixture of both) coming from either nostril. Any of these discharges might indicate damage inside the skull.

5 Note the rate, depth, and nature (easy or difficult, noisy or quiet) of the breathing. Note any odour on the breath. Look and feel gently inside the mouth for anything that might obstruct the airway. If the casualty is wearing dentures, and these are intact and fit firmly, leave them in place. Look for any wound in the mouth or irregularity in the line of the teeth. Check the lips for burns.

6 Note the colour, temperature, and state of the skin: is it pale, flushed, or grey–blue (cyanosis); is it hot or cold, dry or damp? For example, pale, cold, sweaty skin suggests shock; a flushed, hot face suggests fever or heatstroke. A blue tinge indicates lack of oxygen; look for this sign especially in the lips, ears, and face.

7 Loosen clothing around the neck, and look for signs such as a medical warning medallion (p.30) or a hole (stoma) in the windpipe left by a surgical operation. Run your fingers gently along the spine from the base of the skull downwards as far as possible, without disturbing the casualty's position; check for any irregularity, swelling, or tenderness.

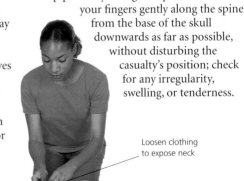

Loosen clothing to expose neck

8 Ask the casualty to breathe deeply, and note whether the chest expands evenly, easily, and equally on both sides. Feel the ribcage to check for deformity, irregularity, or tenderness. Ask if the casualty feels grating sensations on breathing, and listen for unusual sounds. Observe whether breathing causes any pain. Look for bleeding.

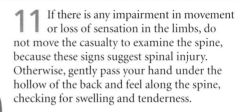

11 If there is any impairment in movement or loss of sensation in the limbs, do not move the casualty to examine the spine, because these signs suggest spinal injury. Otherwise, gently pass your hand under the hollow of the back and feel along the spine, checking for swelling and tenderness.

12 Gently feel the casualty's abdomen to detect any evidence of bleeding, and to identify any rigidity or tenderness of the abdomen's muscular wall.

Feel gently with your whole hand

9 Gently feel along both the collar bones and the shoulders for any deformity, irregularity or tenderness.

10 Check the movements of the elbows, wrists, and fingers by asking the casualty to bend and straighten the arm and hand at each of the joints. Check that the

Support the arm while checking movement

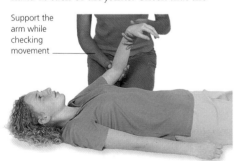

casualty can feel normally with her fingers and that there are no abnormal sensations in the limbs. Note the colour in the fingers: if the fingertips are pale or grey–blue, this may indicate a problem with the circulation. Look for any needle marks on the forearms, and for a medical warning bracelet (p.30). Take the pulse at the wrist or neck (p.42).

13 Feel both sides of the hips, and gently move the pelvis to look for signs of fracture. Check the clothing for any evidence of incontinence or bleeding from orifices.

14 Ask the casualty to raise each leg in turn, and to move her ankles and knees. Look and feel for bleeding, swelling, deformity, or tenderness.

15 Check the movement and feeling in the toes. Look at their skin colour: grey–blue skin may indicate a circulatory disorder or an injury due to cold.

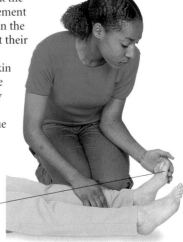

Check toes once you have removed shoes and socks

TREATMENT AND AFTERCARE

Treat each condition found methodically and calmly. Reassure and listen to the casualty. Do not ask a lot of questions or let people crowd the scene. Avoid moving the casualty unnecessarily. If necessary, ensure that someone contacts the casualty's family.

TREATMENT PRIORITIES
The order of priorities is as follows:
● Carry out a primary survey (p.29) and act on your findings, making sure that the casualty's airway is kept open and clear.
● Control bleeding.
● Carry out a secondary survey.
● Treat large wounds and burns.
● Immobilise bone and joint injuries.
● Give appropriate treatment for other injuries and conditions found.
● Regularly monitor and record vital signs – level of response, pulse, and breathing (pp.42–43). Deal with any problems.

ARRANGING AFTERCARE
Decide whether the casualty needs medical aid. If help is needed, send someone else to

> ### ⓘ CAUTION
> ● Any casualty who has impaired consciousness, serious injuries, severe breathing difficulties, or signs of shock (p.120) must not be allowed to go home. Stay with the casualty until help arrives.
> ● Do not give anything by mouth to any casualty who may have internal injuries or to anyone who needs hospital care.
> ● Do not allow the casualty to smoke.

summon it if possible. Stay with the casualty until help arrives, in case the casualty's condition alters or worsens. According to your assessment, you may need to:
● Call a doctor for advice.
● Call an ambulance or arrange transport to hospital.
● Pass care of the casualty to a doctor, nurse, or ambulance crew.
● Take the casualty to a nearby house or shelter to await medical help.
● Allow the casualty to go home, ensuring that he is accompanied if possible. Ask if someone will be at home to meet him.
● Advise the casualty to see a doctor.

Care of personal belongings

If you have to search a casualty's belongings for identification or clues to his condition, do so in front of a reliable witness. Make sure that all of the casualty's clothing and personal belongings go with him to hospital or are handed over to the police.

Searching belongings
In some cases, the only way of finding clues to a casualty's identity or condition is by searching belongings.

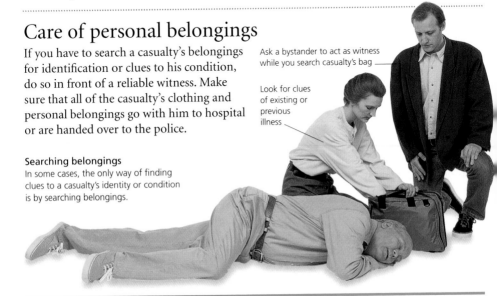

Ask a bystander to act as witness while you search casualty's bag

Look for clues of existing or previous illness

The use of medication

In first aid, administering medication is largely confined to relieving general aches and pains. It usually involves simply helping a casualty to take paracetamol, as described in the relevant sections of this book.

A wide variety of medications can be bought without a doctor's prescription, and you may know and have used many of them. However, when treating a casualty, you must not buy or borrow medication to administer yourself, even if the casualty has forgotten his own medication or you have the type he might normally expect to use.

If you administer, or advise taking, any medication other than those stipulated in this manual when giving first aid, the casualty may be put at risk, and you could face legal or civil action as a consequence.

Whenever a casualty takes medication, it is essential to make sure that:
● It is appropriate for the condition.
● It is not out of date.
● It is taken as advised.
● Any precautions are strictly followed.
● The recommended dose is not exceeded.
● A record is kept of the name and dose and the time and method of administration.

> **❶ CAUTION**
>
> If the necessary medication is not available, seek medical help. The only exception to this principle occurs where there are clear protocols laid down by an employer or voluntary organisation. Such protocols allow trained staff or members to administer medication in specific circumstances, such as giving antidotes to industrial poisons.

PASSING ON INFORMATION

Having summoned medical aid, try to make notes on the incident and on the casualty so that you can pass on this information to medical personnel. The charts overleaf show examples of specific observations, such as level of response, pulse, and breathing. You should make a brief written report to accompany your observations.

A written record of the timing of events is particularly valuable to medical personnel. Note, for example, the length of a period of unconsciousness, the duration of a seizure, the time of any changes in the casualty's condition, and the time of any intervention or treatment. Hand over your report or a copy to medical staff or emergency services.

Record your observations
While waiting for help to arrive, make a note of your observations. The records you keep will be important for the medical staff who take over the care of the casualty.

MAKING A REPORT
Your report should include:
● Casualty's name and address.
● History of the incident or illness.
● Brief description of any injuries.
● Any unusual behaviour.
● Any treatment given, and when.
● Level of response, pulse, and breathing.

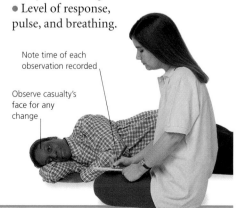

Note time of each observation recorded

Observe casualty's face for any change

FIRST-AID ESSENTIALS

USING OBSERVATION CHARTS

Every time you attend to a casualty, you should monitor and record vital signs – level of response, pulse, and breathing (pp.42–43). This information is important for medical personnel. Note the details on observation charts at regular intervals. Completed charts are shown below; blank charts for use by first aiders are provided on p.280.

On the levels of response chart, place a dot opposite the appropriate score at each time interval. For example, if the casualty does not respond to speech at the first check, place a dot opposite 1 in the first column.

On the pulse and breathing check chart, tick the relevant rates at each time interval; in addition, record the quality of the pulse and breathing as shown.

▶ **See also** MONITORING VITAL SIGNS pp.42–43 ● OBSERVATION CHARTS p.280

LEVEL OF RESPONSE CHART

DATE 24/10/01   CASUALTY'S NAME John Smith

OBSERVATION	RESPONSE/SCORE	Time of observation (minutes)					
		0	10	20	30	40	50
Eyes Observe for reaction while testing other responses.	Open spontaneously 4					●	●
	Open to speech 3				●		
	Open to painful stimulus 2			●			
	No response 1	●	●				
Speech When testing responses, speak clearly and directly, close to casualty's ear.	Responds sensibly to questions 5						●
	Seems confused 4				●	●	
	Uses inappropriate words 3						
	Makes incomprehensible sounds 2			●			
	No response 1	●	●				
Movement Apply painful stimulus: pinch ear lobe or skin on back of hand.	Obeys commands 6					●	●
	Points to pain 5				●		
	Withdraws from painful stimulus 4			●	●		
	Bends limbs in response to pain 3						
	Straightens limbs in response to pain 2						
	No response 1	●	●				
	TOTAL SCORE	3	3	8	11	14	15

Record date and casualty's name on each chart

Place dot opposite appropriate number in each column

Add up the three scores (using the numbers that correspond to each dot) to give a total at each time

PULSE AND BREATHING CHECK CHART

DATE 24/10/01   CASUALTY'S NAME John Smith

PULSE/BREATHING	RATE	Time of observation (minutes)					
		0	10	20	30	40	50
Pulse (beats per minute) Take pulse at wrist or at neck on adult, or at inner arm on baby (p.42). Note the rate, and whether beats are weak (w) or strong (s), regular (reg) or irregular (irreg).	Over 110						
	101–110						
	91–100						
	81–90						
	71–80				✓(w)	✓(s)	✓(s)
	61–70						
	Below 61	✓(w)	✓(w)	✓(w)			
Breathing (breaths per minute) Note rate, and whether breathing is quiet (q) or noisy (n), easy (e) or difficult (diff).	Over 40						
	31–40						
	21–30						
	11–20	✓(q)	✓(q)	✓(q)	✓(e)	✓(e)	✓(e)
	Below 11						

Tick box that matches casualty's pulse rate; use letters given in left-hand column to indicate quality of pulse

Tick box that matches casualty's breathing rate; use letters given in left-hand column to indicate quality of breathing

2

THIS CHAPTER outlines the core procedures that underpin first aid. Techniques that help a first aider to assess a casualty are outlined first. These are followed by a guide to the materials that make up a useful first-aid kit, and how to use them. Applying dressings and bandages is an essential part of first aid: wounds usually require a dressing, and almost all injuries benefit from the support that bandages can give.

Usually, a first aider is not expected to move an injured person, but in some circumstances – for example, when a person is in immediate danger – it may be necessary. Some of the key principles and techniques for handling and moving casualties are described here.

✚ FIRST-AID PRIORITIES

- Assess the casualty's condition.
- Comfort and reassure the casualty.
- Remove clothing if necessary.
- Use a first-aid technique relevant to the injury.
- Use dressings and bandages as needed.
- Monitor and record level of response, pulse, and breathing.
- Apply good handling techniques if moving a casualty.
- Obtain medical aid if necessary. Call an ambulance if you suspect a serious illness or injury.

CONTENTS

TECHNIQUES AND EQUIPMENT

REMOVING CLOTHING

To make a thorough examination of a casualty, obtain an accurate diagnosis, or give treatment, you may have to remove some of his clothing. This should be done with the minimum of disturbance to the casualty and with his agreement if possible. Remove as little clothing as possible and do not damage clothing unless it is absolutely necessary. If you need to cut a garment off a casualty, try to cut along the seams of trousers or sleeves. Try to maintain the casualty's privacy and prevent exposure to cold. Stop if removing clothing increases the casualty's discomfort or pain.

REMOVING CLOTHING IN LOWER BODY INJURIES

1 Support the ankle and carefully remove the shoe. To remove long boots, you may need to slit them down the back seam with a knife.

2 Remove socks by pulling them off gently. If this is not possible, lift each sock away from the leg and cut the fabric with scissors.

3 Gently pull up the trouser leg to expose the calf and knee. Pull trousers down from the waist to remove them or expose the thigh.

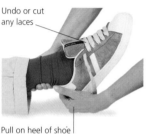

Undo or cut any laces

Pull on heel of shoe

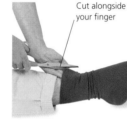

Cut alongside your finger

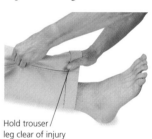

Hold trouser leg clear of injury

REMOVING CLOTHING IN UPPER BODY INJURIES

1 Undo any fastenings on the garment, such as buttons or zips. Gently pull the garment off the casualty's shoulders.

2 Remove the arm on the uninjured side from its sleeve. Pull the garment round to the injured side.

3 Support the injured arm and ease the garment off, keeping the arm as still as possible.

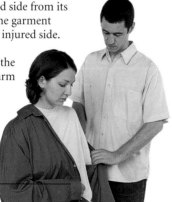

Support injured arm on lap

SPECIAL CASE

SWEATERS AND SWEATSHIRTS
With clothing that cannot be unfastened, begin by easing the arm on the uninjured side out of its sleeve. Next, roll up the garment and stretch it over his head. Finally, slip off the other sleeve of the garment, taking care not to disturb the arm.

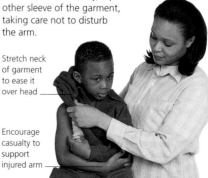

Stretch neck of garment to ease it over head

Encourage casualty to support injured arm

REMOVING HEADGEAR

Protective headgear, such as a riding hat or a motorcyclist's crash helmet, is best left on; it should be removed only if this is strictly necessary (for example, if you cannot maintain an open airway). If the item does need to be removed, the casualty should do this himself if possible; otherwise, you and a helper should remove it. Take care to support the head and neck at all times and keep the head aligned with the spine.

▶ **See also** SPINAL INJURY, pp.165–167

FOR AN OPEN-FACE HELMET

> **⚠ CAUTION**
>
> Do not remove the helmet unless it is absolutely necessary.

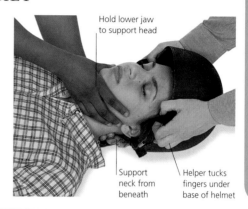

Hold lower jaw to support head

Support neck from beneath

Helper tucks fingers under base of helmet

1 Unfasten or cut through the chinstrap. Support the casualty's head and neck, keeping them aligned with the spine.

2 Ask a helper to grip the sides of the helmet from above, and pull them apart to take pressure off the head. He should then gently lift the helmet upwards and backwards.

FOR A FULL-FACE HELMET

> **⚠ CAUTION**
>
> Do not remove the helmet unless it is absolutely necessary.

1 Undo or cut the straps. Support the neck with one hand and hold the lower jaw firmly. Working from the base of the helmet, ease your fingers underneath the rim. Ask a helper to hold the helmet with both hands.

2 Ask the helper, working from above, to tilt the helmet backwards (try not to move the head at all) and gently lift the front clear of the casualty's chin.

3 Continue to support the casualty's neck and lower jaw. Ask your helper to tilt the helmet forwards slightly so that it will pass over the base of the skull, and then to lift it straight off the casualty's head.

Support head and neck

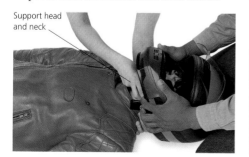

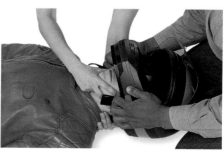

MONITORING VITAL SIGNS

When treating a casualty, you may need to assess and monitor his level of response, pulse, and breathing. You may also need to monitor temperature. These vital signs may help you to identify specific problems and indicate changes in a casualty's condition.

Monitoring should be repeated regularly and your findings recorded on an observation chart and handed over to the medical assistance taking over (p.37).

 See also OBSERVATION CHARTS p.280

CHECKING LEVEL OF RESPONSE

You will need to monitor a casualty's level of response to assess consciousness. Any injury or illness that affects the brain may affect consciousness, and any deterioration is potentially serious.

Assess the casualty's level of response using the AVPU code:
A – Is the casualty *Alert*? Does the casualty open his eyes and respond to questions?

V – Does the casualty responds to *Voice*? Does he answer simple questions and obey commands?
P – Does the casualty respond to *Pain*? Does he open his eyes or move if pinched?
U – Is the casualty *Unresponsive* to any stimulus?
Using this code, you can check whether there is any change in the casualty's condition.

CHECKING PULSE

Each heartbeat creates a wave of pressure as blood is pumped along the arteries (*see* THE HEART AND BLOOD VESSELS, pp.116–117). In places where arteries lie just under the skin surface, such as on the inside of the wrist and at the neck, this pressure wave can be felt as a pulse. The normal pulse rate in adults is 60–80 beats per minute. The rate is faster in children and may be slower in very fit adults. An abnormally fast or slow pulse may be a sign of certain illnesses.

The pulse may be measured at the neck (carotid pulse) or the wrist (radial pulse). In babies, the pulse in the upper arm (brachial pulse) may be easier to find.

When checking a pulse, use your fingers rather than your thumb (which has its own pulse), and press lightly until you can feel the pulse. Record the following points:
- Rate (number of beats per minute).
- Strength (strong or weak).
- Rhythm (regular or irregular).

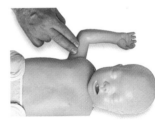

Brachial pulse
Place two fingers on the inner side of the infant's upper arm.

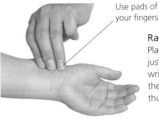

Use pads of your fingers

Radial pulse
Place three fingers just below the wrist creases at the base of the thumb.

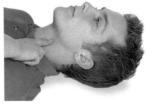

Carotid pulse
Place two fingers on the side of the neck, in the hollow between the windpipe and the large neck muscle.

CHECKING BREATHING

When assessing a casualty's breathing, check the rate of breathing and listen for any breathing difficulties or unusual noises.

The normal breathing rate in adults is 12–16 breaths per minute; in babies and young children it is 20–30 breaths per minute. To check breathing, listen to the breathing and watch the casualty's chest movements. For a baby or young child, it might be easier to place your hand on the chest and feel for breathing. Record the following information:
- Rate (number of breaths per minute).
- Depth (deep or shallow breaths).
- Ease (easy, difficult, or painful breaths).
- Noise (quiet or noisy breathing, and types of noise).

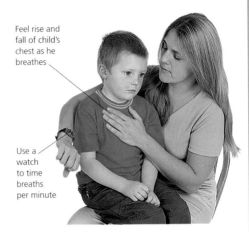

Feel rise and fall of child's chest as he breathes

Use a watch to time breaths per minute

Assessing breathing rate
Watch the chest move and count the number of breaths per minute. For a baby or young child, it may be easier if you place your hand on the chest.

CHECKING TEMPERATURE

To assess body temperature, feel exposed skin and use a thermometer to obtain an accurate reading. Normal body temperature is 37°C (98.6°F). A high temperature (fever) is usually caused by infection. A low body temperature (hypothermia) may result from exposure to cold and/or wet conditions. There are several types of thermometer, including the traditional glass mercury thermometer and digital thermometers. Make sure that you know how to use the particular type of thermometer.

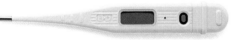

Digital thermometer
This can be used to measure temperature under the tongue or under the armpit. It should be left in place until it makes a beeping sound (about 30 seconds), then the temperature should be read from the display.

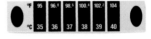

Forehead thermometer
This small heat-sensitive strip is useful for measuring temperature in a young child. Hold the strip in place against the child's forehead for about 30 seconds. A change in colour on the strip indicates the temperature.

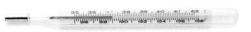

Mercury thermometer
Before using this thermometer you should check that the mercury level is below 37°C (98.6°F). Leave the thermometer in position (under the tongue or in the armpit) for 2–3 minutes before reading.

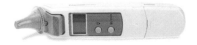

Ear sensor
The tip of this thermometer is placed inside the ear and gives a temperature reading within 1 second. The sensor is easy to use and is especially useful for a sick child. It can be used while the child is asleep.

FIRST-AID MATERIALS

All workplaces, leisure centres, homes, and cars should have first-aid kits. The kits for workplaces or leisure centres must conform to legal requirements; they should also be clearly marked and easily accessible. For a home or a car, you can either buy a kit or assemble first aid items yourself and keep them in a clean, waterproof container. Any first-aid kit must be kept in a dry place, and checked and replenished regularly, so that the items are always ready for use.

The items on these pages form the basis of a first-aid kit for the home. You may wish to add items such as aspirin and paracetamol.

DRESSINGS

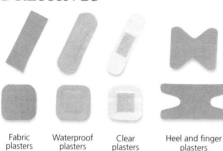

Fabric plasters   Waterproof plasters   Clear plasters   Heel and finger plasters

Adhesive dressings or plasters
These are applied to small cuts and grazes and are made of fabric or waterproof plastic. Waterproof types are best for hand wounds, and hypoallergenic types for anyone who is allergic to the adhesive in normal ones. People who work with food are required to use blue plasters.

Sterile dressings
These consist of a dressing pad attached to a roller bandage, and are sealed in a protective wrapping. They are easy to apply, so are ideal in an emergency. Various sizes are available.

Medium dressing   Large dressing   Extra-large dressing

Sterile eye pads
Eye pads are dressings to protect injured eyes. Some eye pads have bandages attached so that they can be secured to a casualty's head.

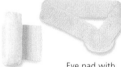

Eye pad   Eye pad with headband

BANDAGES

Self-adhesive roller bandage   Crêpe roller bandage   Open-weave roller bandage

Elasticated roller bandage   Conforming roller bandage   Crêpe conforming roller bandage

Triangular bandages
Made of cloth or strong paper, these items can be used as bandages and slings. If they are sterile and individually wrapped, they may also be used as dressings for large wounds and burns.

Folded paper triangular bandage

Folded cloth triangular bandage

Elasticated tubular bandage   Gauze tubular bandage   Tubular gauze applicator

Roller bandages
These items are used to give support to injured joints, restrict movement, secure dressings in place and maintain pressure on them, and limit swelling.

Tubular bandages
These bandages are seamless tubes of gauze or strong, elasticated material. They are used on joints and on toes or fingers. Gauze types are used with a special applicator.

USEFUL ADDITIONAL ITEMS

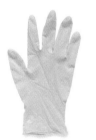

Face shield

Pocket mask

Bandage clip

Safety pins

Pins and clips
These items can be used to secure the ends of bandages.

Gauze pads
Use these as dressings, as padding, or as swabs to clean around wounds.

Disposable gloves
Wear gloves, if available, whenever you dress wounds or when you handle body fluids or other waste materials.

Face protection
Use a plastic face shield (left) or a pocket mask (right) to protect you and the casualty from infections when giving rescue breaths.

Cleansing wipes
Alcohol-free wipes can be used to clean skin around wounds, or to clean your hands if water and soap are not available.

Cotton wool
This material can be used as padding or an absorbent layer over a dressing. Never place it directly on a wound.

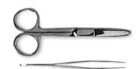

Cardboard tags
Use these items to label casualties of major accidents.

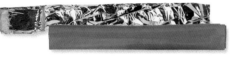

Survival bags

Items for use outdoors
A blanket can protect a casualty from cold. A torch improves visibility, and a whistle can be used to attract attention and summon help. Survival bags are wrapped around casualties to keep them warm and dry.

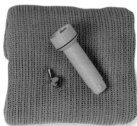

Blanket, torch, and whistle

Adhesive tape
Use tape to secure dressings or the ends of bandages. Some people are allergic to the adhesive, so check first. Hypoallergenic tape is available.

Scissors and tweezers
Choose items that are blunt-ended so that they will not cause injuries.

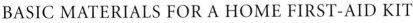

BASIC MATERIALS FOR A HOME FIRST-AID KIT

- Easily identifiable watertight box.
- 20 adhesive dressings (plasters) in assorted sizes.
- Six medium sterile dressings.
- Two large sterile dressings.
- Two extra-large sterile dressings.
- Two sterile eye pads.
- Six triangular bandages.
- Six safety pins.
- Disposable gloves.

USEFUL ADDITIONS
- Two crêpe roller bandages.
- Scissors.
- Tweezers.
- Cotton wool.
- Non-alcoholic wound cleansing wipes.
- Adhesive tape.
- Plastic face shield or pocket face mask.
- Notepad, pencil, and tags.
- Blanket, survival bag, torch, whistle.

DRESSINGS

You should always cover a wound with a dressing because this helps to prevent infection. With severe bleeding, dressings are used to aid the blood-clotting process by exerting pressure on the wound.

Use a pre-packed sterile dressing (opposite) whenever possible. If no sterile dressing is available, any clean, non-fluffy material can be used to improvise a dressing (p.48). Small cuts and grazes can be protected by an adhesive dressing (p.49).

▶ **See also** CUTS AND GRAZES p.134
● FIRST-AID MATERIALS pp.44–45 ● SEVERE BLEEDING p.130

RULES FOR USING DRESSINGS

When handling or applying a dressing, there are a number of rules to follow. These enable you to apply dressings correctly; they also protect the casualty and yourself from infection (*see* GUIDELINES FOR PREVENTING CROSS INFECTION, p.15).
● Always wear disposable gloves, if these are available, before handling any dressing other than a plaster.

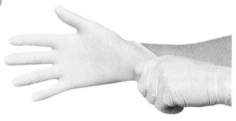

● Always use a dressing that is large enough to cover the wound and extend beyond the wound's edges.
● Hold the dressing at the edges, keeping your fingers well away from the area that will be in contact with the wound.

● Place the dressing directly on top of the wound; do not slide it on from the side.
● Remove and replace any dressing that slips out of position.
● If there is only one sterile dressing, use this to cover the wound, and apply other clean materials on top of the dressing.
● If blood seeps through the dressing, do not remove it; instead, apply another dressing over the top. If blood seeps through a second dressing, remove both dressings completely and then apply a fresh dressing, making sure that you apply pressure over the bleeding point.
● After treating a wound, dispose of gloves, used dressings, and soiled items in a suitable plastic bag. Always keep disposable gloves on until you have finished handling any other contaminated materials.

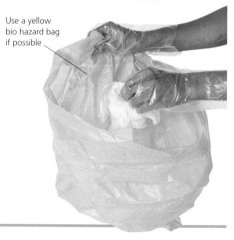

Use a yellow bio hazard bag if possible

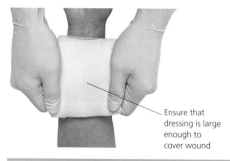

Ensure that dressing is large enough to cover wound

STERILE DRESSINGS

This type of dressing consists of a dressing pad attached to a roller bandage. The pad consists of a piece of gauze backed by a layer of cotton wool.

Sterile dressings are sold individually in various sizes and are sealed in protective wrappings to prevent contamination. Once the seal on this type of dressing has been broken, the dressing is no longer sterile.

> **① CAUTION**
>
> ● If the dressing slips out of place, remove it and apply a new dressing.
>
> ● If bleeding appears through the dressing, apply another on top of the original one. If blood seeps through the second dressing as well, take both dressings off and apply a fresh dressing.
>
> ● Take care not to impair the circulation beyond the dressing.

1 Break the seal and remove the wrapping. Unwind the bandage, taking care not to drop the roll or touch the dressing pad.

2 Unfold the dressing pad, holding the bandage on each side of it. Lay the pad directly on the wound.

Use a pad that is larger than wound

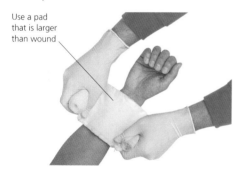

3 Wind the short end (tail) of the bandage once around the limb and the dressing to secure the pad.

Head of bandage

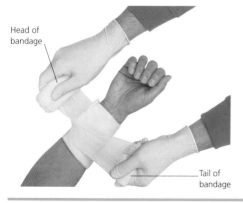

Tail of bandage

4 Wind the other end (head) of the bandage around the limb to cover the whole pad. Leave the tail of the bandage hanging free.

Head of bandage

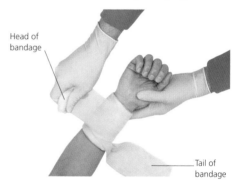

Tail of bandage

5 To secure the bandage, tie the ends in a reef knot (p.58). Tie the knot directly over the pad to exert firm pressure on the wound.

Ensure that bandage covers dressing pad completely

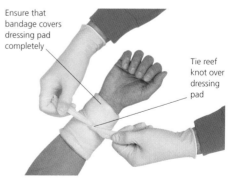

Tie reef knot over dressing pad

6 Once you have secured the bandage, check the circulation in the limb beyond it (p.51). Loosen the bandage if it is too tight.

NON-STERILE DRESSINGS

If a sterile dressing is not available, you can use items such as gauze pads or any clean, non-fluffy material and apply cotton wool on top to absorb blood or other fluids. When using a non-sterile dressing, make sure the item is clean. Wear disposable gloves if possible, and keep your fingers away from the surface of the dressing that will be touching the wound. In order to apply pressure to a wound, secure the dressing with tape or a bandage.

> **⚠ CAUTION**
> - Never apply adhesive tape all the way around a limb or digit, as this can impair circulation.
> - Check that the casualty is not allergic to the adhesive before using adhesive tape; if there is any allergy, use a bandage.

▶ **See also** ROLLER BANDAGES pp.52–53

GAUZE DRESSINGS

1 Holding the gauze pad by the edges, place it directly on to the wound.

2 Add a layer of cotton wool padding on top of the gauze dressing.

3 Secure the gauze and padding with adhesive tape or a roller bandage.

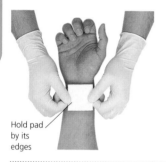

Hold pad by its edges

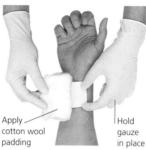

Apply cotton wool padding

Hold gauze in place

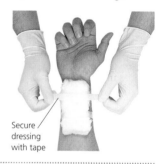

Secure dressing with tape

IMPROVISED DRESSINGS

1 Hold the material by the edges. Open it out and refold it so that the inner surface faces outwards.

2 Place the pad of cloth directly on to the wound. If necessary, cover the pad with more material.

3 Secure the pad with a bandage or a clean strip of cloth, such as a scarf. Tie the ends in a reef knot (p.58).

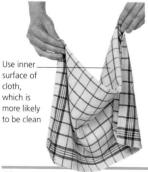

Use inner surface of cloth, which is more likely to be clean

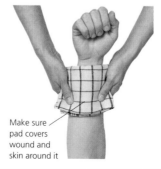

Make sure pad covers wound and skin around it

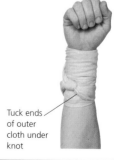

Tuck ends of outer cloth under knot

ADHESIVE DRESSINGS

Plasters are useful for dressing small cuts and grazes. They consist of a gauze or cellulose pad and an adhesive backing, and are often wrapped singly in sterile packs. There are several sizes and special shapes for use on fingertips, heels, and elbows; some types are waterproof. Before you apply a plaster, check that the casualty is

> **❶ CAUTION**
>
> Always ask whether the casualty is allergic to adhesive dressings.

not allergic to adhesive dressings. People who work with food must cover wounds on their hands with waterproof, easily visible, blue plasters.

1 Clean and dry the skin around the wound. Unwrap the plaster and hold it by the protective strips over the backing, with the pad side facing downwards.

2 Peel back the strips to expose the pad, but do not remove them. Without touching the pad surface, place the pad on the wound.

3 Carefully pull away the protective strips, then press the edges of the plaster down.

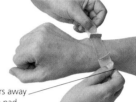

Keep fingers away from sterile pad

COLD COMPRESSES

Cooling an injury such as a bruise or sprain can reduce swelling and pain, although it will not relieve the injury itself. There are two types of compress: cold pads, which are made from material dampened with cold water; and ice packs, which are cold items (such as ice cubes or packs of frozen peas or other vegetables) wrapped in a dry cloth.

COLD PAD

1 Soak a flannel or towel in very cold water. Wring it out lightly and fold it into a pad, then place it firmly on the injury.

2 Re-soak the pad in cold water every 3–5 minutes to keep it cold. Cool the injury for at least 10 minutes.

ICE PACK

1 Partly fill a plastic bag with small ice cubes or crushed ice, or use a pack of frozen vegetables. Wrap the bag in a dry cloth.

> **❶ CAUTION**
>
> To prevent cold injuries, always wrap an ice pack in a cloth; and do not use it for more than 10 minutes at one application.

2 Hold the pack firmly on the area. Cool for 10 minutes, replacing the pack as needed.

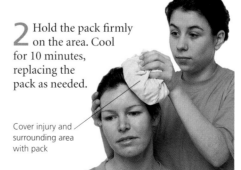

Cover injury and surrounding area with pack

PRINCIPLES OF BANDAGING

There are a number of different first aid uses for bandages: they can be used to secure dressings, control bleeding, support and immobilise limbs, and reduce swelling in an injured part. There are three main types of bandage. Roller bandages secure dressings and support injured limbs. Tubular bandages hold dressings on fingers or toes or support injured joints. Triangular bandages can be used as large dressings; as slings; to secure dressings; or to immobilise limbs. If you have no bandage available, you can improvise one from an everyday item; for example, you can fold a square of fabric, such as a headscarf, diagonally to make a triangular bandage (p.57).

▶ See also ROLLER BANDAGES pp.52–55 ● TUBULAR BANDAGE p.56 ● TRIANGULAR BANDAGES pp.57–62

RULES FOR APPLYING A BANDAGE

● Before applying a bandage, reassure the casualty and explain clearly what you are going to do.
● Make the casualty comfortable, in a suitable sitting or lying position.
● Keep the injured part supported while you are working on it. Ask the casualty or a helper to do this.
● Always work at the front of the casualty, and from the injured side where possible.

● If the casualty is lying down, pass the bandages under the body's natural hollows at the ankles, knees, waist, and neck, then slide the bandages into position by easing them back and forth under the body. For example, to bandage the head or upper trunk, pull a bandage through the hollow under the neck.

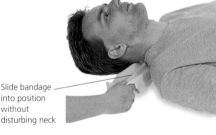

Slide bandage into position without disturbing neck

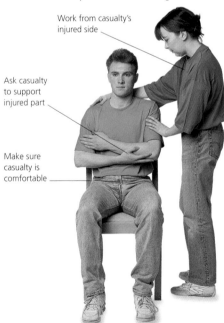

Work from casualty's injured side

Ask casualty to support injured part

Make sure casualty is comfortable

● Apply bandages firmly, but not so tightly that they interfere with circulation to the area beyond the bandage (opposite).
● Leave the fingers or toes on a bandaged limb exposed, if possible, so that you can check the circulation afterwards.
● Use reef knots to tie bandages. Ensure that the knots do not cause discomfort, and do not tie the knot over a bony area. Tuck loose ends under a knot if possible.
● Regularly check the circulation in the area beyond the bandage (opposite). If necessary, unroll the bandage until the blood supply returns, and reapply it more loosely.

IMMOBILISING A LIMB

When applying bandages to immobilise a limb, you also need to use soft, bulky material, such as towels, clothing, or cotton wool, as padding. Place the padding between the legs, or between an arm and the body, so that the bandaging does not displace broken bones or press bony areas against each other. Tie the bandages at intervals along the limb, avoiding the injury site. Secure with reef knots (p.58) on the uninjured side. If both sides of the body are injured, you should tie knots in the middle or where there is least chance of causing further damage.

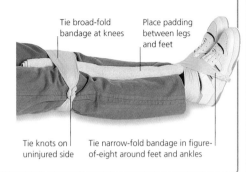

Tie broad-fold bandage at knees

Place padding between legs and feet

Tie knots on uninjured side

Tie narrow-fold bandage in figure-of-eight around feet and ankles

CHECKING CIRCULATION AFTER BANDAGING

When bandaging a limb or using a sling, you must check the circulation in the hand or foot immediately after you have finished bandaging, and every 10 minutes thereafter. These checks are essential because limbs swell after an injury, and a bandage can rapidly become too tight and interfere with blood circulation to the area beyond it. The symptoms of impaired circulation change as first the veins and then the arteries become constricted.

If circulation is impaired there may be:
- A swollen and congested limb.
- Blue skin with prominent veins.
- A feeling that the skin is painfully distended.

Later there may be:
- Pale, waxy skin.
- Cold numbness.
- Tingling, followed by deep pain.
- Inability to move affected fingers or toes.

1 Briefly press one of the nails (inset), or the skin, until it turns pale, then release the pressure. If the colour does not return, or returns slowly, the bandage may be too tight.

2 Loosen a tight bandage by unrolling just enough turns for warmth and colour to return to the skin. The casualty may feel a tingling sensation. Reapply the bandage.

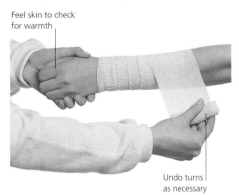

Press until nail goes pale

Check circulation at ends of fingers or toes

Feel skin to check for warmth

Undo turns as necessary

ROLLER BANDAGES

These bandages are made of cotton, gauze, elasticated fabric or linen and are wrapped around the injured part in spiral turns. There are three main types of roller bandage:

- Open-weave bandages, which are used to hold dressings in place. Because of their loose weave they allow good ventilation, but they cannot be used to exert direct pressure on the wound or to give support to joints.
- Elasticated bandages, which mould to the body shape. These are used to secure dressings and support soft tissue injuries.
- Crêpe bandages, which are used to give firm support to injured joints.

SECURING ROLLER BANDAGES

There are several ways to fasten the end of a roller bandage. Safety pins or adhesive tape are usually included in first-aid kits. Specialised kits may contain bandage clips. If you do not have any of these, a simple tuck should keep the bandage end in place.

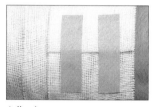

Adhesive tape
The ends of bandages can be folded under and then stuck down with small strips of adhesive tape.

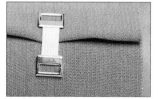

Bandage clip
Metal clips are sometimes supplied with elasticated and crêpe roller bandages for securing the ends.

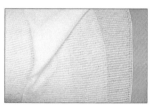

Tucking in the end
If you have no fastening, secure the bandage by passing the end around the limb once and tucking it in.

Safety pin
These pins can secure all types of roller bandage. Fold the end of the bandage under, then tuck your finger between the bandage and the casualty's skin to prevent injury as you insert the pin (right). Make sure that, once fastened, the pin lies flat (far right).

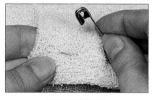

INSERTING PIN

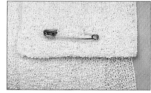

BANDAGE SECURED WITH PIN

CHOOSING THE CORRECT SIZE OF BANDAGE

Before applying a roller bandage, check that it is tightly rolled and of a suitable width for the injured area. Different parts of the body need particular widths of bandage – small areas such as fingers require narrow bandages, while large areas such as limbs need wide ones. It is better for a roller bandage to be too wide than too narrow. The bandages shown on the right are the recommended sizes for an adult. Smaller sizes may be needed for a child.

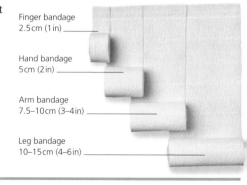

Finger bandage
2.5cm (1in)

Hand bandage
5cm (2in)

Arm bandage
7.5–10cm (3–4in)

Leg bandage
10–15cm (4–6in)

APPLYING A ROLLER BANDAGE

Follow these general rules when you are applying a roller bandage:

● Keep the rolled part of the bandage (the "head") uppermost as you work (the unrolled part is called the "tail").

● Position yourself towards the front of the casualty, on the injured side.

● While you are working, make sure that the injured part is supported in the position in which it will remain after bandaging.

> **ⓘ CAUTION**
>
> Once you have applied the bandage, check the circulation in the limb beyond it (p.51). This is especially important if you are applying an elasticated or crêpe bandage because these mould to the shape of the limb and may become tighter if the limb swells.

1 Place the tail of the bandage below the injury. Working from the inside of the limb outwards, make two straight turns with the bandage to anchor the tail in place.

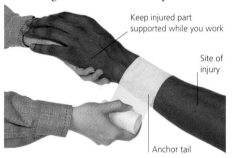

Keep injured part supported while you work

Site of injury

Anchor tail

2 Make a series of spiralling turns with the bandage. Wind it from the inside to the outside of the upper surface of the limb, and work up the limb. Make sure that each new turn covers between one half and two-thirds of the previous turn of bandaging.

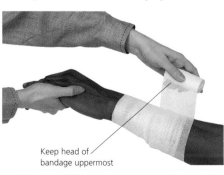

Keep head of bandage uppermost

3 Finish with one straight turn, and secure the end of the bandage (opposite). If the bandage is too short, apply another one in the same way so that the injured area is covered.

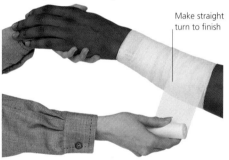

Make straight turn to finish

4 As soon as you have finished, check the circulation beyond the bandage (p.51). If necessary, unroll the bandage until the blood supply returns, and reapply it more loosely.

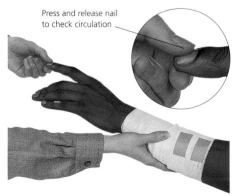

Press and release nail to check circulation

ELBOW AND KNEE BANDAGES

Roller bandages can be used on elbows and knees to hold dressings in place or support soft tissue injuries such as strains or sprains. To ensure that there is effective support, flex the joint slightly, then apply the bandage in a figure-of-eight rather than the standard spiralling turns (p.53). Work from the inside to the outside of the upper surface of the joint. Extend the bandaging far enough on either side of it to exert an even pressure.

1 Support the injured limb, in a comfortable position for the casualty, with the joint partially flexed if possible.

> **⚠ WARNING**
>
> Do not apply the bandage so tightly that the circulation to the limb is impaired.

2 Place the tail of the bandage on the inner side of the joint. Pass the bandage over and around to the outside of the joint. Make one-and-a-half turns, so that the end of the bandage is fixed and the joint is covered.

5 Continue to bandage diagonally above and below the joint in a figure-of-eight. Increase the bandaged area by covering about two-thirds of the previous turn each time.

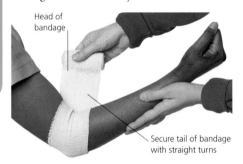

Head of bandage

Secure tail of bandage with straight turns

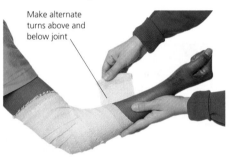

Make alternate turns above and below joint

3 Pass the bandage to the inner side of the limb, just above the joint. Make a turn around the limb, covering the upper half of the bandage from the first turn.

6 To finish bandaging the joint, make two straight turns around the limb, then secure the end of the bandage (p.52).

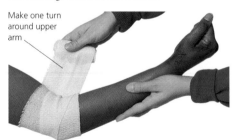

Make one turn around upper arm

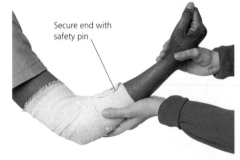

Secure end with safety pin

4 Pass the bandage from the inner side of the upper limb to just below the joint. Make one diagonal turn below the joint to cover the lower half of the bandaging from the first straight turn.

7 Check the circulation beyond the bandage as soon as you have finished, then every 10 minutes (p.51). If the bandage is too tight, unroll it until the blood supply returns and reapply it more loosely.

HAND AND FOOT BANDAGES

A roller bandage may be applied to hold dressings in place on a hand or foot, or to support a wrist or ankle in soft tissue injuries. A support bandage should extend well beyond the injury site to provide pressure over the whole of the injured area. The method shown below for bandaging a hand can also be used on a foot; in this case, begin bandaging at the base of the big toe and leave the heel unbandaged.

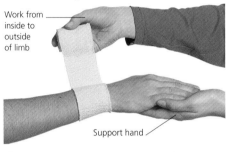

1 Place the tail of the bandage on the inner side of the wrist, by the base of the thumb. Make two straight turns around the wrist.

Work from inside to outside of limb

Support hand

2 Working from the inner side of the wrist, pass the bandage diagonally across the back of the hand to the nail of the little finger.

Position bandage so that top edge touches nail of little finger

Diagonal turn

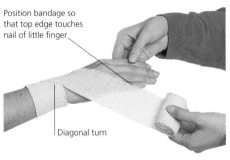

3 Take the bandage under and across the fingers so that the upper edge touches the base of the nail on the index finger. Leave the casualty's thumb free.

Bandage passes around index finger

4 Leaving the thumb free, pass the bandage diagonally across the back of the hand to the outer side of the wrist. Wrap it diagonally around the wrist and over the hand again.

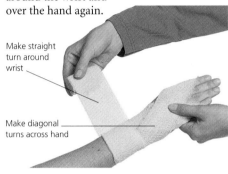

Make straight turn around wrist

Make diagonal turns across hand

5 Repeat the sequence of diagonal turns. Extend the bandaging by covering about two-thirds of the bandage from the previous turn each time. When the hand is covered, finish with two straight turns around the wrist.

6 Secure the end (p.52). As soon as you have finished, check the circulation beyond the bandage (p.51), then recheck every 10 minutes. If necessary, unroll the bandage until the blood supply returns and reapply it more loosely.

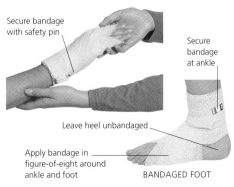

Secure bandage with safety pin

Secure bandage at ankle

Leave heel unbandaged

Apply bandage in figure-of-eight around ankle and foot

BANDAGED FOOT

TECHNIQUES AND EQUIPMENT

55

TUBULAR BANDAGE

These bandages are rolls of seamless, tubular fabric. There are two types: elasticated bandages, used to support joints such as the elbow or ankle; and tubular gauze, designed to cover a finger or toe. The gauze is used with a special applicator, supplied with the bandage. It is suitable for holding dressings

> **! CAUTION**
>
> Do not encircle the finger completely with tape because this may impair circulation.

in place, but cannot exert enough pressure to control bleeding. The steps below illustrate how to apply tubular gauze to a finger.

1 Cut a piece of tubular gauze about two-and-a-half times the length of the injured finger. Slide the whole length of the tubular gauze on to the applicator, then gently slide the applicator over the casualty's finger.

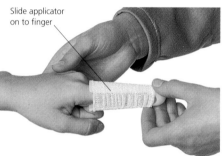

Slide applicator on to finger

2 Holding the end of the gauze on the finger, pull the applicator slightly beyond the fingertip to leave a gauze layer on the finger. Twist the applicator twice to seal the bandage over the end of the finger.

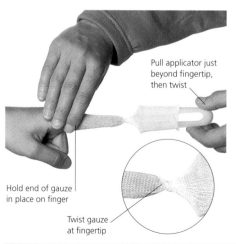

Pull applicator just beyond fingertip, then twist

Hold end of gauze in place on finger

Twist gauze at fingertip

3 While still holding the gauze at the base of the finger, gently push the applicator back over the finger to apply a second layer of gauze. Once all of it has been applied, remove the applicator from the finger.

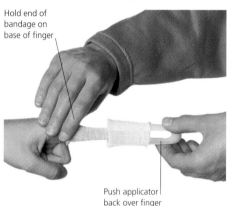

Hold end of bandage on base of finger

Push applicator back over finger

4 Secure the gauze at the base of the finger with adhesive tape. Check the circulation to the finger immediately and recheck every 10 minutes. Ask the casualty if the finger feels cold or tingly. If it does, remove the gauze and reapply it more loosely.

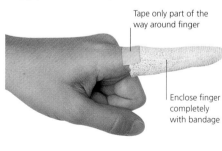

Tape only part of the way around finger

Enclose finger completely with bandage

TRIANGULAR BANDAGES

This type of bandage may be supplied in a sterile pack, as part of a first-aid kit. You can also make one by cutting or folding a square metre of sturdy fabric (such as linen or calico) diagonally in half. The bandage can be used in the following ways:

- Folded into a broad-fold bandage (below) to immobilise and support a limb or to secure a splint or bulky dressing.
- Folded into a narrow-fold bandage (below) to immobilise feet and ankles or hold a dressing in place.

- Used directly from a sterile pack and folded into a pad to form a sterile dressing.
- Opened to form a sling, or to hold a hand, foot, or scalp dressing in place.

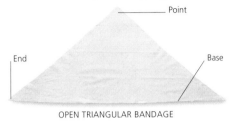

OPEN TRIANGULAR BANDAGE

MAKING A BROAD-FOLD BANDAGE

1 Open out a triangular bandage and lay it flat on a clean surface. Fold the bandage in half horizontally, so that the point of the triangle touches the centre of the base.

2 Fold the triangular bandage in half again, in the same direction, so that the first folded edge touches the base. The bandage should now form a broad strip.

First folded edge aligned with base

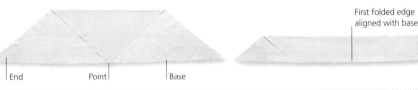

End   Point   Base

MAKING A NARROW-FOLD BANDAGE

1 Fold a triangular bandage to make a broad-fold bandage (above).

2 Fold the bandage horizontally in half again. It should form a long, narrow, thick strip of material.

STORING A TRIANGULAR BANDAGE

Keep triangular bandages in their packs so that they remain sterile until you need them. Alternatively, fold them in the way shown below so that they are ready-folded for use or can simply be shaken open.

1 Start by folding the triangle into a narrow-fold bandage (above). Bring the two ends of the bandage into the centre.

2 Continue folding the ends into the centre until the bandage is a convenient size for storing. Keep the bandage in a dry place.

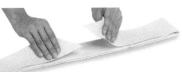

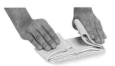

REEF KNOTS

When securing a triangular bandage, always use a reef knot. It is secure and will not slip; it is easy to untie; and it lies flat, so it is more comfortable for the casualty. Avoid tying the knot around or directly over the injury itself, as this may cause discomfort.

TYING A REEF KNOT

1 Pass the left end (dark) over and under the right end (light).

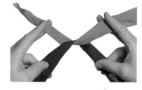

2 Lift both ends of the bandage above the rest of the material.

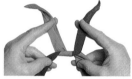

3 Pass the right end (dark) over and under the left end (light).

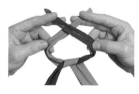

4 Pull the ends to tighten the knot, then tuck them under the bandage.

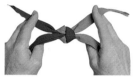

UNTYING A REEF KNOT

1 Pull one end and one piece of bandage firmly so that it straightens.

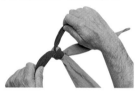

2 Hold the knot and pull the straightened end through it.

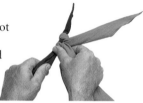

HAND AND FOOT COVER

An open triangular bandage can be used to hold a dressing in place on a hand or foot, but it will not provide enough pressure to control bleeding. The method for covering a hand (below) can also be used for a foot, with the bandage ends tied at the ankle.

1 Lay the bandage flat and fold the base to form a hem. Place the casualty's hand on the bandage, fingers towards the point. Fold the point over the hand.

2 Pass the ends around the wrist in opposite directions and tie them in a reef knot. Pull the point gently to tighten the bandage. Fold the point up over the knot and tuck it in.

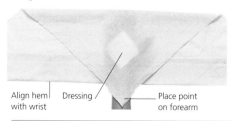

Align hem with wrist | Dressing | Place point on forearm

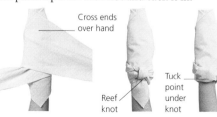

Cross ends over hand

Reef knot

Tuck point under knot

SCALP BANDAGE

A triangular bandage may be used to hold a dressing in position on top of a casualty's head. It cannot, however, provide enough pressure to control bleeding; to hold a dressing in position on a bleeding wound, use a roller bandage (pp.52–53). Before applying a scalp bandage, ask the casualty to sit down, if possible, because this will make it easier for you to reach all parts of the casualty's head.

1 Fold a hem along the base of the bandage. Place the bandage on the casualty's head with the hem underneath and the centre of the base just above his eyebrows.

Fold base of bandage under to form hem

Drape ends behind shoulders

3 Bring the crossed ends to the front of the casualty's head. Tie the ends in a reef knot (opposite) at the centre of the forehead, positioning it over the hem of the bandage. Tuck the free part of each end under the knot.

Position reef knot over hem of bandage

Tuck ends under knot

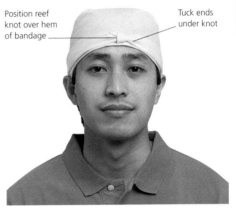

2 Wrap the ends of the bandage securely around the casualty's head, tucking the hem just above his ears. Cross the two ends at the nape of the casualty's neck, over the point of the bandage.

Pass hem above casualty's ears

Cross ends over point

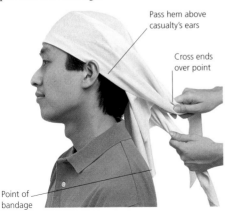

Point of bandage

4 Steady the casualty's head with one hand and draw the point down to tighten the bandage. Then fold the point up over the ends and pin it at the crown of his head. If you do not have a pin, tuck the point over the ends.

Secure point at crown with safety pin

Fold point up over crossed ends

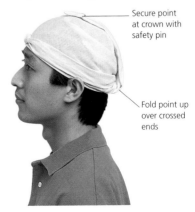

ARM SLING

An arm sling holds the forearm in a horizontal or slightly raised position. It provides support for an injured upper arm, wrist, or forearm, or a simple rib fracture (p.164) and is used for a casualty whose elbow can be bent. An elevation sling (opposite) is used to keep the forearm and hand raised in a higher position.

1 Ensure that the injured arm is supported with its hand slightly raised. Fold the base of the bandage under to form a hem. Place the bandage with the base parallel to the casualty's body and level with her little finger nail. Pass the upper end under the injured arm and pull it around the neck to the opposite shoulder.

Pass end over shoulder and around back of neck

Hold point beyond elbow

2 Fold the lower end of the bandage up over the forearm and bring it to meet the upper end at the shoulder.

Upper end

Lower end of bandage

Point

3 Tie a reef knot (p.58) on the injured side, at the hollow above the casualty's collar bone. Tuck both free ends of the bandage under the knot to pad it.

Tie knot just above collar bone

Ensure sling supports forearm and hand up to little finger

4 Fold the point forwards at the casualty's elbow. Tuck any loose fabric around the elbow, and secure the point to the front with a safety pin. If you do not have a pin, twist the point until the fabric fits the elbow snugly; tuck it into the sling at the back of the arm.

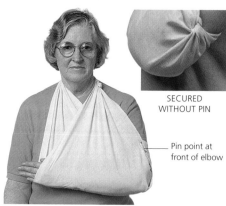

SECURED WITHOUT PIN

Pin point at front of elbow

5 As soon as you have finished, check the circulation in the fingers (p.51). Recheck every 10 minutes. If necessary, loosen and reapply the bandages and sling.

ELEVATION SLING

This form of sling supports the forearm and hand in a raised position, with the fingertips touching the casualty's shoulder. In this way, an elevation sling helps to control bleeding from wounds in the forearm or hand, to minimise swelling in burn injuries, and to support the chest in complicated rib fractures (p.164).

1 Ask the casualty to support his injured arm across his chest, with the fingers resting on the opposite shoulder.

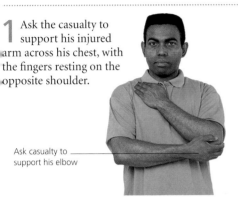

Ask casualty to support his elbow

2 Place the bandage over his body, with one end over the uninjured shoulder. Hold the point just beyond his elbow.

Base of bandage

Hold point beyond elbow of injured side

3 Ask the casualty to let go of his injured arm. Tuck the base of the bandage under his hand, forearm, and elbow.

Support arm as you work

Leave thumb showing

4 Bring the lower end of the bandage up diagonally across his back, to meet the other end at his shoulder.

Bring ends together

Pass lower end of bandage up across back

5 Tie the ends in a reef knot (p.58) at the hollow above the casualty's collar bone. Tuck the ends under the knot to pad it.

6 Twist the point until the bandage fits closely around the casualty's elbow. Tuck the point in just above his elbow to secure it. If you have a safety pin, fold the fabric over the elbow, and fasten the point at the corner.

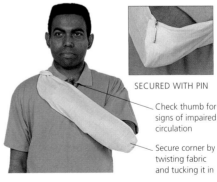

SECURED WITH PIN

Check thumb for signs of impaired circulation

Secure corner by twisting fabric and tucking it in

7 Regularly check the circulation in the thumb (p.51). If necessary, loosen and reapply the bandages and sling.

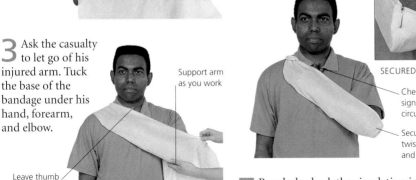

IMPROVISED SLINGS

If you need to support a casualty's injured arm but do not have a triangular bandage, you can improvise a sling by using a square metre of any strong cloth (p.57). You can also improvise by using an item of the casualty's clothing (below).

JACKET CORNER

Undo the casualty's jacket. Fold the lower edge on the injured side up over her arm. Secure the corner of the hem to the jacket breast with a large safety pin. Tuck and pin the excess material closely around the elbow.

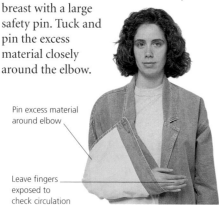

Pin excess material around elbow

Leave fingers exposed to check circulation

BUTTON-UP JACKET

Undo one button of a jacket or coat (or of a waistcoat). Place the hand of the injured arm inside the garment at the gap formed by the unfastened button. Advise the casualty to rest her wrist on the button just beneath the gap.

Unfasten button at centre of chest

Support wrist on lower button

LONG-SLEEVED SHIRT

Lay the injured arm across the casualty's chest. Pin the cuff of the sleeve to the opposite breast of the shirt. To improvise an elevation sling (previous page), pin the sleeve at the casualty's opposite shoulder, to keep her arm raised.

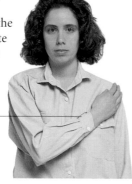

Use a safety pin that is sturdy enough to take weight of arm

BELT OR THIN GARMENT

Use a belt, a tie, or a pair of braces or tights to make a "collar-and-cuff" support. Fasten the item to form a loop. Place it over the casualty's head, then twist it once to form a smaller loop at the front. Place the casualty's hand into the loop.

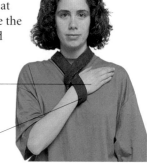

Place hand in loop, where it cannot slip out

Check that cuff is not impeding circulation to hand

CASUALTY HANDLING

As a general rule, when giving first aid you should leave casualties in the position in which you found them until medical help arrives. You should only move a casualty if he is in imminent danger, and even then only if it is safe for you to approach and you have the training and equipment to carry out the move.

This page and the next offer advice on assessing the risk of moving a casualty, and give safety guidelines to help you plan any necessary moves. The subsequent pages illustrate good practice in helping casualties who can walk and in carrying out moves. Note, however, that this information is no substitute for comprehensive training.

Information is given on some of the equipment for moving casualties that is used by emergency services.

> **❶ WARNING**
>
> Do not move a casualty unless there is an emergency situation (below) that demands that you take action.

ASSESSING THE RISK OF MOVING A CASUALTY

Before you consider moving a casualty, you need to decide whether or not the person is in immediate danger and needs to be moved (below). If you do think that it is necessary to move him, you need to find out what help and equipment is available and assess how difficult it might be to carry out the procedure. Consider the following:

● Is the task really necessary? Usually, the casualty can be assessed and treated in the position in which you find him.
● If a move is necessary, can the casualty move himself? Ask the casualty if he feels able to move; in addition, make your own assessment of his condition, using your common sense.
● What is the casualty's weight and size?

● What are his injuries, and will a move make his condition worse?
● Who is available to help with the move? Are you and any helpers properly trained and physically fit?
● Will you need to use protective equipment to enter the area, and do you have such equipment available?
● Is there any equipment available to assist with moving the casualty? Do you have all the items that you need?
● Is there enough space around the casualty to carry out the move?
● What sort of ground will you be crossing with the casualty?

> **SPECIAL CASE**
>
> EMERGENCY SITUATIONS
> There are four emergency situations in which a casualty should be moved quickly out of danger. Do this only if you will not be putting your own life at risk and you have the correct training and equipment. If you do not have these resources, you must call the emergency services instead of attempting to rescue the casualty yourself.
>
> The emergency situations are as follows:
>
> ● When a casualty is in water and in imminent danger of drowning (p.28).
>
> ● When a casualty is in an area on fire or an area that is filling with smoke (pp.24–25).
> ● When a casualty is in danger from a bomb or from gunfire.
> ● When a casualty is in or near to a collapsing building or other structure.
>
> The speed of your response depends on the level of danger, but even in the situations listed above there may be time for you to plan how to move the casualty safely and correctly (p.64).

CASUALTY HANDLING (continued)

ASSISTING A CASUALTY SAFELY

If you need to assist or move a casualty, you need to be aware of the risks that using an incorrect technique might entail. There is the possibility that you might aggravate the casualty's condition, and you or any helpers could also suffer injury. You should always take time to plan the operation carefully in order to minimise these risks.

SAFETY GUIDELINES
Take the following steps to ensure safety:
• Select a method relevant to the situation, the casualty's condition, and the help and equipment that is available.

• Use a team and appoint one person to coordinate the move. Make sure that the team understands the sequence of actions.
• Prepare any equipment available and make sure that the team and equipment is in position before proceeding.
• Always use the correct technique to avoid injuring the casualty, yourself, or helpers.
• Try to ensure the safety and comfort of the casualty, yourself, and any helpers throughout the move.
• Always explain to the casualty what is happening, and encourage the casualty to cooperate as much as possible.

GOOD PRACTICE IN MOVING AND HANDLING

The method that you use to help a casualty will depend on the situation, the casualty's condition, and whether or not you have any helpers or equipment available. Always plan a move carefully and make sure that the casualty and any helpers are prepared for the move. The following sequence of actions when assisting or moving a casualty will help to ensure the safety and comfort of everyone involved:
• Position yourself as close as possible to the casualty's body.

• Adopt a stable base, with your feet shoulder-width apart, so that you remain well-balanced.
• Maintain good posture at all times during the procedure.
• Move smoothly. Use the strongest muscles in your legs and arms to provide the power for the move.

ASSISTING THE EMERGENCY SERVICES

As a first aider, you may be asked to assist the emergency services to move a casualty using specialised equipment. Always adopt the elements of good practice outlined above. However, as part of the emergency service team, you should always follow instructions given by the team.

When a casualty is being rescued by helicopter, there are a number of ground safety rules to follow. Your main task is to control bystanders. Make sure that people are at least 50 m (55 yds) away, and that no-one smokes. Kneel down while the helicopter is landing, making sure that you are well clear of the rotor blades. Once the helicopter has landed, do not approach it, but wait for a member of the crew to meet you. Do not touch any winch lines until they reach the ground; they carry a static electrical charge until they are earthed.

ASSISTING A WALKING CASUALTY

If a casualty is conscious and able to walk, and you need to remove him from danger, you may be able to help him yourself. You can use the method described below to steady the casualty.

If there is a transfer belt available, or if the casualty has a walking aid, you can use these items to give extra stability.

▶ See also CONTROLLING A FALL p.66

SUPPORTING A CASUALTY

1 Stand at the casualty's injured or weaker side. Take hold of the hand nearest to you using the palm-to-palm thumb grip: place your palm under the casualty's palm, and close your fingers and thumb around her thumb. Hold the casualty's arm out straight, slightly in front of her body.

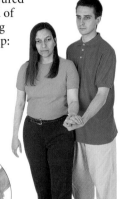

Wrap your thumb around casualty's thumb

2 Pass your other arm around the casualty's waist. Grasp her belt, waistband, or other clothing at her waist to support her.

3 Make sure that the casualty is ready to move. Take small steps, and walk at the casualty's pace. Reassure her throughout.

4 If at any stage the casualty starts to fall, follow the steps for controlling a fall (p.66).

USING A TRANSFER BELT

1 Fasten the transfer belt around the casualty's waist, ensuring that the shaped area of the belt fits centrally at the back.

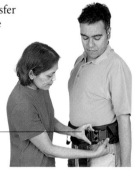

Adjust belt so that it is comfortably tight

2 Stand by the casualty's weaker side, facing the direction of movement.

3 With one hand, hold the casualty's hand nearest to you using the palm-to-palm thumb grip (above).

4 Place your other arm around the casualty's waist, and grasp one handle of the transfer belt. Make sure that you can easily let go of the belt should the casualty fall.

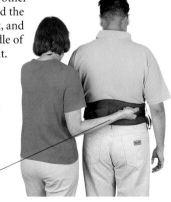

Grasp handle firmly

5 If the casualty starts to fall, let go of the transfer belt and follow the steps for controlling a fall (p.66).

CONTROLLING A FALL

If you can see that a casualty is about to collapse, perhaps because he is fainting, do not try to hold him up; instead, you need to control his fall in order to minimise the risk of injury. You should adopt the following procedure, which allows the casualty to slide gently to the floor without injuring either himself or you.

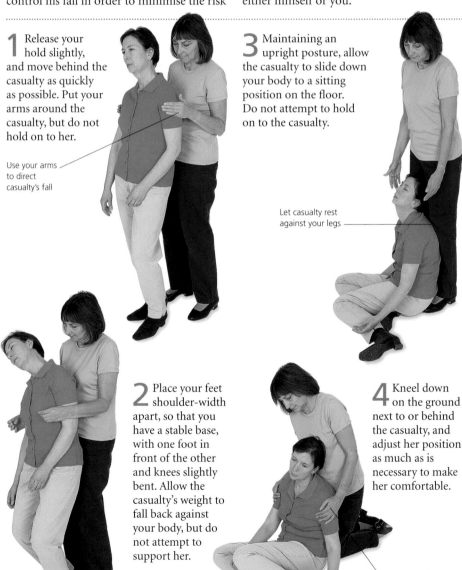

1 Release your hold slightly, and move behind the casualty as quickly as possible. Put your arms around the casualty, but do not hold on to her.

Use your arms to direct casualty's fall

3 Maintaining an upright posture, allow the casualty to slide down your body to a sitting position on the floor. Do not attempt to hold on to the casualty.

Let casualty rest against your legs

2 Place your feet shoulder-width apart, so that you have a stable base, with one foot in front of the other and knees slightly bent. Allow the casualty's weight to fall back against your body, but do not attempt to support her.

Keep one foot in front of the other

4 Kneel down on the ground next to or behind the casualty, and adjust her position as much as is necessary to make her comfortable.

Support and reassure casualty

MOVING FROM CHAIR TO FLOOR

If a seated casualty is feeling faint or unwell, encourage him to sit or lie down on the floor because this may help him to recover. It is much more difficult to move a casualty who has already become unconscious. In this situation, you will need two other people to help you move the casualty out of his seat and lay him down on the floor.

IF THE CASUALTY IS CONSCIOUS

1 Advise the casualty to slide off the chair slightly sideways, so that he is kneeling on one knee.

2 From kneeling, the casualty should move into a half-sitting position and then sit or lie down as appropriate.

IF THE CASUALTY IS UNCONSCIOUS

1 Place a slide sheet (p.69) beneath the casualty's legs and feet.

2 You should kneel at the side of the chair and support the casualty's head throughout the manoeuvre. Ask two helpers to position themselves on either side of the casualty, facing her.

4 Direct the helpers to grasp the casualty's clothing at the back of the hips with their outside hands and to grasp under the casualty's knees with their inside hands.

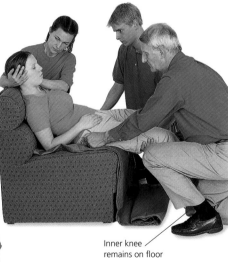

Keep hands on each side of casualty's head to support it

Adjust slide sheet if necessary

Inner knee remains on floor

3 The two helpers should get into a half-kneeling position, with their inner knees on the floor and outer legs bent at a right angle with the foot on the floor.

5 Under your direction, while you continue to support the head, the helpers should slide the casualty on to the sheet by transferring their body weight back on to their heels. They should then ease the casualty into a sitting position on the floor.

6 Move the chair away, then lower the casualty on to the slide sheet and into a lying position.

MOVING A COLLAPSED CASUALTY

If a casualty has collapsed, you may need to turn him over to place him in the recovery position or begin resuscitation. Do not move him from the place where you found him, however, unless he is in a position that may put him or others in danger (such as blocking an exit) or you need to give him life-saving treatment. If you need to move the casualty, try to enlist several helpers. Adopt the procedures below to transfer the casualty to a blanket, carry sheet, or slide sheet. A carry sheet or a blanket is used to lift a casualty. A slide sheet is used to pull a casualty along the floor.

PLACING CASUALTY ON A CARRY SHEET/BLANKET

1 Roll the sheet or blanket lengthways to half its usual width.

2 Space your helpers evenly on each side of the casualty's body, and ask the helpers to roll the casualty on to her side.

3 Place the rolled side of the sheet or blanket against the casualty's back with the roll uppermost and the unrolled part on the opposite side to her body.

4 Lower the casualty back over the roll and on to her other side.

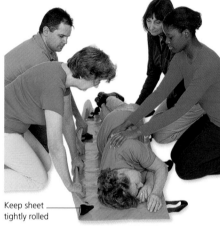

Keep sheet tightly rolled

Ensure the casualty's back is kept straight

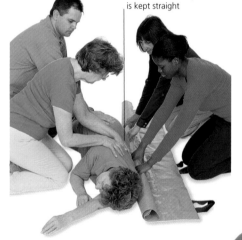

5 Unroll enough of the blanket or sheet to lay the casualty flat, then lower her on to it in the required position. If you are moving the casualty (opposite), you should all take hold of the sheet together and then move the casualty.

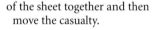

> **! WARNING**
> Try not to move a casualty if you suspect that she has a spinal injury. If you need to move her out of danger, use the "log-roll" technique (p.167).

68

MOVING EQUIPMENT

There are various items designed for moving casualties. The two items described below – the slide sheet and the carry sheet – can be used by non-professional handlers such as first aiders or carers. You will need training in the use of these items. In addition, you should follow the safety guidelines given by the manufacturer.

SLIDE SHEET

This is a large reinforced nylon sheet with a low-friction underside. A slide sheet enables handlers to carry out a variety of moving procedures. These include helping to turn a casualty over, moving a collapsed casualty from a chair to the floor (p.67), sliding a casualty along the floor, and repositioning a casualty in bed.

CARRY SHEET

This sheet has a number of strong fabric handles along the sides for lifting and carrying a casualty in any position. The handles allow the weight of the casualty to be distributed between a team of handlers (six or eight people). Some types of carry sheet have pockets down the sides to allow poles to be inserted. Metal supports that run across the width of the carry sheet may be attached to the poles; these give the casualty additional support.

When the carry sheet is used, handlers should maintain an upright posture, with a straight back and feet shoulder-width apart to provide a stable base.

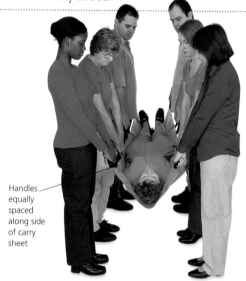

Handles equally spaced along side of carry sheet

CARRY CHAIR

This item is designed for moving a casualty in a seated position, particularly through confined spaces or up and down steps. The basic carry chair has two wheels. More sophisticated chairs are available with "roll-over" wheels. This design allows the chair to be wheeled easily over rough ground and moved up and down stairs.

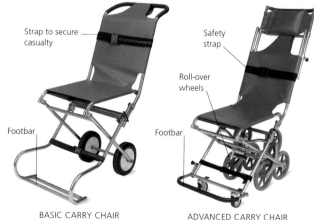

Strap to secure casualty

Footbar

Safety strap

Roll-over wheels

Footbar

BASIC CARRY CHAIR

ADVANCED CARRY CHAIR

STRETCHERS AND BOARDS

These items are commonly used by the emergency services. They are designed for carrying casualties to ambulances, to shelter, or out of danger. A variety of equipment is available, from basic canvas sheets with poles to specialised stretchers for particular rescue situations and boards for casualties with spinal injuries.

ORTHOPAEDIC STRETCHER

This device, also called a "scoop" stretcher, is used to lift a casualty on to a stretcher trolley in the position in which he is found, with minimal movement of the body. It is not designed to carry casualties very far. The stretcher splits in half lengthways. The halves are slid under the casualty, then re-joined. Once the casualty is on the trolley, the halves are separated and removed.

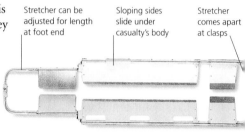

Stretcher can be adjusted for length at foot end

Sloping sides slide under casualty's body

Stretcher comes apart at clasps

SPINAL BOARD

This full-body immobilisation board is for moving a casualty with a suspected spinal injury. The casualty is rolled or slid on to it and then lifted on to a stretcher trolley. The casualty remains on the board during transport and hospital admission.

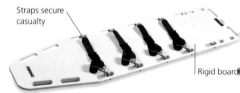

Straps secure casualty

Rigid board

STRETCHER TROLLEY

There are many different kinds of stretcher trolley, which are used for transporting casualties by ambulance. Modern designs of these stretchers use electric or hydraulic systems so that the position of the casualty can be adjusted as necessary to ensure his comfort. The stretcher is loaded on to the ambulance by ramp or trolley lift.

Research continues into new designs that will reduce risks to the handlers.

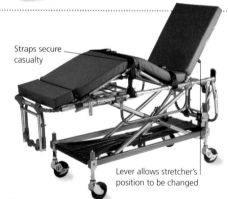

Straps secure casualty

Lever allows stretcher's position to be changed

RESCUE STRETCHERS

These stretchers are used for evacuating casualties from places that are difficult to reach, such as cliffs, mines, and confined spaces. There are many types; all require specific training and practice before use.

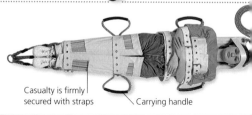

Casualty is firmly secured with straps

Carrying handle

3

TO STAY ALIVE we need an adequate supply of oxygen to enter the lungs and be transferred to all cells in the body through the bloodstream. If a casualty is deprived of oxygen, the brain begins to fail. The casualty will lose consciousness, the heartbeat and breathing will cease, and death results.

RESUSCITATION
To restore oxygen to the brain, the airway must be open so that oxygen can enter the body; breathing must be restored to enable oxygen to enter the bloodstream via the lungs; and blood must circulate to all tissues and organs.

Therefore, the priority in treating any collapsed casualty is to establish an open airway and maintain breathing and circulation. Because there are certain important differences in the treatment for children and infants, this chapter gives separate step-by-step instructions for adults, children, and infants. Techniques for treating an adult, child, or infant who is choking are also given in this chapter.

+ FIRST-AID PRIORITIES

- Maintain an open airway, check breathing, and resuscitate.
- If casualty is choking, relieve airway obstruction if possible.

CONTENTS

LIFE-SAVING PROCEDURES

BREATHING AND CIRCULATION

Oxygen is essential to support life. Without it, cells in the body die – those in the brain survive only a few minutes without oxygen. Oxygen is taken in when we breathe in (*see* THE RESPIRATORY SYSTEM, p.104), and it is then circulated to all the body tissues via the circulatory system (p.118). It is vital to maintain breathing and circulation in order to sustain life.

BREATHING

The process of breathing enables air, which contains oxygen, to be taken into the air sacs (alveoli) in the lungs. Here, the oxygen is transferred across blood vessel walls into the blood, where it combines with blood cells. At the same time, the waste product of breathing, carbon dioxide, is released and exhaled in the breath.

CIRCULATION

When oxygen has been transferred to the blood cells, it has to be circulated to all the body tissues (via blood vessels). The "pump" that maintains this circulation is the heart. Oxygen-rich blood is carried from the lungs to the heart through the pulmonary veins. The heart pumps the oxygen-rich blood to the rest of the body in blood vessels called arteries. Other blood vessels called veins bring deoxygenated blood back from the tissues to the heart (p.118). The heart pumps this blood, via the pulmonary arteries, to the lungs, where it is oxygenated and carbon dioxide is removed.

▶ See also HOW BREATHING WORKS p.105
● THE HEART AND BLOOD VESSELS p.118
● THE RESPIRATORY SYSTEM p.104

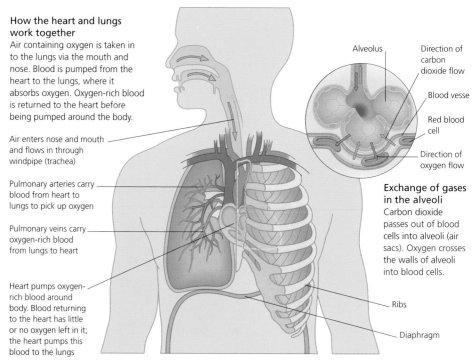

How the heart and lungs work together
Air containing oxygen is taken in to the lungs via the mouth and nose. Blood is pumped from the heart to the lungs, where it absorbs oxygen. Oxygen-rich blood is returned to the heart before being pumped around the body.

Air enters nose and mouth and flows in through windpipe (trachea)

Pulmonary arteries carry blood from heart to lungs to pick up oxygen

Pulmonary veins carry oxygen-rich blood from lungs to heart

Heart pumps oxygen-rich blood around body. Blood returning to the heart has little or no oxygen left in it; the heart pumps this blood to the lungs

Alveolus

Direction of carbon dioxide flow

Blood vesse

Red blood cell

Direction of oxygen flow

Exchange of gases in the alveoli
Carbon dioxide passes out of blood cells into alveoli (air sacs). Oxygen crosses the walls of alveoli into blood cells.

Ribs

Diaphragm

LIFE-SAVING PRIORITIES

The procedures set out in this chapter can maintain a casualty's breathing and circulation until emergency aid arrives.

With an unconscious casualty, your priorities are to maintain an open airway, breathe for the casualty (to get oxygen into the body), and maintain blood circulation (to get oxygen-rich blood to the tissues). In addition, a machine called a defibrillator (pp.82–83) can deliver a controlled electric shock to restore a normal heartbeat. The following factors increase the chances of survival if all elements are complete:

- Help is called quickly.
- Blood circulation is maintained by rescue breathing and chest compressions (together known as cardiopulmonary resuscitation or CPR).
- In an adult casualty with no signs of circulation, a defibrillator is used promptly.
- The casualty reaches hospital quickly for specialised treatment and advanced care.

Chain of survival
Four elements increase the chances of a collapsed adult casualty surviving. If any one of the elements in this chain is missing, the chances are reduced.

Early help
Call an ambulance so that a defibrillator and expert help can be brought to the casualty.

Early CPR
Chest compressions and rescue breaths are used to "buy time" until expert help arrives.

Early defibrillation
A controlled electric shock from a defibrillator is given. This jolts the heart into a normal rhythm.

Early advanced care
Specialised treatment by paramedics and in hospital stabilises the casualty's condition.

IMPORTANCE OF AN OPEN AIRWAY

An unconscious casualty's airway may become narrowed or blocked. This is due to muscular control being lost, allowing the tongue to fall back and block the airway. When this happens, the casualty's breathing becomes difficult and noisy or breathing may become completely impossible.

Lifting the chin and tilting the head back lifts the tongue from the entrance to the air passage, allowing the casualty to breathe.

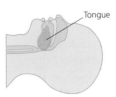 Tongue

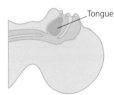 Tongue

Blocked airway
In an unconscious casualty, the tongue falls back, blocking the throat and airway.

Open airway
In the head tilt, chin lift position, the tongue is lifted from the back of the throat: the airway is clear.

BREATHING FOR A CASUALTY

The air we exhale contains about 16 per cent oxygen (5 per cent less than in the air we inhale) in addition to a small amount of carbon dioxide. Exhaled breath therefore contains enough oxygen to supply another person with oxygen – and keep him alive – when it is forced into the casualty's lungs during rescue breathing.

By giving rescue breaths, you can force air into the casualty's air passages. This air reaches the air sacs (alveoli) in the lungs, and oxygen is then transferred to the tiny blood vessels within the lungs.

When you remove your mouth from the casualty's mouth, the chest falls and air containing waste products is exhaled.

UNCONSCIOUS ADULT

The following pages gives instructions for all the techniques that may be needed in the resuscitation of an unconscious adult.

Always approach and treat the casualty from the side, kneeling down next to his head or chest. You will then be in the correct position for doing all the possible stages of resuscitation: opening the casualty's airway; checking breathing and circulation; and giving rescue breaths and chest compressions (together called cardiopulmonary resuscitation or CPR).

At each stage in the process, you will have decisions to make – for example, is the casualty breathing? The steps given here tell you what to do next in each situation.

The first priority is to open the casualty's airway so that he can breathe or you can give effective rescue breaths. If breathing and circulation return at any stage, place the casualty in the recovery position. If he is not breathing and there are no signs of circulation, the correct use of a defibrillator will increase the chance of survival.

HOW TO CHECK RESPONSE

On discovering a collapsed casualty, you should first establish whether he is conscious or unconscious. Do this by gently shaking the casualty's shoulders. Ask "What has happened?" or give a command: "Open your eyes". Speak loudly and clearly.

> **❶ CAUTION**
> Always assume that there is a neck injury and shake the shoulders very gently.

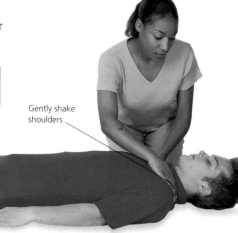

Gently shake shoulders

IF THERE IS A RESPONSE

1 If there is no further danger, leave the casualty in the position in which he was found and summon help if needed.

2 Treat any condition found and monitor vital signs – level of response, pulse, and breathing (pp.42–43).

3 Continue monitoring the casualty either until help arrives or he recovers.

IF THERE IS NO RESPONSE

1 CALL AN AMBULANCE. If possible, leave the casualty in the position in which he was found and open the airway.

2 If this is not possible, turn him onto his back and open the airway.

(▶) Go to HOW TO OPEN THE AIRWAY opposite

HOW TO OPEN THE AIRWAY

1 Kneel by the casualty's head. Place one
hand on his forehead. Gently tilt his head
back. As you do this, the mouth will fall open.

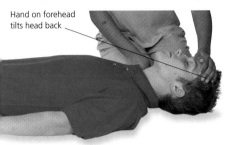

Hand on forehead
tilts head back

3 Place the fingertips of your other hand
under the point of the casualty's chin
and lift the chin.

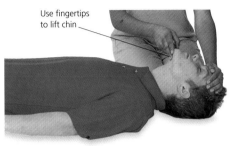

Use fingertips
to lift chin

2 Pick out any obvious obstructions, such
as dislodged dentures or broken teeth,
from the casualty's mouth. Do not do a finger
sweep. Leave well-fitting dentures in place.

4 Check to see if the casualty is now
breathing.

▶ **Go to** HOW TO CHECK BREATHING below

HOW TO CHECK BREATHING

Keeping the airway open, look, listen, and
feel for breathing: look for chest movement,
listen for sounds of breathing, and feel for
breath on your cheek. Do this for no more
than 10 seconds before deciding that
breathing is absent.

Look along chest for
movement indicating
breathing

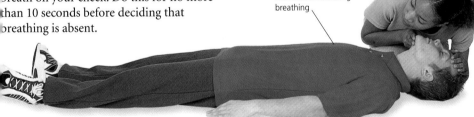

IF THE CASUALTY IS BREATHING

1 Check the casualty for any life-threatening
injuries, such as severe bleeding, and treat
as necessary.

2 Place the casualty in the recovery
position. Monitor vital signs – level of
response, pulse, and breathing (pp.42–43).

▶ **Go to** HOW TO PLACE IN
RECOVERY POSITION pp.84–85

IF THE CASUALTY IS NOT BREATHING

Give two effective rescue breaths and then
check for signs of circulation.

▶ **Go to** HOW TO GIVE RESCUE
BREATHS pp.78–79

UNCONSCIOUS ADULT (continued)

HOW TO GIVE RESCUE BREATHS

1 Make sure that the casualty's airway is still open, by keeping one hand on his forehead and two fingers of the other hand under the tip of his chin.

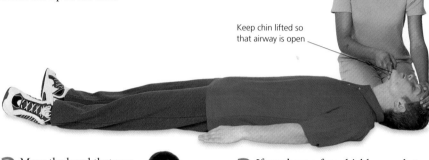

Keep chin lifted so that airway is open

2 Move the hand that was on the forehead down to the nose. Pinch the soft part of the nose with the finger and thumb. Open the casualty's mouth.

3 If you have a face shield or pocket mask (below), place it over the casualty's mouth. Take a deep breath to fill your lungs with air and place your lips around the casualty's mouth, making sure you have a good seal.

Continue to pinch the nose while taking a breath

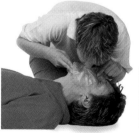

SPECIAL CASE

USING A FACE SHIELD OR POCKET MASK

First aiders may receive training in the use of these aids for hygienic purposes. Face shields are plastic barriers with a reinforced hole to fit over the casualty's mouth. The mask is more substantial and has a valve.

If you are trained to use one of these aids, carry it with you at all times and use it if you need to resuscitate a casualty. If you do not have a mask or shield with you, do not hesitate to give rescue breaths.

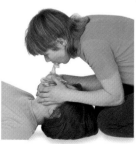

USING A FACE SHIELD   USING A POCKET MASK

4 Blow steadily into the casualty's mouth until the chest rises. This usually takes about 2 seconds.

5 Maintaining head tilt and chin lift, take your mouth off the casualty's mouth and see if his chest falls. If the chest rises visibly as you blow and falls fully when you lift your mouth away, you have given an effective breath. Give two effective breaths, then check for signs of circulation.

▶ **Go to** HOW TO CHECK FOR CIRCULATION p.80

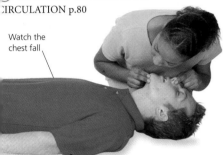

Watch the chest fall

IF YOU CANNOT ACHIEVE EFFECTIVE BREATHS

* Recheck the head tilt and chin lift.
* Recheck the casualty's mouth. Remove any obvious obstructions, but do not do a finger sweep of the mouth.
* Make no more than five attempts to achieve two effective breaths.

If you still cannot achieve two effective breaths, check the casualty for signs of circulation.

▶ **Go to** HOW TO CHECK FOR CIRCULATION p.80

> **① WARNING**
>
> If you know that the casualty has choked, and you cannot achieve effective breaths, you must immediately begin giving chest compressions and rescue breaths to try to relieve the obstruction quickly (*see* HOW TO GIVE CPR, pp.80–81).

SPECIAL CASE

MOUTH-TO-NOSE RESCUE BREATHING

In situations such as rescue from water, or where injuries to the mouth make it impossible to achieve a good seal, you may choose to use the mouth-to-nose method for giving rescue breaths. With the casualty's mouth closed, form a tight seal with your lips around the nose and blow steadily into the casualty's nose. Then allow the mouth to fall open to let the air escape.

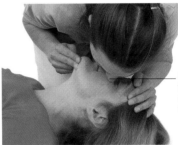

Make a tight seal around the nose

SPECIAL CASE

MOUTH-TO-STOMA RESCUE BREATHING

A casualty who has had the voice-box surgically removed breathes through a stoma (opening) in the front of the neck rather than the mouth and nose. Always check for a stoma before giving rescue breaths. If you find a stoma, close off the mouth and nose with your thumb and fingers and then breathe into the stoma.

Close off casualty's mouth and nose with your thumb and fingers

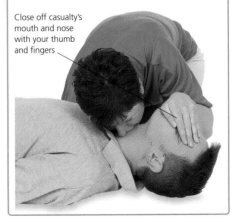

UNCONSCIOUS ADULT (continued)

HOW TO CHECK FOR CIRCULATION

Still kneeling beside the casualty's head, look, listen, and feel for signs of circulation, such as breathing, coughing, or movement. Carry out this check for no more than 10 seconds.

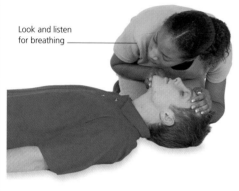

Look and listen for breathing

IF SIGNS OF CIRCULATION ARE ABSENT

Begin giving chest compressions with rescue breaths (cardiopulmonary resuscitation – CPR) immediately.

(▶) **Go to** HOW TO GIVE CPR below

IF YOU ARE SURE YOU HAVE DETECTED SIGNS OF CIRCULATION

1 Continue rescue breathing. After every 10 breaths (about 1 minute), recheck for signs of circulation. If the casualty starts to breathe but remains unconscious, turn him into the recovery position (pp.84–85).

2 Monitor vital signs – level of response, pulse, and breathing (pp.42–43). Be prepared to turn him on to his back again to restart rescue breathing (pp.78–79).

HOW TO GIVE CPR

1 Kneel beside the casualty. With the index and middle fingers of your lower hand, locate one of his lowermost ribs on the side nearest to you. Slide your fingertips along the rib to the point where the lowermost ribs meet at the breastbone. Place your middle finger at this point and your index finger beside it on the lower breastbone.

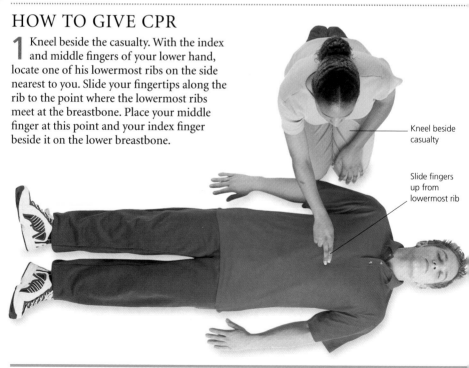

Kneel beside casualty

Slide fingers up from lowermost rib

2 Place the heel of your other hand on the breastbone, and slide it down until it reaches your index finger. This is the point at which you should apply pressure.

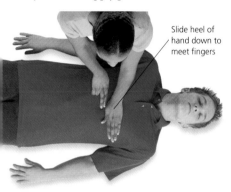

Slide heel of hand down to meet fingers

3 Place the heel of your first hand on top of the other hand, and interlock your fingers.

Keep fingers clear of chest

4 Leaning well over the casualty, with your arms straight, press down vertically on the breastbone and depress the chest by about 4–5 cm (1½–2 in). Release the pressure without removing your hands from his chest.

5 Compress the chest 15 times at a rate of 100 compressions per minute. The time taken for compression and release should be about the same.

6 Tilt the head, lift the chin, and give two rescue breaths (pp.78–79).

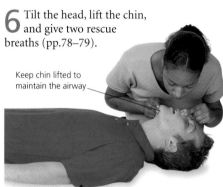

Keep chin lifted to maintain the airway

7 Continue this cycle of alternating 15 chest compressions with two rescue breaths. Check for signs of circulation after 1 minute and then every 3–4 minutes thereafter.

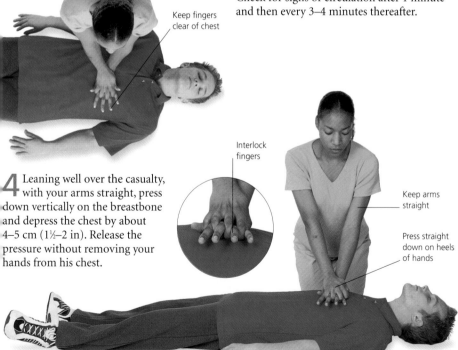

Interlock fingers

Keep arms straight

Press straight down on heels of hands

UNCONSCIOUS ADULT (continued)

HOW TO USE A DEFIBRILLATOR

When the heart stops and there are no signs of circulation, a cardiac arrest has occurred. The most common cause is an abnormal rhythm of the heart known as ventricular fibrillation. This abnormal rhythm can occur when insufficient oxygen reaches the heart or when the heart is damaged as a result of a heart attack. A machine called an automated external defibrillator (AED), or defibrillator, can be used to correct the heart rhythm. Defibrillators are available in many public places, including shopping centres and railway stations. The defibrillator analyses the casualty's heart rhythm and tells you what action to take at each stage. However, you must be trained in its use and be able to carry out CPR (pp.80–81).

In most cases where a defibrillator is called for, you will have already started the life-saving sequence. When the defibrillator arrives, stop what you are doing and start using the defibrillator.

> **❶ CAUTION**
>
> ● Make sure that no-one is touching the casualty because this will interfere with the defibrillator readings.
>
> ● Do not turn off the defibrillator or remove the pads at any point, even if the casualty appears to have recovered.

1 Switch on the defibrillator and check that the electrode leads are plugged in. Remove or cut through clothing covering the chest and quickly wipe away any sweat. Shave chest hair if it is excessive because it will prevent the pads from sticking to the skin.

2 Remove the backing paper from the electrode pads and attach them to the casualty's chest in the position indicated on the pads.

3 The defibrillator will start analysing the heart rhythm: ensure no-one is touching the casualty. Follow the spoken and/or visual prompts (opposite). These will advise you when a shock is indicated, when to check for signs of circulation (p.80), and when to give chest compressions and rescue breaths (*see* HOW TO GIVE CPR, p.80–81).

4 Continue to follow the prompts from the defibrillator until the emergency services arrive and advanced care is available. If at any time the casualty starts breathing, place him in the recovery position (pp.84–85). Leave the defibrillator attached.

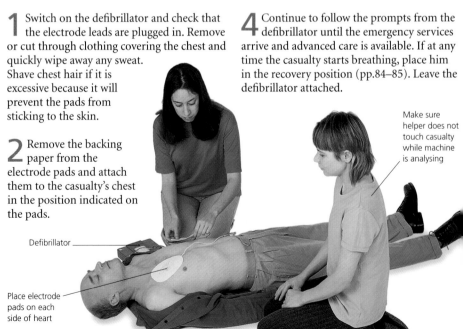

Make sure helper does not touch casualty while machine is analysing

Defibrillator

Place electrode pads on each side of heart

SEQUENCE OF DEFIBRILLATOR INSTRUCTIONS

The defibrillator will give a series of visual and verbal prompts as soon as it is switched on. Some older machines may tell you to check the pulse. In this case, you must in fact check for circulation. Do not waste time trying to find the pulse. Continue to follow the prompts given by the defibrillator until advanced care is available.

- Switch defibrillator on and make sure leads are connected.
- Attach pads to casualty's chest.

Defibrillator gets ready to analyse the casualty's heart. It may state "Stand clear, analysing now" or just "Analysing". Make sure no-one is touching the casualty or the defibrillator will be unable to analyse. Is shock advised?

YES

Defibrillator advises that a shock is needed. The machine charges up; an alarm sounds when the machine is ready.

Defibrillator instructs you to deliver the shock.
- Make sure everyone is clear of the casualty.
- Push the shock button.
Defibrillator delivers the shock and then re-analyses the heart rhythm. You may be prompted to give up to three shocks.

Defibrillator instructs you to check for circulation (older machines may state "check pulse" – always check circulation).
- Check for signs of circulation (p.80) for no more than 10 seconds. Is there a circulation?

YES

- Check airway and breathing (p.77).

NO

- Start CPR (pp.80–81) as instructed. Continue for 1 minute (until machine prompts you to stop).

The defibrillator re-analyses heart rhythm.

NO

Defibrillator advises that no shock is needed.

Defibrillator instructs you to check for circulation (older machines may state "check pulse" – always check circulation).
- Look for signs of circulation (p.80) for no more than 10 seconds. Is there a circulation?

YES

- Check airway and breathing (p.77).

NO

- Start CPR (pp.80–81) Continue for 1 minute (until machine prompts you to stop).

The defibrillator re-analyses heart rhythm.

UNCONSCIOUS ADULT (continued)

HOW TO PLACE IN RECOVERY POSITION

1 Kneel beside the casualty. Remove spectacles and any very bulky objects, such as mobile phones and large bunches of keys, from the pockets. Do not search the pockets for small items.

2 Make sure that both of the casualty's legs are straight.

3 Place the arm that is nearest to you at right angles to the casualty's body, with the elbow bent and the palm facing upwards.

> **⚠ WARNING**
>
> If you suspect a spinal injury, and you cannot maintain an open airway with the casualty in the position in which he was found, or by using the jaw thrust method (p.167), use the guidelines opposite for turning him.

> **⚠ CAUTION**
>
> If the casualty is found lying on his side or front, not all these steps will be necessary to place him in the recovery position.

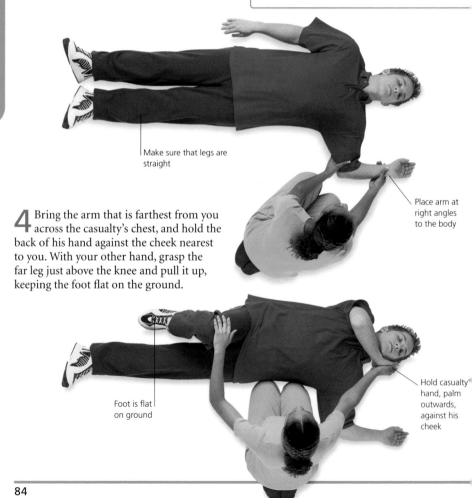

Make sure that legs are straight

Place arm at right angles to the body

4 Bring the arm that is farthest from you across the casualty's chest, and hold the back of his hand against the cheek nearest to you. With your other hand, grasp the far leg just above the knee and pull it up, keeping the foot flat on the ground.

Foot is flat on ground

Hold casualty hand, palm outwards, against his cheek

5 Keeping the casualty's hand pressed against his cheek, pull on the far leg and roll the casualty towards you and on to his side.

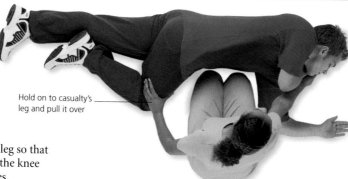

Hold on to casualty's leg and pull it over

6 Adjust the upper leg so that both the hip and the knee are bent at right angles.

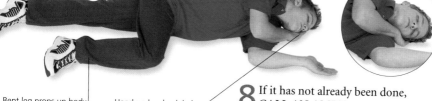

Bent leg props up body and prevents casualty from rolling forwards

Hand under cheek helps to keep airway open

7 Tilt the casualty's head back so that the airway remains open. If necessary, adjust the hand under the cheek to make sure that the head remains tilted and the airway stays open.

8 If it has not already been done, CALL AN AMBULANCE
Monitor and record vital signs – level of response, pulse, and breathing (pp.42–43).

9 If the casualty has to be left in the recovery position for longer than 30 minutes, roll him on to his back, and then turn him on to the opposite side – unless other injuries prevent you from doing this.

SPECIAL CASE

SPINAL INJURY
If you suspect a spinal injury and need to place the casualty in the recovery position to maintain an open airway, try to keep the spine straight using the following guidelines:

- If you are alone, use the technique shown on this page.
- If you have a helper, one of you should steady the head while the other turns the casualty (right).

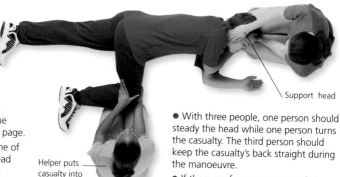

Helper puts casualty into position

Support head

- With three people, one person should steady the head while one person turns the casualty. The third person should keep the casualty's back straight during the manoeuvre.
- If there are four or more people in total, use the log-roll technique (p.167).

85

CHILD RESUSCITATION CHART

The resuscitation method used depends on the child's age and size. In children aged 1–7, respiratory failure (absence of breathing) is the main reason for the heart to stop. Ask a helper to call an ambulance while you treat the child, but if you are alone, resuscitate for 1 minute before calling an ambulance.

For a child aged 8 or over, use the adult resuscitation sequence (pp.75–85).

CHECK CHILD'S RESPONSE
- Try to get a response by asking questions and gently tapping the child's shoulder.
- Is there a response?

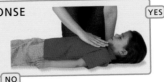

YES → Leave the child in the position found and summon help if needed.

NO

Send a helper to **CALL AN AMBULANCE**.

Check for life-threatening injuries. Place the child in the recovery position (pp.92–93).

OPEN THE AIRWAY; CHECK FOR BREATHING
- Tilt the head back to open the airway (p.88), removing any obvious obstruction. Check for breathing (p.88).
- Is the child breathing?

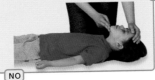

YES →

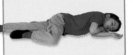

NO

BREATHE FOR CHILD
- Give two effective rescue breaths (p.89).

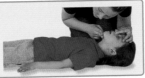

❶ WARNING

If you are alone, carry out rescue breathing and chest compressions for 1 minute before leaving the child to call an ambulance (see WHEN TO CALL AN AMBULANCE, p.74).

ASSESS FOR CIRCULATION
- Check for circulation for no more than 10 seconds (p.90).
- Are there signs of circulation?

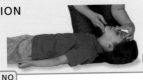

YES →

NO

Continue rescue breathing. After every 20 breaths (about 1 minute) recheck for signs of circulation. If the child starts to breathe but remains unconscious, place her in the recovery position (pp.92–93).

COMMENCE CPR
- Alternate five chest compressions with one rescue breath (pp.90–91).
- Repeat as necessary.

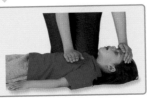

UNCONSCIOUS CHILD (1–7 years)

The following pages give full instructions for resuscitating a child aged 1–7 who is found collapsed. For a child aged 8 or over, use the adult resuscitation procedure (pp.75–85).

Always approach and treat the child from the side, kneeling down next to the head or chest. You will then be in the correct position for doing all the possible stages of resuscitation: opening the airway, checking the breathing and circulation, and giving rescue breaths and chest compressions (together known as cardiopulmonary resuscitation or CPR).

At each stage you will have decisions to make. The steps given here will guide you through each technique, then advise you on what to do next. Your first priority is to ensure that the airway is open and clear so that the child can breathe or you can give effective rescue breaths if needed. If normal breathing and circulation resume, place the child in the recovery position (pp.92–93).

Call an ambulance immediately if a child who has a known heart disease collapses suddenly because early access to advanced care may be life-saving.

HOW TO CHECK FOR RESPONSE

On discovering a collapsed child, you should first establish whether she is conscious or unconscious. Do this by speaking loudly and clearly to the child. Ask "What has happened?" or give a command: "Open your eyes". Place one hand on her shoulder, and gently tap her.

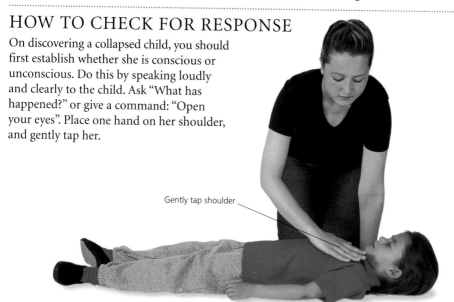

Gently tap shoulder

IF THERE IS A RESPONSE

1 If there is no further danger, leave the child in the position in which she was found and summon help if needed.

2 Treat any condition found and regularly monitor vital signs – level of response, pulse, and breathing (pp.42–43).

3 Continue this until either help arrives or the child recovers.

IF THERE IS NO RESPONSE

1 CALL AN AMBULANCE. If possible, leave the child in the position in which she was found, then open the airway.

2 If this is not possible, turn the child on to her back and open the airway.

(▶) Go to HOW TO OPEN THE AIRWAY, p.88.

UNCONSCIOUS CHILD (continued)

HOW TO OPEN THE AIRWAY

1 Kneel by the child's head. Place one hand on her forehead. Gently tilt her head back. As you do this, the mouth will fall open.

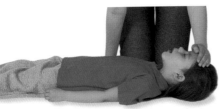

3 Place the fingertips of your other hand under the point of the child's chin and gently lift the chin.

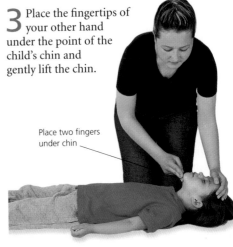

Place two fingers under chin

2 Pick out any obvious obstructions from the mouth. Do not do a finger sweep.

Use fingertips only to remove obstruction

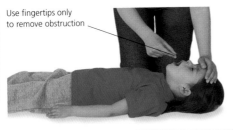

4 Check to see if the child is now breathing.

▶ Go to HOW TO CHECK BREATHING below

HOW TO CHECK BREATHING

Keep the airway open and look, listen, and feel for breathing – look for chest movement, listen for sounds of breathing, and feel for breath on your cheek. Do this for no more than 10 seconds.

Lean right down over casualty

Look for chest movement, indicating breathing

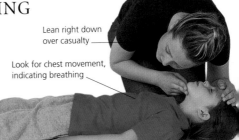

IF THE CHILD IS BREATHING

1 Check for life-threatening injuries such as severe bleeding. Treat as necessary.

2 Place the child in the recovery position. Regularly monitor her vital signs – level of response, pulse, and breathing (pp.42–43).

▶ Go to HOW TO PLACE IN RECOVERY POSITION pp.92–93

IF THE CHILD IS NOT BREATHING

Give two effective rescue breaths (right) and then check for signs of circulation.

▶ Go to HOW TO GIVE RESCUE BREATHS opposite

HOW TO GIVE RESCUE BREATHS

1 Ensure the airway is still open by keeping one hand on the child's forehead and two fingers of the other hand under her chin.

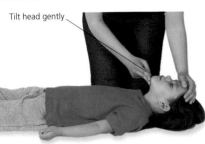

Tilt head gently

2 Pinch the soft part of the child's nose with the finger and thumb of the hand that was on the forehead. Make sure that her nostrils are closed to prevent air from escaping. Open her mouth.

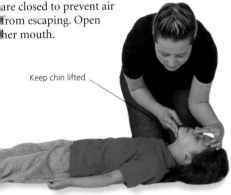

Keep chin lifted

3 Take a deep breath to fill your lungs with air. Place your lips around the child's mouth, making sure that you form an airtight seal.

Make sure that nostrils are tightly closed

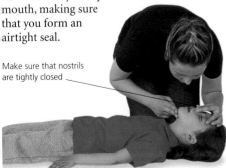

4 Blow steadily into the child's mouth until the chest rises.

5 Maintaining head tilt and chin lift, take your mouth off the child's mouth and see if her chest falls. If the chest rises visibly as you blow and falls fully when you lift your mouth, you have given an effective breath. Give two effective breaths, then check for signs of circulation.

▶ **Go to** HOW TO CHECK FOR CIRCULATION p.90

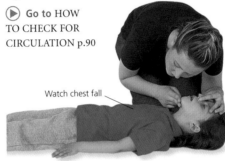

Watch chest fall

IF YOU CANNOT ACHIEVE EFFECTIVE BREATHS

- Recheck the head tilt and chin lift.
- Recheck the child's mouth. Remove any obvious obstructions, but do not do a finger sweep of the mouth.
- Make no more than five attempts to achieve two effective breaths.

If you still cannot achieve two effective breaths, check the child for signs of circulation.

▶ **Go to** HOW TO CHECK FOR CIRCULATION p.90

> **⊘ WARNING**
>
> If you know that the child has choked, and you cannot achieve effective breaths, you must immediately begin giving chest compressions to try to relieve the obstruction quickly (see HOW TO GIVE CPR, p.90).

UNCONSCIOUS CHILD (continued)

HOW TO CHECK FOR CIRCULATION

Still kneeling beside the child's head, look, listen, and feel for signs of circulation, such as breathing, coughing, or movement. Check for these signs of circulation for no more than 10 seconds.

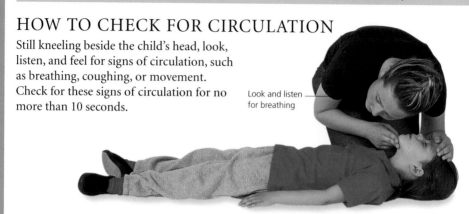

Look and listen for breathing

IF THERE ARE NO SIGNS OF CIRCULATION

Begin chest compressions and rescue breaths (cardiopulmonary resuscitation – CPR) immediately. Continue for 1 minute then CALL AN AMBULANCE

▶ Go to HOW TO GIVE CPR below

IF YOU ARE SURE YOU HAVE DETECTED SIGNS OF CIRCULATION

1 Continue rescue breathing for 1 minute. Then CALL AN AMBULANCE
After every 20 breaths (about 1 minute), check for signs of circulation. If the child starts to breathe but remains unconscious, place her in the recovery position (pp.92–93).

2 Monitor and record vital signs – level of response, pulse, and breathing (pp.42–43). Be prepared to turn the child on to her back again to restart rescue breathing (p.89).

HOW TO GIVE CPR

1 Kneel beside the child. With the fingertips of your lower hand, locate one of her lowermost ribs on the side nearest to you. Slide your fingertips along the rib to the point where the lowermost ribs meet at the breastbone. Place your middle finger at this point and your index finger beside it on the lower breastbone.

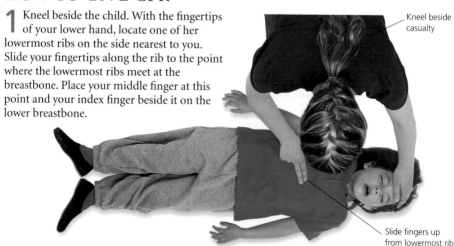

Kneel beside casualty

Slide fingers up from lowermost rib

2 Remember where your fingers are, remove them, and place the same hand on the breastbone and slide it down until it reaches where your fingers were. This is the point at which you will apply pressure.

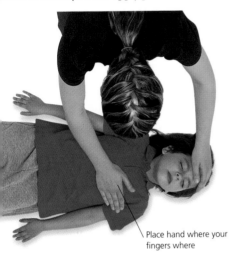

Place hand where your fingers where

3 Use the heel of this hand only to apply pressure – keep your fingers raised so that you do not apply pressure to the child's ribs.

4 Leaning well over the child, with your arms straight, press down vertically on the breastbone and depress the chest by one-third of its depth. Release the pressure without removing your hand.

5 Compress the chest five times, at a rate of 100 compressions per minute. Compression and release should take the same amount of time.

6 Tilt the head, using the hand on the child's forehead, and give one rescue breath (p.89).

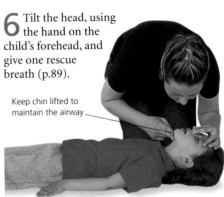

Keep chin lifted to maintain the airway

7 Continue this cycle of alternating five chest compressions with one rescue breath. After you have given 15 chest compressions, give two rescue breaths (p.89). Check for signs of circulation after 1 minute and then every 3–4 minutes thereafter.

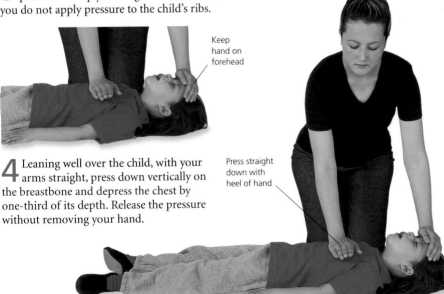

Keep hand on forehead

Press straight down with heel of hand

91

UNCONSCIOUS CHILD (continued)

HOW TO PLACE IN RECOVERY POSITION

1 Kneel beside the child. Remove any spectacles and very bulky objects from the pockets, but do not search for small items.

2 Make sure that both of the child's legs are straight. Place the arm that is nearest to you at right angles to the child's body, with the elbow bent and the palm facing upwards.

> **⚠ WARNING**
>
> If you suspect a spinal injury, and you cannot maintain the airway with the child in the position in which she was found or by using the jaw thrust method (p.167), place her in the recovery position using the guidelines opposite.

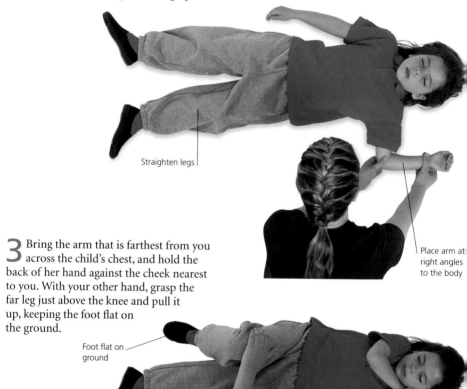

Straighten legs

3 Bring the arm that is farthest from you across the child's chest, and hold the back of her hand against the cheek nearest to you. With your other hand, grasp the far leg just above the knee and pull it up, keeping the foot flat on the ground.

Place arm at right angles to the body

Foot flat on ground

Hold child's hand, palm outwards, against her cheek

> **⚠ CAUTION**
>
> If the child is found lying on her side or front, not all of these steps will be necessary to place her in the recovery position.

4 Keeping the child's hand pressed against her cheek, pull on the far leg and roll the child towards you and on to her side.

Tilt chin so that fluid can drain from mouth

Pull bent leg towards you

Hand supports head

5 Adjust the upper leg so that both the hip and the knee are bent at right angles. Tilt the child's head back so that the airway remains open. If necessary, adjust the hand under the cheek to make sure that the head remains tilted and the airway stays open.

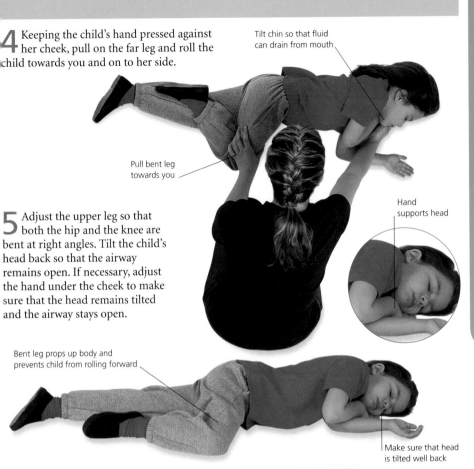

Bent leg props up body and prevents child from rolling forward

Make sure that head is tilted well back

6 If it has not already been done, CALL AN AMBULANCE Monitor and record vital signs – level of response, pulse, and breathing (pp.42–43) – until help arrives.

7 If the child has to be left in the recovery position for longer than 30 minutes, you should roll her on to her back, then turn her on to the opposite side – unless other injuries prevent you from doing this.

SPECIAL CASE

SPINAL INJURY
If you suspect a spinal injury, and need to place the child in the recovery position to maintain an open airway, try to keep the spine straight using the following guidelines:

● If you are alone, use the technique shown on this page.

● If there are two of you, one person should steady the head while the other turns the child.

● With three people, one person should steady the head while one person turns the child. The third person should keep the child's back straight during the manoeuvre.

● If there are four or more people in total, use the log-roll technique (p.167).

INFANT RESUSCITATION CHART

In infants under 1 year, a problem with breathing is the most probable reason for the heart to stop. As soon as you have established that the infant is not breathing, ask a helper to call an ambulance while you treat the infant.

CHECK INFANT'S RESPONSE
- Gently tap or flick the sole of the infant's foot. Never shake an infant.
- Is there a response?

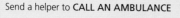

YES — Take the infant with you to summon help if needed.

NO

Send a helper to **CALL AN AMBULANCE**

Check for life-threatening injuries. Hold the infant in the recovery position (p.98).

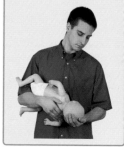

OPEN THE AIRWAY; CHECK FOR BREATHING
- Place one hand on the infant's forehead and very gently tilt the head back. Remove any obvious obstruction. Lift the chin. Check for breathing (p.96).
- Is the infant breathing?

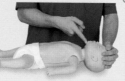

YES

NO

BREATHE FOR THE INFANT
- Give two effective rescue breaths (pp.96–97).

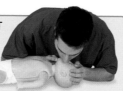

❶ WARNING
If you are alone, carry out rescue breathing and chest compressions for 1 minute before taking the infant with you to call an ambulance (*see* WHEN TO CALL AN AMBULANCE, p.74).

ASSESS FOR CIRCULATION
- Check for signs of circulation for no more than 10 seconds (p.97).
- Are there signs of circulation?

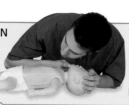

YES — Continue rescue breathing. After every 20 breaths (about 1 minute), recheck for signs of circulation. If the infant starts to breathe but remains unconscious, hold him in the recovery position (p.98).

NO

COMMENCE CPR
- Alternate five chest compressions with one rescue breath (p.98).
- Repeat as necessary.

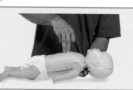

UNCONSCIOUS INFANT (under 1 year)

The following pages give full instructions for resuscitating an infant under 1 year who is found in an apparently lifeless condition. For an older infant, you should use the child resuscitation procedure (pp.86–93).

Always treat the infant from the side. You will then be in the correct position for doing all the possible stages of resuscitation: opening the airway; checking breathing and circulation; and giving rescue breaths and chest compressions (together known as cardiopulmonary resuscitation or CPR).

The steps given here guide you through each technique, then advise you on what to do next. Your first priority is to ensure that the airway is open and clear. If breathing and circulation resume, hold the infant in the recovery position (p.98). Call an ambulance immediately if an infant has known heart disease.

HOW TO CHECK FOR RESPONSE

Gently tap or flick the sole of the infant's foot and call his name to see if he responds. Never shake an infant.

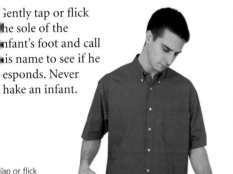

Tap or flick
sole of foot

IF THERE IS A RESPONSE

Take the infant with you to summon help if needed. Monitor vital signs – level of response, pulse, and breathing (pp.42–43) – until help arrives.

IF THERE IS NO RESPONSE

CALL AN AMBULANCE, then open the airway.

▶ Go to HOW TO OPEN THE AIRWAY below

HOW TO OPEN THE AIRWAY

1 Place one hand on the infant's forehead and very gently tilt the head back.

2 Pick out any obvious obstructions from the mouth. Do not do a finger sweep.

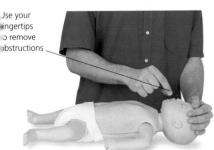

Use your
fingertips
to remove
obstructions

3 Place one fingertip of the other hand under the point of the chin. Gently lift the chin. Do not push on the soft tissues under the chin as this may block the airway.

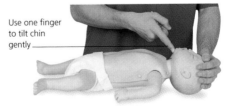

Use one finger
to tilt chin
gently

4 Check to see if the infant is now breathing.

▶ Go to HOW TO CHECK BREATHING p.96

95

UNCONSCIOUS INFANT (continued)

HOW TO CHECK BREATHING

Keep the airway open and look, listen, and feel for breathing – look for chest movement, listen for sounds of breathing, and feel for breath on your cheek. Do this for no more than 10 seconds.

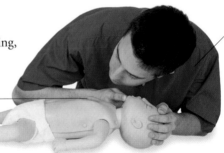

Lean right down over infant

Look for chest movement, which indicates breathing

IF THE INFANT IS BREATHING

1 Check the infant for life-threatening injuries, such as severe bleeding, and treat if necessary.

2 Hold the infant in the recovery position. Regularly monitor vital signs – level of response, pulse, and breathing (pp.42–43).

▶ **Go to** HOW TO HOLD IN RECOVERY POSITION p.98

IF THE INFANT IS NOT BREATHING

Give two effective rescue breaths and then check for signs of circulation.

▶ **Go to** HOW TO GIVE RESCUE BREATHS below

HOW TO GIVE RESCUE BREATHS

1 Make sure that the airway is still open by keeping one hand on the infant's forehead and one fingertip of the other hand under the tip of his chin.

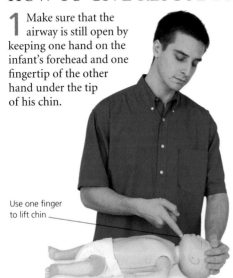

Use one finger to lift chin

2 Take a breath. Place your lips around the infant's mouth and nose to form an airtight seal. If you cannot make a seal around the mouth and nose, close the infant's mouth and make a seal around the nose only.

3 Blow steadily into the infant's lungs until the chest rises.

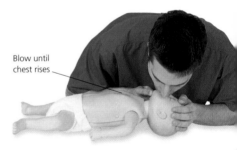

Blow until chest rises

4 Maintaining head tilt and chin lift, take your mouth off the infant's face and see if he chest falls. If the chest rises visibly as you blow and falls fully when you lift your mouth away, you have given an effective breath.

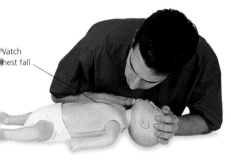

Watch chest fall

5 Give another effective rescue breath and then check for circulation.

(▶) Go to HOW TO CHECK FOR CIRCULATION below.

IF YOU CANNOT ACHIEVE EFFECTIVE BREATHS

- Recheck the head tilt and chin lift.
- Recheck the infant's mouth. Remove any obvious obstructions, but do not do a finger sweep of the mouth.
- Check that you have a firm seal around the mouth and nose.
- Make no more than five attempts to achieve two effective breaths. If you still cannot achieve two effective breaths, check the infant for signs of circulation.

(▶) Go to HOW TO CHECK FOR CIRCULATION below.

HOW TO CHECK FOR CIRCULATION

Look, listen, and feel for signs of circulation, such as breathing, coughing, or movement. Check for these signs of circulation for no more than 10 seconds.

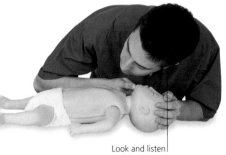

Look and listen for breathing

IF THERE ARE NO SIGNS OF CIRCULATION

Begin chest compressions and rescue breaths (cardiopulmonary resuscitation – CPR) immediately. Continue for 1 minute, then CALL AN AMBULANCE

(▶) Go to HOW TO GIVE CPR p.98

IF YOU ARE SURE YOU HAVE DETECTED SIGNS OF CIRCULATION

1 Continue rescue breaths for 1 minute, then CALL AN AMBULANCE
After every 20 breaths (about 1 minute), check for signs of circulation.

2 If the infant begins to breathe but remains unconscious, hold him in the recovery position.

(▶) Go to HOW TO HOLD IN RECOVERY POSITION p.98

UNCONSCIOUS INFANT (continued)

HOW TO GIVE CPR

1 Place the infant on his back on a flat surface, at about waist height in front of you, or on the floor. Position your upper hand under the infant's shoulder blades. Place three fingertips of your lower hand on the infant's chest so that your index finger is in line with the infant's nipples.

3 Compress the chest five times, at a rate of 100 times per minute. Compression and release should take the same amount of time.

4 After five compressions, maintain head ti and chin lift, and give one rescue breath through the mouth and nose (pp.96–97).

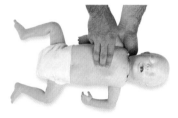

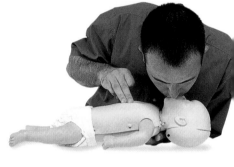

2 Remove your index finger. Using middle and fourth fingers, press down vertically on the infant's breastbone and depress the chest by one-third of its depth. Release the pressure, but keep your fingers on the breastbone.

5 Continue this cycle of alternating five chest compressions with one rescue breath. After you have given 15 chest compressions, give two rescue breaths (p.89). Check for signs of circulation after 1 minute and then every 3–4 minutes thereafter.

Press down firmly and rhythmically

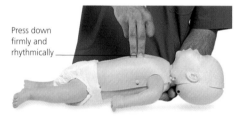

HOW TO HOLD IN RECOVERY POSITION

1 Cradle the infant in your arms with his head tilted downwards. This position prevents him from choking on his tongue or from inhaling vomit.

2 Monitor and record vital signs – level of response, pulse, and breathing (pp.42–43) – until help arrives.

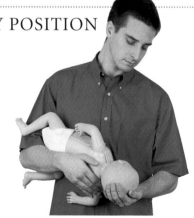

LIFE-SAVING PROCEDURES

CHOKING SUMMARY CHARTS

The following pages explain how to treat a choking adult, child, or infant. The charts below summarise how to treat choking in a conscious casualty. In an adult or a child, always encourage coughing first, and start the procedures described when the casualty shows signs of weakening.

> **❶ WARNING**
>
> If at any stage the casualty becomes unconscious, open the airway, check breathing and, if necessary, begin rescue breaths. If you cannot achieve effective breaths, you must immediately begin giving chest compressions to try to relieve the obstruction quickly (p.80, p.90, p.98).

PROCEDURE FOR ADULT *see* p.100

If the casualty can spreak and breathe

ENCOURAGE HIM OR HER TO TRY TO COUGH UP THE OBSTRUCTION

→

If the obstruction is still present or the casualty is getting weaker

GIVE UP TO FIVE ABDOMINAL THRUSTS
- Check the mouth and remove any obvious obstruction.

→

If the obstruction does not clear after three cycles of abdominal thrusts and checking the mouth

CALL AN AMBULANCE
Continue until help arrives.

PROCEDURE FOR CHILD (1–7 years) *see* p.101

If the casualty can spreak and breathe

ENCOURAGE HIM OR HER TO TRY TO COUGH UP THE OBSTRUCTION

→

If the obstruction is still present or the child is getting weaker

GIVE UP TO FIVE ABDOMINAL THRUSTS
- Check the mouth and remove any obvious obstruction.

→

If the obstruction is still present

GIVE UP TO FIVE MORE ABDOMINAL THRUSTS
- Check the mouth and remove any obvious obstruction.

→

If the obstruction does not clear after three cycles of abdominal thrusts and checking the mouth

CALL AN AMBULANCE
Continue until help arrives.

PROCEDURE FOR INFANT (under 1 year) *see* p.102

GIVE UP TO FIVE BACK SLAPS
- Check the mouth and remove any obvious obstruction.

→

If the obstruction is still present

GIVE UP TO FIVE CHEST THRUSTS
- Check the mouth; remove any obvious obstruction.

→

If the obstruction does not clear after three cycles of back slaps and chest thrusts

CALL AN AMBULANCE
Continue until help arrives.

CHOKING ADULT

A foreign object that is stuck at the back of the throat may block the throat or cause muscular spasm. If blockage of the airway is partial, the casualty should be able to clear it; if it is complete he will be unable to speak, breathe, or cough, and will lose consciousness. Be prepared to begin rescue breaths and chest compressions. The throat muscles may relax, leaving the airway sufficiently open for rescue breathing.

See also UNCONSCIOUS ADULT pp.75–86

RECOGNITION

With partial obstruction:
- Coughing and distress.
- Difficulty speaking.

With complete obstruction:
- Inability to speak, breathe, or cough, and eventual loss of consciousness.

➕ YOUR AIMS

- To remove the obstruction.
- To arrange urgent removal to hospital if necessary.

❗ WARNING

If at any stage the casualty becomes unconscious, open the airway, check breathing, and give rescue breaths (pp.77–79). If you cannot achieve effective breaths, immediately begin giving chest compressions to try to relieve the obstruction quickly (*see* HOW TO GIVE CPR, pp.80–81).

1 If the victim is able to speak, breathe, or cough, encourage him to continue coughing to relieve the obstruction.

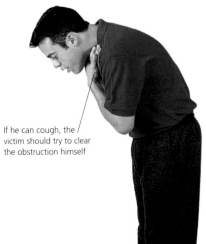

If he can cough, the victim should try to clear the obstruction himself

2 If the victim is becoming weak, or stops breathing or coughing, carry out abdominal thrusts. Stand behind the victim and put both arms around the upper part of the abdomen. Make sure that he is bending forward. Clench your fist and place it (thumb inward) between the navel and the bottom of the breastbone. Grasp your fist with your other hand. Pull sharply inward and upward up to five times.

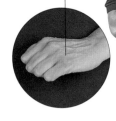

Make a fist with one hand, and position it with thumb side against the abdomen

3 Check his mouth. If the obstruction is still not cleared, repeat step 2 up to three times, checking his mouth after each step.

4 If the obstruction still has not cleared, **CALL AN AMBULANCE** Continue until help arrives or the casualty becomes unconscious.

CHOKING CHILD (1–7 years)

Young children are particularly prone to choking. A child may choke on food, or may put small objects into his mouth and cause a blockage of the airway.

If a child is choking, you need to act quickly. If he loses consciousness, be prepared to begin rescue breaths and chest compressions. The throat muscles may relax, leaving the airway sufficiently open for rescue breathing.

RECOGNITION

With partial obstruction:
● Coughing and distress.
● Difficulty speaking.

With complete obstruction:
● Inability to speak, breathe, or cough, and eventual loss of consciousness.

 See also UNCONSCIOUS CHILD pp.87–93

✚ YOUR AIMS

● To remove the obstruction.
● To arrange urgent removal to hospital if necessary.

1 If the child is breathing, encourage him to cough; this may be enough to clear the obstruction.

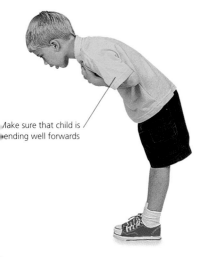

Make sure that child is bending well forwards

2 If the child shows signs of becoming weak, or stops breathing or coughing, carry out abdominal thrusts. Put your arms around the child's upper abdomen. Make sure that he is bending well forward. Place your fist between the navel and the bottom of the breastbone, and grasp it with your other hand. Pull sharply inward and upward up to five times. Stop if the obstruction clears. Check his mouth.

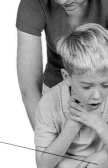

Fist should be just above child's navel

⚠ WARNING

If at any stage the child becomes unconscious, open the airway, check breathing, and give rescue breaths (pp.88–89). If you cannot achieve effective breaths, immediately begin giving chest compressions to try to relieve the obstruction quickly (*see* HOW TO GIVE CPR, pp.90–91).

3 If the obstruction is still not cleared, repeat step 2 up to three times.

4 If the obstruction still has not cleared, CALL AN AMBULANCE
Continue until help arrives or the child becomes unconscious.

CHOKING INFANT (under 1 year)

An infant may readily choke on food or on very small objects in the mouth. The infant will rapidly become distressed, and you need to act quickly to clear any obstruction.

If the infant becomes unconscious, be prepared to give rescue breaths and chest compressions. In an unconscious infant, the throat muscles may relax, leaving the airway sufficiently open for rescue breathing. If rescue breaths fail, chest compressions may clear the obstruction.

RECOGNITION

With partial obstruction:
- Coughing and distress.
- Difficulty crying or making any other noise.

With complete obstruction:
- Inability to breathe or cough, and eventual loss of consciousness.

▶ **See also** UNCONSCIOUS INFANT pp.95–98

✚ YOUR AIMS

- To remove the obstruction.
- To arrange urgent removal to hospital if necessary.

❶ WARNING

If at any stage the infant becomes unconscious, open the airway, check breathing, and give rescue breaths (p.96). If you cannot achieve effective breaths, immediately begin chest compressions to try to relieve the obstruction quickly (*see* HOW TO GIVE CPR, p.98).

1 If the infant is distressed, shows signs of becoming weak, or stops breathing or coughing, lay him face down along your forearm, with his head low, and support his back and head. Give up to five back slaps.

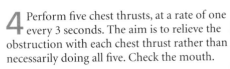

Make sure that head is below level of chest

2 Check the infant's mouth; remove any obvious obstructions with your fingertips. Do not do a finger sweep of the mouth.

3 If this fails to clear the obstruction, turn the infant on to his back and give up to five chest thrusts. Using two fingers, push inwards and upwards (towards the head) against the infant's breastbone, one finger's breadth below the nipple line.

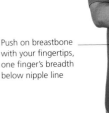

Push on breastbone with your fingertips, one finger's breadth below nipple line

4 Perform five chest thrusts, at a rate of one every 3 seconds. The aim is to relieve the obstruction with each chest thrust rather than necessarily doing all five. Check the mouth.

5 If the obstruction is not cleared, repeat steps 1–4 three times. If the obstruction still has not cleared, take the infant with you to CALL AN AMBULANCE
Continue until help arrives or the infant becomes unconscious.

4

CONTENTS

O XYGEN IS ESSENTIAL TO LIFE. Every time we breathe in, air containing oxygen enters the lungs. This oxygen is then transferred to the blood, to be transported around the body. Breathing and the exchange of oxygen and carbon dioxide (a waste product from body tissues) are described as "respiration", and the structures that enable us to breathe make up the respiratory system.

WHAT CAN GO WRONG
Respiration can be impaired in various ways. The airways may be blocked; the exchange of oxygen and carbon dioxide in the lungs may be affected by inhalation of smoke or fumes; the function of the lungs may be impaired by chest injury; or the breathing mechanism may be affected by conditions such as asthma. Problems with respiration can be life-threatening and require urgent first aid.

✚ FIRST-AID PRIORITIES

● Assess the casualty's condition.

● Identify and remove the cause of the problem and provide fresh air.

● Comfort and reassure the casualty.

● Maintain an open airway, check breathing, and be prepared to resuscitate if necessary.

● Obtain medical aid if necessary. Call an ambulance if you suspect a serious illness or injury.

THE RESPIRATORY SYSTEM

This system comprises the mouth, nose, windpipe (trachea), lungs, and pulmonary blood vessels. Respiration involves the process of breathing and the exchange of gases (oxygen and carbon dioxide) in the lungs and in cells throughout the body.

We breathe in air in order to take oxygen into the lungs, and we breathe out to expel the waste gas carbon dioxide, a by-product of respiration.

When we breathe, air is drawn through the nose and mouth into the airway and the lungs. In the lungs, oxygen is taken from air sacs (alveoli) into the pulmonary capillaries. At the same time, carbon dioxide is released from the capillaries into the alveoli. This gas is then expelled as we breathe out.

An average man's lungs can hold approximately 6 litres (10 pints) of air; a woman's lungs can hold about 4 litres (7 pints).

Structure of the respiratory system
The lungs form the central part of the respiratory system. Together with the circulatory system, they perform the vital function of gas exchange in order to distribute oxygen around the body and remove carbon dioxide.

Lungs are two spongy organs that occupy a large part of chest cavity

Pleural membrane has two layers, separated by a lubricating fluid, which surround and protect each of the lungs

Capillary

Alveolus

Epiglottis

Larynx

Windpipe (trachea) extends from larynx to two main bronchi

Main bronchi branch from base of windpipe (trachea) into each lung and divide into smaller airways (bronchioles)

Bronchioles are small air passages that branch from bronchi and eventually open into alveoli (air sacs) within lungs

Rib

Intercostal muscles span spaces between ribs

Section through alveoli
A network of tiny blood vessels (capillaries) surrounds each alveolus (air sac). The thin walls of both structures allow oxygen to diffuse into the blood and carbon dioxide to leave it.

Diaphragm is a sheet of muscle that separates chest and abdominal cavities

How breathing works

The breathing process consists of the actions of breathing in (inspiration) and breathing out (expiration), followed by a pause. Pressure differences between the lungs and the air outside the body determine whether air is drawn in or expelled. When the air pressure in the lungs is lower than outside, air is drawn in; when pressure is higher, air is expelled. The pressure within the lungs is altered by the movements of the two main sets of muscles involved in breathing: the intercostal muscles and the diaphragm.

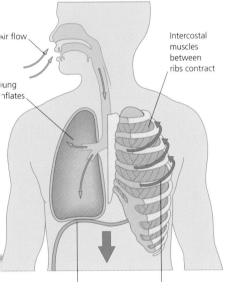

Air flow

Intercostal muscles between ribs contract

Lung inflates

Diaphragm contracts and moves down

Ribs rise and swing outwards

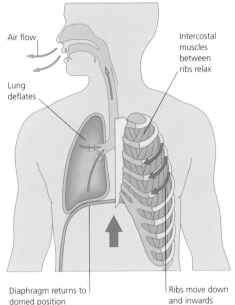

Air flow

Intercostal muscles between ribs relax

Lung deflates

Diaphragm returns to domed position

Ribs move down and inwards

Breathing in
The intercostal muscles (the muscles between the ribs) and the diaphragm contract, causing the chest cavity to expand, and the lungs expand to fill the space. As a result, the pressure inside the lungs is reduced, and air is drawn into the lungs.

Breathing out
The intercostal muscles relax, and the ribcage returns to its resting position, while the diaphragm relaxes and resumes its domed shape. As a result, the chest cavity becomes smaller, and pressure inside the lungs increases. Air flows out of the lungs to be exhaled.

How breathing is controlled

Breathing is regulated by a set of nerve cells in the brain called the respiratory centre. This centre responds to changes in the level of carbon dioxide in the blood. When the level rises, the respiratory centre responds by stimulating the intercostal muscles and the diaphragm to contract, and a breath occurs. Our breathing rate can be altered consciously under normal conditions. It also changes in response to abnormal levels of carbon dioxide, or to low levels of oxygen, or with stress, exercise, injury, or illness.

HYPOXIA

This condition arises when insufficient oxygen reaches body tissues from the blood. There are a number of causes (below), ranging from suffocation or poisoning to impaired lung or brain function. The condition is accompanied by a variety of symptoms, depending on the degree of hypoxia. If not treated quickly, hypoxia is potentially fatal because a sufficient level of oxygen is vital for the normal function of all the body organs and tissues.

In a healthy person, the amount of oxygen in the air is more than adequate for the body tissues to function normally. However, in a person who is ill or injured, a reduction in oxygen reaching the tissues results in deterioration of body function.

Mild hypoxia reduces a casualty's ability to think clearly, but the body responds to this by increasing the rate and depth of breathing (previous page). However, if the oxygen supply to the brain cells is cut off for as little as 3 minutes, the brain cells will begin to die. All the conditions covered in this chapter can result in hypoxia.

RECOGNITION

In moderate and severe hypoxia, there may be:
- Rapid breathing.
- Breathing that is distressed or gasping.
- Difficulty speaking.
- Grey–blue skin (cyanosis). At first, this will affect the extremities such as the lips, nailbeds, and earlobes, but, as the hypoxia worsens, cyanosis will affect the whole body.
- Anxiety.
- Restlessness.
- Headache.
- Nausea and possibly vomiting.
- Cessation of breathing if the hypoxia is not quickly reversed.

See also ANAPHYLACTIC SHOCK p.123
- ASTHMA p. 115 ● BURNS TO THE AIRWAY p.197 ● CROUP p.116 ● DROWNING p.109
- HANGING AND STRANGULATION p.108
- INHALATION OF FUMES p.110
- PENETRATING CHEST WOUND p.112
- STROKE p.183

CONDITIONS CAUSING LOW BLOOD OXYGEN (HYPOXIA)

Condition	Causes
Insufficient oxygen in inspired air	Suffocation by smoke or gas ● Changes in atmospheric pressure, for example at high altitude or in a depressurised aircraft
Airway obstruction	Blocking or swelling of the airway ● Hanging or strangulation ● Something covering the mouth and nose ● Asthma ● Choking ● Anaphylaxis
Conditions affecting the chest wall	Crushing, for example by a fall of earth or sand or pressure from a crowd ● Chest wall injury with multiple rib fractures or constricting burns
Impaired lung function	Lung injury ● Collapsed lung ● Lung infections, such as pneumonia
Damage to the brain or nerves that control respiration	A head injury or stroke that damages the breathing centre in the brain ● Some forms of poisoning ● Paralysis of nerves controlling the muscles of breathing, as in spinal cord injury
Impaired oxygen uptake by the tissues	Carbon monoxide or cyanide poisoning ● Shock

AIRWAY OBSTRUCTION

The airway may be obstructed internally, for example by an object that is stuck at the back of the throat, or externally. The main causes of obstruction are:

- Inhalation of a foreign object such as food or false teeth – choking.
- Blockage by the tongue when a casualty is unconscious.
- Blockage from blood or vomit.
- Internal swelling of the throat occurring with burns, scalds, stings, or anaphylaxis.
- Injuries to the face or jaw.
- Asthma.
- External pressure on the neck, as in hanging or strangulation (p.108).

Dry peanuts, which can swell up when in contact with body fluids, pose a particular danger in young children because they can obstruct one of the bronchi.

Airway obstruction requires prompt action from the first aider; be prepared to give rescue breaths and chest compressions if the casualty stops breathing (see LIFE-SAVING PROCEDURES, pp.71–102).

The information on this page is appropriate for all causes of airway obstruction, but if you need detailed instructions for specific situations, refer to the relevant pages.

▶ See also ASTHMA p. 115 ● BURNS TO THE AIRWAY p.197 ● CHOKING ADULT p.100 ● CHOKING INFANT p.102 ● CHOKING CHILD p.101 ● DROWNING p.109 ● HANGING AND STRANGULATION p.108 ● INHALATION OF FUMES p.110

✚ YOUR AIMS

- To remove the obstruction.
- To restore normal breathing.
- To arrange transport to hospital.

⓵ WARNING

If the casualty is unconscious, open the airway and check for breathing; be prepared to give rescue breaths and chest compressions if necessary (see LIFE-SAVING PROCEDURES, pp.71–102).

CALL AN AMBULANCE

1 Remove the obstruction if it is external or visible in the mouth.

2 If the casualty is conscious and breathing normally, reassure her, but keep her under observation. Monitor and record vital signs – level of response, pulse, and breathing (pp.42–43). Be prepared to give rescue breaths and chest compressions if necessary (see LIFE-SAVING PROCEDURES, pp.71–102).

3 Even if the casualty appears to have made a complete recovery, call a doctor or take or send the casualty to hospital.

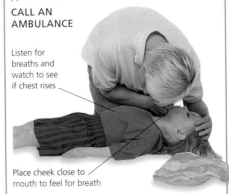

Listen for breaths and watch to see if chest rises

Place cheek close to mouth to feel for breath

HANGING AND STRANGULATION

If pressure is exerted on the outside of the neck, the airway is squeezed and the flow of air to the lungs is cut off. The main causes of such pressure are:

- Hanging – suspension of the body by a noose around the neck.
- Strangulation – constriction or squeezing around the neck or throat.

Sometimes, hanging or strangulation may occur accidentally – for example, by ties or clothing becoming caught in machinery. Hanging may cause a broken neck; for this reason, a casualty in this situation must be handled extremely carefully.

RECOGNITION

- A constricting article around the neck.
- Marks around the casualty's neck.
- Rapid, difficult breathing; impaired consciousness; grey–blue skin (cyanosis).
- Congestion of the face, with prominent veins and, possibly, tiny red spots on the face or on the whites of the eyes.

▶ **See also** LIFE-SAVING PROCEDURES pp.71–102 ● SPINAL INJURY pp.165–167

✚ YOUR AIMS

- To restore adequate breathing.
- To arrange urgent removal to hospital.

❶ CAUTION

- Do not move the casualty unnecessarily, in case of spinal injury.
- Do not destroy or interfere with any material that has been constricting the neck, such as knotted rope; police may need it as evidence.

1 Quickly remove any constriction from around the casualty's neck. Support the body while you do so if it is still hanging. Be aware that the body may be very heavy.

2 Lay the casualty on the ground. Open the airway and check breathing. If she is not breathing, be prepared to give rescue breaths and chest compressions if necessary (*see* LIFE-SAVING PROCEDURES, pp.71–102). If she is breathing, place her in the recovery position.

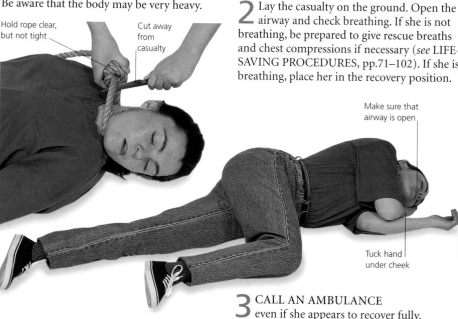

Hold rope clear, but not tight

Cut away from casualty

Make sure that airway is open

Tuck hand under cheek

3 CALL AN AMBULANCE even if she appears to recover fully.

DROWNING

Death by drowning occurs when air cannot get into the lungs, usually because a small amount of water has entered the lungs. This may also cause spasm of the throat.

When a drowning person is rescued, water may gush from the mouth. This water is from the stomach and should be left to drain of its own accord. Do not attempt to force water from the stomach because the casualty may vomit and then inhale it.

A casualty from a drowning incident should always receive medical attention even if he seems to recover at the time. Any water entering the lungs causes them to become irritated, and the air passages may begin to swell several hours later – a condition known as secondary drowning.

The casualty may also need to be treated for hypothermia (pp.206–208).

▶ See also HYPOTHERMIA pp.206–208
● LIFE-SAVING PROCEDURES pp.71–102
● WATER RESCUE p.28

✚ YOUR AIMS
● To restore adequate breathing.
● To keep the casualty warm.
● To arrange urgent removal to hospital.

1 If you are rescuing the casualty from the water to safety, keep her head lower than the rest of the body to reduce the risk of her inhaling water (p.28).

2 Lay the casualty down on her back on a rug or coat. Open the airway and check breathing; be prepared to give rescue breaths and chest compressions if necessary (*see* LIFE-SAVING PROCEDURES, pp.71–102). If the casualty is breathing, place her in the recovery position (pp.84–85).

3 Treat the casualty for hypothermia; remove wet clothing if possible and cover her with dry blankets. If the casualty regains full consciousness, give her a warm drink.

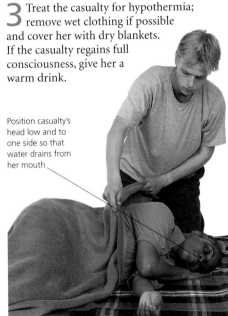

Position casualty's head low and to one side so that water drains from her mouth

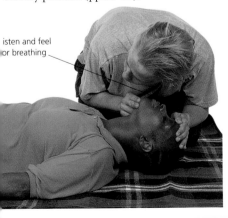

Listen and feel for breathing

4 CALL AN AMBULANCE even if she appears to recover fully.

❶ WARNING
Water in the lungs and the effects of cold can increase resistance to rescue breaths and chest compressions: you may have to do both at a slower rate than normal.

INHALATION OF FUMES

The inhalation of smoke, gases (such as carbon monoxide), or toxic vapours can be lethal. A casualty who has inhaled fumes is likely to have low levels of oxygen in his body tissues (see HYPOXIA, p.106) and therefore needs urgent medical attention. Do not attempt to carry out a rescue if it is likely to put your own life at risk; fumes that have built up in a confined space may quickly overcome anyone who is not wearing protective equipment.

SMOKE INHALATION

Any person who has been enclosed in a confined space during a fire should be assumed to have inhaled smoke. Smoke from burning plastics, foam padding, and synthetic wall coverings is likely to contain poisonous fumes. Casualties should also be examined for other injuries due to the fire.

INHALATION OF CARBON MONOXIDE

Carbon monoxide is a poisonous gas that i produced by burning. It acts directly on red blood cells, preventing them from carrying oxygen to the body tissues. If the gas is inhaled in large quantities – for example, from smoke or vehicle exhaust fumes in a confined space – it can very quickly prove fatal. However, lengthy exposure to even a small amount of carbon monoxide – for example, due to a leakage of fumes from a defective heater or flue – may also result in severe, or possibly fatal, poisoning.

Carbon monoxide has no taste or smell, so take care if you suspect a leak.

▶ See also BURNS TO THE AIRWAYS, p.197 ● FIRES p.24 ● HYPOXIA p.106 ● LIFE-SAVING PROCEDURES pp.71–102

EFFECTS OF FUME INHALATION

Gas	Source	Effects
Carbon monoxide	Exhaust fumes of motor vehicles ● Smoke from most fires ● Back-draughts from blocked chimney flues ● Emissions from defective gas or paraffin heaters	*Prolonged exposure to low levels:* Headache ● Confusion ● Aggression ● Nausea and vomiting ● Incontinence *Brief exposure to high levels:* Grey–blue skin coloration with a faint red tinge ● Rapid, difficult breathing ● Impaired consciousness, leading to unconsciousness
Smoke	Fires: smoke is a bigger killer than fire itself. Smoke is low in oxygen (which is used up by the burning of the fire) and may contain toxic fumes from burning materials	Rapid, noisy, difficult breathing ● Coughing and wheezing ● Burning in the nose or mouth ● Soot around the mouth and nose ● Unconsciousness
Carbon dioxide	Tends to accumulate and become dangerously concentrated in deep enclosed spaces, such as coal pits, wells, and underground tanks	Breathlessness ● Headache ● Confusion ● Unconsciousness
Solvents and fuels	Glues ● Cleaning fluids ● Lighter fuels ● Camping gas and propane-fuelled stoves. Solvent abusers may use a plastic bag to concentrate the vapour (especially with glues)	Headache and vomiting ● Impaired consciousness ● Airway obstruction from using a plastic bag or from choking on vomit may result in death ● Cardiac arrest is potential cause of death, and this may occur following inhalation of the very cold gases that are released from pressurised containers

✚ YOUR AIMS

● To restore adequate breathing.
● To obtain urgent medical attention and call the emergency services.

❶ CAUTION

If entering a garage filled with vehicle exhaust fumes, open the doors wide and let the gas escape before entering.

1 CALL FOR EMERGENCY HELP
Ask for both fire and ambulance services. If the casualty's clothing is still burning, try to extinguish the flames (p.25).

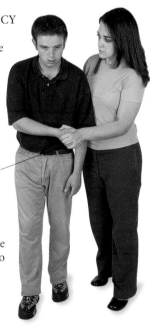

Support the casualty

2 If it is necessary to escape from the source of the fumes, move the casualty into fresh air (*see* CASUALTY HANDLING, pp.63–64).

3 Support the casualty and encourage him to breathe normally. Treat any obvious burns (pp.192–197) or other injuries.

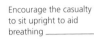

Encourage the casualty to sit upright to aid breathing

4 Stay with the casualty until help arrives. Monitor and record vital signs – level of response, pulse, and breathing (pp. 42–43).

❶ WARNING

If the casualty is unconscious, open the airway and check breathing; be prepared to give rescue breaths and chest compressions if necessary (*see* LIFE-SAVING PROCEDURES, pp.71–102). If he is breathing, place him in the recovery position (pp.84–85).

Listen for breathing

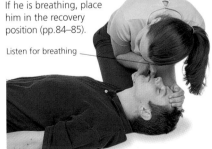

Monitor his pulse

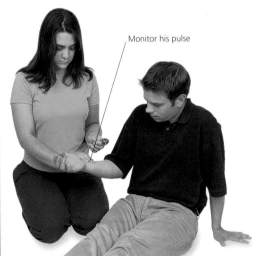

PENETRATING CHEST WOUND

The heart and lungs, and the major blood vessels around them, lie within the chest (thorax), protected by the breastbone and the 12 pairs of ribs that make up the ribcage. The ribcage extends far enough downwards to protect organs such as the liver and spleen in the upper part of the abdomen.

If a sharp object penetrates the chest wall, there may be severe internal damage within the chest and the upper abdomen. The lungs are particularly susceptible to injury, either by being damaged themselves or from wounds that perforate the two-layered membrane (pleura) surrounding and protecting each lung. Air can then enter between the membranes and exert pressure on the lung, and the lung may collapse – a condition called pneumothorax.

Pressure around the affected lung may build up to such an extent that it also affects the uninjured lung. As a result, the casualty becomes increasingly breathless. This build-up of pressure may prevent the heart from refilling with blood properly, impairing the

circulation and causing shock – a condition known as a tension pneumothorax. Sometimes, blood collects in the pleural cavity and puts pressure on the lungs.

> **RECOGNITION**
>
> ● Difficult and painful breathing, possibly rapid, shallow, and uneven.
> ● Casualty feels an acute sense of alarm.
> ● Features of hypoxia (p.106), including grey–blue skin coloration (cyanosis).
>
> *There may also be:*
> ● Coughed-up frothy, red blood.
> ● A crackling feeling of the skin around the site of the wound, caused by air collecting in the tissues.
> ● Blood bubbling out of the wound.
> ● Sound of air being sucked into the chest as the casualty breathes in.
> ● Veins in the neck becoming prominent.

▶ **See also** HYPOXIA, p.106 ● LIFE-SAVING PROCEDURES p.71–102 ● SHOCK pp.120–121

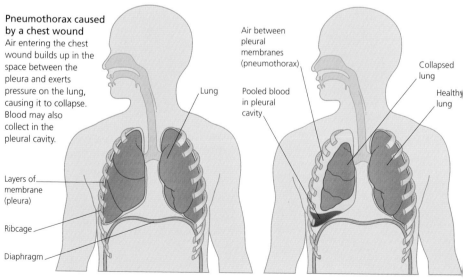

Pneumothorax caused by a chest wound
Air entering the chest wound builds up in the space between the pleura and exerts pressure on the lung, causing it to collapse. Blood may also collect in the pleural cavity.

Layers of membrane (pleura)

Ribcage

Diaphragm

Lung

NORMAL LUNGS

Air between pleural membranes (pneumothorax)

Pooled blood in pleural cavity

Collapsed lung

Healthy lung

PNEUMOTHORAX

- To seal the wound and maintain breathing.
- To minimise shock.
- To arrange urgent removal to hospital.

1 Put on disposable gloves if available. Encourage the casualty to lean towards the injured side and use the palm of his hand to cover the wound.

Completely cover the wound to stop air from being drawn into the chest cavity

2 Place a sterile dressing or non-fluffy clean pad over the wound and surrounding area. Cover with a plastic bag, foil, or kitchen film. Secure firmly with adhesive tape on three edges, or with bandages around the chest, so that the dressing is taut.

Leave fourth side untaped to allow air under pressure during expiration to escape

3 CALL AN AMBULANCE While waiting for help, continue to support the casualty in the same position as long as he remains conscious.

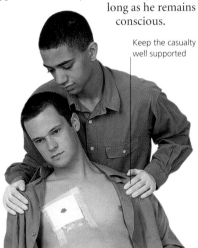

Keep the casualty well supported

4 Monitor and record vital signs – level of response, pulse, and breathing (pp.42–43) – until medical help arrives.

! WARNING

If the casualty becomes unconscious, open the airway and check breathing; be prepared to give rescue breaths and chest compressions, if necessary (see LIFE-SAVING PROCEDURES, pp.71–102). If breathing, place him in the recovery position (pp.84–85), lying on his injured side to help the healthy lung to work effectively.

Keep head tilted back, supported by hand

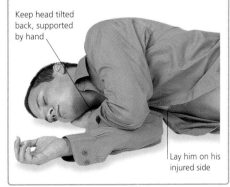

Lay him on his injured side

HYPERVENTILATION

Excessive breathing (hyperventilation) is commonly a manifestation of acute anxiety and may accompany a panic attack. It may occur in susceptible individuals who have recently experienced an emotional or psychological shock.

Hyperventilation causes an abnormal loss of carbon dioxide from the blood, leading to chemical changes within the blood. These changes lead to symptoms such as unnaturally fast breathing, dizziness, and trembling and tingling in the hands. As breathing returns to normal, these symptoms will gradually subside.

RECOGNITION

● Unnaturally fast, deep breathing.

There may also be:
● Attention-seeking behaviour.
● Dizziness or faintness.
● Trembling or marked tingling in the hands.
● Cramps in the hands and feet.

 See also PANIC ATTACK p.242

YOUR AIMS

● To remove the casualty from the cause of distress.
● To reassure the casualty and calm her down.

1 When speaking to the casualty, be firm but kind and reassuring.

2 If possible, lead the casualty away to a quiet place where she may be able to regain control of her breathing more easily and quickly. If this is not possible, ask any bystanders to leave.

3 If the casualty is not able to regain control of her breathing, ask her to rebreathe her own exhaled air from a paper bag. Tell her to breathe in and out slowly, using the bag, about 10 times and then breathe without the bag for 15 seconds. She should continue to alternate this cycle of breathing with and without the bag until the need to breathe rapidly has passed.

Ensure bag covers nose and mouth

4 Encourage the casualty to see her doctor about preventing and controlling panic attacks in the future.

ASTHMA

In an asthma attack, the muscles of the air passages in the lungs go into spasm and the linings of the airways swell. As a result, the airways become narrowed, which makes breathing difficult.

Sometimes there is a recognised trigger for an attack, such as an allergy, a cold, a particular drug, or cigarette smoke. At other times, there is no obvious trigger. Many sufferers have sudden attacks at night.

People with asthma usually deal with their own attacks, using a "reliever" inhaler at the first sign of an attack. Most reliever inhalers have blue caps. A plastic diffuser, or "spacer", can be fitted to an inhaler to help the casualty breathe in the medication more effectively. Preventer inhalers usually have brown or white caps and are used regularly by people with asthma to help prevent attacks. However, preventer inhalers are not an effective treatment for asthma attacks and should not be used in this situation.

RECOGNITION
● Difficulty in breathing, with a very prolonged breathing-out phase.

There may also be:
● Wheezing as the casualty breathes out.
● Difficulty speaking and whispering.
● Features of hypoxia (p.106), such as a grey–blue tinge to the lips, earlobes, and nailbeds (cyanosis).
● Distress and anxiety.
● Cough.
● In a severe attack, exhaustion. Rarely, the casualty loses consciousness and stops breathing.

YOUR AIMS
● To ease breathing.
● To obtain medical help if necessary.

1 Keep calm and reassure the casualty. Get her to take a puff of her reliever inhaler. It should relieve the asthma attack within a few minutes. Ask her to breathe slowly and deeply.

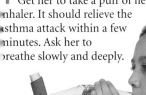

Inhaler

Use a spacer with the inhaler, if the child has one

2 Let her adopt the position that she finds most comfortable – often sitting down. Do not make the casualty lie down.

3 A mild asthma attack should ease within 3 minutes. If it does not, ask the casualty to take another dose from the same inhaler.

● CAUTION
If this is the first attack, or if the attack is severe and any one of the following occurs:
● the inhaler has no effect after 5 minutes,
● the casualty is getting worse,
● breathlessness makes talking difficult,
● she is becoming exhausted,

CALL AN AMBULANCE

Help her to use her inhaler every 5–10 minutes. Monitor and record her breathing and pulse every 10 minutes (pp.42–43).

● WARNING
If the casualty loses consciousness, open the airway and check breathing; be prepared to give rescue breaths and chest compressions if necessary (*see* LIFE-SAVING TECHNIQUES, pp.71–102).

CALL AN AMBULANCE

If the casualty is breathing, place her in the recovery position (pp.84–85). Monitor her vital signs – level of response, pulse, and breathing (pp.42–43) – until help arrives.

CROUP

An attack of severe breathing difficulty in very young children is known as croup. It is caused by inflammation in the windpipe and larynx. Croup can be alarming but usually passes without lasting harm. Attacks of croup usually occur at night and may recur before the child settles.

EPIGLOTTITIS RISK

If an attack of croup persists or is severe, and is accompanied by fever, call an ambulance. There is a small risk that the child is suffering from a rare, croup-like condition called epiglottitis, in which the epiglottis (p.104), a small, flap-like structure in the throat, becomes infected and swollen and may block the airway completely. The child then needs urgent medical attention.

RECOGNITION

● Distressed breathing in a young child.
There may also be:
● A short, barking cough.
● A crowing or whistling noise, especially on breathing in (stridor).
● Blue–grey skin (cyanosis).
● In severe cases, the child using muscles around the nose, neck, and upper arms in trying to breathe.
Suspect epiglottitis if:
● A child is sitting bolt upright and is in respiratory distress.
● The child has a high temperature.

✚ YOUR AIMS

● To comfort and support the child.
● To obtain medical help if necessary.

1 Sit the child up on your knee, supporting her back. Calmly reassure the child. Try not to panic because this will only alarm her and is likely to make the attack worse.

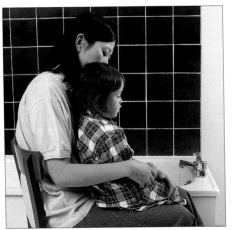

2 Create a steamy atmosphere: either take the child into the bathroom and run the hot tap or shower, or go into the kitchen and boil some water. Sit her down and encourage her to breathe in the steam; this should ease her breathing. Take care to keep the child clear of running hot water or steam.

3 Call a doctor or, if croup is severe, CALL AN AMBULANCE

4 When the child is put back to bed, create a humid atmosphere in her bedroom – for example, by hanging a wet towel over a radiator in the room. The humidity may prevent an attack from recurring.

❶ CAUTION

Do not put your fingers down the child's throat. This can cause the throat muscles to go into spasm and block the airway.

5

T HE HEART AND the network of blood
vessels are collectively known as the
circulatory (cardiovascular) system.
This system keeps the body supplied
with blood, which carries oxygen and
nutrients to all body tissues.

The circulatory system may be
disrupted in two main ways: severe
bleeding and fluid loss may cause the
volume of blood to fall, depriving the
organs of oxygen; or age or disease may
cause the system to break down. The
techniques described in this section show
how a first aider can help to maintain an
adequate blood supply to a casualty's
heart and brain. In minor incidents,
first aid should ensure the casualty's
recovery. In serious cases, such as a
heart attack, your action may be vital
in preserving life until help arrives.

CONTENTS

+ FIRST-AID PRIORITIES

- Assess the casualty's condition.
- Comfort and reassure the casualty.
- Position the casualty to improve the blood supply to the vital organs.
- Loosen tight clothing to ease breathing and improve circulation.
- Maintain an open airway, check breathing, and be prepared to resuscitate if necessary.
- Obtain medical aid if necessary. Call an ambulance if you suspect a serious illness or injury.

THE HEART AND BLOOD VESSELS

The circulatory system consists of the heart and the blood vessels. These structures supply the body with a constant flow of blood, which brings oxygen and nutrients to the tissues and carries waste products away.

Blood is pumped around the body by rhythmic contractions (beats) of the heart muscle. The blood runs through a network of vessels, divided into three types: arteries, veins, and capillaries. The force that is exerted by the blood flow through the main arteries is called blood pressure. It varies with the strength and phase of the heartbeat, the elasticity of the arterial walls, and the volume and thickness of the blood.

How blood circulates
Oxygen-rich (oxygenated) blood passes from the lungs to the heart, then travels to body tissues via the arteries. Blood that has given up its oxygen (deoxygenated blood) returns to the heart through the veins.

Brachial artery

Aorta carries oxygenated blood to body tissues

Vena cava carries deoxygenated blood from body tissues to heart

Radial artery

Femoral artery

Carotid artery

Jugular vein

Brachial vein

Pulmonary arteries carry deoxygenated blood to lungs

Pulmonary veins carry oxygenated blood from lungs to heart

Heart pumps blood around body

Radial vein

Femoral vein

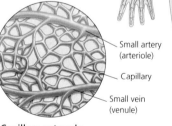

Small artery (arteriole)

Capillary

Small vein (venule)

Capillary networks
Networks of fine blood vessels (capillaries) link arteries and veins within body tissues. Oxygen and nutrients pass from the blood into the tissues; waste products pass from the tissues into the blood, through capillaries.

Superior vena cava

Inferior vena cava

Aorta

Heart muscle

Coronary artery

Coronary vein

The heart
This muscular organ pumps blood around the body and then to the lungs to pick up oxygen. Coronary blood vessels supply the heart muscle with oxygen and nutrients.

KEY
 Vessels carrying oxygenated blood

Vessels carrying deoxygenated blood

How the heart functions

The heart pumps blood by muscular contractions called heartbeats, which are controlled by electrical impulses generated in the heart. Each beat has three phases: diastole, when blood enters the heart; atrial systole, when blood is squeezed out of the atria (collecting chambers); and ventricular systole, when blood leaves the heart.

In diastole, the heart relaxes. Oxygen-rich (oxygenated) blood from the lungs flows via the pulmonary veins into the left atrium. Blood that has given up its oxygen to body tissues (deoxygenated blood) flows from the venae cavae (large veins) to the right atrium.

In atrial systole, the two atria contract and the valves between the atria and the ventricles (pumping chambers) open so that blood flows into the ventricles.

During ventricular systole, the ventricles contract. The thick-walled left ventricle forces blood into the aorta (main artery), which carries it to the rest of the body. The right ventricle pumps blood into the pulmonary artery, which carries it to the lungs to collect more oxygen.

Blood flow through the heart

The heart's right side pumps deoxygenated blood from the body to the lungs. The left side pumps oxygenated blood to the whole of the body.

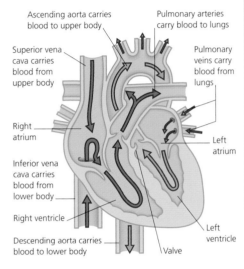

Ascending aorta carries blood to upper body

Pulmonary arteries carry blood to lungs

Superior vena cava carries blood from upper body

Pulmonary veins carry blood from lungs

Right atrium

Left atrium

Inferior vena cava carries blood from lower body

Right ventricle

Left ventricle

Descending aorta carries blood to lower body

Valve

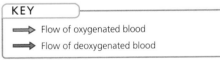

KEY

⟹ Flow of oxygenated blood

⟹ Flow of deoxygenated blood

Composition of blood

There are about 6 litres (10 pints), or 1 litre per 13 kg of body weight (1 pint per stone), of blood in the average adult body. Roughly 55 per cent of the blood is clear yellow fluid (plasma). In this fluid are suspended the red and white blood cells and the platelets, all of which make up the other 45 per cent.

The blood cells

Red blood cells contain haemoglobin, a red pigment that enables the cells to carry oxygen. White blood cells play a role in defending the body against infection. Platelets help blood to clot.

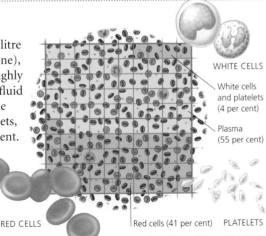

WHITE CELLS

White cells and platelets (4 per cent)

Plasma (55 per cent)

RED CELLS

Red cells (41 per cent)

PLATELETS

119

SHOCK

This life-threatening condition occurs when the circulatory system (which distributes oxygen to the body tissues and removes waste products) fails and, as a result, vital organs such as the heart and brain are deprived of oxygen. It requires immediate emergency treatment to prevent permanent organ damage and death.

Shock can be made worse by fear and pain. Whenever there is a risk of shock developing, reassuring the casualty and making him comfortable may be sufficient to prevent him from deteriorating.

CAUSES OF SHOCK

The most common cause of shock is severe blood loss. If this exceeds 1.2 litres (2 pints), which is about one-fifth of the normal blood volume, shock will occur. This degree of blood loss may result from wounds. It may also be caused by hidden bleeding from internal organs (p.122), blood escaping into a body cavity, or bleeding from damaged blood vessels due to a closed fracture (p.151). Loss of other body fluids can also result in shock. Conditions that can cause heavy fluid loss include diarrhoea, vomiting, blockage in the intestine, and severe burns.

In addition, shock may occur when there is adequate blood volume but the heart is unable to pump the blood. This problem can be due to severe heart disease, heart

attack, or acute heart failure. Other causes of shock include overwhelming infection, lack of certain hormones, low blood sugar (hypoglycaemia), hypothermia, severe allergic reaction (anaphylactic shock), drug overdose, and spinal cord injury.

▶ See also ANAPHYLACTIC SHOCK p.123
● LIFE-SAVING PROCEDURES pp.71–102
● SEVERE BLEEDING pp.130–131 ● SEVERE BURNS AND SCALDS pp.194–195

RECOGNITION

Initially:
● A rapid pulse.
● Pale, cold, clammy skin; sweating.

As shock develops:
● Grey–blue skin (cyanosis), especially inside the lips. A fingernail or earlobe, if pressed, will not regain its colour immediately.
● Weakness and dizziness.
● Nausea, and possibly vomiting.
● Thirst.
● Rapid, shallow breathing.
● A weak, "thready" pulse. When the pulse at the wrist disappears, about half of the blood volume will have been lost.

As the brain's oxygen supply weakens:
● Restlessness and aggressiveness.
● Yawning and gasping for air.
● Unconsciousness.

Finally, the heart will stop.

EFFECTS OF BLOOD OR FLUID LOSS

Approximate volume lost	Effects on the body
0.5 litre (about 1 pint)	Little or no effect; this is the quantity normally taken in a blood-donor session
Up to 2 litres (3.5 pints)	Hormones such as adrenaline are released, quickening the pulse and inducing sweating ● Small blood vessels in non-vital areas, such as the skin, shut down to divert blood and oxygen to the vital organs ● Shock becomes evident
2 litres (3.5 pints) or more (over a third of the normal volume in the average adult)	As blood or fluid loss approaches this level, the pulse at the wrist may become undetectable ● Casualty will usually lose consciousness ● Breathing may cease and the heart may stop

1 Treat any possible cause of shock that you can detect, such as severe bleeding (pp.130–131) or serious burns (p.194).

2 Lay the casualty down on a blanket to insulate her from the cold ground. Constantly reassure her.

3 Raise and support her legs to improve the blood supply to the vital organs. Take care if you suspect a fracture.

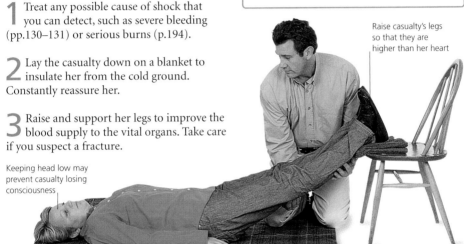

Raise casualty's legs so that they are higher than her heart

Keeping head low may prevent casualty losing consciousness

4 Loosen tight clothing at the neck, chest, and waist to reduce constriction in these areas.

5 Keep the casualty warm by covering her body and legs with coats or blankets.
CALL AN AMBULANCE

6 Monitor and record vital signs – level of response, pulse, and breathing (pp.42–43). If the person becomes unconscious, open the airway and check breathing; be prepared to give rescue breaths and chest compressions if necessary (*see* LIFE-SAVING PROCEDURES, pp.71–102).

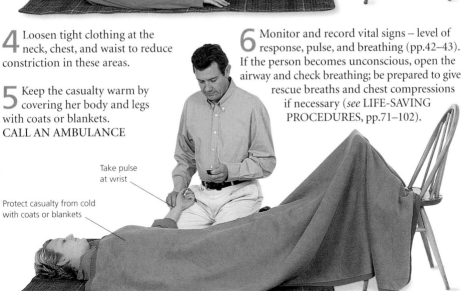

Take pulse at wrist

Protect casualty from cold with coats or blankets

INTERNAL BLEEDING

Bleeding inside body cavities may follow an injury, such as a fracture or a penetrating wound, but can also occur spontaneously – for example, bleeding from a stomach ulcer. The main risk from internal bleeding is shock (pp.120–121). In addition, blood can build up around organs such as the lungs or brain and exert damaging pressure on them.

You should suspect internal bleeding if a casualty develops signs of shock without obvious blood loss. Check for any bleeding from body openings (orifices) such as the ear, mouth, urethra, or anus (below).

 See also CEREBRAL COMPRESSION p.181
● CRUSH INJURY p.133

 Treat as for SHOCK pp.120–121

> ## RECOGNITION
>
> ● Initially, pale, cold, clammy skin. If bleeding continues, skin may turn blue–grey (cyanosis).
> ● Rapid, weak pulse.
> ● Thirst.
> ● Rapid, shallow breathing.
> ● Confusion, restlessness, and irritability.
> ● Possible collapse and unconsciousness.
> ● Bleeding from body openings (orifices).
> ● In cases of violent injury, "pattern bruising" – an area of discoloured skin with a shape that matches the pattern of clothes, crushing objects, or restraining objects (such as a seat belt).
> ● Pain.
> ● Information from the casualty that indicates recent injury or illness; previous similar episodes of internal bleeding; or use of drugs to control a medical condition such as thrombosis (in which unwanted clots form in blood vessels).

POSSIBLE SIGNS OF INTERNAL BLEEDING

Signs of bleeding vary depending on the site of the blood loss, but the most obvious feature is a discharge of blood from a body opening (orifice). Blood loss from any orifice is significant and can lead to shock (pp.120–121). In addition, bleeding from some orifices can indicate a serious underlying injury or illness.

Site	Appearance of blood	Cause of blood loss
Mouth	Bright red, frothy, coughed-up blood	Bleeding in the lungs
	Vomited blood, red or dark reddish-brown, resembling coffee grounds	Bleeding within the digestive system
Ear	Fresh, bright red blood	Injury to the inner or outer ear ● Perforated eardrum
	Thin, watery blood	Leakage of fluid from around brain due to head injury
Nose	Fresh, bright red blood	Ruptured blood vessel in the nostril
	Thin, watery blood	Leakage of fluid from around brain due to head injury
Anus	Fresh, bright red blood	Piles ● Injury to the anus or lower intestine
	Black, tarry, offensive-smelling stool (melaena)	Disease or injury to the intestine
Urethra	Urine with a red or smoky appearance and occasionally containing clots	Bleeding from the bladder, kidneys, or urethra
Vagina	Either fresh or dark blood	Menstruation ● Miscarriage ● Pregnancy or recent childbirth ● Disease of, or injury to, the vagina or uterus

ANAPHYLACTIC SHOCK

This condition is a severe allergic reaction affecting the whole body. In susceptible individuals, it may develop within seconds or minutes of contact with a trigger factor and is potentially fatal. Possible triggers include the following:

- Skin or airborne contact with particular materials.
- The injection of a specific drug.
- The sting of a certain insect.
- The ingestion of a food such as peanuts.

In an anaphylactic reaction, chemicals are released into the blood that widen (dilate) blood vessels and constrict (narrow) air passages. Blood pressure falls dramatically, and breathing is impaired. The tongue and throat can swell, increasing the risk of

hypoxia (p.106). The amount of oxygen reaching the vital organs is severely reduced.

A casualty with anaphylactic shock needs emergency treatment with an injection of epinephrine (adrenaline). First aid priorities are to ease breathing and minimise shock until specialised help arrives.

RECOGNITION

- Anxiety.
- Widespread red, blotchy skin eruption.
- Swelling of the tongue and throat.
- Puffiness around the eyes.
- Impaired breathing, ranging from a tight chest to severe difficulty; the casualty may wheeze and gasp for air.
- Signs of shock (pp.120–121).

YOUR AIM

- To arrange urgent removal to hospital.

1 CALL AN AMBULANCE
Give any information you have on the cause of the casualty's condition.

2 Check whether the casualty is carrying the necessary medication – a syringe or an auto-injector of epinephrine (adrenaline) for self-administration. Help her to use it. If the casualty is unable to administer the medication, and you have been trained to use an auto-injector, give it to her yourself.

3 If the casualty is conscious, help her to sit up in the position that most relieves any breathing difficulty.

4 Treat the casualty for shock (pp.120–121) if necessary.

WARNING

If the casualty becomes unconscious, open the airway and check breathing; be prepared to give rescue breaths and chest compressions if necessary (*see* LIFE-SAVING PROCEDURES, pp.71–102). If the casualty is breathing, place her in the recovery position (pp.84–85).

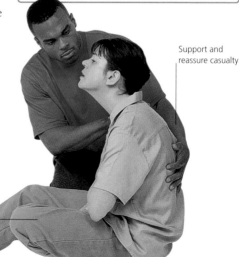

Support and reassure casualty

Sitting position should help to ease casualty's breathing

ANGINA PECTORIS

The term "angina pectoris" means literally "a constriction of the chest". Angina occurs when coronary arteries, which supply the heart muscle with blood, become narrowed and cannot carry sufficient blood to meet increased demands during exertion or excitement. An attack forces the casualty to rest; the pain should ease soon afterwards.

RECOGNITION
- Vice-like central chest pain, often spreading to the jaw and down one or both arms.
- Pain easing with rest.
- Shortness of breath.
- Weakness, which is often sudden and extreme.
- Feeling of anxiety.

✚ YOUR AIMS
- To ease strain on the heart by ensuring that the casualty rests.
- To obtain medical help if necessary.
- To help the casualty with any medication.

❶ WARNING

If the pain persists, or returns, suspect a heart attack (opposite)

CALL AN AMBULANCE

Treat by giving the casualty a full-dose (300mg) aspirin tablet to chew. Constantly monitor and record vital signs – level of response, pulse, and breathing (pp.42–43).

If the casualty becomes unconscious, open the airway and check breathing; be prepared to give rescue breaths and chest compressions if necessary (see LIFE-SAVING PROCEDURES, pp.71–102).

1 Help the casualty to sit down. Make sure that she is comfortable and reassure her. This action should help her breathing.

2 If the casualty has medication for angina, such as tablets or a pump-action or aerosol spray, let her administer it herself. If necessary, help her to take it.

Supervise and support casualty as she takes medication

3 Encourage the casualty to rest, and keep any bystanders away. The attack should ease within a few minutes.

ACUTE HEART FAILURE

In heart failure, the heart muscle is over-strained or damaged and cannot pump sufficient blood to the body tissues. Fluid may also build up in the lungs, leading to breathing difficulties. A possible cause of heart failure is a clot in a coronary artery (coronary thrombosis). Attacks of acute heart failure occur suddenly, often at night.

RECOGNITION
- Severe breathlessness.
- Often, but not always, signs and symptoms of heart attack (opposite).

▶ **Treat as for HEART ATTACK opposite**

124

HEART ATTACK

A heart attack is most commonly caused by sudden obstruction of the blood supply to part of the heart muscle – for example, because of a clot in a coronary artery (coronary thrombosis). The main risk is that the heart will stop beating.

The effects of a heart attack depend largely on how much of the heart muscle is affected; many casualties recover completely. Drugs such as aspirin, and medications that dissolve the clot, are used to limit the extent of damage to the heart muscle.

> See also LIFE-SAVING PROCEDURES
> pp.71–102

RECOGNITION

- Persistent, vice-like central chest pain, often spreading to the jaw and down one or both arms. Unlike angina pectoris (opposite), the pain does not ease when the casualty rests.
- Breathlessness, and discomfort occurring high in the abdomen, which may feel similar to severe indigestion.
- Collapse, often without any warning.
- Sudden faintness or dizziness.
- A sense of impending doom.
- "Ashen" skin, and blueness at the lips.
- A rapid, weak, or irregular pulse.
- Profuse sweating.
- Extreme gasping for air ("air hunger").

+ YOUR AIMS

- To encourage the casualty to rest.
- To arrange urgent removal of the casualty to hospital.

⊘ WARNING

If the casualty becomes unconscious, open the airway and check breathing; be prepared to give rescue breaths and chest compressions if needed (see LIFE-SAVING PROCEDURES, pp.71–102).

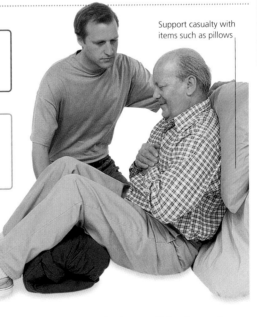

Support casualty with items such as pillows

1 Make the casualty as comfortable as possible to ease the strain on his heart. A half-sitting position, with the casualty's head and shoulders well supported and his knees bent, is often best.

2 CALL AN AMBULANCE
State that you suspect a heart attack. If the casualty asks you to do so, call his own doctor as well.

3 If the casualty is fully conscious, give him a full-dose (300 mg) aspirin tablet and advise him to chew it slowly.

4 If the casualty has medicine for angina, such as tablets or a pump-action or aerosol spray, help him to take it. Encourage the casualty to rest.

5 Constantly monitor and record vital signs – level of response, pulse, and breathing (pp.42–43) – until help arrives.

FAINTING

A faint is a brief loss of consciousness caused by a temporary reduction of the blood flow to the brain. Fainting may be a reaction to pain, exhaustion, lack of food, or emotional stress. It is also common after long periods of physical inactivity, such as standing or sitting still, especially in a warm atmosphere. This inactivity causes blood to pool in the legs, reducing the amount of blood reaching the brain.

When a person faints, the pulse rate becomes very slow. However, the rate soon

picks up and returns to normal. A casualty who has fainted usually makes a rapid and complete recovery.

▶ See also LIFE-SAVING PROCEDURES pp.71–102

✚ YOUR AIMS

● To improve blood flow to the brain.
● To reassure the casualty as she recovers and make her comfortable.

1 When a casualty feels faint, advise her to lie down. Kneel down, raise her legs, and support her ankles on your shoulders; this helps to improve the blood flow to the brain.

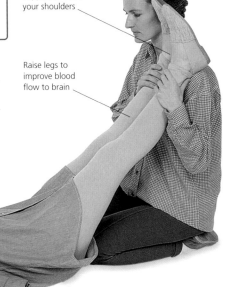

Support ankles on your shoulders

Raise legs to improve blood flow to brain

Watch face for signs of recovery

2 Make sure that the casualty has plenty of fresh air; ask someone to open a window. In addition, ask any bystanders to stand clear.

3 As she recovers, reassure her and help her to sit up gradually. If she starts to feel faint again, advise her to lie down again, and raise and support her legs until she recovers fully.

❶ WARNING

If the casualty does not regain consciousness quickly, open the airway and check breathing; be prepared to give rescue breaths and chest compressions if necessary (see LIFE-SAVING PROCEDURES, pp.71–102).

CALL AN AMBULANCE

6

B REAKS IN THE SKIN or the body surfaces are known as wounds. Open wounds allow blood and other fluids to be lost from the body and enable germs to enter. In a closed wound, bleeding is confined within the body tissues and is most easily recognised by bruising. Wounds can be daunting, particularly if there is a lot of bleeding, but prompt action will reduce the amount of blood loss and minimise shock.

UNDERSTANDING TREATMENT
The way in which an injury is inflicted and the force that is exerted determine the effect of the wound on the body and influence its treatment. Recommended treatments for all types of wound are covered in this chapter. When you are treating any wound, it is important to follow good hygiene procedures to guard both yourself and the casualty against cross-infection (p.15).

FIRST-AID PRIORITIES

- Assess the casualty's condition.
- Comfort and reassure the casualty.
- Take care with hygiene.
- Control blood loss by applying pressure and elevating the injured part.
- Minimise shock.
- Obtain medical help, if necessary. Call an ambulance if you suspect a serious illness or injury.

CONTENTS

WOUNDS AND BLEEDING

SEVERE BLEEDING

When bleeding is severe, it can be dramatic and distressing. Shock is likely to develop, and the casualty may lose consciousness. If bleeding is not controlled, the casualty's heart could stop. Bleeding at the face or neck may impede the air flow to the lungs.

When treating severe bleeding, check first whether there is an object embedded in the wound; take care not to press on the object.

▶ **See also** LIFE-SAVING PROCEDURES pp.71–102 ● SHOCK pp.120–121

IF NO OBJECT IS EMBEDDED IN WOUND

✚ YOUR AIMS

- To control bleeding.
- To prevent and minimise the effects of shock.
- To minimise infection.
- To arrange urgent removal to hospital.

1 Put on disposable gloves if available. Remove or cut clothing as necessary to expose the wound (p.40).

2 Apply direct pressure over the wound with your fingers or palm, preferably over a sterile dressing or non-fluffy, clean pad (but do not waste any time by looking for a dressing). You can ask the casualty to apply direct pressure herself.

3 Raise and support the injured limb above the level of the casualty's heart to reduce blood loss. Handle the limb very gently if you suspect that there is a fracture.

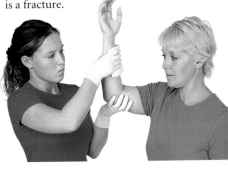

4 Help the casualty to lie down on a blanket, if available, to protect her from the cold. If you suspect that shock may develop, raise and support her legs so that they are above the level of her heart.

Keep injured part raised

Hold dressing firmly over wound

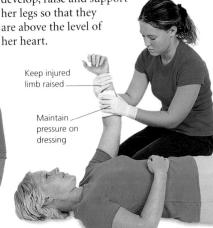

Keep injured limb raised

Maintain pressure on dressing

5 Secure the dressing with a bandage that is tight enough to maintain pressure, but not so tight that it impairs the circulation.

6 If further bleeding occurs, apply a second dressing on top of the first. If blood seeps through this dressing, remove both dressings and apply a fresh one, ensuring that pressure is applied accurately to the point of bleeding.

7 Support the injured part in a raised position with a sling and/or bandaging.

8 CALL AN AMBULANCE
Monitor and record vital signs – level of response, pulse, and breathing (pp.42–43). Watch for signs of shock (pp.120–121), and check the dressings for seepage. Check the circulation beyond the bandage (p.51).

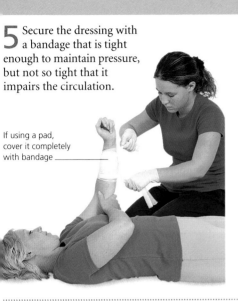

If using a pad, cover it completely with bandage

> **⊘ CAUTION**
> Do not allow the casualty to eat, drink, or smoke.

IF AN OBJECT IS EMBEDDED IN WOUND

> **➕ YOUR AIMS**
> ● To control bleeding without pressing the object into the wound.
> ● To prevent and minimise the effects of shock.
> ● To minimise infection.
> ● To arrange urgent removal to hospital.

4 Build up padding on either side of the object. Carefully bandage over the object without pressing on it.

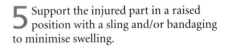

Take care not to press on object

1 Put on disposable gloves if available. Press firmly on either side of the embedded object to push the edges of the wound together.

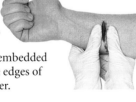

2 If the injury is to a casualty's limb, raise and support the limb above the level of her heart to reduce the blood loss.

3 Help the casualty to lie down on a blanket, if available, to protect her from the cold. If you suspect that shock may develop, raise and support her legs so that they are above the level of her heart.

5 Support the injured part in a raised position with a sling and/or bandaging to minimise swelling.

6 CALL AN AMBULANCE
Monitor and record vital signs – level of response, pulse, and breathing (pp.42–43). Watch for signs of shock (pp.120–121), and check the dressing for seepage. Check the circulation beyond the bandage (p.51).

CUTS AND GRAZES

Bleeding from small cuts and grazes is easily controlled by pressure and elevation. An adhesive dressing is normally all that is necessary, and the wound will heal by itself in a few days. Medical aid need only be sought in the following circumstances:
- If the bleeding does not stop.
- If there is a foreign object embedded in the cut (opposite).
- If the wound is at particular risk of infection (such as a human or animal bite, or a puncture by a dirty object).
- If an old wound shows signs of becoming infected (p.136).

TETANUS

This is a dangerous infection caused by the bacterium *Clostridium tetani*, which lives in soil as spores. If tetanus bacteria enter a wound, they may multiply in the damaged and swollen tissues and may release a poisonous substance (toxin) that spreads through the nervous system, causing muscle spasms and paralysis.

The disorder can be prevented by immunisation, and people are normally given a course of tetanus immunisation during childhood. However, immunisation may need to be repeated in adulthood.

+ YOUR AIM
- To minimise the risk of infection.

1 Wash your hands thoroughly, and put on disposable gloves if available.

2 If the wound is dirty, clean it by rinsing lightly under running water, or use an alcohol-free wipe. Pat the wound dry using a gauze swab and cover with sterile gauze.

3 Elevate the injured part above the level of the heart, if possible. Avoid touching the wound directly. Support the affected limb with one hand.

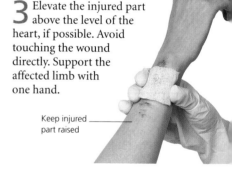

Keep injured part raised

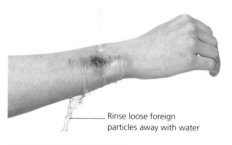

Rinse loose foreign particles away with water

4 Clean the surrounding area with soap and water; use clean swabs for each stroke. Pat dry. Remove the wound covering and apply an adhesive dressing. If there is a special risk of infection, advise the casualty to see her doctor.

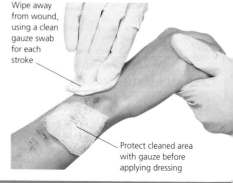

Wipe away from wound, using a clean gauze swab for each stroke

Protect cleaned area with gauze before applying dressing

! CAUTION
Always ask about tetanus immunisation.

Seek medical advice if:
- The casualty has never been immunised.
- The casualty is uncertain about the timing and number of injections that have been given.
- It is more than 10 years since the casualty's last injection.

FOREIGN OBJECT IN A CUT

It is important to remove foreign objects, such as small pieces of glass or grit, from wounds before beginning treatment. If such items remain in a wound, they may cause infection or delayed healing in the short term and discoloration in the long term. The best way to remove superficial pieces of glass or grit is with tweezers if you have them. Alternatively, carefully pick the pieces off the wound or rinse them off with cold water. Do not try to remove objects that are firmly embedded in the wound because you may damage the surrounding tissue and aggravate bleeding. Instead, apply dressings or bandages around them.

▶ **See also** EMBEDDED FISH-HOOK p.213
● SPLINTER p.212

+ YOUR AIMS

● To control bleeding without pressing the object into the wound.
● To minimise the risk of infection.
● To arrange transport to hospital if necessary.

1 Put on disposable gloves if available. Control any bleeding by applying pressure on either side of the object and raising the injured part above the level of the heart.

2 Cover the wound with gauze to minimise the risk of infection.

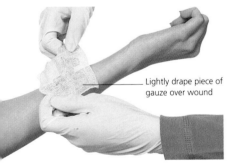

Lightly drape piece of gauze over wound

3 Build up padding around the object until you can bandage over it without pressing down. Carefully hold the padding in place until the bandaging is complete.

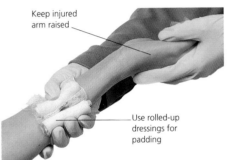

Keep injured arm raised

Use rolled-up dressings for padding

4 Arrange to take or send the casualty to hospital if necessary.

SPECIAL CASE

LARGE OBJECTS
If the object is particularly large, and you cannot pad high enough to bandage over it without pressing on it, bandage around the object.

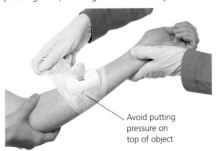

Avoid putting pressure on top of object

! CAUTION

Always ask about tetanus immunisation.

Seek medical advice if:
● The casualty has never been immunised.
● The casualty is uncertain about the timing and number of injections that have been given.
● It is more than 10 years since the casualty's last injection.

BRUISING

This is caused by bleeding into the skin or into tissues beneath the skin. It can either develop rapidly or emerge a few days later. Bruises that appear rapidly will benefit from first aid. Bruising can also indicate deep injury. Elderly people and those taking anticoagulant drugs can bruise very easily.

▶ See also INTERNAL BLEEDING p.122

✚ YOUR AIM
- To reduce blood flow to the injury, and thus minimise swelling.

1 Raise and support the injured part in a comfortable position.

2 Apply firm pressure to the bruise using a cold compress (p.49). Keep the compress in place for at least 5 minutes.

INFECTED WOUND

Any open wound can become contaminated with microorganisms (germs). The germs may come from the source of the injury, from the air, from the breath or the fingers, or from particles of clothing embedded in a wound (as may occur in gunshot wounds). Bleeding flushes some dirt away; remaining germs may be destroyed by the white blood cells. However, if dirt or dead tissue remain in a wound, infection may spread through the body. Tetanus is also a risk.

Any wound that does not begin to heal within 48 hours is likely to be infected. A casualty with a wound that is at high risk of infection may need treatment with antibiotics and/or anti-tetanus injections (*see* CUTS AND GRAZES, p.134).

RECOGNITION
- Increasing pain and soreness at the site of the wound.
- Swelling, redness, and a feeling of heat around the injury.
- Pus within, or oozing from, the wound.
- Swelling and tenderness of the glands in the neck, armpit, or groin.
- Faint red trails on the skin that lead to the glands in the neck, armpit, or groin.
- In casualties who have advanced infection, signs of fever such as sweating, thirst, shivering, and lethargy.

▶ See also BLEEDING AND TYPES OF WOUND pp.128–129 ● CUTS AND GRAZES p.134

✚ YOUR AIMS
- To prevent further infection.
- To obtain medical aid if necessary.

1 Put on disposable gloves if available. Cover the wound with a sterile dressing or a clean, non-fluffy pad and bandage in place. Do not bandage too tightly.

2 Raise and support the injured part using a sling and/or bandaging. This will help to reduce any swelling around the wound.

3 Tell the casualty to see his doctor. If the infection appears to be advanced (with signs of fever such as sweating, shivering, thirst, and lethargy), call a doctor or take or send the casualty to hospital.

SCALP AND HEAD WOUNDS

The scalp has many small blood vessels running close to the skin surface, so any cut can result in profuse bleeding. This bleeding will often make a scalp wound appear worse than it is. In some cases, however, a scalp wound may form part of a more serious underlying injury, such as a skull fracture, or may be associated with a head or neck injury. For these reasons, you should examine a casualty with a scalp wound very carefully, particularly if it is possible that signs of a serious head injury are being masked by alcohol or drug intoxication. If you are in any doubt, follow the treatment for head injury (p.179). In addition, bear in mind the possibility of a neck (spinal) injury.

▶ See also HEAD INJURY p.179 ● SHOCK pp.120–121 ● SPINAL INJURY pp.165–167

✚ YOUR AIMS

● To control blood loss.
● To arrange transport to hospital.

❗ WARNING

If the casualty becomes unconscious, open the airway and check breathing; be prepared to give rescue breaths and chest compressions if necessary (see LIFE-SAVING PROCEDURES, pp.71–102).

1 Put on disposable gloves if available. If there are any displaced flaps of skin at the injury site, carefully replace them over the wound. Reassure the casualty.

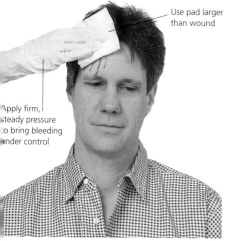

Use pad larger than wound

Apply firm, steady pressure to bring bleeding under control

2 Cover the wound with a sterile dressing or a clean, non-fluffy pad. Apply firm, direct pressure on the pad. This measure will help to control bleeding and reduce blood loss, minimising the risk of shock.

3 Secure the dressing with a roller bandage. (For minor bleeding, you can keep the pad in place with a triangular bandage.)

Apply bandage that secures pad and maintains pressure

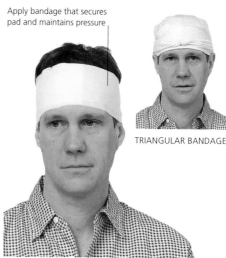

TRIANGULAR BANDAGE

4 Help the casualty to lie down, with his head and shoulders slightly raised. Then take or send the casualty to hospital in the final treatment position. Regularly monitor and record vital signs – level of response, pulse, and breathing (pp.42–43).

EYE WOUND

The eye can be bruised or cut by direct blows or by sharp, chipped fragments of metal, grit, and glass.

All eye injuries are potentially serious because of the risk to the casualty's vision. Even superficial grazes to the surface (cornea) of the eye can lead to scarring or infection, with the possibility of permanent deterioration of vision.

RECOGNITION
- Intense pain and spasm of the eyelids.
- Visible wound and/or bloodshot appearance.
- Partial or total loss of vision.
- Leakage of blood or clear fluid from a wound.

▶ **See also** FOREIGN OBJECT IN THE EYE p.21

＋ YOUR AIMS
- To prevent further damage.
- To arrange transport to hospital.

❶ CAUTION
Do not touch or attempt to remove an embedded foreign object in the eye (p.214).

1 Help the casualty to lie on her back, and hold her head to keep it as still as possible. Tell her to keep both eyes still; movement of the "good" eye will cause movement of the injured one, which may damage it further.

2 Ask the casualty to hold a sterile dressing o a clean, non-fluffy pad over the affected eye. If it will take some time to obtain medical help, secure the pad in place with a bandage.

Keep head supported

Use a large, soft pad that covers eye

3 Take or send the casualty to hospital in the treatment position.

BLEEDING FROM THE EAR

This is usually due to a burst (perforated) eardrum, caused by, for example, a foreign object pushed in the ear, a blow to the side of the head, or an explosion. Symptoms include a sharp pain, then earache, deafness, and possible dizziness. Watery blood is a serious sign: it shows that the skull is fractured and fluid is leaking from around the brain.

▶ **See also** FOREIGN OBJECT IN THE EAR p.215 ● HEAD INJURY p.179

＋ YOUR AIM
- To arrange transport to hospital.

❶ CAUTION
Do not tilt the casualty's head if you suspect a skull fracture.

1 Help the casualty into a half-sitting position, with his head tilted to the injured side to allow blood to drain away.

2 Put on gloves if available. Hold a sterile dressing or a clean, non-fluffy pad lightly in place on the ear. Send or take the casualty to hospital in the treatment position.

NOSEBLEED

leeding from the nose most commonly ccurs when tiny blood vessels inside the ostrils are ruptured, either by a blow to the ose, or as a result of sneezing, picking, or lowing the nose. Nosebleeds may also ccur as a result of high blood pressure. A nosebleed can be dangerous if the sualty loses a lot of blood. In addition, if bleeding follows a head injury, the blood may appear thin and watery. The latter is a very serious sign because it indicates that the skull is fractured and fluid is leaking from around the brain.

▶ **See also** FOREIGN OBJECT IN THE NOSE p.215 ● HEAD INJURY p.179

1 Ask the casualty to sit down. Advise her to tilt her head forwards to allow the blood drain from the nostrils.

2 Ask the casualty to breathe through her mouth (this will also have a calming ffect) and to pinch the soft part of the nose. eassure and help er if necessary.

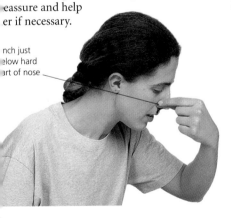

nch just elow hard art of nose

SPECIAL CASE

CHILDREN
A young child may be worried by a nosebleed. Reassure her and give her a bowl to spit or dribble into.

Pinch child's nose

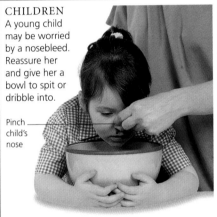

3 Tell the casualty to keep pinching her nose. Advise her not to speak, swallow, cough, spit, or sniff because she may disturb blood clots that have formed in the nose. Give her a clean cloth or tissue to mop up any dribbling.

4 After 10 minutes, tell the casualty to release the pressure. If the bleeding has not stopped, tell her to reapply the pressure for two further periods of 10 minutes.

5 Once the bleeding has stopped, and with the casualty still leaning forwards, clean around her nose with lukewarm water.

6 Advise the casualty to rest quietly for a few hours. Tell her to avoid exertion and, in particular, not to blow her nose, because these actions will disturb any clots.

BLEEDING FROM THE MOUTH

Cuts to the tongue, lips, or lining of the mouth range from trivial injuries to more serious wounds. The cause is usually the casualty's own teeth or dental extraction.

Bleeding from the mouth may be profuse and can be alarming. In addition, there is a danger that blood may be inhaled into the lungs, causing problems with breathing.

✚ YOUR AIMS
- To control bleeding.
- To safeguard the airway by preventing any inhalation of blood.

1 Ask the casualty to sit down, with her head forwards and tilted slightly to the injured side, to allow blood to drain from her mouth.

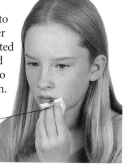

Apply pressure on wound to control bleeding

SPECIAL CASE

BLEEDING SOCKET
To control bleeding from a tooth socket, take a gauze pad that is thick enough to stop the casualty's teeth meeting, place it across the empty socket, and tell her to bite down on it.

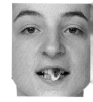

❗ CAUTION
- If the wound is large, or if bleeding persists beyond 30 minutes or recurs, seek medical or dental advice.
- Do not wash the mouth out because this may disturb a clot.

2 Put on gloves if available. Place a gauze pad over the wound. Ask the casualty to squeeze the pad between finger and thumb and press on the wound for 10 minutes.

3 If bleeding persists, replace the pad. Tell the casualty to let the blood dribble out; if swallowed, it may induce vomiting. Advise her to avoid drinking anything hot for 12 hours.

KNOCKED-OUT TOOTH

If a secondary (adult) tooth is knocked out, it should be replanted in its socket as soon as possible. If this is not possible, ask the casualty to keep the tooth inside her cheek or place the tooth in a small container of milk to prevent it from drying out.

✚ YOUR AIM
- To replant the tooth as soon as possible.

❗ CAUTION
Do not clean the tooth as you may damage the tissues, reducing the chance of reimplantation.

1 Put on disposable gloves if available. Gently push the tooth into the socket. Keep it in place by pressing a gauze pad between the bottom and top teeth.

2 Ask the casualty to hold the tooth firmly in place. Send her to a dentist or hospital.

WOUND TO THE PALM

The palm of the hand has several large blood vessels, which is why a wound to the palm may cause profuse bleeding. There is also a risk that a deep wound to the palm may sever tendons and nerves in the hand and result in loss of feeling or movement in the fingers. If a casualty has a foreign object embedded in a wound, it will be impossible for the casualty to clench his fist. In such cases, you should treat the injury using the method described on p.135.

▶ See also FOREIGN OBJECT IN A CUT p.135
● SHOCK pp.120–121

＋ YOUR AIMS
- To control blood loss and the effects of shock.
- To minimise the risk of infection.
- To arrange transport to hospital.

1 Put on disposable gloves if available. Press a sterile dressing or clean pad firmly into the palm, and ask the casualty to clench his fist over it. If he finds it difficult to press hard, tell him to grasp his fist with his uninjured hand.

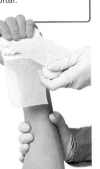

2 Bandage the casualty's fingers so that they are clenched over the pad. Tie the ends of the bandage over the top of the fingers.

Leave thumb free

Raise and support arm

3 Support the casualty's arm in an elevation sling (p.61) to keep it raised. Arrange to take or send him to hospital.

WOUND AT A JOINT CREASE

Major blood vessels pass across the inside of the elbow and knee. If severed, these vessels will bleed copiously. The steps given below help to control bleeding and shock; however, they also impede the flow of blood to the lower part of the limb, so you must ensure adequate circulation to this area.

▶ See also FOREIGN OBJECT IN A CUT p.135
● SHOCK pp.120–121

＋ YOUR AIMS
- To control blood loss.
- To prevent and minimise the effects of shock.
- To arrange transport to hospital.

1 Put on disposable gloves if available. Press a sterile dressing or clean, non-fluffy pad on the injury. Bend the joint firmly to hold the pad in place and keep pressure on the wound.

2 Raise and support the limb. If possible, help the casualty to lie down with his legs raised and supported.

3 Take or send the casualty to hospital in the final treatment position. Every 10 minutes, check the circulation beyond the injury. If necessary, briefly release the pressure on the wound to restore normal blood flow to the lower part of the limb, then reapply pressure.

ABDOMINAL WOUND

A stab wound, gunshot, or crush injury to the abdomen may cause serious or even life-threatening wounds. Organs and major blood vessels deep inside the body may be punctured, lacerated, or ruptured. The severity of a wound may be evident from symptoms such as external bleeding and protruding abdominal contents. More commonly, there is hidden internal injury and bleeding, which may be fatal if there is any delay in emergency treatment. In addition, abdominal wounds carry a high risk of shock and infection.

▶ **See also** INTERNAL BLEEDING p.122
● SHOCK pp.120–121

✚ YOUR AIMS
● To minimise shock.
● To minimise the risk of infection.
● To arrange urgent removal to hospital.

3 CALL AN AMBULANCE
Treat the casualty for shock (pp.120–121) Monitor and record vital signs – level of response, pulse, and breathing (pp.42–43).

1 Put on disposable gloves if available. Help the casualty to lie down on a firm surface, preferably on a blanket. Loosen any tight clothing, such as a belt or a shirt.

Raise and support casualty's knees to ease strain on injury

Undo belt

2 Put a dressing over the wound, and secure it in place with a bandage or adhesive tape. If blood seeps through the dressing, apply another dressing or pad on top.

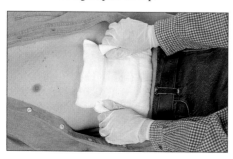

❶ WARNING
● If a casualty with an open wound coughs or vomits, press firmly on the dressing to prevent the contents of the abdomen from pushing through the wound and being exposed.

● Do not touch any protruding intestine. Cover the area with a clean plastic bag or kitchen film to prevent the intestine surface from drying out. Alternatively, apply a sterile dressing.

● If the casualty becomes unconscious, open the airway and check breathing; be ready to give rescue breaths and chest compressions if needed (see LIFE-SAVING PROCEDURES, pp.71–102). If he is breathing, put him in the recovery position (pp.84–85), supporting the abdomen.

VAGINAL BLEEDING

Bleeding from the vagina is most likely to be menstrual bleeding, and the woman often has abdominal cramps. However, it can also indicate a more serious condition such as miscarriage; pregnancy; recent abortion or childbirth; internal disease or infection; or injury as a result of sexual assault (below). If the bleeding is severe, shock may develop. The history of the condition is vital to diagnosis, and has some bearing on the first aid that you give. Be sensitive to the woman's feelings. She may feel embarrassed or may resent a male presence. Male first aiders should, if possible, seek the help of a female chaperone.

▶ See also MISCARRIAGE p.237 ● SHOCK pp.120–121

✚ YOUR AIMS

- To make the woman comfortable and to reassure her.
- To observe her and treat for shock.
- To arrange removal to hospital if necessary.

❗ WARNING

If bleeding continues and is severe:
CALL AN AMBULANCE
Treat for shock (pp.120–121). Monitor and record level of response, pulse, and breathing (pp.42–43).

1 Remove the woman, if possible, to a place with some privacy. Otherwise, arrange for screening to be set up around her.

2 Find a sanitary pad or a clean towel and give it to her to use.

3 Make the casualty as comfortable as possible, in whichever position she prefers. If she chooses to sit up, prop her up with rolled-up clothing or cushions.

4 If the casualty knows that her cramps are due to a menstrual period, she may take painkillers or her own medication.

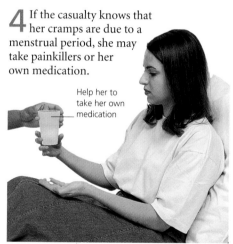

Help her to take her own medication

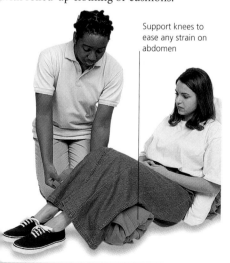

Support knees to ease any strain on abdomen

SPECIAL CASE

SEXUAL ASSAULT

If a woman has been sexually assaulted, it is vital to preserve the evidence if possible. Gently advise her to refrain from washing or using the toilet until a forensic examination has been performed by a police doctor, but do not insist. If she wishes to remove clothing, keep it intact in a clean plastic bag if possible. A woman who has recently been assaulted may feel threatened by a male rescuer; a man should seek help from another woman.

BLEEDING VARICOSE VEIN

Veins contain one-way valves that keep the blood flowing towards the heart. If these valves fail, blood collects behind them and makes the veins swell. This problem, called varicose veins, usually develops in the legs.

A varicose vein has taut, thin walls and is often raised, producing typically knobbly skin over the affected area. The vein can be burst by a gentle knock, and this may resul in profuse bleeding. Shock will quickly develop if bleeding is not controlled.

See also SHOCK pp.120–121

✚ YOUR AIMS

- To bring blood loss under control.
- To minimise shock.
- To arrange urgent removal to hospital.

1 Put on disposable gloves if available. Help the casualty to lie down on her back, then raise and support the injured leg as high as possible. This measure will help to reduce the amount of bleeding.

2 Carefully expose the site of the bleeding. Apply firm, direct pressure on the area, using a sterile dressing, or a clean, non-fluffy pad, until the blood loss is under control.

Support leg on your shoulder during treatment

3 Remove garments such as garters or elastic-topped stockings because these garments may cause bleeding to continue.

4 Put a large, soft pad over the dressing; bandage it firmly enough to exert even pressure, but not so tightly that the circulation is impaired.

Bandage over dresssing

Keep leg high

5 CALL AN AMBULANCE
Keep the injured leg raised and supportec until the ambulance arrives. Monitor and record vital signs – level of response, pulse, an breathing (pp.42–43). Check the casualty's circulation beyond the bandage (p.51).

7

THE SKELETON is the supporting framework around which the body is constructed. It is jointed in many places, and muscles attached to the bones enable us to move. Most of our movements are controlled at will and coordinated by impulses that travel from the brain via the nerves to every muscle and joint in the body.

DIAGNOSING TYPES OF INJURY
Because it is sometimes difficult to distinguish between bone, joint, and muscle injuries, the chapter begins with an overview of how bones, muscles, and joints function and how damage occurs. First-aid treatments for most injuries, from major fractures to sprains and dislocations, are included here. Skull fracture is covered in the chapter on nervous system problems (p.176) because of the potential damage this injury can have on the brain.

✚ FIRST-AID PRIORITIES

- Assess the casualty's condition.
- Comfort and reassure the casualty.
- Steady and support the injured part.
- Enhance the support with padding, bandages, and splints if necessary.
- Minimise shock.
- Obtain medical aid if necessary. Call an ambulance if you suspect a serious injury.

CONTENTS

THE SKELETON

The body is built on a framework of bones called the skeleton. This structure supports the muscles, blood vessels, and nerves of the body. Many bones of the skeleton also protect important organs such as the brain and heart. At many points on the skeleton, bones articulate with each other by means of joints. These are supported by ligaments and moved by muscles that are attached to the bones by tendons.

The skeleton

There are 206 bones in the skeleton, providing a protective framework for the body. The skull, spine, and ribcage protect vital body structures; the pelvis supports the abdominal organs; and the bones and joints of the arms and legs enable the body to move.

Breastbone (sternum)

Twelve pairs of ribs form ribcage, which protects vital organs in chest and moves with lungs during breathing

Spine, which is formed from 33 bones (vertebrae), protects spinal cord and enables back to move

Pelvis is attached to lower part of spine and protects lower abdominal organs

Scaphoid

Wrist bones (carpals)

Hand bone (metacarpal)

Finger bone (phalanx)

BONES OF HAND

Skull protects brain and supports structures of face

Jawbone (mandible) is hinged and enables mouth to open and close

Collar bone (clavicle)

Shoulder blade (scapula)

Collar bones and shoulder blades form the shoulder girdle, to which arms are attached

Upper arm bone (humerus)

Ulna

Radius

Forearm bones

Hip joint is point at which leg bones are connected to pelvis

Thigh bone (femur)

Kneecap (patella)

Lower leg bones

Shin bone (tibia)

Splint bone (fibula)

Ankle bones (tarsals)

Foot bones (metatarsals)

Toe bones (phalanges)

Heel bone (calcaneus)

THE SPINE

The spine, or backbone, has a number of functions. It supports the head, makes the upper body flexible, helps to support the body's weight, and protects the spinal cord (p.177). The spine is a column made up of 33 bones called vertebrae, which are connected by joints. Between individual vertebrae are discs of fibrous tissue, called intervertebral discs, which help to make the spine flexible and cushion it from jolts. Muscles and ligaments attached to the vertebrae stabilise the spine and control the movements of the back.

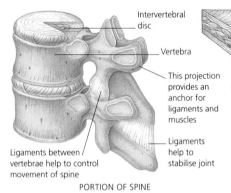

Cervical spine (7 bones)

Thoracic spine (12 bones)

Lumbar spine (5 bones)

Sacrum (5 fused bones)

Coccyx (4 fused bones)

Intervertebral disc

Vertebra

This projection provides an anchor for ligaments and muscles

Ligaments between vertebrae help to control movement of spine

Ligaments help to stabilise joint

PORTION OF SPINE

Fibrous covering

Gelatinous core

SECTION OF INTERVERTEBRAL DISC

Structures that make the spine flexible
The joints connecting the vertebrae, and the discs between vertebrae, allow the spine to move. There is only limited movement between adjacent vertebrae, but together the vertebrae, discs, and ligaments allow a range of movements in the spine as a whole.

Spinal column
The vertebrae form five groups. The cervical vertebrae support the head and neck. The thoracic vertebrae form an anchor for the ribs. The lumbar vertebrae help to support the body's weight and give stability. The sacrum supports the pelvis, and the coccyx forms the end of the spine.

THE SKULL

This bony structure protects the brain and the top of the spinal cord. It also supports the eyes and other facial structures.

The skull is made up of several bones, most of which are fused at joints called sutures. Within the bone are air spaces (sinuses), which lighten the skull. The bones covering the brain form a dome called the cranium. Several other bones form the eye sockets, nose, cheeks, and jaws.

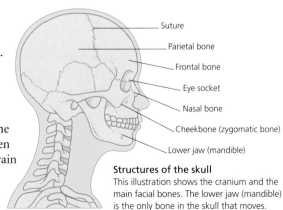

Suture

Parietal bone

Frontal bone

Eye socket

Nasal bone

Cheekbone (zygomatic bone)

Lower jaw (mandible)

Structures of the skull
This illustration shows the cranium and the main facial bones. The lower jaw (mandible) is the only bone in the skull that moves.

BONES, MUSCLES, AND JOINTS

The bones

Bone is a living tissue containing large amounts of calcium and phosphorus; these minerals make it hard, rigid, and strong. Bones can be long, short, or flat. From birth to early adulthood, bones grow by continually laying down calcium on the outside. Bones are also able to generate new tissue after an injury such as a fracture.

Age and certain diseases can weaken bones, making then brittle and susceptible to breaking or crumbling, either under stress or spontaneously. Inherited problems, or bone disorders such as rickets, cancer, and infections, can cause bones to become distorted and weakened. Damage to the bones during adolescence can shorten a bone or impair movement. In older people, a disorder called osteoporosis can cause the bones to lose density, making them brittle and prone to fractures.

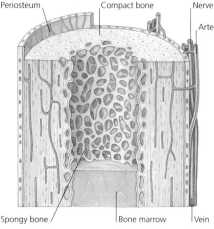

Periosteum — Compact bone — Nerve — Artery — Spongy bone — Bone marrow — Vein

Parts of a bone
Each bone is covered by a membrane (periosteum), which contains nerves and blood vessels. Under this membrane is a layer of compact, dense bone; at the core is spongy bone. In some bones, there is a cavity at the centre containing soft tissue called bone marrow.

The muscles

Muscles cause various parts of the body to move. Skeletal (voluntary) muscles control movement and posture. They are attached to bones by bands of strong, fibrous tissue (tendons), and many operate in groups. As one group of muscles contracts, its paired group relaxes. Involuntary muscles operate the internal organs, such as the heart, and work constantly, even while we are asleep. They are controlled by the autonomic nervous system (p.177).

Straightening the arm
The triceps muscle, at the back of the upper arm, shortens (contracts) to pull down the bones of the forearm. The biceps muscle, at the front of the arm, relaxes.

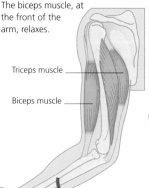

Triceps muscle

Biceps muscle

Bending the arm
The biceps muscle at the front of the arm shortens (contracts), pulling the bones of the forearm upwards to bend the arm. At the same time, the triceps muscle (at the back of the arm) relaxes and lengthens.

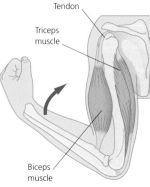

Tendon

Triceps muscle

Biceps muscle

The joints

A joint is a place at which one bone meets another. In a few joints (immovable joints), the bone edges fit firmly together or are fused. Immovable joints are found in the skull and pelvis. Most joints are movable, and there are several types (below). In these joints, the bone ends are joined by fibrous tissue called ligaments, which form a capsule around the joint. The capsule lining (synovial membrane) produces fluid to lubricate the joint; the ends of the bones are also protected by smooth cartilage. Muscles that move the joint are attached to the bones by tendons. The degree and type of movement depends on the way the ends of the bones fit together, the strength of the ligaments, and the arrangement of muscles.

Pivot joint
One bone rotates within a fixed collar formed by another, as at the base of the skull.

Ball-and-socket joint
This allows movement in all directions. Examples are the hip and shoulder joints.

Saddle joint
Bone ends meet at right angles in this joint. The only example is at the base of the thumb.

Ellipsoidal joint
In this type of joint, movement can occur in most directions. The wrist is an example.

Hinge joint
This type allows bending and straightening in only one plane, as in the knees and elbows.

Bone
Synovial membrane
Ligament
Synovial fluid
Cartilage

Plane joint
Surfaces of this type of joint are almost flat and slide over each other. This joint is found in the wrist and foot.

Structures of a movable joint
Cartilage covers the bone ends and minimises friction. Bands of tissue (ligaments) hold the ends together. The joint is enclosed in a lubricant-filled capsule.

FRACTURES

A fracture is a break or crack in a bone. Generally, considerable force is needed to break a bone, unless it is diseased or old. However, bones that are still growing are supple and may split, bend, or crack – hence the term greenstick fracture.

Both direct and indirect force can cause bones to fracture. A bone may break at the point where a heavy blow is received – for example, when struck by a car (direct force). Fractures may also result from a twist or a wrench (indirect force).

RECOGNITION

There may be:

- Deformity, swelling, and bruising at the fracture site.
- Pain, and difficulty in moving the area.
- Shortening, bending, or twisting of a limb.
- Coarse grating (crepitus) of the bone ends that can be heard or felt, but must not be sought.
- Signs of shock, especially if the fracture is to the thigh bone or pelvis.
- Difficulty in moving a limb normally or at all (for example, inability to walk).
- A wound, possibly with bone ends protruding.

STABLE AND UNSTABLE FRACTURES

A fracture may be stable or unstable. In a stable injury, the broken bone ends do not move, either because they are incompletely broken or they are jammed together. Such injuries are common at the wrist, shoulder, ankle, and hip. Usually, they can be gently handled without causing further damage.

In an unstable injury, the broken bone ends can easily move out of position. As a result, there is a risk that they may cause damage to blood vessels, nerves, and organs. Unstable injuries can occur if the bone is completely broken or the ligaments are torn (ruptured). Such injuries should be handled very carefully to avoid further damage.

OPEN AND CLOSED FRACTURES

In an open fracture, one of the broken bone ends may pierce the skin surface, or there may be a wound at the fracture site. An open fracture carries a high risk of becoming infected.

In a closed fracture, the skin above the fracture is intact. However, bones may be displaced (unstable) and cause damage to other internal tissues in the area. If the bone ends pierce organs or major blood vessels, the casualty may have internal bleeding and suffer shock (pp.120–121).

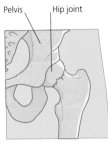

Pelvis | Hip joint

Stable injury
Although the bone is fractured, the ends of the injury remain in place. The risk of bleeding or further damage is minimal.

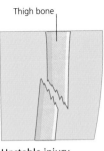

Thigh bone

Unstable injury
In this type of fracture, the broken bone ends can easily be displaced by movement or muscle contraction.

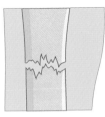

Closed fracture
The skin is not broken, although the bone ends may damage nearby tissues and blood vessels. Internal bleeding is a risk.

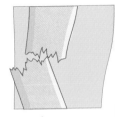

Open fracture
Bone is exposed at the surface where it breaks the skin. The casualty is likely to suffer bleeding and shock. Infection is a risk.

▶ See also CRUSH INJURY p.133 ● INTERNAL BLEEDING p.122 ● SHOCK pp.120–121

CLOSED FRACTURE

- To prevent movement at the injury site.
- To arrange removal to hospital, with comfortable support during transport.

Support above and below injury

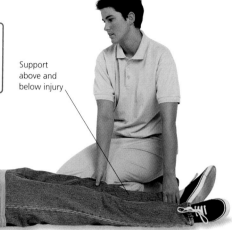

1 Advise the casualty to keep still. Support the injured part with your hands, or ask a helper to do this, until it is immobilised.

2 For firmer support, bandage the injured part to an unaffected part of the body. Make sure the bandage is tied on the uninjured side. For upper limb fractures, immobilise the arm against the trunk (pp.60–62). For lower limb fractures, bandage the uninjured leg to the injured one if removal to hospital is likely to be delayed.

Tie bandage on uninjured side

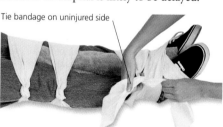

3 Arrange to transport the casualty to hospital as necessary. Treat for shock (pp.120–121) if necessary by raising the legs. However, do not raise the injured limb if this causes the casualty more pain.

4 Check the circulation beyond a bandage (p.51) every 10 minutes. If the circulation is impaired, loosen the bandages.

❗ CAUTION
- Do not move the casualty until the injured part is secured and supported, unless she is in danger.
- Do not allow the casualty to eat, drink, or smoke as a general anaesthetic may be needed.

SPECIAL CASE

APPLYING TRACTION
If a fractured limb is bent or angled so that it cannot be immobilised, gentle traction may be needed to pull it straight. This action overcomes the pull of the muscles and helps to reduce pain and bleeding at the fracture site.

To apply traction, pull steadily in the line of the bone until the limb is straight. Pull only in a straight line and hold until the limb is immobilised. Do not persist if traction causes intolerable pain.

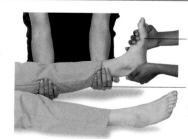

Pull injured limb if necessary

Ask a helper to support the limb

FRACTURES (continued)

OPEN FRACTURE

+ YOUR AIMS
- To prevent blood loss, movement, and infection at the site of injury.
- To arrange removal to hospital, with comfortable support during transport.

SPECIAL CASE

PROTRUDING BONE
If bone is protruding, build up pads of clean, soft, non-fluffy material around the bone, until you can bandage over the pads, to protect it from any pressure.

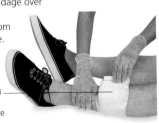

Hold padding in place with roller bandage

1 Put on gloves, if available. Loosely cover the wound with a large, clean, non-fluffy pad or sterile dressing. Apply pressure to control bleeding (p.130), but do not press on a protruding bone.

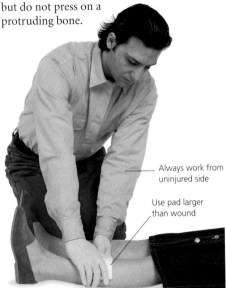

Always work from uninjured side

Use pad larger than wound

2 Carefully place clean padding over and around the dressing.

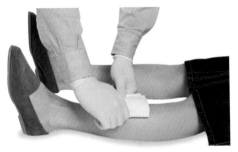

3 Secure the dressing and padding with a bandage. Bandage firmly but not so tightly that it impairs the circulation.

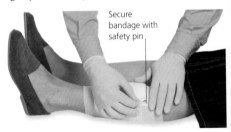

Secure bandage with safety pin

4 Immobilise the injured part as for a closed fracture (p.151), and arrange to transport the casualty to hospital.

5 Treat for shock (pp.120–121) if necessary. Monitor and record vital signs – level of response, pulse, and breathing (pp.42–43). Check the circulation beyond the bandage (p.51) every 10 minutes.

❶ CAUTION
- Do not move the casualty until the injured part is secured and supported, unless she is in danger.
- Do not allow the casualty to eat, drink, or smoke, as a general anaesthetic may be needed.
- Do not press down directly on a protruding bone end.

DISLOCATED JOINT

his is a joint injury in which the bones e partially or completely pulled out of osition. Dislocation can be caused by a rong force wrenching the bone into an bnormal position or by violent muscle ontraction. This very painful injury most ften affects the shoulder, jaw, or joints in ne thumbs or fingers. Dislocations may e associated with torn ligaments (*see* PRAINS AND STRAINS, pp.154–155), r with damage to the synovial membrane, /hich lines the joint capsule (p.149).

In some cases, joint dislocation can ave serious consequences. If vertebrae in ne spine are dislocated, the spinal cord can e damaged. Dislocation of the shoulder or ip may damage the major nerves that

RECOGNITION

There may be:
● "Sickening", severe pain, and difficulty in moving the area.
● Swelling and bruising around the joint.
● Shortening, bending, or twisting of the area.

supply the limbs and result in paralysis. A severe dislocation of any joint may also fracture the bones involved.

In many cases, it can be difficult to distinguish a dislocation from a closed fracture (p.151). If you are in any doubt, treat the injury as a fracture.

⏵ See also FRACTURES pp.150–152 ● SHOCK pp.120–121 ● STRAINS AND SPRAINS pp.154–155

✚ YOUR AIMS

● To prevent movement at the injury site.
● To arrange transport to hospital, with comfortable support during transport.

❗ CAUTION

● Do not try to reposition a dislocated bone into its socket because this may cause further injury.
● Do not move the casualty until the injured part is secured and supported, unless he is in danger.
● Do not allow the casualty to eat, drink, or smoke, as a general anaesthetic may be needed.

1 Advise the casualty to keep still. Support the injured art, in a position of naximum comfort or the casualty, efore you mmobilise it.

Ask casualty to support injured part

2 Immobilise the injured part with padding, bandages, and slings (pp.60–62). For firm support, bandage the injured part to an unaffected part of the body.

Use a broad-fold bandage to immobilise the injured part against the chest

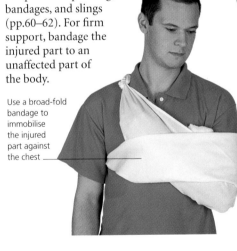

3 Arrange to transport the casualty to hospital. Treat for shock if necessary. Monitor and record vital signs – level of response, pulse, and breathing (pp.42–43).

4 Check the circulation beyond the bandages (p.51) every 10 minutes. If the circulation is impaired, loosen the bandages.

STRAINS AND SPRAINS

The softer structures around bones and joints – the ligaments, muscles, and tendons – may be injured in several ways. Injuries to these soft tissues are commonly called strains and sprains. They occur when the tissues are overstretched and partially or completely torn (ruptured) by violent or sudden movements. For this reason strains and sprains are frequently associated with sporting activities.

MUSCLE AND TENDON INJURY

Muscles and tendons may be strained, ruptured, or bruised. A strain occurs when the muscle is overstretched and may be partially torn. This often occurs at the junction of the muscle and the tendon that joins the muscle to a bone. In a rupture, a muscle or tendon is torn completely; this may occur in the main bulk of the muscle or in the tendon. Deep bruising may be

extensive in parts of the body where there is a large bulk of muscle. Injuries in these areas are usually accompanied by bleeding into the surrounding tissues, which can lead to pain, swelling, and bruising.

Strains and sprains should be treated initially by the "RICE" procedure:

R – *Rest* the injured part.
I – Apply *Ice* or a cold compress.
C – *Compress* the injury.
E – *Elevate* the injured part.

This treatment may be sufficient to relieve the symptoms, but if you are in any doubt as to the severity of the injury, treat it as a fracture (pp.150–152).

LIGAMENT INJURY

One common form of ligament injury is a sprain. This is the tearing of a ligament at or near a joint. It is often due to a sudden or unexpected wrenching motion that pulls the bones in the joint too far apart and tears the surrounding tissues.

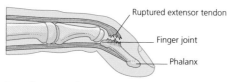

Ruptured extensor tendon

Finger joint

Phalanx

Torn finger tendon
Tendons attach muscle to bone across a joint. If a hard object strikes the end of the finger, the sudden bending may tear the extensor tendon, which passes over the top of the finger joint, from its attachment.

Sprained ankle
This is due to overstretching or tearing of a ligament – the fibrous cords that connect bones at a joint. In this example, one of the ligaments in the ankle is partially torn

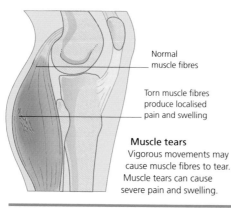

Normal muscle fibres

Torn muscle fibres produce localised pain and swelling

Muscle tears
Vigorous movements may cause muscle fibres to tear. Muscle tears can cause severe pain and swelling.

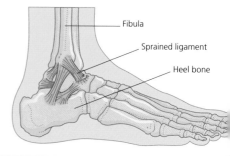

Fibula

Sprained ligament

Heel bone

1 Advise the casualty to sit or lie down. Support the injured part in a comfortable position.

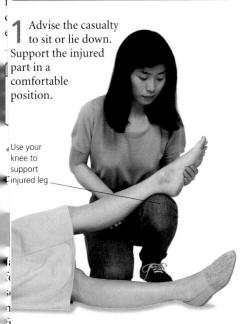

Use your knee to support injured leg

2 If the injury has just happened, cool the area by applying an ice pack or cold compress (p.49). This will help to reduce swelling, bruising, and pain.

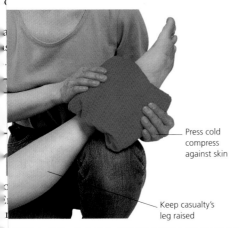

Press cold compress against skin

Keep casualty's leg raised

3 Apply gentle, even pressure (compression) to the injured part by surrounding the area with a thick layer of soft padding, such as cotton wool or plastic foam, and securing this layer of padding with a bandage. Check the circulation beyond the bandaging (p.51) every 10 minutes.

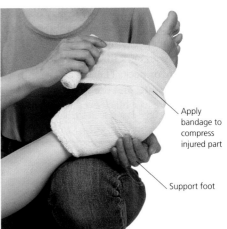

Apply bandage to compress injured part

Support foot

4 Raise (elevate) and support the injured part to reduce the flow of blood to the injury. This action will help to minimise bruising in the area.

Keep limb elevated at a comfortable level

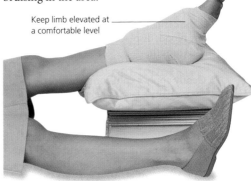

5 If the pain is severe, or the casualty is unable to use the injured part, take or send the casualty to hospital. Otherwise, advise the casualty to rest and to see her doctor if necessary.

FRACTURED COLLAR BONE

The collar bones (clavicles) form "struts" between the shoulder blades and the top of the breastbone to help support the arms. It is rare for a collar bone to be broken by a direct blow. Usually, a fracture results from an indirect force transmitted from an impact at the shoulder or passing along the arm, for example from a fall on to an outstretched arm. Collar bone fractures often occur in young people as a result of sports activities. The broken ends of the collar bone may be displaced, causing swelling and bleeding in the surrounding tissues as well as distortion of the shoulder.

> See also UPPER ARM INJURY p.160

RECOGNITION

There may be:
- Pain and tenderness, increased by movement.
- Swelling and deformity of the shoulder.
- Attempts by the casualty to relax muscles and relieve pain; she may support the arm at the elbow, and incline the head to the injured side.

YOUR AIMS

- To immobilise the injured shoulder and arm.
- To arrange transport to hospital.

1 Help the casualty to sit down. Lay the affected arm diagonally across her chest with her fingertips resting against the opposite shoulder. Ask her to support the elbow with her other hand.

Remove any restricting clothing, such as a bra strap, if it is causing discomfort

Injury makes casualty incline head to injured side

Ask casualty to support elbow

2 Support the arm on the affected side in an elevation sling (p.62).

3 Gently place some soft padding, such as a small towel or folded clothing, between the arm and the body to make the casualty more comfortable.

4 Secure the arm to the chest with a broad-fold bandage (p.57) tied around the chest and over the sling.

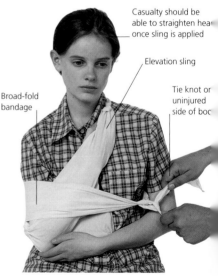

Casualty should be able to straighten head once sling is applied

Elevation sling

Tie knot on uninjured side of body

Broad-fold bandage

5 Arrange to take or send the casualty to hospital in a sitting position.

SHOULDER INJURY

fall on to the shoulder or an outstretched
m, or a wrenching force, may pull the
ad of the arm bone (humerus) out of the
int socket. At the same time, ligaments
ound the shoulder joint may be torn.
his painful injury is called dislocation of
e shoulder. Some people have repeated
slocations and may need a strengthening
eration on the affected shoulder.
A fall on to the point of the shoulder may
mage the ligaments bracing the collar
ne at the shoulder. Other shoulder
juries include damage to the joint capsule
d to the tendons around the shoulder;
ese injuries tend to be common in older

people. To treat a shoulder injury, follow
the RICE procedure – *rest* the affected part,
apply *ice, compress,* and *elevate* (p.154).

▶ **See also** DISLOCATED JOINT p.153

YOUR AIMS
● To support and immobilise the injured limb.
● To arrange removal to hospital.

Help the casualty to sit down. Gently place
the arm on the affected side across her
ody in the position that is most comfortable.

Place a triangular bandage between the
arm and the chest, in preparation for
ing an arm sling (p.60).

Insert soft padding, such as a folded towel
or clothing, between the arm and the
est, inside the bandage.

ng is draped under the arm

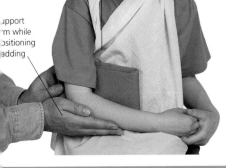

upport
m while
ositioning
adding

4 Finish tying the
arm sling so
that the arm and its
padding are well
supported.

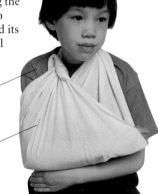

Site of injury

Keep bandage
clear of injury site

5 Secure the limb to the chest by tying a
broad-fold bandage (p.57) around the
chest and over the sling.

6 Arrange to take or send the casualty to
hospital in a sitting position.

UPPER ARM INJURY

The most serious form of upper arm injury is a fracture of the long bone in the upper arm (humerus). The bone may be fractured across the centre by a direct blow. However, it is much more common, especially in elderly people, for the arm bone to break at the shoulder end, usually in a fall.

A fracture at the top of the bone is usually a stable injury (p.150), so the broken bone ends stay in place. For this reason, it may not be immediately apparent that the bone is broken, although the arm is likely to be painful. There is a possibility that the casualty will cope with the pain and leave the fracture untreated for some time.

RECOGNITION

There may be:
● Pain, increased by movement.
● Tenderness and deformity over the site of a fracture.
● Rapid swelling.
● Bruising, which may develop more slowly.

▶ **See also** FRACTURES pp.150–152

＋ YOUR AIMS

● To immobilise the arm.
● To arrange transport to hospital.

1 Ask the casualty to sit down. Gently place the forearm horizontally across her body in the position that is most comfortable. Ask her to support her elbow if possible.

2 Place soft padding beneath the injured arm. Then tie the arm and its padding in an arm sling to support it (p.60).

3 Secure the arm by tying a broad-fold bandage (p.57) around the chest and over the sling. Try to avoid bandaging over the fracture site if possible. Arrange to take or send the casualty to hospital.

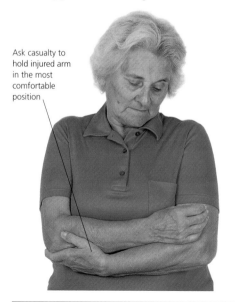

Ask casualty to hold injured arm in the most comfortable position

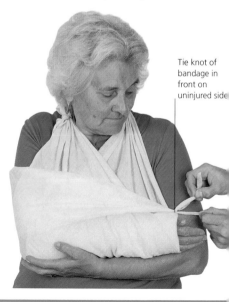

Tie knot of bandage in front on uninjured side

ELBOW INJURY

ractures or dislocations at the elbow usually esult from a fall on to the hand. Children ften fracture the upper arm bone just bove the elbow. This is an unstable fracture p.150), and the bone ends may damage lood vessels. Circulation in the arm needs o be checked regularly. In any elbow injury, he elbow will be stiff and difficult to traighten. Never try to force it to bend.

RECOGNITION

There may be:
- Pain, increased by movement.
- Tenderness over the site of a fracture.
- Swelling, bruising, and deformity.
- Fixed elbow.

▶ See also UPPER ARM INJURY opposite

FOR AN ELBOW THAT CAN BEND

+ YOUR AIMS

- To immobilise the arm without further injury to the joint.
- To arrange transport to hospital.

▶ Treat as for UPPER ARM INJURY opposite

❶ CAUTION

Check the pulse in the affected wrist regularly (p.42). If the pulse is not present, gently straighten the elbow until the pulse returns. Support the arm in this position.

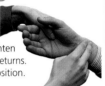

FOR AN ELBOW THAT CANNOT BEND

+ YOUR AIMS

- To immobilise the arm without further injury to the joint.
- To arrange urgent removal to hospital.

❶ WARNING

- Do not try to move the injured arm.
- Do not attempt to apply bandages if help is on its way.

1 Help the casualty to lie down. Place padding, such as cushions or towels, round the elbow for comfort and support.

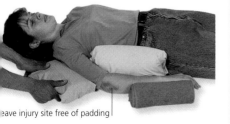

eave injury site free of padding

2 CALL AN AMBULANCE
Check the pulse (p.42) in the injured rm until medical help arrives.

SPECIAL CASE

PREPARING FOR TRANSPORT
Put padding between the injured limb and body. Then use three folded triangular bandages to immobilise the injured limb against the trunk, at the wrist and hips (1), then above (2) and below (3) the elbow.

Tie bandages firmly on the non-injured side

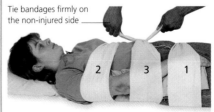

FOREARM AND WRIST INJURIES

The bones of the forearm (radius and ulna) can be fractured by an impact such as a heavy blow or a fall on to an outstretched hand. As the bones have little fleshy covering, the broken ends may pierce the skin, producing an open fracture (p.152).

At the wrist, the most common form of fracture is a Colles' fracture, which is a break at the end of the radius. This injury often occurs in older women. In a young adult, a fall may break one of the small wrist bones (carpals).

The wrist joint is rarely dislocated but is often sprained. It can be difficult to distinguish between a sprain and a fracture, especially if the tiny scaphoid bone (at the base of the thumb) is injured.

RECOGNITION

There may be:
- Pain, increased by movement.
- Swelling, bruising, and deformity.
- In an open fracture, a wound and bleeding.

▶ **See also** DISLOCATED JOINT p.153
- FRACTURES pp.150–152

✚ YOUR AIMS

- To immobilise the arm.
- To arrange transport to hospital.

1 Ask the casualty to sit down. Gently steady and support the injured forearm by placing it across his body. Expose and treat any wound that you find, wearing disposable gloves if available.

2 Place a triangular bandage between the chest and the injured arm, as for an arm sling (p.60). Surround the forearm in soft padding, such as a small towel or a thick layer of cotton wool.

3 Fasten the arm sling around the arm and its padding using a reef knot (p.58). Tie the knot at the hollow of the casualty's collar bone on the injured side.

4 If the journey to hospital is likely to be prolonged, secure the arm to the body by tying a broad-fold bandage (p.57) over the sling. Position the bandage close to the elbow. Then take or send the casualty to hospital.

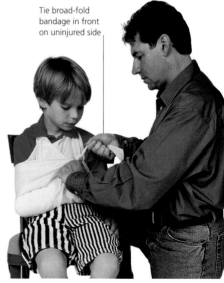

Tie broad-fold bandage in front on uninjured side

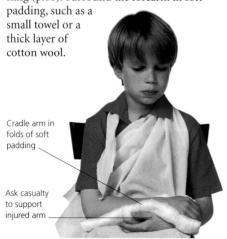

Cradle arm in folds of soft padding

Ask casualty to support injured arm

HAND AND FINGER INJURIES

The bones and joints in the hand can suffer various types of injury. Minor fractures are usually caused by direct force. The most common type – a fracture of the knuckle between the little finger and the hand – often results from a misdirected punch.

Multiple fractures, affecting many or all of the bones in the hand, are usually caused by crushing injuries. The fractures may be open, with severe bleeding and swelling, needing immediate first-aid treatment.

The joints in the fingers or thumb are sometimes dislocated or sprained as a result of a fall on to the hand (for example, while someone is skiing or ice skating).

> ## RECOGNITION
>
> There may be:
> - Pain, increased by movement.
> - Swelling, bruising, and deformity.
> - In an open fracture, a wound and bleeding.

Always compare the suspected fractured hand with the normal hand because finger fractures result in deformities that may not be immediately obvious.

▶ **See also** CRUSH INJURY p.133
● DISLOCATED JOINT p.153 ● FRACTURES
pp.150–152 ● WOUND TO THE PALM p.141

YOUR AIMS
- To immobilise and elevate the hand.
- To arrange transport to hospital.

1 If there is any bleeding, put on disposable gloves, if available. Apply a clean, non-fluffy dressing to the wound.

2 Remove any rings before the hand begins to swell, and keep the hand raised to reduce swelling. Protect the injured area by wrapping the hand in folds of soft padding.

3 Gently support the affected arm across the casualty's body by applying an elevation sling (p.61).

4 If necessary, secure the arm to the casualty's body by tying a broad-fold bandage (p.57) around the chest and over the sling. Then arrange to take or send the casualty to hospital.

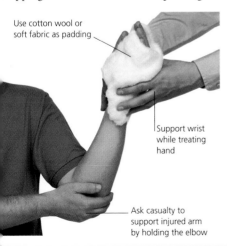

Use cotton wool or soft fabric as padding

Support wrist while treating hand

Ask casualty to support injured arm by holding the elbow

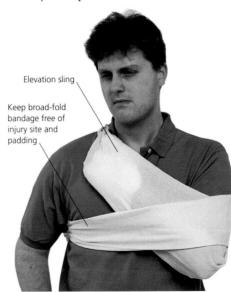

Elevation sling

Keep broad-fold bandage free of injury site and padding

INJURY TO THE RIBCAGE

One or more ribs can be fractured by direct force to the chest from a blow or a fall, or by a crush injury (p.133). If there is an open wound over the fracture, or if a fractured rib pierces a lung, the casualty's breathing may be seriously impaired.

An injury to the chest can cause an area of fractured ribs to become detached from the rest of the chest wall, producing a "flail chest" injury. The detached area moves in when the casualty breathes in, and out as he breathes out. This "paradoxical" breathing causes severe respiratory difficulties.

Fractures of the lower ribs may injure internal organs such as the liver and spleen and cause internal bleeding (p.122).

RECOGNITION

Depending on the severity, there may be:
- Sharp pain at the site of a fracture.
- Pain on taking a deep breath.
- Shallow breathing.
- An open wound over the fracture, through which you may hear air being "sucked" into the chest cavity.
- "Paradoxical" breathing.
- Features of internal bleeding (p.122) and shock (pp.120–121).

▶ **See also** ABDOMINAL WOUND p.142
- PENETRATING CHEST WOUND p.112
- SHOCK pp.120–121

✚ YOUR AIMS
- To support the chest wall.
- To arrange transport to hospital.

❶ CAUTION

If you need to place the casualty in the recovery position (pp.84–85), lay him on his injured side. This position allows the lung on the uninjured side to work to its full capacity.

1 For fractured ribs, support the arm on the injured side in an arm sling (p.60) and take or send him to hospital. If there is a penetrating chest wound, lean the casualty towards the affected side, and cover and seal the wound along three edges (p.113).

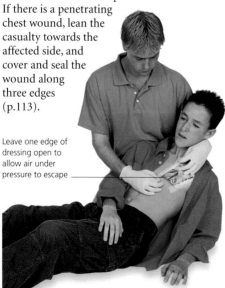

Leave one edge of dressing open to allow air under pressure to escape

2 Help the casualty to settle into the most comfortable position inclined towards the injured side. Support the arm on that side in an elevation sling (p.61). **CALL AN AMBULANCE**

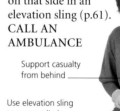

Support casualty from behind

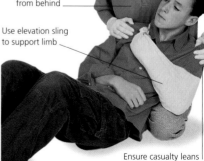

Use elevation sling to support limb

Ensure casualty leans towards injured side

SPINAL INJURY

njuries to the spine can involve one or
more parts of the back and/or neck: the
bones (vertebrae), the discs of tissue that
separate the vertebrae, the surrounding
muscles and ligaments, or the spinal cord
and the nerves that branch off from it.

The most serious risk associated with
spinal injury is damage to the spinal cord.
Such damage can cause loss of power and/or
sensation below the injured area. The spinal
cord or nerve roots can suffer temporary
damage if they are pinched by displaced or
dislocated discs or by fragments of broken
bone. If the cord is partly or completely
severed, the damage may be permanent.

WHEN TO SUSPECT SPINAL INJURY
The most important indicator is the
mechanism of the injury. Always suspect
spinal injury if abnormal forces have been
exerted on the back or neck, and particularly
if the casualty complains of any interference
with feeling or movement.

If the incident involved violent forward
or backward bending, or twisting of the
spine, you must assume that the casualty

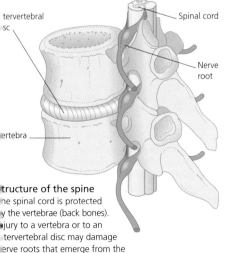

Structure of the spine
The spinal cord is protected
by the vertebrae (back bones).
Injury to a vertebra or to an
intervertebral disc may damage
nerve roots that emerge from the
spinal cord or damage the cord itself.

Labels: Intervertebral disc • Spinal cord • Nerve root • Vertebra

---

> **RECOGNITION**

When the vertebrae are damaged, there may be:
- Pain in the neck or back at the injury site; this
may be masked by other, more painful injuries.
- A step, irregularity, or twist in the normal
curve of the spine.
- Tenderness in the skin over the spine.

When the spinal cord is damaged, there may be:
- Loss of control over limbs; movement may be
weak or absent.
- Loss of sensation, or abnormal sensations such
as burning or tingling. The casualty may say that
limbs feel stiff, heavy, or clumsy.
- Loss of bladder and/or bowel control.
- Breathing difficulties.

---

has a spinal injury. You must take particular
care to avoid unnecessary movement of the
head and neck at all times.

Although spinal cord injury may occur
without any damage to the vertebrae, spinal
fracture vastly increases the risk. The areas
that are most vulnerable are the bones in
the neck and those in the lower back.

SOME CAUSES OF SPINAL INJURY
Any of the following circumstances should
alert you to a possible spinal injury:
- Falling from a height.
- Falling awkwardly while doing
gymnastics or trampolining.
- Diving into a shallow pool and hitting
the bottom.
- Being thrown from a horse or motorbike.
- Being in a collapsed rugby scrum.
- Sudden deceleration in a motor vehicle.
- A heavy object falling across the back.
- Injury to the head or the face.

See also HEAD INJURY p.179 • IMPAIRED
CONSCIOUSNESS p.178 • MECHANICS OF
INJURY p.31

Continued on next page

SPINAL INJURY (continued)

FOR A CONSCIOUS CASUALTY

✚ YOUR AIMS

- To prevent further injury.
- To arrange urgent removal to hospital.

ⓘ CAUTION

- Do not move the casualty from the position in which you found her unless she is in danger.
- If the casualty has to be moved, use the log-roll technique (opposite). Alternatively, an orthopaedic stretcher (p.70) may be used.

ⓘ WARNING

If you suspect neck injury, ask a helper to place rolled-up blankets, towels, or items of clothing on either side of the casualty's head and neck, while you keep her head in the neutral position.
   Continue to support the casualty's head and neck throughout until emergency medical services take over.

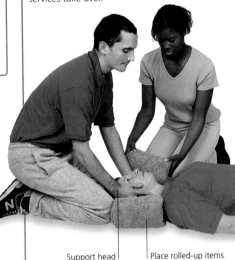

Support head throughout | Place rolled-up items against head and neck

1 Reassure the casualty and advise her not to move.
CALL AN AMBULANCE

2 Kneel behind the casualty's head. Grasp the sides of the casualty's head firmly, with your hands over the ears. Do not completely cover her ears – she should still be able to hear you. Steady and support her head in the neutral head position, in which the head, neck, and spine are aligned. This is the least harmful head position for a casualty with a suspected spinal injury.

Rest arms on legs to keep them steady

3 Continue to support the casualty's head in the neutral position until emergency medical services take over, no matter how long this may be. Get help to monitor and record vital signs – level of response, pulse, and breathing (pp.42–43).

Hold casualty's head straight to steady the neck, but do not completely cover her ears

ᶠOR AN UNCONSCIOUS CASUALTY

- To maintain an open airway.
- To resuscitate the casualty if necessary.
- To prevent further spinal damage.
- To arrange urgent removal to hospital.

1 Kneel behind the casualty's head. Grasp the sides of her head firmly with your ᴴands over the ears. Steady and support her ᴴead in the neutral head position, in which ᵗhe head, neck, and spine are aligned.

2 If necessary, open the casualty's airway using the jaw thrust method. Place your ᴴands on each side of her face with your ᶠingertips at the angles of her jaw. Gently lift ᵗhe jaw to open the ᵃirway. Take care ᶰot to tilt the ᵃsualty's neck.

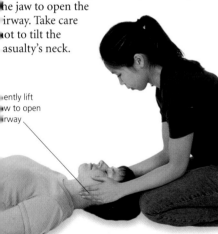

ᵍently lift
ᵃw to open
ᵃirway

SPECIAL CASE

LOG-ROLL TECHNIQUE
This technique should be used if you have to turn a casualty with a spinal injury. Ideally, you need five helpers but the move can be done with three. While you support the casualty's head and neck, ask your helpers to straighten her limbs gently. Then, ensuring that everyone works together, direct your helpers to roll the casualty. Keep the casualty's head, trunk, and toes in a straight line at all times.

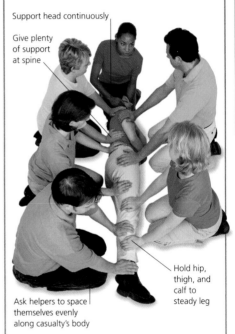

Support head continuously

Give plenty of support at spine

Hold hip, thigh, and calf to steady leg

Ask helpers to space themselves evenly along casualty's body

3 Check the casualty's breathing. If she is breathing, continue to support ᴴer head. Ask a helper to ᶜALL AN AMBULANCE.
ᶠ you are alone and you need to leave the ᶜasualty to call an ambulance, and if ᵗhe casualty is unable to maintain an ᵒpen airway, you should place her in the ᵉecovery position (pp.84–85) before ʸou leave her.

4 If the casualty is not breathing, and there are no signs of circulation, give rescue breaths and chest compressions (*see* LIFE-SAVING PROCEDURES, pp.71–102). If you need to turn the casualty, use the log-roll technique (above).

5 Monitor and record vital signs – level of response, pulse, and breathing (pp.42–43) – until medical help arrives.

BACK PAIN

Pain may occur in the spine itself or in the muscles and ligaments around it. In most instances, back pain is the result of a minor problem. However, pain may be a sign of an underlying serious disorder.

CAUSES OF BACK PAIN

The most common cause of back pain is overstretching of the ligaments or muscles as the result of a fall or strenuous activity. Other common causes of back pain are "whiplash" injuries, which lead to neck pain, and pregnancy and menstruation, which often produce pain in the lower part of the back. More serious causes of back pain include a damaged disc in the spine, which may irritate or pinch the spinal cord or nerves, and kidney disease.

RECOGNITION

There may be:
- Dull to severe pain in the back or neck, which is usually increased by movement.
- Pain travelling down any of the limbs, possibly together with tingling and numbness.
- Spasm of the muscles, causing the neck or back to be held rigid or bent.
- Tenderness in the muscles.

Medical help will be necessary if the back pain is accompanied by muscle spasms, fever, headaches, vomiting, nausea, impaired consciousness, incontinence, or any loss of sensation or movement.

 See also SPINAL INJURY pp.165–167

+ YOUR AIMS
- To relieve pain.
- To obtain medical aid if necessary.

⊘ CAUTION
If the casualty has severe back pain, help him to lie down, and call a doctor.

SPECIAL CASE

NECK PAIN
You can make a temporary neck collar to relieve neck pain using folded newspaper covered by a bandage or scarf. Place the centre of the collar at the front of the casualty's neck, below the chin. Pass the loose ends around her neck and tie at the front. Ensure that breathing is not impeded.

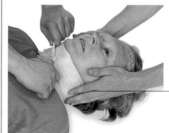

Support head while applying collar

1 Advise the casualty to lie down flat in the most comfortable position for him, either on the ground or on a firm mattress.

2 Advise him to lie as still as possible until the pain eases. Assist the casualty to take his own painkillers. If the symptoms persist, call his doctor or send him to hospital.

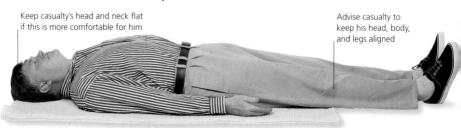

Keep casualty's head and neck flat if this is more comfortable for him

Advise casualty to keep his head, body, and legs aligned

FRACTURED PELVIS

Injuries to the pelvis are usually caused by direct force, such as in a car crash or by crushing. For example, the impact of a car dashboard on a knee can force the head of the thigh bone through the hip socket.

A fracture of the pelvic bones may be complicated by injury to tissues and organs inside the pelvis, such as the bladder and the urinary passages. In addition, internal bleeding associated with the fracture may be severe. This is because there are major organs and blood vessels in the pelvis. Shock often develops as a result of this bleeding, and should be treated promptly.

RECOGNITION

There may be:

- Inability to walk or even stand, although the legs appear uninjured.
- Pain and tenderness in the region of the hip, groin, or back, which increases with movement.
- Blood at the urinary outlet, especially in a male casualty. The casualty may not be able to pass urine or may find this painful.
- Signs of shock and internal bleeding.

See also INTERNAL BLEEDING p.122
- SHOCK pp.120–121

YOUR AIMS

- To minimise the risk of shock.
- To arrange urgent removal to hospital.

CAUTION

Do not bandage the casualty's legs together if this causes any more pain. In such cases, surround the injured area with soft padding such as clothing or towels.

1 Help the casualty to lie down on his back. Keep his legs straight and flat or, if it is more comfortable, help him to bend his knees slightly and support them with padding, such as a cushion or folded clothing.

2 Place padding between the bony points of the knees and the ankles. Immobilise the legs by bandaging them together with folded triangular bandages; secure the feet and ankles (1), then the knees (2).

3 CALL AN AMBULANCE
Treat the casualty for shock (pp.120–121).

4 Monitor and record vital signs – level of response, breathing, and pulse (pp.42–43) – until help arrives.

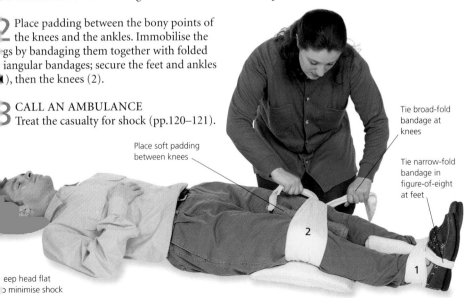

Tie broad-fold bandage at knees

Tie narrow-fold bandage in figure-of-eight at feet

Place soft padding between knees

Keep head flat to minimise shock

HIP AND THIGH INJURIES

The most serious injury of the thigh bone (femur) is a fracture. It takes a considerable force, such as a traffic incident or a fall from a height, to fracture the shaft of the femur. This is a serious injury because the broken bone ends can pierce major blood vessels, causing heavy blood loss, and shock (pp.120–121) may result.

Fracture of the neck of the femur is common in elderly people, particularly women, whose bones become less dense and more brittle with age. This fracture is sometimes a stable injury in which the bone ends are impacted together (see FRACTURES, pp.150–152). The casualty may be able to walk with a fractured neck of femur for some period of time before the fracture is discovered. In the hip joint, the most serious, though much less common, type of injury is dislocation.

▶ **See also** DISLOCATED JOINT p.153
● FRACTURES pp.150–152 ● SHOCK pp.120–12

RECOGNITION

There may be:
● Pain at the site of the injury.
● Inability to walk.
● Signs of shock.
● Shortening of the leg and turning outwards of the knee and foot, as powerful muscles move the broken bone ends over each other.

✚ YOUR AIMS

● To immobilise the lower limb.
● To arrange urgent removal to hospital.

❶ WARNING

● Do not allow the casualty to eat, drink, or smoke, because he may need to have a general anaesthetic in hospital.
● Do not raise the casualty's legs, even if he shows any signs of shock, because you may cause further internal damage.

1 Help the casualty to lie down. If possible, ask a helper to gently steady and support the injured limb.

2 Gently straighten the casualty's lower leg. If necessary, apply traction (p.151) at the ankle to help straighten the leg.

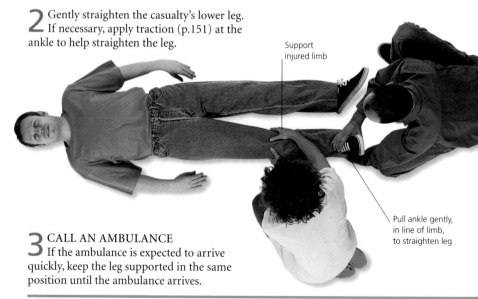

Support injured limb

Pull ankle gently, in line of limb, to straighten leg

3 CALL AN AMBULANCE
If the ambulance is expected to arrive quickly, keep the leg supported in the same position until the ambulance arrives.

4 If the ambulance is not expected to arrive quickly, immobilise the leg by splinting it the uninjured one. Gently bring the sound mb alongside the injured one. Position andages at the ankles and feet (1), then the lees (2). Add bandages above (3) and below) the fracture site. Insert soft padding etween the legs to prevent the bony parts om rubbing against each other, then tie the andages on the uninjured side.

5 Take any steps possible to treat the casualty for shock (pp.120–121): insulate im from the cold with blankets or clothing, ut do not raise his legs.

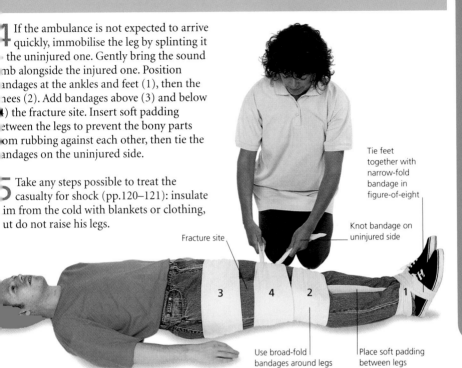

Tie feet together with narrow-fold bandage in figure-of-eight

Knot bandage on uninjured side

Fracture site

Use broad-fold bandages around legs

Place soft padding between legs

SPECIAL CASE

PREPARING FOR TRANSPORT

If the journey to hospital is likely to be long and rough, more sturdy support for the leg and feet will be needed. Use a purpose-made malleable splint or a long, solid object, such as a fence post, that will reach from the armpit to the foot.

Place the splint against the injured side. Insert padding between the legs and between the splint and the casualty's body. Tie the feet together with

a narrow-fold bandage (1). Secure the splint to the body with broad-fold bandages at the chest (2), pelvis (3), knees (4), above and below the fracture site (5 and 6), and at one extra point (7). Do not bandage over the fracture.

Once the casualty's leg is fully immobilised, she should be moved on to the stretcher using the log-roll technique (p.167).

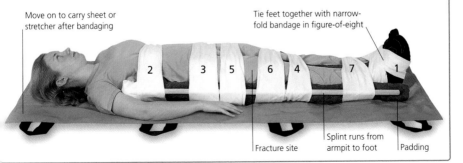

Move on to carry sheet or stretcher after bandaging

Tie feet together with narrow-fold bandage in figure-of-eight

Fracture site

Splint runs from armpit to foot

Padding

KNEE INJURY

The knee is the hinge joint between the thigh bone (femur) and shin bone (tibia). It is capable of bending, straightening, and, in the bent position, slight rotation.

The knee joint is supported by strong muscles and ligaments and protected at the front by a disc of bone called the kneecap (patella). The surfaces of the major bones are protected by discs of cartilage. These structures may be damaged by direct blows, violent twists, or sprains. Possible knee injuries include fracture of the patella, sprains, and damage to the cartilage.

A knee injury may make it impossible for the casualty to bend the joint, and you

RECOGNITION

There may be:

● Pain, spreading from the injury to become deep-seated in the joint.

● If the bent knee has "locked", acute pain on attempting to straighten the leg.

● Rapid swelling at the knee joint.

should ensure that the casualty does not tr to walk on the injured leg.

Bleeding or fluid in the knee joint may cause marked swelling around the knee.

▶ **See also** STRAINS AND SPRAINS pp.154–155

✚ YOUR AIMS

● To protect the knee in the most comfortable position.

● To arrange removal of the casualty to hospital.

⚠ WARNING

● Do not attempt to straighten the knee forcibly. Displaced cartilage or internal bleeding may make it impossible to straighten the knee joint safely.

● Do not allow the casualty to eat, drink, or smoke, because she may need a general anaesthetic in hospital.

● Do not allow the casualty to walk.

1 Help the casualty to lie down, preferably on a blanket to insulate her from the ground. Place soft padding, such as a pillow, blanket, or coat, under her injured knee to support it in the most comfortable position.

2 Wrap soft padding around the joint. Secure with bandages that extend from mid-thigh to the middle of the lower leg.

3 Arrange removal of the casualty to hospital. The casualty needs to remain in the treatment position and should therefore be transported in an ambulance.

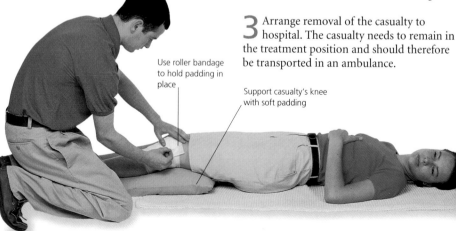

Use roller bandage to hold padding in place

Support casualty's knee with soft padding

LOWER LEG INJURY

njuries to the lower leg include fractures of he shin bone (tibia) and the splint bone fibula), and tearing of the soft tissues muscles, ligaments, and tendons).

Fractures of the tibia are usually due to a eavy blow (for example, from the bumper f a moving vehicle). As there is little flesh ver the tibia, a fracture is more likely to roduce a wound. The fibula can be broken y the twisting that sprains an ankle.

RECOGNITION

There may be:
- Localised pain.
- Swelling, bruising, and deformity of the leg.
- An open wound.

▶ **See also** STRAINS AND SPRAINS pp.154–155

+ YOUR AIMS
- To immobilise the leg.
- To arrange urgent removal to hospital.

1 Help the casualty to lie down, and carefully teady and support the njured leg. If there s an open wound, gently expose the wound and treat leeding. Apply adding to protect the njury.

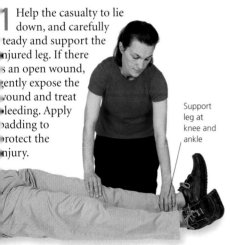

Support leg at knee and ankle

2 CALL AN AMBULANCE
Support the injured leg with your hands o prevent any movement of the fracture site. Do this until the ambulance arrives.

❶ CAUTION

If the casualty's journey to hospital is likely to be long and rough, place soft padding on the outside of the injured leg, from the knee to the foot. Secure legs with broad-fold bandages as described above.

3 If the ambulance is delayed, support the injured leg by splinting it to the other leg. Bring the uninjured limb alongside the injured one and slide bandages under both legs. Position bandages at the feet and ankles (1), then knees (2). Add bandages above (3) and below (4) the fracture. Insert padding between the lower legs. Then tie the bandages firmly, knotting them on the uninjured side.

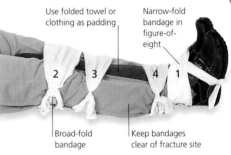

Use folded towel or clothing as padding

Narrow-fold bandage in figure-of-eight

Broad-fold bandage

Keep bandages clear of fracture site

SPECIAL CASE

SUSPECTED FRACTURE NEAR ANKLE
Place separate bandages above the ankle and around the feet, rather than one figure-of-eight.

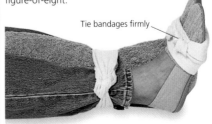

Tie bandages firmly

ANKLE INJURY

If the ankle is broken, treat it as a fracture of the lower leg (p.173). A more common injury is a sprain (p.154), usually caused by a wrench to the ankle. This problem can be treated by the RICE procedure: *rest* the affected part, apply *ice*, *compress* with bandaging, and *elevate*.

See also STRAINS AND SPRAINS pp.154–15

+ YOUR AIMS
- To relieve pain and swelling.
- To obtain medical aid if necessary.

❶ CAUTION

If you suspect a broken bone, tell the casualty not to put weight on the leg. Secure and support the lower leg (p.173), and take or send the casualty to hospital.

1 Rest, steady, and support the ankle in the most comfortable position.

2 If the injury has only recently occurred, apply an ice pack or a cold compress (p.49) to the site to reduce swelling.

3 Wrap the ankle in thick padding and bandage firmly. Raise and support the injured limb. Advise the casualty to rest the ankle and to see a doctor if pain persists.

FOOT AND TOE INJURIES

Fractures affecting the many small bones of the foot are usually caused by crushing injuries. These fractures are best treated in hospital. When giving first aid, concentrate on relieving symptoms such as swelling.

RECOGNITION
- Difficulty in walking.
- Stiffness of movement.
- Bruising and swelling.

+ YOUR AIMS
- To minimise swelling.
- To arrange transport to hospital.

1 Quickly raise and support the foot to reduce blood flow to the area, which will minimise swelling.

2 Apply an ice pack or cold compress (p.49). This will also help to relieve swelling.

3 Arrange to take or send the casualty to hospital. If she is not being transported by ambulance, try to ensure that the foot remains elevated during travel.

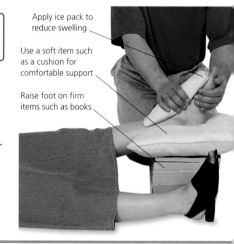

Apply ice pack to reduce swelling

Use a soft item such as a cushion for comfortable support

Raise foot on firm items such as books

8

THE NERVOUS SYSTEM is the most complex system in the body. Its control centre, the brain, is the source of consciousness, thought, speech, and memory. It also receives and interprets sensory information, which is carried by the nerves, and controls other body systems. When we are fully conscious, we are awake, alert, and aware of our surroundings. However, if consciousness is impaired, even survival mechanisms, such as the cough reflex to keep the airway clear, may not function.

TREATMENT PRIORITIES

Because many of the problems described in this chapter can produce impaired consciousness, they need immediate attention. Your priority as a first aider is to monitor and maintain the vital functions of breathing and circulation.

✚ FIRST-AID PRIORITIES

- Assess the casualty's condition.
- Comfort and reassure the casualty.
- Maintain an open airway, check breathing, and be prepared to resuscitate if necessary.
- Protect the casualty from harm.
- Look for and treat any injuries associated with the condition.
- Obtain medical aid if necessary. Call an ambulance if you suspect a serious illness or injury.

CONTENTS

NERVOUS SYSTEM PROBLEMS

NERVOUS SYSTEM PROBLEMS

THE NERVOUS SYSTEM

This is the body's information-gathering, storage, and control system. It consists of a central processing unit – the brain – and a complex network of nerve cells and fibres.

There are two main parts to the nervous system: the central nervous system, consisting of the brain and spinal cord, and the peripheral nervous system, which consists of all the nerves connecting the brain and

the spinal cord to the rest of the body. In addition, the autonomic (involuntary) nervous system controls body functions such as digestion, heart rate, and breathin

The central nervous system receives and analyses information from all parts c the body. The nerves carry message in the form of high-speed electrica impulses, between the brain and th rest of the nervous system.

Structure of the nervous system
The system consists of the brain, spinal cord, and a dense network of nerves that carry electrical impulses between the brain and the rest of the body.

Spinal cord carries nerve impulses between brain and rest of body

Spinal nerves (31 pairs) emerge from spinal cord and extend through vertebral column

Body of vertebra

Spinal nerve

Spinal cord

Brain

Cranial nerves (12 pairs) extend directly from underside of the brain; most supply the head, face, neck, and shoulders

Vagus nerve, longest of the cranial nerves, supplies organs in chest anc abdomen; it controls heart rate

Radial nerve controls muscles that straighten elbow and fingers

Sciatic nerve serves hip and hamstring muscles

Nerve fibre

Myelin sheath

Nerve fascicl

Tibial nerve supplies calf muscles

Spinal-cord protection
The spinal cord is protected by the bony vertebral (spinal) column. Nerves branching from the cord emerge between adjacent vertebrae.

Cross section through nerv
Each nerve is made up of bundl of nerve fibres called fascicles. A protective fatty substance called myelin surrounds and insulates larger nerve fibres.

Central nervous system

The brain and the spinal cord make up the central nervous system (CNS). This system contains billions of interconnected nerve cells (neurons) and is enclosed by three membranes (meninges). A clear fluid called cerebrospinal fluid flows around the brain and spinal cord. It functions as a shock absorber, provides oxygen and nutrients, and removes waste products.

The brain has three main structures: the cerebrum, which is concerned with thought, sensation, and conscious movement; the cerebellum, which coordinates movement, balance, and posture; and the brain stem, which controls basic functions such as breathing.

The main function of the spinal cord is to convey signals between the brain and the peripheral nervous system (below).

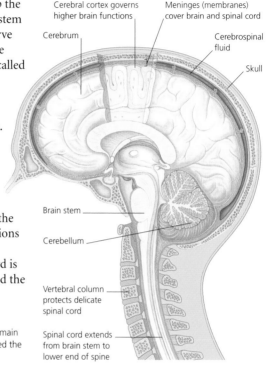

Cerebral cortex governs higher brain functions

Cerebrum

Meninges (membranes) cover brain and spinal cord

Cerebrospinal fluid

Skull

Brain stem

Cerebellum

Vertebral column protects delicate spinal cord

Spinal cord extends from brain stem to lower end of spine

Brain structure
The brain is enclosed within the skull. It has three main parts: the cerebrum, which has an outer layer called the cortex; the cerebellum; and the brain stem.

Peripheral nervous system

This part of the nervous system consists of two sets of paired nerves – the cranial and spinal nerves – connecting the CNS to the body. The cranial nerves emerge in 12 pairs from the underside of the brain. The 31 pairs of spinal nerves branch off at intervals from the spinal cord, passing into the rest of the body. Nerves comprise bundles of nerve fibres that can relay both incoming (sensory) and outgoing (motor) signals.

Autonomic nervous system

Some of the cranial nerves, and several small spinal nerves, work as the autonomic nervous system. This system is concerned with vital body functions such as heart rate and breathing. The system's two parts, the sympathetic and parasympathetic systems, counterbalance each other. The sympathetic system prepares the body for action by releasing hormones that raise the heart rate and reduce the blood flow to the skin and intestines. The parasympathetic system releases hormones with a calming effect.

IMPAIRED CONSCIOUSNESS

There is no absolute dividing line between consciousness and unconsciousness. People may be fully aware and awake (conscious), completely unresponsive to any stimulus (unconscious), or at any level between these two extremes. For example, a casualty may be "groggy" or respond only to loud sounds or to pain. Impaired consciousness is the term used when a casualty is anything less than fully conscious.

AVPU CODE

You can assess consciousness by checking the casualty's level of response to stimuli using the AVPU code.

A – Is the casualty *Alert*? Does he open his eyes and respond to questions?

V – Does the casualty respond to *Voice*? Does he answer simple questions and obey commands?

P – Does the casualty respond to *Pain*? Does he open his eyes or move if pinched?

U – Is the casualty *Unresponsive* to any stimulus?

You should record your findings on the observation charts (p.280).

CAUSES OF IMPAIRED CONSCIOUSNES

The main causes of impaired consciousnes are structural damage to the brain or a lack of nutrients – oxygen and glucose (sugar) – reaching the brain. Structural damage may occur with a head injury or a brain tumour. Low oxygen (hypoxia) or low blood sugar (hypoglycaemia) may occur with any condition that reduces blood flow to the brain, such as stroke, shock, fainting, or a heart attack. It can also occur if blood flow is normal but there is insufficient oxygen or glucose in the blood – for example, due to poisoning, or a chemical imbalance caused by diabetes mellitus. Epilepsy can produce impaired consciousness due to abnormal electrical activity in the brain.

▶ See also DIABETES MELLITUS p.240
● HEAD INJURY opposite ● HYPOXIA p.106
● LIFE-SAVING PROCEDURES pp.71–102
● SPINAL INJURY pp.165–167

YOUR AIMS

- To maintain an open airway.
- To assess and record level of response.
- To arrange urgent removal to hospital if necessary.

⚠ WARNING

- If you suspect that a casualty may have a neck (spinal) injury, handle his head very carefully. To open the airway, use the jaw thrust method (p.167): kneel behind the casualty's head and place your hands on each side of his face, with your fingertips at the angles of his jaw; gently lift the jaw.
- Do not move the casualty unnecessarily.

1 Perform a quick check of consciousness by checking the level of response using th AVPU code (above). If the person is "groggy" but responds to sound or pain, support him in a comfortable, resting position and watch for any change in his level of response.

2 If the casualty is unconscious, follow the procedure for treating an unconscious casualty (*see* LIFE-SAVING PROCEDURES, pp.71–102).
CALL AN AMBULANCE

3 While waiting for medical help to arrive, monitor and record vital signs – level of response, pulse, and breathing (pp.42–43). Treat any associated injuries.

HEAD INJURY

All head injuries are potentially serious and require proper assessment because they can result in impaired consciousness (opposite). Injuries may be associated with damage to the brain tissue or to blood vessels inside the skull, or with a skull fracture.

A head injury may produce concussion, which is a brief period of unconsciousness followed by complete recovery. Some head injuries may produce compression of the brain (cerebral compression), which is life-threatening. It is therefore important to be able to recognise possible signs of cerebral compression (below) – in particular, a deteriorating level of response.

A head wound should alert you to the risk of deeper, underlying damage, such as a skull fracture, which may be serious. Bleeding inside the skull may also occur and lead to compression. Clear fluid or watery blood leaking from the ear or nose are signs of serious injury.

Any casualty with an injury to the head should be assumed to have a neck (spinal) injury as well and be treated accordingly (see SPINAL INJURY, p.165–167).

⚠ WARNING

Handle the casualty's head very carefully because of the risk of neck (spinal) injury. Open the airway, using the jaw thrust method (p.167), and check breathing.

Gently lift the jaw to open the airway

If the position in which the casualty was found prevents maintenance of an open airway or you fail to open it using the jaw thrust, place her in the recovery position (pp.84–85). If you have helpers, use the "log-roll" technique (p.167).

▶ See also CEREBRAL COMPRESSION p.181 ● CONCUSSION p.180 ● LIFE-SAVING PROCEDURES pp.71–102 ● SCALP AND HEAD WOUNDS p.137 ● SKULL FRACTURE p.182 ● SPINAL INJURY pp.165–167

RECOGNITION

Concussion	Cerebral compression	Skull fracture
● Brief period of impaired consciousness following a blow to the head.	● Deteriorating level of response – may progress to unconsciousness.	● Wound or bruise on the head.
There may also be:	*There may also be:*	● Soft area or depression on the scalp.
● Dizziness or nausea on recovery.	● History of recent head injury.	● Bruising/swelling behind one ear.
● Loss of memory of any events that occurred at the time of, or immediately preceding, the injury.	● Intense headache.	● Bruising around one or both eyes.
	● Noisy breathing, becoming slow.	● Loss of clear fluid or watery blood from the nose or an ear.
● Mild, generalised headache.	● Slow, yet full and strong, pulse.	● Blood in the white of the eye.
	● Unequal pupil size.	● Distortion or lack of symmetry of the head or face.
	● Weakness and/or paralysis down one side of the face and/or body.	● Deteriorating level of response – may progress to unconsciousness.
	● High temperature; flushed face.	
	● Drowsiness.	
	● Noticeable change in personality or behaviour, such as irritability.	

CONCUSSION

The brain is free to move a little within the skull, and can thus be "shaken" by a blow to the head. This shaking is called concussion. Among the more common causes of concussion are traffic incidents, sports injuries, falls, and blows received in fights.

Concussion produces widespread but temporary disturbance of normal brain activity. However, it is not usually associated with any lasting damage to the brain. The casualty will suffer impaired consciousness, but this only lasts for a short time (usually only a few minutes) and is followed by a full recovery. By definition, concussion can only be confidently diagnosed once the casualty has completely recovered.

A casualty who has been concussed should be monitored and advised to obtain medical aid if symptoms such as headache or blurred vision develop later.

▶ See also CEREBRAL COMPRESSION opposite ● LIFE-SAVING PROCEDURES pp.71–102 ● SPINAL INJURY pp.165–167

RECOGNITION

● Brief period of impaired consciousness following a blow to the head.

There may also be:

● Dizziness or nausea on recovery.
● Loss of memory of events at the time of, or immediately preceding, the injury.
● Mild, generalised headache.

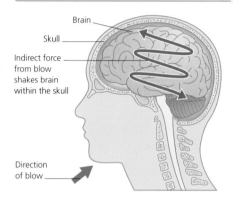

Brain
Skull
Indirect force from blow shakes brain within the skull
Direction of blow

Mechanism of concussion
Concussion usually occurs as a result of a blow to the head. This "shakes" the brain within the skull, resulting in a temporary disturbance of brain function.

✚ YOUR AIMS

● To ensure the casualty recovers fully and safely.
● To place the casualty in the care of a responsible person.
● To obtain medical aid if necessary.

❶ WARNING

If the casualty does not recover fully, OR if there is a deteriorating level of response after an initial recovery

CALL AN AMBULANCE

❶ CAUTION

All casualties who have had a head injury should also be treated for a neck injury (see SPINAL INJURY, pp.165–167).

1 Treat the casualty as for impaired consciousness (p.178).

2 Monitor and record vital signs – level of response, pulse, and breathing (pp.42–43). Even if the casualty appears to recover fully, watch him for subsequent deterioration in his level of response.

3 When the casualty has recovered, place him in the care of a responsible person. If a casualty has been injured on the sports field, never allow him to "play on" without first obtaining medical advice.

4 Advise the casualty to go to hospital if he later develops headache, nausea, vomiting, or excessive sleepiness following a blow to the head.

CEREBRAL COMPRESSION

Compression of the brain – a condition called cerebral compression – is very serious and almost invariably requires surgery. Cerebral compression occurs when there is a build-up of pressure on the brain. This pressure may be due to one of several different causes, such as an accumulation of blood within the skull or swelling of injured brain tissues.

Cerebral compression is usually caused by a head injury. However, it can also be due to other causes, such as stroke (p.183), infection, or a brain tumour. The condition may develop immediately after a head injury, or it may appear a few hours or even days later. For this reason, you should always try to find out whether the casualty has a recent history of a head injury.

▶ **See also** LIFE-SAVING PROCEDURES pp.71–102 ● SPINAL INJURY pp.165–167

Compression caused by bleeding
Bleeding may occur within the skull following a head injury or a disorder such as a stroke. The escaped blood may put pressure on tissues in the brain.

RECOGNITION

● Deteriorating level of response – casualty may become unconscious.

There may also be:
● History of a recent head injury.
● Intense headache.
● Noisy breathing, becoming slow.
● Slow, yet full and strong pulse.
● Unequal pupil size.
● Weakness and/or paralysis down one side of the face or body.
● High temperature; flushed face.
● Drowsiness.
● Noticeable change in personality or behaviour, such as irritability or disorientation.

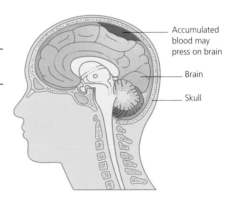

Accumulated blood may press on brain

Brain

Skull

YOUR AIM

● To arrange urgent removal of the casualty to hospital.

⚠ WARNING

If the casualty is unconscious, open the airway using the jaw thrust method (p.167) and check breathing; be prepared to give rescue breaths and chest compressions if necessary (*see* LIFE-SAVING PROCEDURES, pp.71–102).

CALL AN AMBULANCE

If the casualty is breathing, try to maintain the airway in the position the casualty was found.

1 CALL AN AMBULANCE
If the casualty is conscious, keep him supported in a comfortable resting position and reassure him.

2 Regularly monitor and record the casualty's vital signs – level of response, pulse, and breathing (pp.42–43) – until medical help arrives.

⚠ CAUTION

Do not allow the casualty to eat, drink, or smoke because a general anaesthetic may need to be given in hospital.

SKULL FRACTURE

If a casualty has a head wound, be alert for a possible skull fracture. An affected casualty may have impaired consciousness.

A skull fracture is serious because there is a risk that the brain may be damaged either directly by fractured bone from the skull or by bleeding inside the skull. Clear fluid (cerebrospinal fluid) or watery blood leaking from the ear or nose are signs of serious injury.

Suspect a skull fracture in any casualty who has received a head injury resulting in impaired consciousness. Bear in mind that a casualty with a possible skull fracture may also have a neck (spinal) injury and should be treated accordingly (*see* SPINAL INJURY, pp.165–167).

▶ **See also** LIFE-SAVING PROCEDURES pp.71–102 ● SCALP AND HEAD WOUNDS p.137 ● SPINAL INJURY pp.165–167

➕ YOUR AIMS
- To maintain an open airway.
- To arrange urgent removal of the casualty to hospital.

❗ WARNING
If the casualty is unconscious, open the airway using the jaw thrust method (p.167) and check breathing; be prepared to give rescue breaths and chest compressions if needed (*see* LIFE-SAVING PROCEDURES, pp.71–102).
CALL AN AMBULANCE

1 If the casualty is conscious, help her to lie down. Do not turn the head in case there is a neck injury.

2 Control any bleeding from the scalp by applying pressure around the wound. Look for and treat any other injuries. **CALL AN AMBULANCE**

3 If there is discharge from an ear, cover the ear with a sterile dressing or clean pad, lightly secured with a bandage (*see* BLEEDING FROM THE EAR, p.138). Do not plug the ear.

4 Monitor and record vital signs – level of response, pulse, and breathing (pp.42–43) – until medical help arrives.

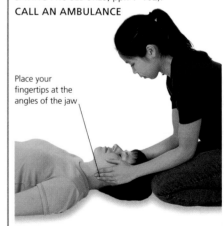

Place your fingertips at the angles of the jaw

If the position in which the casualty was found prevents maintenance of an open airway or you fail to open it using the jaw thrust, place her in the recovery position (pp.84–85). If you have helpers, use the "log-roll" technique (p.167).

STROKE

he term "stroke" describes a condition in which the blood supply to part of the brain s suddenly and seriously impaired by a lood clot or a ruptured blood vessel. It is itally important that the casualty is taken o hospital quickly. If the stroke is due to a lot, drugs can then be given to limit the xtent of the damage to the brain tissue nd promote recovery.

Strokes occur more commonly in later fe and in people who suffer from high lood pressure or some other circulatory isorder. The effect of a stroke depends on ow much, and which part, of the brain is ffected. In some cases, the condition can e fatal; however, many people make a omplete recovery from a stroke.

RECOGNITION

There may be:
- Problems with speech and swallowing.
- If asked to show teeth, only one side of mouth will move or movement will be uneven.
- Loss of power or movement in the limbs.
- Sudden, severe headache.
- Confused, emotional mental state that could be mistaken for drunkenness.
- Sudden or gradual loss of consciousness.

See also LIFE-SAVING PROCEDURES pp.71–102

YOUR AIMS

- To maintain an open airway.
- To arrange urgent removal of the casualty to hospital.

WARNING

If the casualty is unconscious, open the airway and check breathing; be prepared to give rescue breaths and chest compressions if necessary (*see* LIFE-SAVING PROCEDURES, pp.71–102).

If she is breathing, place her in the recovery position (pp.184–185).

CALL AN AMBULANCE

Monitor and record vital signs – level of response, pulse, and breathing (pp.42–43) – until medical help arrives.

CAUTION

Do not give the casualty anything to eat or drink because a stroke may make it difficult to swallow.

1 If the casualty is conscious, help her to lie down with her head and shoulders slightly raised and supported. Incline her head to the affected side, and place a towel on her shoulder to absorb any dribbling.
CALL AN AMBULANCE

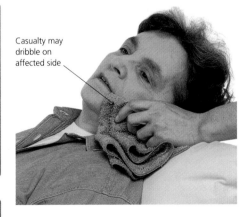

Casualty may dribble on affected side

2 Loosen any clothing that might impair the casualty's breathing. Continue to reassure her. Monitor and record vital signs – level of response, pulse, and breathing (pp.42–43) – until medical help arrives.

SEIZURES IN ADULTS

A seizure – also called a convulsion or fit – consists of involuntary contractions of many of the muscles in the body. The condition is due to a disturbance in the electrical activity of the brain. Seizures usually result in loss or impairment of consciousness. The most common cause is epilepsy. Other causes include head injury, some brain-damaging diseases, shortage of oxygen or glucose in the brain, and the intake of certain poisons, including alcohol.

Epileptic seizures are due to recurrent, major disturbances of brain activity. These seizures can be sudden and dramatic. Just before a seizure, a casualty may have a brief warning period (aura) with, for example, a strange feeling or a special smell or taste.

No matter what the cause of the seizure, care must always include maintaining an open, clear airway and monitoring the casualty's vital signs – level of response, pulse, and breathing. You will also need to protect the casualty from further harm during a seizure and arrange appropriate aftercare once he has recovered.

RECOGNITION

Generally:
- Sudden unconsciousness.
- Rigidity and arching of the back.
- Convulsive movements.

In epilepsy the following sequence is common:
- The casualty suddenly falls unconscious, often letting out a cry.
- He becomes rigid, arching his back.
- Breathing may cease. The lips may show a grey–blue tinge (cyanosis) and the face and neck may become red and puffy.
- Convulsive movements begin. The jaw may be clenched and breathing may be noisy. Saliva may appear at the mouth and may be blood-stained if the lips or tongue have been bitten. There may be loss of bladder or bowel control.
- Muscles relax and breathing becomes normal; the casualty recovers consciousness, usually within a few minutes. He may feel dazed, or act strangely. He may be unaware of his actions.
- After a seizure, the casualty may feel tired and fall into a deep sleep.

▶ See also IMPAIRED CONSCIOUSNESS p.17
- LIFE-SAVING PROCEDURES pp.71–102

✚ YOUR AIMS

- To protect the casualty from injury.
- To give care when consciousness is regained.
- To arrange removal of the casualty to hospital if necessary.

1 If you see the casualty falling, try to ease her fall (*see* CONTROLLING A FALL, p.66). Make space around her; ask bystanders to move away. Remove potentially dangerous items, such as hot drinks and sharp objects. Note the time when the seizure started.

2 If possible, protect the casualty's head by placing soft padding underneath it. Loosen clothing around her neck.

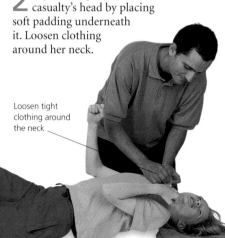

Loosen tight clothing around the neck

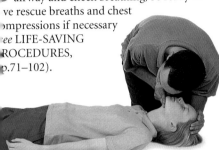

3 When the seizure has ceased, open the airway and check breathing; be ready to give rescue breaths and chest compressions if necessary (see LIFE-SAVING PROCEDURES, p.71–102).

(see LIFE-SAVING PROCEDURES, p.71–102).

4 If she is breathing, place her in the recovery position. Monitor and record vital signs – level of response, pulse, and breathing (pp.42–43). Note the duration of the seizure.

! CAUTION

● Do not move the casualty unless she is in immediate danger.
● Do not put anything in her mouth or use force to restrain her.

! WARNING

If any of the following apply
CALL AN AMBULANCE

● The casualty is unconscious for more than 10 minutes.
● The seizure continues for more than 5 minutes.
● The casualty is having repeated seizures or having her first seizure.
● The casualty is not aware of any reason for the seizure.

ABSENCE SEIZURES

Some people experience a mild form of epilepsy, with small seizures during which they appear distant and unaware of their surroundings. These episodes, called "absence seizures", tend to affect children more than adults. There is unlikely to be any convulsive movement or loss of consciousness, but a full seizure may follow.

RECOGNITION

● Sudden "switching off"; the casualty may stare blankly ahead.
● Slight or localised twitching or jerking of the lips, eyelids, head, or limbs.
● Odd "automatic" movements, such as lip-smacking, chewing, or making noises.

+ YOUR AIM

● To protect the casualty until she is fully recovered.

1 Help the casualty to sit down in a quiet place. Make space around her; remove any potentially dangerous items, such as hot drinks and sharp objects.

2 Talk to the casualty in a calm and reassuring way. Do not pester her with questions. Stay with her until you are sure that she is fully recovered.

3 If the casualty does not recognise or have any awareness of her condition, advise her to consult her own doctor as soon as possible.

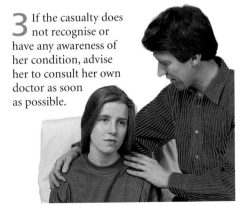

SEIZURES IN CHILDREN

In young children, seizures – sometimes called fits or convulsions – are most often the result of a raised body temperature associated with a throat or ear infection or other infectious disease. This type of seizure is known as a febrile convulsion and is a reaction of the brain to high body temperature. Epilepsy is another possible cause of seizures in infants and children.

Although seizures can be alarming, they are rarely dangerous if properly dealt with. For safety's sake, however, the child should be seen at a hospital to rule out any serious underlying condition.

▶ See also UNCONSCIOUS CHILD pp.86–93

RECOGNITION

● Violent muscle twitching, with clenched fists and an arched back.

There may also be:

● Obvious signs of fever: hot, flushed skin, and perhaps sweating.

● Twitching of the face with squinting, fixed, or upturned eyes.

● Breath-holding, with red, "puffy" face and neck or drooling at the mouth.

● Loss or impairment of consciousness.

✚ YOUR AIMS

● To protect the child from injury.
● To cool the child.
● To reassure the parents or carer.
● To arrange removal to hospital.

1 Position pillows or soft padding around the child so that even violent movement will not result in injury.

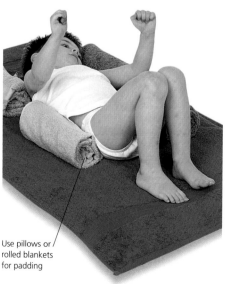

Use pillows or rolled blankets for padding

2 Remove any covering or clothes. Ensure a good supply of cool, fresh air (but be careful not to overcool the child).

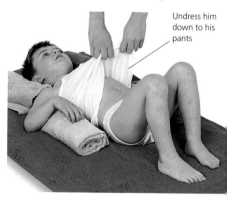

Undress him down to his pants

3 Sponge the child's skin with tepid water to help cooling; start at his forehead and work down his body.

4 Once the seizures have stopped, keep the airway open by placing the child in the recovery position (pp.92–93) if necessary. **CALL AN AMBULANCE**

5 Reassure the child and parents or carer. Monitor and record vital signs – level of response, pulse, and breathing (pp.42–43) – until medical help arrives.

MENINGITIS

This is a disorder in which the linings that surround the brain and the spinal cord (the meninges) become inflamed. It can be caused by several different types of bacteria or viruses, and can occur at any age.

Meningitis is potentially a very serious illness, and the casualty may deteriorate very fast. Prompt treatment in hospital with antibiotic drugs is vital. Without immediate treatment, meningitis may cause permanent disability, such as deafness or brain damage, and it can even be fatal.

For this reason, it is important that you are able to recognise the symptoms of meningitis – these may include high fever, severe headache, and a distinctive rash. With early diagnosis and treatment, most people make a full recovery.

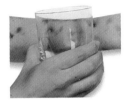

Testing for meningitis
Press a glass over a skin rash. If the rash does not fade under the glass, suspect meningitis.

RECOGNITION

The symptoms and signs include the following, but usually not all are present at the same time:

● High temperature or fever.
● Vomiting, which is often violent, or loss of appetite.
● Severe headache.
● Neck stiffness (the casualty cannot touch his chest with his chin).
● Joint or muscle pains.
● Drowsiness.
● Confusion or disorientation.
● Dislike of bright light.
● Seizures.
● Skin rash of small red/purple "pin prick" spots that may spread to look like fresh bruising. (The rash is more difficult to see on dark skin.) This rash does not fade when the side of a glass is pressed against it.

In babies and young children there may also be:
● Drowsiness or restlessness and high-pitched crying.
● Reluctance to feed.
● In babies, slight tenderness and swelling of the soft parts of the skull.

✚ YOUR AIM

● To obtain urgent medical aid.

❶ WARNING

If a doctor cannot be contacted or is likely to be delayed

CALL AN AMBULANCE

If the casualty is ill and becoming worse, even if he has already seen a doctor, seek urgent medical attention again.

1 If you are concerned that an individual may have meningitis, seek medical advice immediately. Do not wait for all the symptoms and signs listed above to appear because casualties with meningitis may not always develop all of these.

2 When calling the doctor or ambulance, describe the symptoms and say that you are concerned that it may be meningitis. Be prepared to insist on medical attention.

3 While waiting for the doctor or ambulance, reassure the casualty and keep him cool.

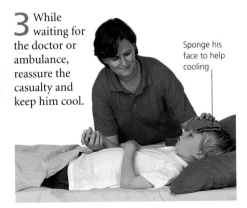

Sponge his face to help cooling

HEADACHE

A headache may accompany any illness, particularly a feverish ailment such as flu. It may develop for no reason but can often be traced to tiredness, tension, stress, or undue heat or cold. Mild "poisoning" caused by a stuffy or fume-filled atmosphere, or by excess alcohol or any other drug, can also induce a headache. However, a headache may also be the most prominent symptom of meningitis or stroke.

▶ See also MENINGITIS p.187 ● STROKE p.1

✚ YOUR AIMS
● To relieve the pain.
● To obtain medical aid if necessary.

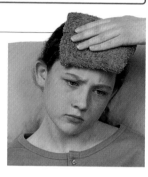

Cold compress may give relief

1 Help the casualty to sit or lie down in a quiet place. Apply a cold compress to the head (p.49).

❗ CAUTION
Always seek urgent medical advice if the pain:
● Develops very suddenly.
● Is severe and incapacitating.
● Is accompanied by fever or vomiting.
● Is recurrent or persistent.
● Is accompanied by loss of strength or sensation or by impaired consciousness.
● Is accompanied by a stiff neck.
● Follows a head injury.

2 An adult may take two paracetamol tablets, a child the recommended dose of paracetamol syrup. Do not give a child aspiri

MIGRAINE

Many people are prone to migraine attacks – severe, "sickening" headaches. Attacks can be triggered by a variety of causes, such as allergy, stress, or tiredness. Other triggers include lack of sleep, missed meals, alcohol, and some foods, such as cheese or chocolate. Migraine sufferers usually know how to recognise and deal with attacks. They may carry their own medication.

RECOGNITION
● Before the attack there may be a warning period, with disturbance of vision in the form of flickering lights and/or a "blind patch".
● Intense throbbing headache, which is sometimes on just one side of the head.
● Abdominal pain, nausea, and vomiting.
● Inability to tolerate bright light or loud noise.

✚ YOUR AIMS
● To relieve the pain.
● To obtain medical aid if necessary.

1 Help the casualty to take any medication that she may have for migraine attacks.

2 Advise the casualty to lie down or sleep for a few hours in a quiet, dark room. Provide her with some towels and a container in case she vomits.

3 If this is the first attack, advise the casualty to see her doctor.

9

THIS CHAPTER DEALS with the effects of injuries and illnesses caused by environmental factors such as extremes of heat and cold.

The skin protects the body and helps to maintain body temperature within a normal range. It can be damaged by fire, hot liquids, or caustic substances. Such injuries are often sustained in incidents such as explosions or chemical spillages.

The effects of temperature extremes can also impair skin and other body functions. Injuries may be localised – as in frostbite or sunburn – or generalised, as in heat exhaustion or hypothermia. Very young children and elderly people are most susceptible to problems caused by extremes of temperature.

FIRST-AID PRIORITIES

- Assess the casualty's condition.
- Comfort and reassure the casualty.
- Obtain medical aid if necessary. Call an ambulance if you suspect a serious illness or injury.

BURNS
- Protect yourself and the casualty from danger.
- Assess the burn, prevent further damage, and relieve symptoms.

EXTREME TEMPERATURES
- Protect the casualty from heat or cold.
- Restore normal body temperature.

CONTENTS

ENVIRONMENTAL INJURIES

THE SKIN

One of the largest organs, the skin plays key roles in protecting the body from injury and infection and in maintaining a constant body temperature.

The skin consists of two layers of tissue – an outer layer (epidermis) and an inner layer (dermis) – which lie on a layer of fatty tissue (subcutaneous fat). The top part of the epidermis is made up of dead, flattened skin cells, which are constantly shed and replaced by new cells made in the lower part of this layer. The epidermis is protected by an oily substance called sebum, secreted from glands called sebaceous glands, which keeps the skin supple and waterproof.

The lower layer of the skin, the dermis, contains the blood vessels, nerves, muscles, sebaceous glands, sweat glands, and hair roots (follicles). The ends of sensory nerves within the dermis register sensations from the body's surface, such as heat, cold, pain, and even the slightest touch. Blood vessels supply the skin with nutrients and help to regulate body temperature by preserving or releasing heat (opposite).

Structure of the skin
The skin is made up of two layers: the thin, outer epidermis and the thicker dermis beneath it. Most of the structures of the skin, such as blood vessels, nerves, and hair roots, are contained within the dermis.

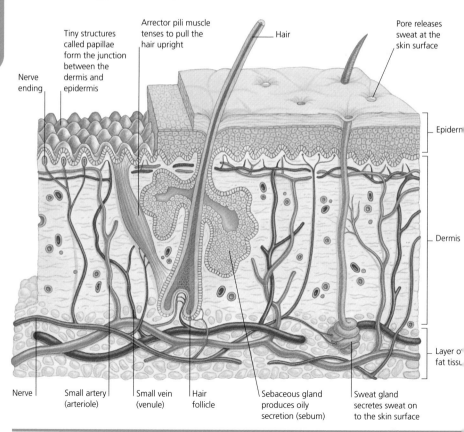

Tiny structures called papillae form the junction between the dermis and epidermis

Nerve ending

Arrector pili muscle tenses to pull the hair upright

Hair

Pore releases sweat at the skin surface

Epidermis

Dermis

Layer of fat tissue

Nerve

Small artery (arteriole)

Small vein (venule)

Hair follicle

Sebaceous gland produces oily secretion (sebum)

Sweat gland secretes sweat on to the skin surface

Maintaining body temperature

One of the major functions of the skin is to help maintain the body temperature within its optimum range of 36–37°C (97–99°F). Body temperature is constantly monitored by a "thermostat" that lies deep within the brain. If the temperature of blood passing through this thermostat falls or rises to a level outside the optimum range, various mechanisms are activated to either warm or cool the body as necessary.

HOW THE BODY KEEPS WARM

When the body becomes too cold, changes take place to prevent heat from escaping. Blood vessels at the body surface narrow (constrict) to keep warm blood in the main part (core) of the body. The activity of the sweat glands is reduced, and hairs stand on end to "trap" warm air close to the skin.

In addition to the mechanisms that prevent heat loss, other body systems act to produce more warmth. The rate of metabolism is increased. Heat is also generated by muscle activity, which may be either voluntary (for example, during physical exercise) or, in cold conditions, involuntary (shivering).

HOW THE BODY LOSES HEAT

In hot conditions, the body activates a number of mechanisms to encourage heat loss and thus prevent the body temperature from becoming too high. Blood vessels that lie in or just under the skin widen (dilate). As a result, blood flow to the body surface increases and more heat is lost. In addition, the sweat glands become more active and secrete more sweat. This sweat then cools the skin as it evaporates.

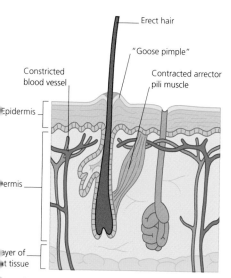

How skin responds to low body temperature
Blood vessels narrow (constrict) to reduce blood flow to the skin. The arrector pili muscles contract, making the hairs stand upright and trap warm air close to the skin.

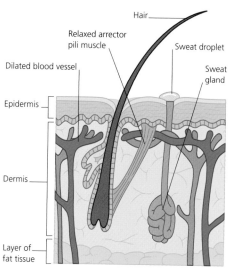

How skin responds to high body temperature
Blood vessels widen (dilate), making the skin look flushed, and heat is lost. Sweat glands become active and produce sweat, which evaporates to cool the skin.

ASSESSING A BURN

When skin is damaged by burning, it can no longer function effectively as a natural barrier against infection. In addition, body fluid may be lost because tiny blood vessels in the skin leak tissue fluid (serum). This fluid either collects under the skin to form blisters or leaks through the skin surface.

By assessing a burn before you start treatment, you can judge whether there are likely to be any related injuries, significant fluid loss, or infection.

WHAT TO ASSESS

While assessing a burn, it is important to consider the circumstances in which the burn has occurred; whether or not the airway is likely to have been affected; and the extent, location, and depth of the burn.

There are many possible causes of burns (below). By establishing the cause of the burn, the first aider may be able to identify any other potential problems that could result from the incident. For example, a fire in an enclosed space is likely to have produced poisonous carbon monoxide gas; other toxic fumes may have been released

if burning material was involved. If the casualty's airway has been affected in any way, he may have difficulty breathing and will need urgent medical attention and admission to hospital.

The extent of the burn will indicate whether or not shock is likely to develop. Shock is life-threatening condition and occurs whenever there is a major loss of body fluids. In a burn over a large area of the body, fluid loss will be significant and the risk of shock high.

If the burn is on a limb, fluid may collect in the tissues, causing swelling and pain. This build-up of fluid is particularly serious if the limb is being constricted, for example by clothing or footwear.

Burns allow germs to enter the skin and thus carry a serious risk of infection. To determine the degree of risk, you need to assess the depth of the burn (opposite): the deeper the burn, the higher the risk.

▶ See also BURNS TO THE AIRWAY p.197
● INHALATION OF FUMES pp.110–111
● SHOCK pp.120–121

TYPES OF BURN AND POSSIBLE CAUSES

Type of burn	Causes
Dry burn	Flames ● Contact with hot objects, such as domestic appliances or cigarettes ● Friction – for example, in rope burns
Scald	Steam ● Hot liquids, such as tea and coffee, or hot fat
Electrical burn	Low-voltage current, as used by domestic appliances ● High-voltage currents, as carried in mains overhead cables ● Lightning strikes
Cold injury	Frostbite ● Contact with freezing metals ● Contact with freezing vapours, such as liquid oxygen or liquid nitrogen
Chemical burn	Industrial chemicals, including inhaled fumes and corrosive gases ● Domestic chemicals and agents, such as paint stripper, caustic soda, weedkillers, bleach, oven cleaner, or any other strong acid or alkali
Radiation burn	Sunburn ● Over-exposure to ultraviolet rays from a sunlamp ● Exposure to a radioactive source, such as an X-ray

)epth of burns

urns are classified according to the depth
f skin damage. There are three depths:
ıperficial, partial-thickness, and full-
ıickness. A casualty may suffer one or
ıore depths of burn in a single incident.

A superficial burn involves only the
utermost layer of skin, the epidermis.
his type of injury usually heals well if first
d is given promptly and if blisters do not
ırm. Sunburn is one of the most common
ʻpes of superficial burn. Other causes
ıclude minor domestic incidents.

Partial-thickness burns destroy the
epidermis and are very painful. The skin
becomes red and blistered. These burns
usually heal well, but they can be serious
if large areas of the body are affected. If
they cover more than 20 per cent of the
body, they may be fatal.

In full-thickness burns, pain sensation
is usually lost, which may mislead you and
the casualty about the severity of the injury.
The skin may look waxy, pale, or charred.
These burns need urgent medical attention.

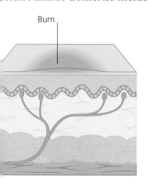

ıperficial burn
ıis type of burn involves only the
ıtermost layer of skin. Superficial
ırns are characterised by redness,
ʋelling, and tenderness.

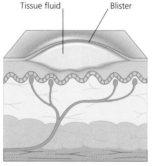

Partial-thickness burn
This affects the epidermis, and the
skin becomes red and raw. Blisters
form over the skin due to fluid
released from the damaged tissues.

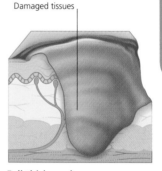

Full-thickness burn
With this type of burn, all the layers
of the skin are affected; there may
be some damage to nerves, fat
tissue, muscles, and blood vessels.

Labels: Burn | Tissue fluid | Blister | Damaged tissues

;urns that need hospital treatment

ʻ the casualty is a child, call a doctor or
ke the child to hospital, however small the
ırn appears. For other people, medical
tention should be sought for any serious
ırn. Such burns include:
All full-thickness burns.
All burns involving the face, hands, feet,
r genital area.
All burns that extend right around an
ʻm or a leg.

● All partial-thickness burns larger than
1 per cent of the body surface (an area the
size of the palm of the casualty's hand).
● All superficial burns larger than 5 per cent
of the casualty's body surface (equivalent to
five palm areas).
● Burns with a mixed pattern of varying
depths.

If you are unsure about the severity of
any burn, seek medical attention.

SEVERE BURNS AND SCALDS

Take great care when treating burns that are deep or extensive. The longer the burning continues, the more severe the injury will be. If the casualty has been burnt in a fire, you should assume that smoke or hot air has also affected the respiratory system (*see* BURNS TO THE AIRWAY, p.197).

The priorities are to begin rapid cooling of the burn and to check breathing. A casualty with a severe burn or scald injury will almost certainly be suffering from shock and will need hospital care.

The possibility of non-accidental injury must always be considered, no matter what the age of the casualty. Ensure you record all details accurately. Retain any removed clothing in case of future investigation.

RECOGNITION

There may be:
- Pain.
- Difficulty breathing.
- Signs of shock (pp.120–121).

▶ **See also** BURNS TO THE AIRWAY p.197
- FIRES pp.24–25 ● LIFE-SAVING PROCEDURE:
pp.71–102 ● SHOCK pp.120–121

➕ YOUR AIMS

- To stop the burning and relieve pain.
- To maintain an open airway.
- To treat associated injuries.
- To minimise the risk of infection.
- To arrange urgent removal to hospital and to gather information for the emergency services.

⚠ WARNING

Watch for signs of difficulty breathing; be prepared to give rescue breaths and chest compressions if necessary (*see* LIFE-SAVING PROCEDURES, pp.71–102).

1 Help the casualty to lie down. If possible, try to prevent the burnt area from coming into contact with the ground.

2 Douse the burn with plenty of cold liqui for at least 10 minutes, but do not delay the casualty's removal to hospital.
CALL AN AMBULANCE

3 Continue cooling the affected area until the pain is relieved.

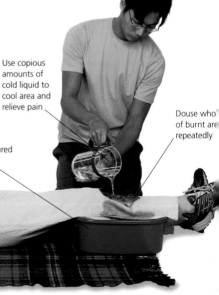

Use copious amounts of cold liquid to cool area and relieve pain

Douse who of burnt are repeatedly

Place bowl under injured leg to catch water

4 Put on disposable gloves if available. Gently remove any rings, watches, belts, shoes, or smouldering clothing before the tissues begin to swell. Carefully remove burnt clothing, unless it is sticking to the burn.

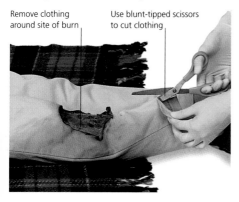

Remove clothing around site of burn

Use blunt-tipped scissors to cut clothing

5 Cover the injured area with a sterile dressing to protect it from infection. If a sterile dressing is not available, use a folded triangular bandage, part of a sheet, or kitchen film (discard the first two turns from the roll and apply it lengthways over the burn). A clean plastic bag can be used to cover a hand or foot; secure it with a bandage or adhesive tape applied over the plastic, not the skin.

❶ CAUTION

● Do not over-cool the casualty because you may lower the body temperature to a dangerous level. This is a particular hazard for babies and elderly people.

● Do not remove anything sticking to the burn; you may cause further damage and introduce infection into the burnt area.

● Do not touch or otherwise interfere with the burnt area.

● Do not burst any blisters.

● Do not apply lotions, ointment, fat, or adhesive tape to the burnt area.

SPECIAL CASE

BURNS TO THE FACE
If the casualty has a facial burn, do not cover the injury; you could cause the casualty distress and obstruct the airway. Keep cooling the area with water to relieve the pain until help arrives.

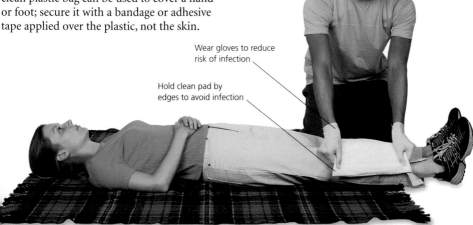

Wear gloves to reduce risk of infection

Hold clean pad by edges to avoid infection

6 Gather and record details of the casualty's injuries. Regularly monitor and record her vital signs – level of response, pulse, and breathing (pp.42–43).

7 While waiting for help to arrive, reassure the casualty and treat her for shock (pp.120–121) if necessary.

MINOR BURNS AND SCALDS

Small, superficial burns and scalds are often due to domestic incidents, such as touching a hot iron or spilling boiling water on the skin. Most minor burns can be treated successfully by first aid and will heal naturally. However, you should advise the casualty to see a doctor if you are at all concerned about the severity of the injury (*see* ASSESSING A BURN, pp.192–193).

Some time after a burn, blisters may form. These thin "bubbles" are caused by tissue fluid (serum) leaking into the burnt area

just beneath the skin's surface. You should never break a blister because you may introduce infection into the wound.

 See also ASSESSING A BURN pp.192–193

RECOGNITION

- Reddened skin.
- Pain in the area of the burn.

Later there may be:

- Blistering of the affected skin.

➕ YOUR AIMS

- To stop the burning.
- To relieve pain and swelling.
- To minimise the risk of infection.

❗ CAUTION

- Do not break blisters or otherwise interfere with the injured area.
- Do not apply adhesive dressings or adhesive tape to the skin; the burn may be more extensive than it first appears.
- Do not apply ointments or fats; they may damage tissues and increase the risk of infection.

1 Flood the injured part with cold water for at least 10 minutes to stop the burning and relieve the pain. This is more effective than using sprays. If water is not available, any cold, harmless liquid, such as milk or canned drinks, can be used.

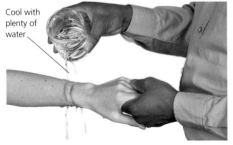

Cool with plenty of water

2 Put on disposable gloves if available. Gently remove any jewellery, watches, belts, or constricting clothing from the injured area before it begins to swell.

3 Cover the area with a sterile dressing or a clean, non-fluffy pad, and bandage loosely in place. A plastic bag or kitchen film makes a good temporary covering. Apply kitchen film lengthways to prevent constriction of the area if the tissues swell.

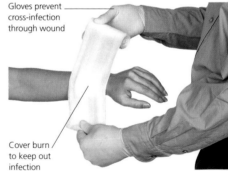

Gloves prevent cross-infection through wound

Cover burn to keep out infection

SPECIAL CASE

BLISTERS

A blister usually needs no treatment. However, if the blister breaks or is likely to burst, apply a non-adhesive dressing that extends well beyond the edges of the blister. Leave in place until the blister subsides.

BURNS TO THE AIRWAY

Burns to the face, and within the mouth or throat, are very serious because the air passages rapidly become swollen. Usually, signs of burning will be evident. However, you should always suspect damage to the airway if burns have been sustained in a confined space because the casualty is likely to have inhaled hot air or gases.

There is no specific first-aid treatment for an extreme case; the swelling will rapidly block the airway, and there is a serious risk of suffocation. Immediate and specialised medical aid is required.

RECOGNITION

There may be:
- Soot around the nose or mouth.
- Singeing of the nasal hairs.
- Redness, swelling, or actual burning of the tongue.
- Damage to the skin around the mouth.
- Hoarseness of the voice.
- Breathing difficulties.

▶ **See also** LIFE-SAVING PROCEDURES pp.71–102 ● SHOCK pp.120–121

✚ YOUR AIMS

- To maintain an open airway.
- To arrange urgent removal to hospital.

❶ WARNING

If the casualty becomes unconscious, open the airway and check breathing; be prepared to give rescue breaths and chest compressions if necessary (*see* LIFE-SAVING PROCEDURES, pp.71–102). If he is breathing, place him in the recovery position (pp.84–85).

1 CALL AN AMBULANCE
Tell the control officer that you suspect burns to the airway.

2 Take any steps possible to improve the casualty's air supply, such as loosening clothing around his neck.

3 Offer ice or small sips of cold water to reduce swelling and/or pain.

4 Reassure the casualty. Monitor and record his vital signs – level of response, pulse, and breathing (pp.42–43) – until help arrives.

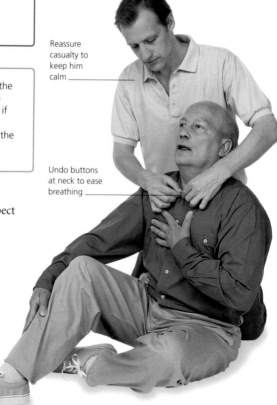

Reassure casualty to keep him calm

Undo buttons at neck to ease breathing

197

ELECTRICAL BURN

Burns may occur when electricity passes through the body. Much of the visible damage occurs at the points of entry and exit of the current. However, there may also be a track of internal damage. The position and direction of entry and exit wounds will alert you to the likely site and extent of hidden injury, and to the degree of shock that the casualty may suffer.

Burns may be caused by a lightning strike or by low- or high-voltage electric current. An electric shock can also cause cardiac arrest. If the casualty is unconscious, your immediate priority, once you are sure the area is safe, is to open the casualty's airway and check for breathing and circulation.

● See also ELECTRICAL INJURIES pp.26–27
● LIFE-SAVING PROCEDURES pp.71–102
● SEVERE BURNS AND SCALDS pp.194–195
● SHOCK pp.120–121

RECOGNITION

There may be:
● Unconsciousness.
● Full-thickness burns, with swelling, scorching, and charring, at the points of entry and exit.
● Signs of shock.
● A brown, coppery residue on the skin if the casualty has been a victim of "arcing" high-voltage electricity. (Do not mistake this residue for injury.)

✚ YOUR AIMS

● To treat the burns and shock.
● To arrange urgent removal to hospital.

❶ WARNING

If the casualty is unconscious, open the airway and check breathing; be prepared to give rescue breaths and chest compressions if necessary (see LIFE-SAVING PROCEDURES, pp.71–102).

1 Before touching the casualty, you must make sure that contact with the electrical source is broken (pp.26–27).

2 Flood the sites of injury, at the entry and exit points of the current, with plenty of cold water to cool the burns.

3 Put on disposable gloves if available. Place a sterile dressing, a clean, folded triangular bandage, or some other clean, non-fluffy material over the burns to protect them against airborne infection. CALL AN AMBULANCE

4 Reassure the casualty and treat him for shock (pp.120–121).

❶ CAUTION

Do not approach a victim of high-voltage electricity until you are officially informed that the current has been switched off and isolated.

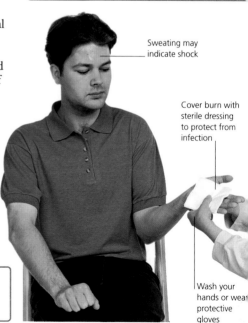

Sweating may indicate shock

Cover burn with sterile dressing to protect from infection

Wash your hands or wear protective gloves

CHEMICAL BURN

Certain chemicals may irritate, burn, or penetrate the skin, causing widespread and sometimes fatal damage. Unlike burns caused by heat, signs of chemical burns develop slowly, but the first aid is similar.

Most strong, corrosive chemicals are found in industry, but chemical burns can also occur in the home, especially from dishwasher products (the most common cause of alkali burns in children), oven cleaners, and paint stripper.

Chemical burns are always serious, and the casualty may need urgent hospital treatment. If possible, note the name or brand of the burning substance. Before treating the casualty, ensure your own safety and that of others because some chemicals give off poisonous fumes.

See also CHEMICALS ON THE SKIN p.221
● INHALATION OF FUMES pp.110–111

RECOGNITION

There may be:
● Evidence of chemicals in the vicinity.
● Intense, stinging pain.
● Later, discoloration, blistering, peeling, and swelling of the affected area.

YOUR AIMS

● To make the area safe and inform the relevant authority.
● To disperse the harmful chemical.
● To arrange transport to hospital.

CAUTION

● Never attempt to neutralise acid or alkali burns unless trained to do so.
● Do not delay starting treatment by searching for an antidote.

1 Make sure that the area around the casualty is safe. Ventilate the area to disperse fumes, and, if possible, seal the chemical container. Remove the casualty if necessary.

2 Flood the burn with water for at least 20 minutes to disperse the chemical and stop the burning. If treating a casualty on the ground, ensure that the water does not collect underneath her.

3 Gently remove any contaminated clothing while flooding the injury.

4 Arrange to take or send the casualty to hospital. Make sure that the airway is open. Monitor vital signs – level of response, pulse, and breathing (pp.42–43). Pass on details of the chemical to medical staff. If in the workplace, notify the safety officer and/or emergency services.

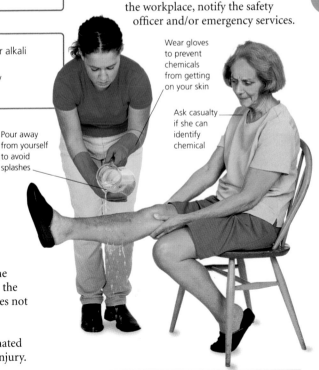

Wear gloves to prevent chemicals from getting on your skin

Ask casualty if she can identify chemical

Pour away from yourself to avoid splashes

CHEMICAL BURN TO THE EYE

Splashes of chemicals in the eye can cause serious injury if not treated quickly. They can damage the surface of the eye, resulting in scarring and even blindness.

The priority for the first aider is to wash out (irrigate) the eye so that the chemical is diluted and dispersed. When irrigating the eye, be careful that the contaminated rinsing water does not splash you or the casualty. Before beginning to treat the casualty, put on protective gloves if available.

RECOGNITION

There may be:
- Intense pain in the eye.
- Inability to open the injured eye.
- Redness and swelling around the eye.
- Copious watering of the eye.
- Evidence of chemical substances or containers in the immediate area.

➕ YOUR AIMS

- To disperse the harmful chemical.
- To arrange transport to hospital.

❗ CAUTION

Do not allow the casualty to touch the injured eye or forcibly remove a contact lens.

1 Put on protective gloves if available. Hold the casualty's affected eye under gently running cold water for at least 10 minutes. Take care to irrigate the eyelid thoroughly both inside and out. You may find it easier to pour the water over the eye using an eye irrigator or a glass.

2 If the eye is shut in a spasm of pain, gently but firmly pull the eyelids open. Be careful that contaminated water does not splash the uninjured eye.

3 Ask the casualty to hold a sterile eye dressing or a clean, non-fluffy pad over the injured eye. If it will be some time before the casualty receives medical attention, bandage the pad loosely in position.

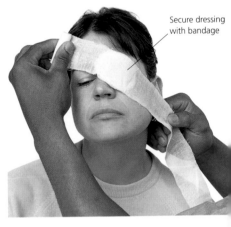

Secure dressing with bandage

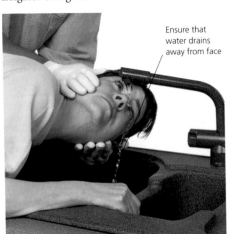

Ensure that water drains away from face

4 Identify the chemical if possible. Then arrange to take or send the casualty to hospital.

FLASH BURN TO THE EYE

This condition occurs when the surface (cornea) of the eye is damaged by exposure to ultraviolet light, such as prolonged glare from sunlight reflected off snow. Symptoms usually develop gradually, and recovery can take up to a week. Flash burns can also be caused by glare from a welder's torch.

RECOGNITION

● Intense pain in the affected eye(s).

There may also be:
● A "gritty" feeling in the eye(s).
● Sensitivity to light.
● Redness and watering of the eye(s).

✚ YOUR AIMS

● To prevent further damage.
● To arrange transport to hospital.

⊘ CAUTION

Do not remove any contact lenses.

1 Reassure the casualty. Ask him to hold an eye pad to each injured eye. If it is likely to take some time to obtain medical attention, lightly bandage the pad(s) in place.

2 Arrange to take or send the casualty to hospital.

CS SPRAY INJURY

This solvent spray is used by police forces for riot control and self-protection, and is sometimes used by unauthorised people as a weapon in assaults. It irritates the eyes and upper airways and may cause vomiting.

The effects usually wear off within about 15 minutes, although the eyes may remain sore for longer than this.

If CS spray is used on a person who has asthma, it may induce an attack.

RECOGNITION

There may be:
● Watering of the eyes.
● Uncontrollable coughing and sneezing.
● Burning sensation in the skin and throat.
● Chest tightness and difficulty with breathing.

▶ **See also** ASTHMA p.115

✚ YOUR AIM

● To get the casualty into fresh air.

⊘ CAUTION

● Washing out (irrigating) the eyes is not usually necessary and may prolong the irritation.
● Do not rub any area affected by the spray.

1 Move the casualty to a well-ventilated area and reassure him that the symptoms will soon disappear – he may be very agitated. Try to stop the casualty from rubbing his eyes.

2 If the casualty's eyes are painful, fan them to help speed up the vaporisation of any remaining CS chemical.

3 If a large amount of the chemical is inhaled at close quarters, arrange to take or send the casualty to hospital.

SUNBURN

This type of burn can be caused by over-exposure to the sun or a sunlamp. At high altitudes, it can occur even on an overcast summer day. Some medicines trigger severe sensitivity to sunlight. Rarely, sunburn can be caused by exposure to radioactivity.

Most sunburn is superficial; in severe cases, the skin is lobster-red and blistered and the casualty may suffer heatstroke.

RECOGNITION

- Reddened skin.
- Pain in the area of the burn.

Later there may be:

- Blistering of the affected skin.

▶ **See also** HEATSTROKE p.204

✚ YOUR AIMS

- To move the casualty out of the sun.
- To relieve discomfort and pain.

❶ WARNING

If there is extensive blistering, or other skin damage, seek medical advice.

1 Cover the casualty's skin with light clothing or a towel. Help her to move into the shade or, preferably, indoors.

2 Cool her skin by sponging with cold water, or by soaking the affected area in a cold bath, for 10 minutes.

3 Encourage the casualty to have frequent sips of cold water.

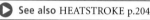
Tell casualty to sip water

4 If the burns are mild, calamine or an after-sun preparation may soothe them. For severe sunburn, obtain medical aid.

PRICKLY HEAT

This is a highly irritating, prickly red rash that most commonly occurs in hot weather. It develops when sweat glands are blocked by bacteria and dead skin cells. The rash particularly affects areas where sweat is trapped and cannot evaporate, such as the feet. People who often have prickly heat also tend to be susceptible to heatstroke.

RECOGNITION

There may be:

- Prickling or burning sensation.
- Rash of tiny red spots or blisters.

▶ **See also** HEATSTROKE p.204

✚ YOUR AIM

- To relieve discomfort and pain.

1 Encourage the person to stay in cool conditions as much as possible.

2 Cool the skin by gently sponging with cold water.

HEAT EXHAUSTION

his disorder is caused by loss of salt and ater from the body through excessive weating. It usually develops gradually. Heat xhaustion usually affects people who are ot acclimatised to hot, humid conditions. eople who are unwell, especially those ith illnesses that cause vomiting and iarrhoea, are more susceptible than others developing heat exhaustion.

A dangerous and common cause of heat xhaustion is the excessively high body mperature, and other physical changes, at result from certain drugs taken for leasure, such as Ecstasy. The user sweats rofusely, due to prolonged overactivity, en dehydration develops, leading to heat

RECOGNITION

As the condition develops, there may be:
- Headache, dizziness, and confusion.
- Loss of appetite and nausea.
- Sweating, with pale, clammy skin.
- Cramps in the arms, legs, or the abdominal wall.
- Rapid, weakening pulse and breathing.

exhaustion. These effects, coupled with the drug's effect on the temperature-regulating centre in the brain, can lead to heatstroke and even cause death.

> See also HEATSTROKE p.204 ● LIFE-SAVING PROCEDURES pp.71–102

YOUR AIMS

- To replace lost body fluids and salt.
- To cool the casualty down if necessary.
- To obtain medical aid if necessary.

1 Help the casualty to a cool place. Get him to e down with raised legs.

2 Give him plenty of water; follow, possible, with a eak salt solution ne teaspoon salt per litre water).

pport sualty's head he drinks ater

3 Even if the casualty recovers quickly, ensure that he sees a doctor. If the casualty's responses deteriorate, place him in the recovery position (pp.84–85). CALL AN AMBULANCE

4 Monitor and record vital signs – level of response, pulse, and breathing (pp.42–43). Be prepared to give rescue breaths and chest compressions if necessary (see LIFE-SAVING PROCEDURES, pp.71–102).

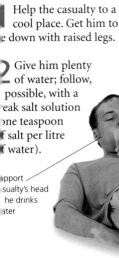

Raise his feet to improve blood flow to brain

Place cushion under his feet for comfort

HEATSTROKE

This condition is caused by a failure of the "thermostat" in the brain, which regulates body temperature. The body becomes dangerously overheated, usually due to a high fever or prolonged exposure to heat. Heatstroke can also result from use of drugs such as Ecstasy. In some cases, heatstroke follows heat exhaustion when sweating ceases, and the body then cannot be cooled by the evaporation of sweat.

Heatstroke can develop with little warning, causing unconsciousness within minutes of the casualty feeling unwell.

RECOGNITION

There may be:
- Headache, dizziness, and discomfort.
- Restlessness and confusion.
- Hot, flushed, and dry skin.
- Rapid deterioration in the level of response.
- Full, bounding pulse.
- Body temperature above 40°C (104°F).

▶ See also DRUG POISONING p.222
- LIFE-SAVING PROCEDURES pp.71–102
- CHECKING TEMPERATURE p.43

➕ YOUR AIMS
- To lower the casualty's body temperature as quickly as possible.
- To arrange urgent removal to hospital.

1 Quickly move the casualty to a cool place. Remove as much of his outer clothing as possible.
CALL AN AMBULANCE

2 Wrap the casualty in a cold, wet sheet and keep the sheet wet until his temperature falls to 38°C (100.4°F) under the tongue, or 37.5°C (99.5°F) under the armpit. If no sheet is available, fan the casualty, or sponge him with cold water.

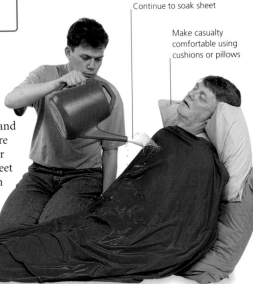

Continue to soak sheet

Make casualty comfortable using cushions or pillows

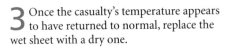

Wrap casualty in wet sheet

3 Once the casualty's temperature appears to have returned to normal, replace the wet sheet with a dry one.

4 Monitor and record vital signs – level of response, pulse, and breathing (pp.42–43) – until help arrives. If his temperature rises again, repeat the cooling process.

❗ WARNING

If the casualty becomes unconscious, open the airway and check breathing; be prepared to give rescue breaths and chest compressions if necessary (*see* LIFE-SAVING PROCEDURES, pp.71–102). If the casualty is breathing, place him in the recovery position (pp.84–85).

FROSTBITE

With this condition, the tissues of the extremities – usually the fingers and toes – freeze due to low temperatures. In severe cases, this freezing can lead to permanent loss of sensation and, eventually, gangrene (tissue death) as the blood vessels become permanently damaged.

Frostbite usually occurs in freezing or cold and windy conditions. People who cannot move around are particularly susceptible. In many cases, frostbite is accompanied by hypothermia (pp.206–208), and this should be treated accordingly.

▶ See also HYPOTHERMIA pp.206–208

✚ YOUR AIMS

● To warm the affected area slowly to prevent further tissue damage.
● To arrange transport to hospital.

1 If possible, move the casualty into warmth before you thaw the affected part (*see* CASUALTY HANDLING, pp.63–64).

2 Gently remove gloves, rings, and any other constrictions, such as boots. Warm the affected part with your hands, in your lap, or in the casualty's armpits. Avoid rubbing the affected area because this can damage skin and other tissues.

3 Place the affected part in warm water at around 40°C (104°F). Dry carefully, and apply a light dressing of fluffed-up, dry gauze bandage.

Use water that is warm but not hot

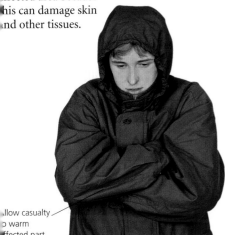
Allow casualty to warm affected part

4 Raise and support the affected limb to reduce swelling. An adult casualty may take two paracetamol tablets for intense pain. Take or send the casualty to hospital.

❶ CAUTION

● Do not put the affected part near direct heat.
● Do not attempt to thaw the affected part if there is danger of it refreezing.
● Do not allow the casualty to smoke.

HYPOTHERMIA

This develops when the body temperature falls below 35°C (95°F). The effects vary depending on the speed of onset and the level to which the body temperature falls. Moderate hypothermia can usually be completely reversed. Severe hypothermia – when the core body temperature falls below 30°C (86°F) – is often, although not always, fatal. However, no matter how low body temperature is, it is always worth persisting with life-saving procedures until a doctor arrives to assess the casualty.

WHAT CAUSES HYPOTHERMIA

Hypothermia may develop over several days in poorly heated houses. Infants, homeless people, elderly people, and those who are thin and frail are particularly vulnerable. Lack of activity, chronic illness, and fatigue all increase the risk; alcohol and drugs can exacerbate the condition.

Hypothermia can also be caused by prolonged exposure to cold out of doors

> **RECOGNITION**
>
> As hypothermia develops there may be:
> - Shivering, and cold, pale, dry skin.
> - Apathy, disorientation, or irrational behaviour; occasionally, belligerence.
> - Lethargy or impaired consciousness.
> - Slow and shallow breathing.
> - Slow and weakening pulse. In extreme cases, the heart may stop.

(p.208). Moving air has a much greater cooling effect than still air so a high "wind-chill factor" can substantially increase the risk of a person developing hypothermia.

Death from immersion in cold water ma[y] be caused by hypothermia, not drowning. When surrounded by cold water, the body cools 30 times faster than in dry air, and body temperature falls rapidly.

▶ **See also** ● DROWNING p.109 ● LIFE-SAVING PROCEDURES pp.71–102

TREATMENT WHEN INDOORS

> **➕ YOUR AIMS**
> - To prevent the casualty losing more body heat.
> - To rewarm the casualty slowly.
> - To obtain medical aid if necessary.

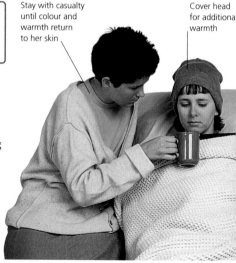

Stay with casualty until colour and warmth return to her skin

Cover head for additiona[l] warmth

1 For a casualty who has been brought in from outside, quickly replace any wet clothing with warm, dry garments.

2 The casualty can be rewarmed by bathing if she is young, fit, and able to climb into the bath unaided. The water should be warm but not too hot – about 40°C (104°F).

3 Put the casualty in a bed and ensure that she is well covered. Give her warm drinks, soup, or high-energy foods such as chocolate to help rewarm her.

HYPOTHERMIA IN THE ELDERLY

An elderly person may develop hypothermia slowly over a number of days. Elderly people often have inadequate food or heating and are more likely to suffer from chronic illness that impairs their mobility.

When treating an elderly person with hypothermia, be careful to warm her slowly. Cover her with layers of blankets in a room at about 25°C (77°F). If the casualty is warmed too rapidly, blood may be diverted suddenly from the heart and brain to the body surfaces.

Always call a doctor because hypothermia may disguise the symptoms of, or accompany, a stroke, a heart attack, or an underactive thyroid gland (hypothyroidism).

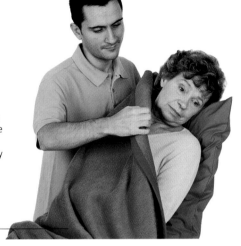

Warm an elderly casualty gradually

⚠ CAUTION

● Do not allow an elderly casualty to have a bath to warm her up – the sudden warming may cause blood to divert suddenly from the heart and brain to the body surfaces.

● Do not place any heat sources, such as hot water bottles or fires, next to the casualty because these may also mobilise blood too rapidly. In addition, they may burn the casualty.

● Do not give the casualty alcohol because this will worsen the hypothermia.

● Handle the casualty gently because, in severe cases, rushed treatment or movement may cause the heart to stop.

4 Regularly monitor and record the casualty's vital signs – level of response, pulse, breathing, and temperature (pp.42–43).

5 It is important to call a doctor if you have any doubts about the casualty's condition. If hypothermia occurs in an elderly person or a baby, you must always obtain medical aid for the casualty.

SPECIAL CASE

HYPOTHERMIA IN INFANTS

A baby's mechanisms for regulating body temperature are under-developed, so she may develop hypothermia in a cold room. The baby's skin may look healthy but feel cold, and she may be limp, unusually quiet, and refuse to feed. Rewarm a cold baby gradually, by wrapping her in blankets and warming the room. You should always call a doctor if you suspect a baby has hypothermia.

Cover head with a hat to prevent heat from being lost

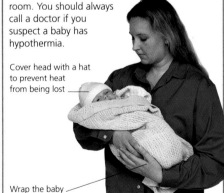

Wrap the baby in a blanket

Continued on next page

HYPOTHERMIA (continued)

TREATMENT WHEN OUTDOORS

➕ YOUR AIMS

- To prevent the casualty from losing more body heat.
- To rewarm the casualty.
- To obtain help.

❶ CAUTION

Do not give the casualty alcohol because it dilates superficial blood vessels and allows heat to escape, making hypothermia worse.

❶ WARNING

If the casualty becomes unconscious, open the airway and check breathing; be prepared to give rescue breaths and chest compressions if necessary (*see* LIFE-SAVING PROCEDURES, pp.71–102).

1 Take the casualty to a sheltered place as quickly as possible.

2 Remove wet clothing. Shield the casualty from the wind. Insulate him with extra clothing or blankets and cover his head. Do not give him your clothes.

3 Protect the casualty from the ground and the elements. Put him in a dry sleeping bag, cover him with blankets or newspapers and enclose him in a plastic or foil survival bag, if available.

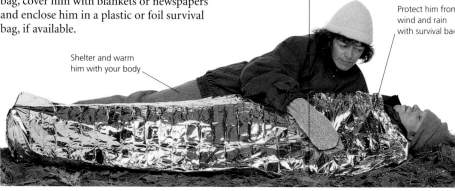

Lay casualty on a thick layer of dry insulating material, such as pine branches, heather, or bracken

Protect him from wind and rain with survival bag

Shelter and warm him with your body

4 Send for help. In an ideal situation, two people should go together for help. However, it is important that you do not leave the casualty alone; someone must remain with him at all times.

5 To help rewarm a casualty who is conscious, give him warm drinks, and high-energy foods such as chocolate, if you have such drinks or foods available.

6 When help arrives, the casualty should be taken to hospital by stretcher.

SPECIAL CASE

WHEN NO HELP IS AVAILABLE
If you are alone with the casualty, try to attract attention by using a whistle, flashing a torch, or lighting a fire.

10

OBJECTS THAT FIND their way into the body, either through a wound in the skin or via an orifice (such as the ear, nose, or eye), are known as "foreign objects". Such items range from specks of dirt or grit in the eye to small objects that young children may push into their noses and ears. Foreign objects do not usually cause serious problems for the casualty, but they can be painful and distressing. Calm, reassuring treatment from the first aider is essential.

TREATMENT PROCEDURES

This chapter begins with an overview of the structure of the sensory organs: the skin, eyes, ears, mouth, and nose. This is followed by advice on how to remove objects from the skin and orifices, including what to do when something has been swallowed or inhaled. First aid for a person with an object embedded in a wound is given in Chapter 6, Wounds and Bleeding (pp.127–144).

+ FIRST-AID PRIORITIES

- Assess the casualty's condition.
- Comfort and reassure the casualty.
- Establish whether or not a foreign object can be removed safely.
- Prevent further damage.
- Obtain medical aid if necessary. Call an ambulance if you suspect a serious illness or injury.

CONTENTS

FOREIGN OBJECTS

THE SENSORY ORGANS

The skin

The body is covered and protected by the skin. This is one of the body's largest organs and is made up of two layers: the outer epidermis and an inner layer, the dermis. The skin forms a barrier against harmful substances and germs. It is also an important sense organ, containing nerves that ensure the body is sensitive to heat, cold, pain, and touch.

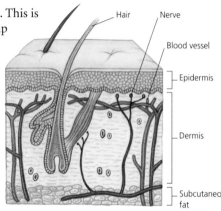

Structure of the skin
The skin consists of the thin epidermis and the thicker dermis, which sit on a layer of fat (subcutaneous fat). Blood vessels, nerves, muscles, oil (sebaceous) glands, sweat glands, and hair roots (follicles) lie in the dermis.

The eyes

These complex organs allow us to see the world around us. Each eye consists of a coloured part (iris) with a small opening (pupil) that allows rays of light to enter the eye. The size of the pupil changes according to the amount of light entering the eye.

Light rays are focused by the transparent lens on to a "screen" (retina) at the back of the eye. Cells in the retina convert this information into electrical impulses that travel, via the optic nerve, to the part of the brain where the impulses are analysed.

The eyes are protected by the bony sockets in the skull. The eyelids, and delicate membranes called conjunctiva, protect the front of the eyes.

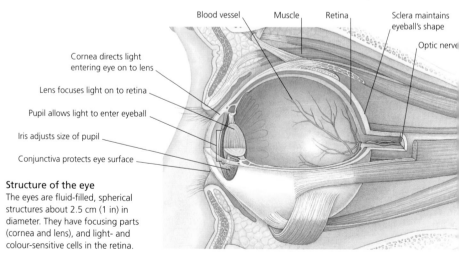

Structure of the eye
The eyes are fluid-filled, spherical structures about 2.5 cm (1 in) in diameter. They have focusing parts (cornea and lens), and light- and colour-sensitive cells in the retina.

The ears

As well as being the organs of hearing, the ears also play an important role in balance. The visible part of each ear is the auricle, which funnels sounds into the ear canal to vibrate the eardrum. Fine hairs in the ear canal filter out dust, and glands secrete ear wax to trap any other small particles. The vibrations of the eardrum pass across the middle ear to the hearing apparatus (cochlea) in the inner ear. This structure converts the vibrations into nerve impulses and transmits them to the brain via the auditory nerve. The vestibular apparatus within the inner ear is involved in balance.

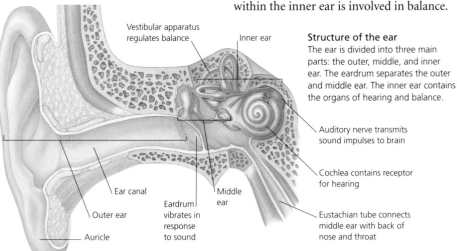

Vestibular apparatus regulates balance

Inner ear

Ear canal

Eardrum vibrates in response to sound

Outer ear

Middle ear

Auricle

Structure of the ear
The ear is divided into three main parts: the outer, middle, and inner ear. The eardrum separates the outer and middle ear. The inner ear contains the organs of hearing and balance.

Auditory nerve transmits sound impulses to brain

Cochlea contains receptor for hearing

Eustachian tube connects middle ear with back of nose and throat

The mouth and nose

These cavities form the entrances to the digestive and respiratory tracts respectively. The nasal cavities connect with the throat. They are lined with blood vessels and with membranes that secrete mucus to trap debris as it enters the nose. Food enters the digestive tract via the mouth, which leads into the gullet (oesophagus). The epiglottis, a flap at the back of the throat, prevents food from entering the windpipe (trachea).

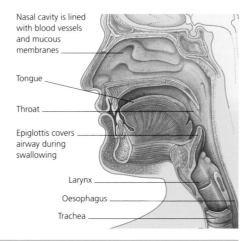

Nasal cavity is lined with blood vessels and mucous membranes

Tongue

Throat

Epiglottis covers airway during swallowing

Larynx

Oesophagus

Trachea

Structure of the nose and mouth
The nostrils lead into the two nasal cavities, which are lined with mucous membranes and blood vessels. The nasal cavities connect directly with the top of the throat.

SPLINTER

Small splinters of wood, metal, or glass may enter the top layer of skin. They carry a risk of infection because they are rarely clean. The areas most frequently affected are the hands, knees, and feet. Usually, a splinter can be successfully withdrawn from the skin using sterile tweezers. However, if the splinter is deeply embedded in the skin, lies over a joint, or is difficult to remove, you should leave it in place and advise the casualty to consult a doctor.

▶ **See also** FOREIGN OBJECT IN A CUT p.135
● INFECTED WOUND p.136

✚ YOUR AIMS

● To remove the splinter.
● To minimise the risk of infection.

1 Sterilise a pair of tweezers by holding them in a flame and then letting them cool. Put on disposable gloves if available. Gently clean around the splinter with soap and warm water.

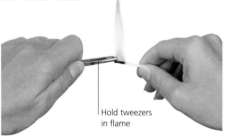

Hold tweezers in flame

2 Grasp the splinter with the tweezers as close to the skin as possible, and draw it out at the angle at which it went in.

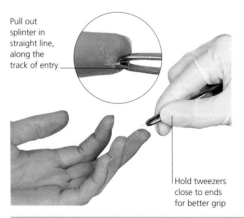

Pull out splinter in straight line, along the track of entry

Hold tweezers close to ends for better grip

SPECIAL CASE

EMBEDDED SPLINTER
If a splinter is embedded or difficult to dislodge, do not probe the area with a sharp object such as a needle or you may introduce infection. Pad around the splinter until you can bandage over it without pressing down, and seek medical advice.

3 Carefully squeeze the wound to encourage a little bleeding. This will help to flush out any remaining dirt.

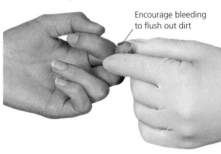

Encourage bleeding to flush out dirt

4 Clean the area, pat it dry, and apply an adhesive dressing (plaster) to minimise the risk of infection.

❶ CAUTION

Always ask about tetanus immunisation.

Seek medical advice if:
● The casualty has never been immunised.
● The casualty is uncertain about the timing and number of injections that have been given.
● It is more than 10 years since the casualty's last injection.

EMBEDDED FISH-HOOK

A fish-hook that is embedded in the skin is difficult to remove because of the barb at the end of the hook. If possible, you should ensure that the hook is removed by a health professional. Only attempt to remove a hook yourself if medical aid is not readily available. Embedded fish-hooks may carry a risk of infection, including tetanus.

WHEN MEDICAL AID IS NOT READILY AVAILABLE

YOUR AIM

● To remove the fish-hook without causing the casualty any further injury and pain.

WARNING

Do not try to pull out a fish-hook unless you can cut off the barb. If you cannot, seek medical help.

1 Put on disposable gloves if available. If the barb is visible, use wirecutters to cut it away; carefully withdraw the hook by its eye.

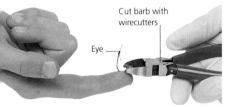

Cut barb with wirecutters

Eye

2 Clean the wound, then pad around it with gauze and bandage it.

SPECIAL CASE

BARB NOT VISIBLE
Push the hook further in until the barb emerges. Cut off the barb, and remove the hook (*see left*). If you cannot do this, seek medical help.

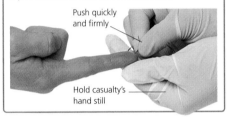

Push quickly and firmly

Hold casualty's hand still

CAUTION

Always ask about tetanus immunisation.

Seek medical advice if:

● The casualty has never been immunised.

● The casualty is uncertain about the timing and number of injections that have been given.

● It is more than 10 years since the casualty's last injection.

WHEN MEDICAL AID IS READILY AVAILABLE

YOUR AIMS

● To obtain medical aid.
● To minimise the risk of infection.

1 Put on disposable gloves if available. Ask the casualty to sit down and support the injured area. Cut off the fishing line as close as possible to the hook.

2 Build up pads of gauze around the hook until you can bandage over it without pushing it in further.

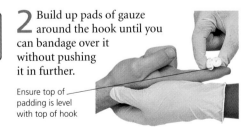

Ensure top of padding is level with top of hook

3 Bandage over the padding and the hook; take care not to press down on the hook. Ensure that the casualty receives medical attention as soon as possible.

FOREIGN OBJECT IN THE EYE

A speck of dust, a loose eyelash, or even a contact lens can float on the white of the eye. Usually, such objects can easily be rinsed off. However, you must not touch anything that sticks to the eye, penetrates the eyeball, or rests on the coloured part of the eye (iris and pupil) because this may damage the eye. Instead, make sure that the casualty gets medical attention quickly.

RECOGNITION

There may be:
- Blurred vision.
- Pain or discomfort.
- Redness and watering of the eye.
- Eyelids screwed up in spasm.

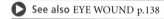 See also EYE WOUND p.138

+ YOUR AIM
- To prevent injury to the eye.

! CAUTION

Do not touch anything that is sticking to, or embedded in, the eyeball or over the coloured part of the eye. Cover the eye (*see* EYE WOUND, p.138) and take or send the casualty to hospital.

1 Advise the casualty to sit down facing the light; tell her not to rub her eye.

2 Stand behind the casualty. Gently separate her eyelids with your finger and thumb. Examine every part of her eye.

Ask her to look right, left, up, and down

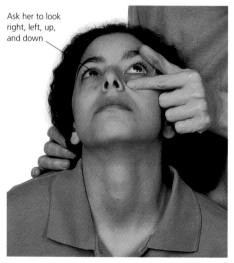

3 If you can see a foreign object on the white of the eye, wash it out by pouring clean water from a glass or by using a sterile eyewash.

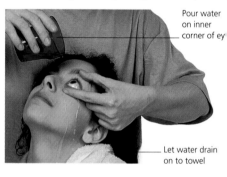

Pour water on inner corner of eye

Let water drain on to towel

4 If this is unsuccessful, lift the object off with a moist swab or the damp corner of a tissue or clean handkerchief. If you still cannot remove the object, seek medical help.

SPECIAL CASE

OBJECT UNDER UPPER EYELID
Ask the casualty to grasp her lashes and pull the upper lid over the lower lid. Blinking under water may also make the object float off.

Lower lashes may brush particle clear

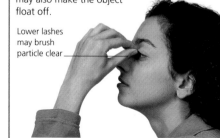

FOREIGN OBJECT IN THE EAR

If a foreign object becomes lodged in the ear, it may cause temporary deafness by blocking the ear canal. In some cases, a foreign object may damage the eardrum.

Young children frequently push objects into their ears; adults may leave cotton wool in an ear after cleaning it. Insects can fly or crawl into the ear and may cause alarm.

YOUR AIMS

- To prevent injury to the ear.
- To remove a trapped insect if it is moving.
- To arrange transport to hospital if a foreign object is lodged in the ear.

1 Arrange to take or send the casualty to hospital as soon as possible. Do not try to remove a lodged foreign object yourself.

2 Reassure the casualty during the journey or until medical help arrives.

❶ CAUTION

Do not attempt to remove any object that is lodged in the ear. You may cause serious injury and push the foreign object in even further.

SPECIAL CASE

INSECT INSIDE THE EAR
Reassure the casualty, and ask her to sit down. Gently flood the ear with tepid water so that the insect floats out. If this flooding does not remove the insect, take or send the casualty to hospital.

Support head, with affected ear uppermost

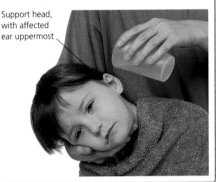

FOREIGN OBJECT IN THE NOSE

Young children may push small objects up their noses. Foreign objects can block the nose and cause infection. Sharp objects may damage the tissues, and "button" batteries can cause burns and bleeding. Do not try to remove a foreign object; you may cause injury or push it further into the airway.

RECOGNITION

There may be:
- Difficult or noisy breathing through the nose.
- Swelling of the nose.
- Smelly or blood-stained discharge, indicating that an object may have been lodged for a while.

YOUR AIM

- To arrange transport to hospital.

❶ CAUTION

Do not attempt to remove the foreign object, even if you can see it.

1 Try to keep the casualty quiet and calm. Tell him to breathe through his mouth at a normal rate. Advise him not to poke inside his nose to try to remove the object himself.

2 Arrange to take or send the casualty to hospital, where the object can safely be removed by hospital staff.

INHALED FOREIGN OBJECT

Small, smooth objects can slip past the protective mechanisms in the throat and enter the air passages leading to the lungs (*see* THE RESPIRATORY SYSTEM, p.104).

Dry peanuts, which can swell up when in contact with body fluids, pose a particular danger in young children. Peanuts can be inhaled into the lungs, resulting in serious damage. In addition, some individuals are allergic to nuts, and may suffer anaphylactic shock (p.123) after swallowing them.

RECOGNITION

There may be:
● Some sign or noise of choking, which quickly passes.
● Persistent dry coughing.
● Difficulty breathing.

▶ **Treat as for** CHOKING ADULT p.100
● CHOKING CHILD p.101 ● CHOKING INFANT p.102

SWALLOWED FOREIGN OBJECT

Small objects such as coins, safety pins, or buttons are most commonly swallowed by young children. Often they travel straight through the digestive tract, but there is a risk that they may enter the respiratory tract and cause choking. Button batteries, which are used in some toys, watches, and hearing aids, are dangerous if swallowed because they contain corrosive chemicals. They can cause severe damage, and even death, if not removed. A large or sharp object may damage the digestive tract.

+ YOUR AIM
● To obtain medical aid if necessary.

1 Reassure the casualty and try to find out exactly what she has swallowed.

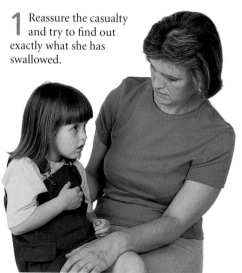

❶ WARNING

If the casualty has swallowed something large or sharp, or has difficulty breathing or swallowing

CALL AN AMBULANCE
Reassure the casualty while waiting for medical help to arrive.

❶ CAUTION
Do not allow the casualty to eat, drink, or smoke because a general anaesthetic may need to be given in hospital.

2 If the swallowed object is small and smooth, take or send the casualty to hospital or to a doctor. Always seek urgent medical advice if you know or suspect that a casualty has swallowed a battery.

11

POISONING IS USUALLY non-intentional. It may result from exposure to or ingestion of toxic substances, including drugs and alcohol, chemicals, and contaminated food. Some cases of poisoning are intentional, as in cases of attempted suicide. The effects of a poison vary depending on the type and amount of the substance absorbed. However, in most cases of poisoning, medical aid will be needed.

BITES AND STINGS

Although insect stings and stings from marine creatures such as jelly fish can spoil a picnic or seaside outing, they are often minor injuries that can be treated successfully with first aid. However, multiple insect stings can produce a serious reaction that requires urgent medical help. Animal and human bites also always require medical attention because the mouth harbours many types of microorganisms (germs).

✚ FIRST-AID PRIORITIES

- Assess the casualty's condition.
- Identify the poisonous substance.
- Ensure the safety of yourself and the casualty.
- Comfort and reassure the casualty.
- Obtain medical aid if necessary. Call an ambulance if you suspect a serious illness or injury.

CONTENTS

POISONING, BITES, AND STINGS

SWALLOWED POISONS

Chemicals that are swallowed may harm the digestive tract, or cause more widespread damage if they enter the bloodstream and are transported to other parts of the body.

Hazardous chemicals include common household substances. For example, bleach, dishwasher detergent, and paint stripper are poisonous or corrosive if swallowed. Drugs, whether they are prescribed or bought over the counter, are also potentially harmful if they are taken in overdose. The effects of poisoning depend on the substance that has been swallowed.

▶ See also CHEMICAL BURN p.199 ● DRUG POISONING p.222 ● INHALATION OF FUMES p.110 ● LIFE-SAVING PROCEDURES pp.71–102

RECOGNITION

Depends on the poison, but there may be:
● Vomiting, sometimes bloodstained.
● Impaired consciousness.
● Pain or burning sensation.
● Empty containers in the vicinity.
● History of ingestion/exposure.

✚ YOUR AIMS

● To maintain the airway, breathing, and circulation.
● To remove any contaminated clothing.
● To identify the poison.
● To arrange urgent removal to hospital.

1 If the casualty is conscious, ask her what she has swallowed, and try to reassure her.

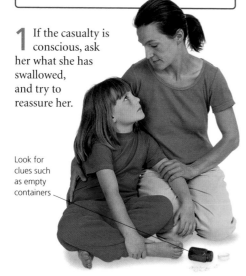

Look for clues such as empty containers

2 CALL AN AMBULANCE
Give as much information as possible about the swallowed poison. This information will assist doctors to give appropriate treatment once the casualty reaches hospital.

SPECIAL CASE

BURNED LIPS
If the casualty's lips are burned by corrosive substances, give her frequent sips of cold milk or water while waiting for medical help to arrive.

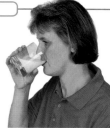

❶ WARNING

● Never attempt to induce vomiting.
● If the casualty becomes unconscious, open the airway and check breathing; be prepared to give rescue breaths and chest compressions if necessary (*see* LIFE-SAVING PROCEDURES, pp.71–102). If she is breathing, place her in the recovery position (pp.92–93).

● Use a face shield or pocket mask (p.79) for rescue breathing if there are any chemicals on the casualty's mouth.

CHEMICALS ON THE SKIN

Hazardous chemicals that are spilt on the skin can cause irritation or burns. In addition, certain substances are absorbed through the skin and may cause widespread damage inside the body.

The most dangerous chemicals are found in industry, but domestic items such as dishwasher products, oven cleaners, and paint strippers are also potentially harmful.

Burns caused by chemicals may require urgent hospital treatment.

RECOGNITION

There may be:
- Intense, stinging pain.
- Evidence of chemical substances or containers in the immediate area.
- Discoloration, blistering, peeling, and swelling of the affected area occurring at once or some time later.

 Treat as for CHEMICAL BURN p.199

INHALED GASES

Inhaling chemical fumes or sprays is potentially harmful and may lead to breathing problems, confusion, and collapse. Some factories use gases that are harmful if they are inhaled accidentally. Chlorine gas is stored at swimming pools and is hazardous if released. Poisonous gases may also be released in the chemical reaction that occurs when different cleaning products are used together, for example bleach and disinfectant.

RECOGNITION

Depends on the gas but there may be:
- Headache.
- Noisy, distressed breathing.
- Confusion.
- Impaired consciousness.

 Treat as for CS SPRAY INJURY p.201 or INHALATION OF FUMES p.110

POISONS IN THE EYE

Many chemicals – both liquids and gases – used in the home and the workplace can irritate the eyes. The membranes covering the eye absorb chemicals rapidly, and this can lead to damage to the eyes within minutes of a chemical being in contact.

Particular chemicals can damage the surface of the eye, and these may cause permanent scarring of the eye and even blindness. For these reasons, immediate first aid is needed to wash out any chemicals splashed in the eye. This should be followed by medical treatment.

RECOGNITION

There may be:
- Intense pain in the eye.
- Inability to open the injured eye.
- Redness and swelling around the eye.
- Copious watering of the eye.

 Treat as for CHEMICAL BURN TO THE EYE p.200 or CS SPRAY INJURY p.201

221

DRUG POISONING

Poisoning can result from an overdose of either prescribed drugs or drugs that are bought over the counter. It can also be caused by drug abuse or drug interaction. The effects vary depending on the type of drug and how it is taken (below). When you call the emergency services, give as much information as possible. While waiting for help to arrive, look for containers that might help you to identify the drug.

▶ **See also** LIFE-SAVING PROCEDURES pp.71–102

RECOGNITION

Category	Drug	Effects of poisoning
Painkillers	Aspirin (swallowed)	Upper abdominal pain, nausea, and vomiting • Ringing in the ears • "Sighing" when breathing • Confusion and delirium • Dizziness
	Paracetamol (swallowed)	Little effect at first, but abdominal pain, nausea, and vomiting may develop • Irreversible liver damage may occur within 3 days (malnourishment and alcohol increase the risk)
Nervous system depressants and tranquillisers	Barbiturates and benzodiazepines (swallowed)	Lethargy and sleepiness, leading to unconsciousness • Shallow breathing • Weak, irregular, or abnormally slow or fast pulse
Stimulants and hallucinogens	Amphetamines (including Ecstasy) and LSD (swallowed); cocaine (inhaled)	Excitable, hyperactive behaviour, wildness, and frenzy • Sweating • Tremor of the hands • Hallucinations, in which the casualty may claim to "hear voices" or "see things"
Narcotics	Morphine, heroin (commonly injected)	Small pupils • Sluggishness and confusion, possibly leading to unconsciousness • Slow, shallow breathing, which may stop altogether • Needle marks, which may be infected
Solvents	Glue, lighter fuel (inhaled)	Nausea and vomiting • Headaches • Hallucinations • Possibly, unconsciousness • Rarely, cardiac arrest

✚ YOUR AIMS

● To maintain breathing and circulation.
● To arrange removal to hospital.

⚠ WARNING

● If the casualty is unconscious, open the airway and check breathing; be prepared to give rescue breaths and chest compressions if necessary (see LIFE-SAVING PROCEDURES, pp.72–p.102). If breathing, place in recovery position (pp.84–85).

CALL AN AMBULANCE
● Do not induce vomiting.

1 If the casualty is conscious, help him into a comfortable position and ask what he has taken. Reassure him while you talk to him

2 CALL AN AMBULANCE
Monitor and record vital signs – level of response, pulse, and breathing (pp.42–43) – until medical help arrives.

3 Keep samples of any vomited material. Look for evidence that might help to identify the drug, such as empty containers. Give these samples and containers to the paramedic or ambulance crew.

ALCOHOL POISONING

Alcohol (chemical name, ethanol) is a drug that depresses the activity of the central nervous system – in particular, the brain. Prolonged or excessive intake can severely impair all physical and mental functions, and the person may sink into deep unconsciousness.

There are several risks to the casualty from alcohol poisoning:
- An unconscious casualty risks inhaling and choking on vomit.
- Alcohol widens (dilates) the blood vessels. This means that the body loses heat, and hypothermia may develop.
- A casualty who smells of alcohol may be misdiagnosed and not receive appropriate treatment for an underlying cause of unconsciousness, such as a head injury, stroke, or heart attack.

RECOGNITION

There may be:
- A strong smell of alcohol
- Empty bottles or cans.
- Impaired consciousness: the casualty may respond if roused, but will quickly relapse.
- Flushed and moist face.
- Deep, noisy breathing.
- Full, bounding pulse.
- Unconsciousness.

In the later stages of unconsciousness:
- Dry, bloated appearance to the face.
- Shallow breathing.
- Weak, rapid pulse.
- Dilated pupils that react poorly to light.

See also HYPOTHERMIA p.206 ● LIFE-SAVING PROCEDURES pp.72–102

YOUR AIMS
- To maintain an open airway.
- To assess for other conditions.
- To seek medical help if necessary.

WARNING
- If the casualty is unconscious, open the airway and check breathing; be prepared to give rescue breaths and chest compressions if necessary (*see* LIFE-SAVING PROCEDURES, pp.72–p.102). If the casualty is breathing, place him in the recovery position (pp.84–85).

CALL AN AMBULANCE
- Do not induce vomiting.

1 Cover the casualty with a coat or blanket to protect him from the cold.

2 Assess the casualty for any injuries, especially head injuries, or other medical conditions.

3 Monitor and record vital signs – level of response, pulse, and breathing (pp.42–43) – until the casualty recovers or is placed in the care of a responsible person.

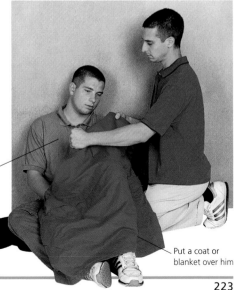

Watch casualty in case he becomes unconscious

Put a coat or blanket over him

FOOD POISONING

This is usually caused by consuming food or drink that is contaminated with bacteria or viruses. Some food poisoning is caused by poisons (toxins) from bacteria already in the food. The salmonella or *E. coli* group of bacteria, which are found mainly in meat, are common causes of food poisoning. Symptoms may develop rapidly (within hours), or they may not occur until a day or so after eating contaminated food.

Toxic food poisoning is frequently caused by poisons produced by the staphylococcus group of bacteria. Symptoms usually develop rapidly, possibly within 2–6 hours of eating the affected food.

One of the dangers of food poisoning is loss of body fluids. The dehydration that results from this fluid loss can be serious if the fluids are not replaced quickly enough. Dehydration is especially serious in the very young and the very old, and, in some cases, treatment may be required in hospital.

See also SHOCK pp.120–121 ● VOMITING AND DIARRHOEA p.247

> ### RECOGNITION
> *There may be:*
> - Nausea and vomiting.
> - Cramping abdominal pains.
> - Diarrhoea (possibly bloodstained).
> - Headache or fever.
> - Features of shock (p.120).
> - Impaired consciousness.

> ### ✚ YOUR AIMS
> - To encourage the casualty to rest.
> - To give the casualty plenty of bland fluids to drink.
> - To obtain medical aid if necessary.

> ### ❶ WARNING
> If the casualty's condition worsens,
> **CALL AN AMBULANCE**

1 Advise the casualty to lie down and rest. Help her if necessary.

2 Give the casualty plenty of bland fluids to drink and a bowl to use if she vomits. Call a doctor for advice.

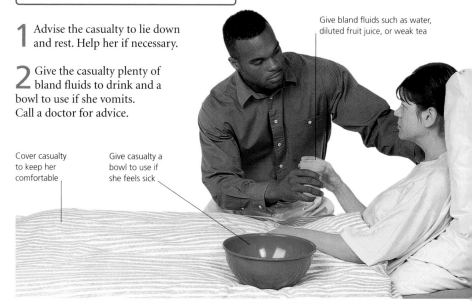

Give bland fluids such as water, diluted fruit juice, or weak tea

Cover casualty to keep her comfortable

Give casualty a bowl to use if she feels sick

POISONOUS PLANTS AND FUNGI

Many young children eat plant leaves or brightly coloured berries, but serious poisoning as a result rarely occurs. However, ingesting even small amounts of foxglove or wild arum can cause nausea, vomiting, and stomach cramps; and large amounts are potentially fatal. Seizures may occur after ingesting laburnum seeds.

Serious poisoning as a result of eating mushrooms is also rare. Mushrooms found in the garden may cause nausea, vomiting, and, occasionally, hallucinations. Death cap mushrooms cause vomiting and severe, watery diarrhoea between 6 and 12 hours after ingestion and can be fatal.

Mushrooms and plants that cause severe poisoning
Death cap mushrooms and wild arum berries grow in woodland and hedgerows during late summer and autumn. Foxgloves flower in spring, and laburnum produces seed pods in summer.

RECOGNITION

There may be:
- Nausea and vomiting.
- Cramping abdominal pains.
- Diarrhoea.
- Seizures.
- Impaired consciousness.

▶ **See also** LIFE-SAVING PROCEDURES pp.71–102 ● SEIZURES pp.184–186 ● VOMITING AND DIARRHOEA p.247

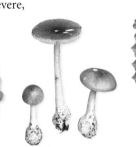
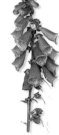
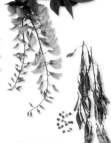

WILD ARUM   DEATH CAP MUSHROOMS   FOXGLOVE   LABURNUM

➕ YOUR AIMS

- To identity the poisonous plant, if possible.
- To manage any seizures.
- To obtain medical aid if necessary.

❗ WARNING

- If the casualty is unconscious, open the airway and check breathing. Be prepared to give rescue breaths and chest compressions, if necessary (*see* LIFE-SAVING PROCEDURES, pp.71–102). If the casualty is breathing, put him in the recovery position (pp.84–85).

CALL AN AMBULANCE
Monitor casualty until medical help arrives.
- Do not induce vomiting.

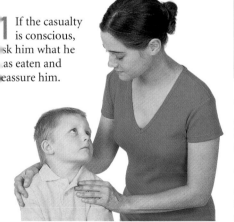

1 If the casualty is conscious, ask him what he has eaten and reassure him.

2 Try to identify the poisonous plant, and find out which part of it has been eaten. Get medical advice at once so that the appropriate treatment can be given.

3 Keep any small pieces of the plant that you have found, together with samples of vomited material, to show to the doctor or to send with the casualty to hospital.

INSECT STING

Usually, a sting from a bee, wasp, or hornet is painful rather than dangerous. An initial sharp pain is followed by mild swelling, redness, and soreness.

However, multiple insect stings can produce a serious reaction. A sting in the mouth or throat is potentially dangerous because swelling can obstruct the airway. With any bite or sting, it is important to watch for signs of an allergic reaction, which may lead to anaphylactic shock (p.123).

RECOGNITION
- Pain at the site of the sting.
- Redness and swelling around the site of the sting.

▶ **See also** ANAPHYLACTIC SHOCK p.123
● LIFE-SAVING PROCEDURES pp.71–102

✚ YOUR AIMS
- To relieve swelling and pain.
- To arrange removal to hospital if necessary.

❗ WARNING
If the casualty shows signs of anaphylactic shock, such as impaired breathing or swelling of the face and neck,

CALL AN AMBULANCE

SPECIAL CASE

STINGS TO THE MOUTH AND THROAT
If a casualty has been stung in the mouth, there is a risk that swelling of tissues in the mouth and/or throat may occur, causing the airway to become blocked. To help prevent this from happening, give the casualty an ice cube to suck or else give her a glass of cold water to sip. If swelling starts to develop,

CALL AN AMBULANCE

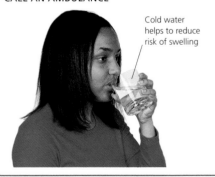

Cold water helps to reduce risk of swelling

1 Reassure the casualty. If the sting is visible, brush or scrape it off sideways with your fingernail or the blunt edge of a knife. Do not use tweezers because more poison may be injected into the casualty.

Brush sting off with a fingernail or blunt edge

2 Raise the affected part if possible, and apply an ice pack or cold compress (p.49). Advise the casualty to see her doctor if the pain and swelling persist.

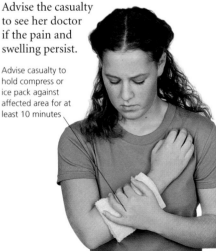

Advise casualty to hold compress or ice pack against affected area for at least 10 minutes

OTHER BITES AND STINGS

Bites from certain species of scorpion and spider can cause serious illness and may even be fatal if not treated promptly. These species are not found in the UK, but bites may occur while travelling overseas.

Bites or stings in the mouth or throat are dangerous because swelling can obstruct the airway. Be alert to an allergic reaction, which may lead to anaphylactic shock (p.123).

RECOGNITION

Depends on the species but generally:
- Pain, redness, and swelling at site of sting.
- Nausea and vomiting.
- Headache.

▶ **See also** ANAPHYLACTIC SHOCK p.123
- LIFE-SAVING PROCEDURES pp.71–102

+ YOUR AIMS
- To relieve the pain and swelling.
- To arrange removal to hospital, if necessary.

❶ WARNING

If the casualty has been stung by a scorpion or a red back or funnel web spider, or if the casualty is showing signs of anaphylactic shock,

CALL AN AMBULANCE

1 Help the casualty to sit or lie down, and reassure her.

2 Raise the affected part if possible. Apply an ice pack or cold compress (p.49).

3 Monitor vital signs – level of response, pulse, and breathing (pp.42–43). Watch for signs of an allergy, such as wheezing.

SPECIAL CASE

STINGS TO THE MOUTH AND THROAT
Give the casualty an ice cube to suck or cold water to drink. If swelling starts to develop,

CALL AN AMBULANCE

TICK BITE

Ticks are tiny, spider-like creatures found in grass or woodlands. They attach themselves to passing animals (including humans) and bite into the skin to suck blood. When sucking blood, a tick swells to about the size of a pea, and it can then be seen easily. Ticks can carry disease and cause infection, so they should be removed as soon as possible.

+ YOUR AIM
- To remove the tick.

1 Using fine-pointed tweezers, grasp the tick's head close to the casualty's skin.

2 Use a to-and-fro action to lever the head out. Try to avoid breaking the tick and leaving the buried head behind.

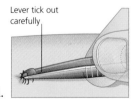

Lever tick out carefully

3 Advise the casualty to see a doctor. Take the tick; it may be required for analysis.

SNAKE BITE

The only poisonous snake native to mainland Britain is the adder, and its bite is rarely fatal. However, more exotic snakes – some of them poisonous – are kept as pets. While a snake bite is not usually a serious injury, it can be frightening. Reassurance is vital; if the casualty keeps still, the spread of venom (poison) through the body may be delayed. Note the snake's appearance to help doctors give the correct antivenom. If it is safe to do so, put the snake in a secure container; bear in mind that venom is active even if the snake is dead. If the snake is not captured, notify the police.

RECOGNITION

Depends on the species, but there may be:
- A pair of puncture marks.
- Severe pain, redness, and swelling at the site of the bite.
- Nausea and vomiting.
- Disturbed vision.
- Increased salivation and sweating.
- Laboured breathing; in extreme cases, breathing may stop altogether.

▶ **See also** LIFE-SAVING PROCEDURES pp.71–102

➕ YOUR AIMS

- To prevent the spread of venom in the body.
- To arrange urgent removal to hospital.

❶ WARNING

- Do not apply a tourniquet, slash the wound with a knife, or suck out the venom.
- If the casualty become unconscious, open the airway and check breathing; be prepared to give rescue breaths and chest compressions if necessary (*see* LIFE-SAVING PROCEDURES, pp.71–102).

1 Help the casualty to lie down. Reassure her, and tell her to keep calm and still. CALL AN AMBULANCE

2 Gently wash the wound and pat dry with clean swabs.

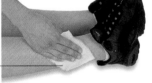

Clean wound with gauze swab

3 Lightly compress the limb above the wound with a roller bandage. Use triangular bandages to immobilise the affected area (p.57).

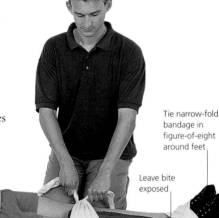

Tie narrow-fold bandage in figure-of-eight around feet

Leave bite exposed

Keep heart above the level of wounded part

Broad-fold bandage | Soft padding | Roller bandag

STINGS FROM SEA CREATURES

Jellyfish, Portuguese man-of-war, corals, and sea anemones cause painful stings. Their venom is contained in stinging cells that stick to the skin. Most marine species found in temperate regions of the world are not dangerous, but some tropical species can cause severe poisoning. Occasionally, death results from paralysis of the chest muscles, and, very rarely, from anaphylaxis.

▶ **See also** ANAPHYLACTIC SHOCK p.269

✚ YOUR AIMS
- To relieve pain and discomfort.
- To arrange removal to hospital if necessary.

1 Reassure the casualty and encourage him to sit or lie down.

2 Hold an ice pack or cold compress (p.49) against the skin for 10 minutes to relieve pain and swelling; raise the affected part.

⚠ WARNING
If the injury is severe or there is a serious reaction,
CALL AN AMBULANCE

SPECIAL CASE
TROPICAL JELLYFISH
Pour copious amounts of vinegar or sea water over the injury to incapacitate the stinging cells. Lightly compress the limb above the sting with a roller bandage, and immobilise the injured limb (opposite).

CALL AN AMBULANCE
Keep the casualty completely still until help arrives.

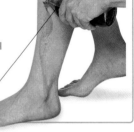

Pour vinegar directly on to wound

MARINE PUNCTURE WOUND

Many marine creatures have spines, which provide a mechanism against attack from predators, but which can cause painful wounds in humans if they are trodden on. Sea urchins and weever fish have sharp spines that can become embedded in the sole of the foot. Wounds may become infected if the spines are not removed.

✚ YOUR AIMS
- To relieve pain and discomfort.
- To minimise the risk of infection.
- To arrange transport of the casualty to hospital.

⚠ CAUTION
Do not bandage the wound.

1 Help the casualty to immerse the injured part in water as hot as he can tolerate for about 30 minutes.

2 Take or send the casualty to hospital so that the spines can be safely removed.

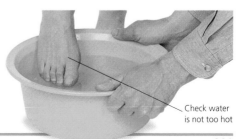

Check water is not too hot

ANIMAL BITE

Bites from sharp, pointed teeth cause deep puncture wounds that can carry bacteria and other microorganisms (germs) far into the tissues. Human bites also crush the tissue. Hitting someone's teeth with a bare fist can produce a bite. Any bite that breaks the skin needs prompt first aid and medical attention because of the risk of infection.

The most serious infection risk is rabies, a potentially fatal viral infection of the nervous system. The virus is carried in the saliva of infected animals. If bitten overseas, where the risk of rabies is greatest, the

casualty must receive anti-rabies injections. Tetanus is also a potential risk following any animal bite. There is probably only a small risk of hepatitis B or C viruses being transmitted through a human bite – and an even smaller risk of transmission of the HIV (AIDS) virus. However, seek medical advice if you are concerned.

> ▶ **See also** CUTS AND GRAZES p.134
> ● INFECTED WOUND p.136 ● SEVERE
> BLEEDING pp.130–131 ● SHOCK pp.120–121

＋YOUR AIMS

- To control bleeding.
- To minimise the risk of infection, both to the casualty and yourself.
- To obtain medical aid if necessary.

❶ CAUTION

Always ask about tetanus immunisation.

Seek medical advice if:

- The casualty has never been immunised.
- The casualty is uncertain about the timing or number of injections that have been given.
- It is more than 10 years since the casualty's last injection.

1 Put on disposable gloves, if available. Wash the bite wound thoroughly with soap and warm water in order to minimise the risk of infection.

2 Pat dry with clean gauze swabs and cover with an adhesive dressing (plaster) or a small sterile dressing.

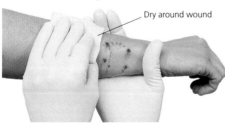
Dry around wound

SPECIAL CASE

DEEP WOUND
If the wound is deep, control bleeding by applying direct pressure and raising the injured part. Cover the wound with a non-fluffy pad, or a sterile dressing, and bandage firmly in place to control bleeding. Arrange to take or send the casualty to hospital.

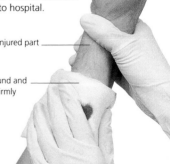

Raise injured part ___

Cover wound and ___
bandage firmly

3 Arrange to take or send the casualty to hospital if the wound is large or deep.

❶ WARNING

If you suspect rabies, arrange to take or send the casualty to hospital immediately.

12

CHILDBIRTH IS A NATURAL and often lengthy process: when a woman goes into labour, there is usually plenty of time to get her to hospital before her baby arrives. In the rare event of a baby arriving quickly, a first aider should not try to deliver the baby – the birth will happen naturally without intervention. Your role is to comfort and listen to the wishes of the mother and care for her and her newborn baby.

Miscarriage, however, is a potentially serious problem because there is a risk of severe bleeding. A woman who is miscarrying needs urgent medical help.

MEDICAL PROBLEMS

Many everyday conditions, such as fever and cramp, and more serious ones, such as diabetes-related hypoglycaemia, develop quickly. They need prompt treatment and respond well to first aid. However, a minor complaint can be the start of serious illness, so you should always consult a doctor if you are in doubt about the casualty's condition.

✚ FIRST-AID PRIORITIES

- Assess the casualty's condition.
- Comfort and reassure the casualty.
- Obtain medical aid if necessary. Call an ambulance if you suspect a serious illness.

CONTENTS

CHILDBIRTH AND MEDICAL PROBLEMS

CHILDBIRTH

The process of giving birth normally begins at about the 40th week of pregnancy. The entire process is called labour, and there are three distinct stages: in the first, the uterus contracts and the baby gets in position for birth; in the second, the baby is born; lastly, in the third, the afterbirth (placenta and umbilical cord) is expelled.

FIRST STAGE OF LABOUR

In the first stage of labour, the woman's body prepares for the birth. A mucous plug, which protects the uterus from infection, is expelled. This is called the "show". It occurs some time before contractions of the uterus begin. The start of the contractions, together with the pressure of the baby's head, causes the cervix (neck of the uterus) to widen (dilate). The contractions become stronger and more frequent until the cervix is fully dilated – about 10cm (4in) in diameter. This process may take several hours. At some point in this stage of labour, the amniotic sac breaks and the "waters" (amniotic fluid) leak out from the vagina.

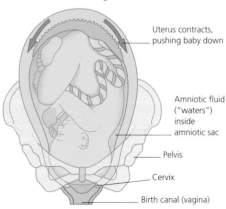

Uterus contracts, pushing baby down

Amniotic fluid ("waters") inside amniotic sac

Pelvis

Cervix

Birth canal (vagina)

Preparations for birth
Muscular contractions begin to spread through the uterus as waves every 2–5 minutes. The intervals between the contractions become shorter as the first stage progresses. At the same time, the cervix gradually widens.

SECOND STAGE OF LABOUR

Once the cervix is fully dilated, the baby's head presses down on the mother's pelvic floor, triggering an urge for the mother to push. The birth canal (vagina) stretches as the baby travels through it. The head emerges and the baby is delivered. This stage usually lasts for up to 1 hour.

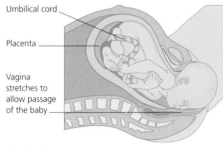

Umbilical cord

Placenta

Vagina stretches to allow passage of the baby

The birth
With the cervix fully dilated, the flexible tissues of the vagina (birth canal) stretch to allow the head to emerge. In most cases, the baby turns to face the mother's back as it travels down the vagina.

THIRD STAGE OF LABOUR

The placenta (the organ that nourishes an unborn baby) and the umbilical cord are expelled from the uterus a short time after the baby' birth. The uterus contracts, closing down the area where the placenta was attached; this reduces bleeding.

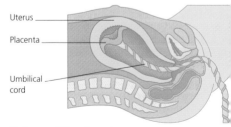

Uterus

Placenta

Umbilical cord

Delivery of the placenta
The placenta comes away from the wall of the uterus 10–30 minutes after the birth of the baby. It moves down the vagina and is pushed out of the mother's body by contractions of the uterus.

CHILDBIRTH: FIRST STAGE

n the first stage of labour, the woman will begin to have contractions – waves of ntense pain that peak and then gradually ade away. The amniotic fluid ("waters") hat cushioned the baby will be discharged t some point during this stage.

Although most pregnant women are ware of what happens during labour, a voman who goes into labour unexpectedly nay be very anxious. You will need to eassure her; she will then be more able to emember any coping techniques that she as learned. If you think that the baby may e born before any other help can be ummoned, try to gather together a few ssential items of equipment for the birth:

disposable gloves, mask to cover your mouth and nose (a handkerchief or similar can be used), a plastic sheet, a bowl of hot water for washing, sanitary towels, clean, warm towels, and a blanket.

YOUR AIMS
● To obtain medical aid or arrange for the woman to be taken to hospital.
● To reassure the woman and make her comfortable.

1 Call for a midwife or a doctor. If the contractions are rapidly becoming more frequent, or if the hospital is some distance away and cannot be reached quickly CALL AN AMBULANCE Give the control officer any information that you have that may affect the labour, and any details of the place where the mother had planned to give birth.

2 Help the mother to sit or lie on the floor in a position that is comfortable for her. Lay cushions or pillows on the floor to support her body if necessary.

3 Stay calm and encourage the mother to breathe deeply, or to use any other methods that she prefers, to cope with the pain. Massaging her lower back can help.

Use heel of your hand to massage lower back

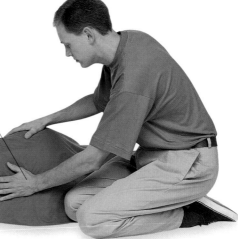

CHILDBIRTH: SECOND STAGE

During the second stage of labour, the baby is delivered (born). At the start of this stage, the cervix (neck of the womb) will be fully dilated (open) and the mother will begin to feel an overwhelming urge to push.

You need to have prepared a comfortable, clean environment for the delivery (*see* CHILDBIRTH: FIRST STAGE, p.233). You also need to take measures to ensure hygiene and prevent infection.

The number of people present at the delivery should be kept to a minimum, but do not exclude anyone whom the mother wishes to be present. You may want to enlist the help of a female friend or relative.

The delivery usually happens naturally. However, as a first aider it will be your responsibility to ensure the baby's comfort and protection once it has been born.

PREVENTING INFECTION
It is extremely important to ensure good hygiene before and during the delivery in order to reduce the risk of the mother, the baby, or yourself contracting an infection. The following precautions should be taken if possible:

RECOGNITION

● Mother experiences an urge to push.
● Strong, frequent contractions due to activity of the uterus.
● Stinging or burning sensation in the vagina as the walls are stretched.
● Emergence of the baby's head at the vaginal opening.
● Rapid delivery of the baby's body.

● Keep anyone with a sore throat, cold, or any other infection well away.
● Wear a mask to cover your mouth and nose. If you do not have a mask, you can improvise by tying a piece of clean fabric, such as a clean handkerchief or a folded triangular bandage, over your face.
● If you are wearing a jacket, remove it. Roll up long sleeves. Wear a plastic apron to cover your clothes if possible.
● Wash your hands and forearms, and scrub your nails thoroughly, for about 5 minutes.
● Put on disposable gloves, if these are available.
● After the baby has been delivered, wash your hands again.

YOUR AIMS

● To ensure that the mother is comfortable.
● To prevent infection in the mother, baby, and yourself.
● To care for the baby during and after delivery.

❶ CAUTION

● Do not allow the mother to eat because there is a risk that she may vomit. If she is thirsty, allow her to take sips of water.
● Do not pull on the baby's head or shoulders during delivery.
● Do not pull on or cut the umbilical cord.
● Do not smack the baby.

1 Cover the area beneath the mother's body with plastic sheeting, newspaper, or towels for warmth and to absorb body fluids.

2 Help her into a comfortable position; a half-sitting position, with the knees raised, may be best. Make sure that her back and shoulders are well supported.

3 Make sure that the midwife or doctor is on the way. If an ambulance has been called, check that all important details have been passed on to the ambulance service, such as the expected delivery date, any medical needs, and the name of the hospital where the mother had planned to give birth.

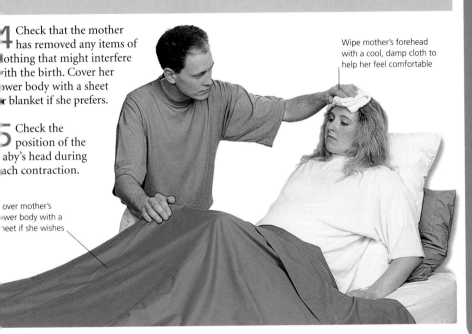

4 Check that the mother has removed any items of clothing that might interfere with the birth. Cover her lower body with a sheet or blanket if she prefers.

5 Check the position of the baby's head during each contraction.

Cover mother's lower body with a sheet if she wishes

Wipe mother's forehead with a cool, damp cloth to help her feel comfortable

6 Once the widest part of the baby's head has emerged at the mother's vaginal opening, advise the mother to stop pushing and start panting.

7 If there is a membrane covering the baby's face, gently move it aside so that he can breathe normally.

8 The baby's shoulders will soon appear. Allow the baby to be expelled naturally. This happens quickly, and you should be ready to hold the baby.

9 Lift the baby away from the vaginal opening. Handle the baby carefully, as newborn babies are very slippery. Pass him to the mother, and lay him on her stomach.

① WARNING

If the umbilical cord is wrapped around the baby's neck, you should first check that it is loose, then very carefully pull it over the head to protect the baby from strangulation.

10 The baby may start to cry at this point. If this does not happen, you must check the airway, breathing, and circulation; be prepared to give the baby rescue breaths and chest compressions if necessary (*see* UNCONSCIOUS INFANT, pp.95–98).

11 Dry the baby with a clean cloth. Wrap him carefully in another cloth or a blanket, and give him back to the mother. When laying the baby down, keep him on his side so that any fluid or mucus can drain easily from his nose and mouth.

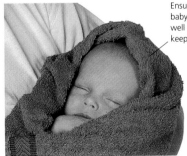

Ensure that baby's head is well covered to keep him warm

CHILDBIRTH: THIRD STAGE

In the third stage of labour, the afterbirth (the placenta and the umbilical cord) is delivered. This stage usually takes place 10–30 minutes after the baby has been born. As the placenta comes away from the wall of the uterus, further contractions occur to constrict the blood vessels in the uterus lining and minimise bleeding. Although the baby has been delivered, the mother still needs your help.

You should collect the afterbirth in a plastic bag so that medical staff can examine it. The umbilical cord, which may continue to pulsate, should be left uncut

until medical help arrives. At the end of the third stage, you should encourage the mother to put the baby to her breast and begin feeding him. This action will also help to reduce blood loss by stimulating uterine contractions.

▶ **See also** SHOCK pp.120–121

✚ YOUR AIMS
- To support the mother while she is delivering the afterbirth.
- To preserve the afterbirth.

❶ WARNING
- Do not pull on the umbilical cord as the afterbirth is being expelled.
- Do not cut the umbilical cord, even when the afterbirth has been delivered.
- Severe bleeding (post-partum or after-delivery haemorrhage) can occur if the uterus does not contract sufficiently when the placenta is detached. Tell the emergency services, and treat the mother for shock (pp.120–121).

1 Reassure the mother while she is delivering the afterbirth.

2 Keep the placenta and umbilical cord intact, preferably in a plastic bag. A midwife will cut the umbilical cord. The midwife will also examine the afterbirth to check that all of it has been expelled; if even a small piece of afterbirth remains inside the uterus, bleeding may continue and infection may develop.

3 It is normal for the mother to bleed slightly as the placenta is expelled. Gently massaging her abdomen, just below the navel, aids the expulsion of the afterbirth, helps the uterus to contract, and stops the bleeding.

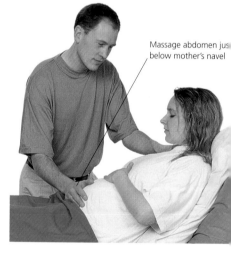
Massage abdomen just below mother's navel

4 Provide warm water, clean towels, and sanitary pads for the mother. Help her to use them if necessary.

5 If bleeding from the uterus is severe, CALL AN AMBULANCE and treat the mother for shock (pp.120–121).

MISCARRIAGE

A miscarriage is the loss of an unborn baby (fetus or embryo) before the 24th week of pregnancy. The main symptoms are lower abdominal pain and vaginal bleeding. There is a risk of severe bleeding and shock. Some pregnant women experience a "threatened miscarriage", with vaginal bleeding but no loss of the baby; but any woman who seems to be miscarrying must be seen by a doctor.

An affected woman may be frightened and very distressed. Offer as much help as you can without being intrusive. A woman who suspects that she is miscarrying may feel reluctant to confide in a stranger, particularly a man, so a male first aider should seek help from a female chaperone.

See also SHOCK pp.120–121 ● VAGINAL BLEEDING p.143

RECOGNITION

There may be:
● Cramp-like pains in the lower abdomen or pelvic area.
● Vaginal bleeding, which may possibly be sudden and profuse.
● Signs of shock (pp.120–121).
● Passage of the fetus or embryo and other tissue from the uterus.

YOUR AIMS

● To reassure and comfort the woman.
● To obtain medical aid.

1 Reassure the woman. Help her into a comfortable lying or sitting position, with legs bent up. Support her body and legs with pillows.

2 Give the woman a sanitary pad or a clean towel for the bleeding. Even if the bleeding or pain is only slight, call a doctor.

3 Monitor and record vital signs – level of response, pulse, and breathing (pp.42–43).

4 If any material is expelled from the vagina, collect it in a plastic bag and give it to the medical services so that it can be examined by a doctor. Keep the material out of the woman's sight, if possible, unless she specifically asks to see it.

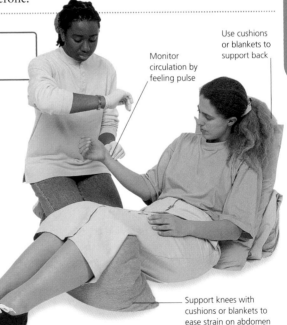

Use cushions or blankets to support back

Monitor circulation by feeling pulse

Support knees with cushions or blankets to ease strain on abdomen

ⓘ WARNING

If the bleeding or pain is severe,

CALL AN AMBULANCE

While waiting for medical help, treat the woman for shock if necessary (pp.120–121).

ALLERGY

An allergic reaction is an abnormal physical sensitivity to a "trigger" substance that is usually harmless, such as a food, a chemical, a drug, or pollen. It occurs when the immune system, which normally fights infection, "attacks" the trigger substance. Allergies may produce various respiratory, digestive, and skin conditions. Examples include asthma (p.115); hay fever; abdominal pain (p.245); vomiting and diarrhoea (p.247); "nettle rash" (urticaria); and dermatitis. Some people are at risk of a life-threatening reaction called anaphylactic shock (p.123).

RECOGNITION

Features vary depending on the trigger and the person. There may be one or more of the following symptoms:

- Red, itchy rash or raised areas of skin (wheals).
- Wheezing and difficulty in breathing.
- Abdominal pain.
- Vomiting and diarrhoea.

▶ **See also** ANAPHYLACTIC SHOCK p.123
- ASTHMA p.115 ● VOMITING AND DIARRHOEA p.247

✚ YOUR AIMS

- To assess the severity of the allergic reaction.
- To treat symptoms if they are only mild.
- To obtain medical aid if necessary.

❶ WARNING

If the casualty is distressed, or has difficulty in breathing,

CALL AN AMBULANCE

1 Assess the casualty's signs and symptoms, and ask him whether he knows that he suffers from an allergy.

2 Treat any symptoms, and help the casualty to take any medication that he has.

3 Advise the casualty to arrange to consult his doctor. If you are at all concerned about the casualty's condition, you should call a doctor yourself.

HICCUPS

This condition is caused by repeated spasms in which the diaphragm (the sheet of muscle that separates the chest cavity from the abdominal cavity) contracts suddenly and, at the same time, the windpipe partially closes. Hiccups is a common problem.

Attacks usually last for only a few minutes, but occasionally they may be prolonged, tiring, and painful. To relieve hiccups, you need to raise the level of carbon dioxide in the blood for a few moments; this should cause normal breathing to resume.

✚ YOUR AIMS

- To help normal breathing to resume.
- To obtain medical aid if necessary.

1 Advise the casualty to sit quietly and hold his breath for as long as possible.

2 If the hiccups persist, advise the casualty to place a paper (not plastic) bag over his nose and mouth and to rebreathe the expired air for a few minutes.

3 If the casualty's hiccups continue for more than a few hours, you should call a doctor for advice.

FEVER

sustained body temperature above the normal level of 37°C (98.6°F) is known as ever. It is usually caused by a bacterial or iral infection, and may be associated with measles, chickenpox, meningitis, earache, sore throat, or local infections such as an abscess. Infection may have been acquired during recent overseas travel.

Moderate fever is not harmful, but a fever above 40°C (104°F) can be dangerous and may trigger seizures in very young children (p.186). If you are in any doubt about the casualty's condition, call a doctor.

RECOGNITION

- Raised temperature.
- Initial pallor.
- A "chilled" feeling – goose pimples, shivering, and chattering teeth.
- Later, hot, flushed skin, and sweating.
- Headache.
- Generalised "aches and pains".

See also HEATSTROKE p.204 ● MENINGITIS p.187 ● OVERSEAS TRAVEL HEALTH pp.249–250 ● SEIZURES IN CHILDREN p.186

YOUR AIMS

- To bring down the fever.
- To obtain medical aid if necessary.

CAUTION

If you are concerned about the casualty's condition, call a doctor.

1 Keep the casualty cool and comfortable, preferably in bed with a light covering. Give him plenty of cool, bland drinks to replace body fluids lost through sweating.

2 An adult may take two paracetamol tablets or her own painkillers. A child may take the recommended dose of paracetamol syrup (not aspirin).

VERTIGO

This disorder is a disturbance of the sense of balance. Vertigo produces an abnormal sensation of movement: the casualty feels "giddy", as if he is spinning.

The usual causes include infections of the middle or inner ear, and psychological disorders such as acute anxiety. Occasionally, the cause is a more serious condition, such as Ménière's disease (an inner ear disorder).

RECOGNITION

- Sensation of spinning.
- Possible nausea and vomiting.

YOUR AIMS

- To relieve any symptoms.
- To obtain medical aid if necessary.

1 Advise the casualty to adopt a comfortable sitting or lying position, and note any change in his condition. Ask if he has had attacks of vertigo before.

2 If the casualty has special medication prescribed for vertigo or nausea, advise him to take it; you may need to help him to take the medication.

3 Call a doctor if the casualty is very distressed or if he requests it. Stay with the casualty until the doctor arrives and note any further changes in his condition.

DIABETES MELLITUS

In this condition, the body fails to produce sufficient amounts of insulin, a chemical that regulates blood sugar (glucose) levels. As a result, sugar builds up in the blood and can cause hyperglycaemia (below). People with diabetes mellitus have to control their blood sugar with diet and insulin injections or tablets; too much insulin or too little sugar can cause hypoglycaemia (opposite). The chart below enables you to compare these two conditions. If a known diabetic casualty appears unwell, give sugar. This will rapidly correct hypoglycaemia and will do little harm in hyperglycaemia.

COMPARING HYPERGLYCAEMIA AND HYPOGLYCAEMIA

Category		Hyperglycaemia	Hypoglycaemia
History	Recent eating habits	Eaten excessively	Undereaten or missed meals
	Amount of insulin used	Not enough for amount of food eaten	Too much for amount of food eaten
	Speed of onset of symptoms	Gradual	Rapid
Symptoms	Thirst	Present	Absent
	Hunger	Absent	Present
	Vomiting	Common	Uncommon
	Urination	Excessive	Normal
Signs	Odour on the breath	Fruity/sweet	Normal
	Breathing	Rapid	Normal
	Pulse	Rapid and weak	Rapid and strong
	Skin	Warm and dry	Pale and cold, with sweating
	Seizures	Uncommon	Common
	Level of consciousness	Drowsy	Rapid loss of consciousness

HYPERGLYCAEMIA

High blood sugar (hyperglycaemia) over a long period can result in unconsciousness. Usually, the casualty will drift into this state over a few days. Hyperglycaemia requires urgent treatment in hospital.

RECOGNITION
- Warm, dry skin; rapid pulse and breathing.
- Fruity/sweet breath and excessive thirst.
- If untreated, drowsiness, then unconsciousness.

✚ YOUR AIM
- To arrange urgent removal of the casualty to hospital.

1 CALL AN AMBULANCE
If the casualty is unconscious, place him in the recovery position (pp.84–85).

2 Monitor and record vital signs – level of response, pulse, and breathing (pp.42–43).

HYPOGLYCAEMIA

When the blood-sugar level falls below normal (hypoglycaemia), brain function is affected. This problem is characterised by a rapidly deteriorating level of response. Hypoglycaemia can occur in people with diabetes mellitus and, more rarely, appear with an epileptic seizure or after an episode of binge drinking. It can also complicate heat exhaustion or hypothermia.

People with diabetes mellitus may carry their own blood-testing kits with which to check their blood-sugar levels, and are usually well prepared for emergencies. For example, many diabetic people carry sugar lumps or a tube of glucose in gel form in case they feel they are having a "hypo".

If the hypo attack is at an advanced stage, consciousness may be impaired or lost and you must get emergency help.

RECOGNITION

There may be:
- A history of diabetes; the casualty may recognise the onset of a "hypo" attack.
- Weakness, faintness, or hunger.
- Palpitations and muscle tremors.
- Strange actions or behaviour; the casualty may seem confused or belligerent.
- Sweating and cold, clammy skin.
- Pulse may be rapid and strong.
- Deteriorating level of response.
- Diabetic's warning card, glucose gel, tablets, or an insulin syringe in casualty's possessions.

See also HEAT EXHAUSTION p.203
● HYPOTHERMIA pp.206–208 ● LIFE-SAVING PROCEDURES pp.71–102 ● SEIZURES IN ADULTS pp.184–185

YOUR AIMS
- To raise the sugar content of the blood as quickly as possible.
- To obtain medical aid if necessary.

WARNING
- If consciousness is impaired, do not give the casualty anything to eat or drink.
- If the casualty is unconscious, open the airway and check breathing; be ready to give rescue breaths and chest compressions if necessary (*see* LIFE-SAVING PROCEDURES, pp.71–102). If he is breathing, place him in the recovery position.

CALL AN AMBULANCE
Monitor and record the vital signs – level of response, pulse, and breathing (pp.42–43).

1 Help the casualty to sit or lie down. Give her a sugary drink, sugar lumps, chocolate, or other sweet food; alternatively, if she has her own glucose gel, help her to take it.

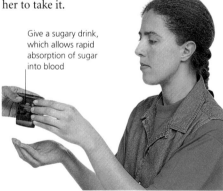

Give a sugary drink, which allows rapid absorption of sugar into blood

2 If the casualty responds quickly, give more food or drink, and let her rest until she feels better. Advise her to see her doctor even if she feels fully recovered. If her condition does not improve, monitor level of response (p.42) and look for other possible causes.

PANIC ATTACK

A panic attack is a sudden bout of extreme anxiety. The casualty has severe physical symptoms, such as hyperventilation and palpitations (a feeling of an abnormal or fast heart rate), as well as being distressed. Panic attacks can occur for no obvious cause or in situations that are not normally stressful. If a casualty is very anxious, check for a history of panic attacks, and ask if he has any intense fear (phobia), such as a terror of spiders or of being in a crowd.

RECOGNITION

There may be:
- Hyperventilation (over-breathing).
- Muscular tension, producing headache, backache, and a feeling of pressure in the chest.
- Extreme apprehension and fear of dying.
- Trembling, sweating, and dry mouth.
- High pulse rate and sometimes palpitations.

▶ See also HYPERVENTILATION p.114

YOUR AIMS
- To remove any obvious cause of panic.
- To help the casualty regain self-control.

CAUTION
- Do not slap the casualty's face.
- Do not try to restrain the casualty.

1 Try to find out and remove the cause of the fear. Take the casualty to a quiet area. Reassure him and explain that he is having a panic attack if he does not already know.

2 Encourage the casualty to breathe more slowly. If he is hyperventilating, advise him to breathe into a paper bag to help control the symptoms (*see* HYPERVENTILATION, p.114). Stay with the casualty until he has recovered. Advise him to seek medical help.

DISTURBED BEHAVIOUR

There are many reasons why a casualty may behave in an abnormal or aggressive way. Some people become irrational in stressful situations. Disturbed behaviour can also be due to alcohol or drug abuse; the use of certain prescribed drugs; or certain physical disorders, such as hypoglycaemia, epilepsy, or head injuries. Other possible causes include mental disorders such as anxiety, psychosis, and dementia.

▶ See also DRUG POISONING p.222
- HEAD INJURY p.179 - HYPOGLYCAEMIA p.241

YOUR AIMS
- To help the casualty resume normal behaviour.
- To obtain medical aid if necessary.

CAUTION
- If the casualty is aggressive, do not put yourself in danger. Make sure that you can retreat rapidly if necessary.
- Do not try to restrain the casualty.

1 Talk calmly to the casualty and, if you can, try to find out the cause of the problem. Do not argue with the casualty, because this may worsen the situation.

2 Call a doctor (if possible, the casualty's own). If necessary, call the police.

EARACHE

This common condition results from inflammation of the tissues inside the ear or from blockage in the ear. It may be accompanied by partial or total hearing loss, which is usually temporary.

The most usual cause, particularly in children, is an ear infection associated with a cold, tonsillitis, or flu. Pain can also be caused by a boil, a foreign object stuck in the ear canal, or another condition such as an abscess in a nearby tooth. In addition, earache often occurs on aeroplane journeys due to changes in cabin air pressure during ascent and descent.

Occasionally, infection causes pus to collect in the middle ear. The eardrum may then rupture, allowing the pus to drain from the ear; this will temporarily ease the pain.

▶ **See also** FOREIGN OBJECT IN THE EAR p.215 ● TOOTHACHE p.244

✚ YOUR AIMS

- To relieve pain.
- To obtain medical aid if necessary.

❶ CAUTION

If there is a discharge, fever, or marked hearing loss, obtain medical help.

1 An adult may take two paracetamol tablets or her own painkillers. A child may take the recommended dose of paracetamol syrup (not aspirin).

2 Make the casualty comfortable. Give her a source of heat, such as a hot-water bottle wrapped in a towel, to hold against the affected ear. If lying flat makes the pain worse, prop her up with pillows.

SPECIAL CASE

AIR TRAVEL
If earache occurs during air travel, help the casualty to equalise the pressure in her ears by making the ears "pop". Advise her to swallow with her mouth open; alternatively, tell her to close her mouth, hold her nose tightly closed, and "blow" her nose. If this does not help, reassure the casualty that the pain will go away when the pressure inside the middle ear is reduced as the aircraft lands.

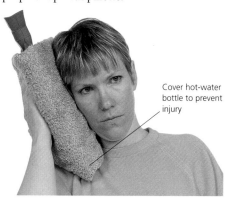

Cover hot-water bottle to prevent injury

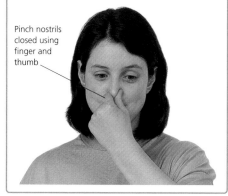

Pinch nostrils closed using finger and thumb

3 Advise the casualty to see her doctor. If you are worried about her condition (particularly if the casualty is a child), obtain medical help.

TOOTHACHE

Pain may occur either in the teeth or in the gums. Persistent toothache is usually caused by a decayed tooth and can be made worse by hot or cold food or drinks.

Throbbing toothache indicates an infection at the root of a tooth. Infection can also cause swelling of the gums in the painful area and bad breath. Pain in the teeth can sometimes be due to disorders affecting the facial nerves, such as sinusitis, or an ear infection.

▶ See also EARACHE p.243

+ YOUR AIMS
- To relieve pain.
- To ensure that the casualty consults a dentist.

1 An adult may take two paracetamol tablets to relieve the pain. A child may take the recommended dose of paracetamol syrup (not aspirin).

2 Make the casualty comfortable. If lying down makes the toothache worse, prop her up with pillows.

3 To help relieve pain, give the casualty a hot-water bottle wrapped in a towel to hold against her face, and/or give her a rolled-up plug of cotton wool soaked in oil of cloves to hold against the affected tooth.

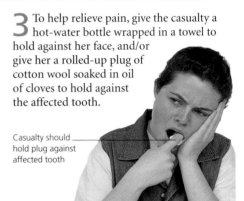

Casualty should hold plug against affected tooth

4 Advise the casualty to make an early appointment with her dentist.

SORE THROAT

The most common type of sore throat is a rough or "raw" feeling, which is caused by inflammation. This problem is often the first sign of a cough or cold, and usually passes within a day or two. A more serious condition, called tonsillitis, occurs when the tonsils, at the back of the throat, become infected with bacteria or a virus. The tonsils are swollen and red, and ulcers or white spots of pus may be seen. Swallowing may be difficult, and the glands at the angle of the jaw may be enlarged and sore.

▶ See also FEVER p.239

+ YOUR AIMS
- To relieve pain.
- To obtain medical aid if necessary.

1 Give the casualty plenty of fluids to drink, to ease the pain and stop the throat from becoming dry.

2 An adult may take two paracetamol tablets or his own painkillers. A child may take the recommended dose of paracetamol syrup (not aspirin).

3 If you suspect that the casualty has tonsillitis, advise her to see a doctor as soon as possible.

ABDOMINAL PAIN

Pain in the abdomen often has a relatively minor cause, such as food poisoning. However, it can occasionally be a sign of a serious disorder affecting the organs and other structures in the abdomen.

Distension (widening) or obstruction of the intestine causes colic – pain that comes and goes in "waves". It often makes the casualty double up in agony and may be accompanied by vomiting. If the appendix bursts, or the intestine is damaged, the contents of the intestine can leak into the abdominal cavity, causing inflammation of the cavity lining. This life-threatening condition, called peritonitis, causes sudden, intense pain, which is made worse by movement or pressure on the abdomen, and will lead to shock (pp.120–121).

APPENDICITIS
An inflamed appendix (appendicitis) is especially common in children. Symptoms include pain (often starting in the centre of the abdomen and moving to the lower right-hand side), nausea, vomiting, bad breath, and fever. If the appendix bursts, peritonitis will develop. The treatment is urgent surgical removal of the appendix.

See also FOOD POISONING p.224

YOUR AIMS
- To relieve pain and discomfort.
- To obtain medical aid if necessary.

1 Make the casualty comfortable, and prop her up if breathing is difficult. Give her a container to use if she is vomiting.

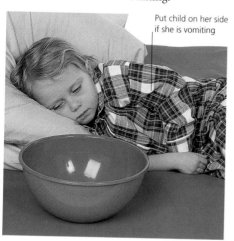

Put child on her side if she is vomiting

2 Give the casualty a hot-water bottle wrapped in a towel for her to place against her abdomen.

SPECIAL CASE

WINDED CASUALTY
A blow to the upper abdomen may stun a local nerve junction, causing a temporary breathing problem called "winding". To treat a winded casualty, help him to sit down, and loosen clothing at the chest and waist. The casualty should recover rapidly.

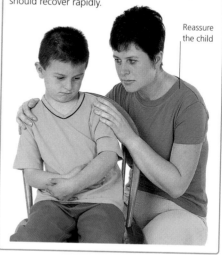

Reassure the child

3 If the pain is severe, or occurs with fever and vomiting, call a doctor. Do not give medicine or allow her to eat, drink, or smoke, because a general anaesthetic may be needed.

HERNIA

A hernia, commonly called a rupture, is a soft swelling in the abdomen or the groin. It occurs when a small loop of intestine, or other tissue, pushes through a weak area of muscle in the abdominal wall. The disorder may result from increased muscle pressure due to persistent coughing, straining during bowel movements, or lifting heavy weights.

A hernia may or may not be painful. If the casualty has a painless lump, no first aid is necessary; simply reassure the casualty and advise him to see a doctor as soon as possible. However, vomiting and severe

RECOGNITION

There may be:
- Bulge or swelling in abdominal wall or groin, which may disappear when the casualty lies flat.
- Dragging or aching sensation in the abdomen or groin.
- Pain in the abdomen or groin.
- Vomiting.

pain indicate that part of the intestine has become trapped and deprived of blood (a condition called strangulated hernia). This problem needs urgent surgery.

YOUR AIMS
- To reassure the casualty.
- To relieve any discomfort.
- To obtain medical aid.

❗ CAUTION
- Do not attempt to push the swelling back or allow the casualty to do so. This may increase the risk of damage to the intestine.
- Do not give the casualty any medicines or allow him to eat, drink, or smoke, because a general anaesthetic may need to be given in hospital.

1 If the casualty is in pain, help him to sit down, and support him in the position he finds most comfortable by propping him up with cushions or pillows.

2 Call a doctor or, if the pain is severe, CALL AN AMBULANCE

3 While you are waiting for medical aid, continue to reassure the casualty. Monitor his vital signs – level of response, pulse, and breathing (pp.42–43) – until help arrives.

Support casualty behind with a pillow

Casualty with abdominal pain may prefer to bend his knees

Support the knees with a folded pillow or rolled-up jacket

VOMITING AND DIARRHOEA

These problems are usually due to irritation of the digestive system. This can be caused by unusual or rich foods; alcohol; certain medications; contaminated foods or drinks; or an allergic reaction.

Vomiting and diarrhoea may occur either separately or together. Both conditions can cause the body to lose vital fluids and salts, resulting in dehydration. When they occur together, the risk of dehydration is increased and can be serious, especially in infants, young children, and elderly people.

The main aim of treatment is to help restore the lost fluids and salts. Water is sufficient in most cases, but non-fizzy, "isotonic" glucose drinks are ideal if they are available. Alternatively, add salt (1 teaspoonful per litre) and sugar (4–5 teaspoonfuls per litre) to water or to diluted orange juice.

▶ **See also** DRUG POISONING p.222 ● FOOD POISONING p.224 ● SWALLOWED POISONS p.220

✛ YOUR AIMS
● To reassure the casualty.
● To restore lost fluids and salts.

❶ CAUTION
If you are worried about the casualty's condition, particularly if the vomiting or diarrhoea is persistent, call a doctor.

1 Reassure the casualty if he is vomiting. Afterwards, give him a warm, damp cloth to wipe his face.

2 Give the casualty plenty of clear fluids to sip slowly and often.

3 If the casualty's appetite returns, give only easily digested, non-spicy foods for the first 24 hours.

STITCH

This common condition is a form of cramp that occurs in the trunk or the sides of the chest. A stitch is usually associated with exercise. The most likely cause of the cramp is an accumulation of chemical waste products, such as lactic acid, in the muscles during physical exertion. The pain of a stitch can be like that of angina pectoris (p.124), but it is usually sharper.

RECOGNITION
● Cramp-like pains in the side of the chest and muscles of the trunk.
● History of recent physical exertion.

▶ **See also** ABDOMINAL PAIN p.245 ● ANGINA PECTORIS p.124

✛ YOUR AIM
● To help relieve the symptoms.

1 Help the casualty to sit down, and reassure him. The pain will usually ease quickly.

2 If the pain does not disappear within a few minutes, or if you are concerned about the casualty's condition, call a doctor.

CRAMP

This condition is a sudden, painful spasm in one or more muscles. Cramp commonly occurs during sleep. It can also develop after strenuous exercise, due to a build-up of chemical waste products in the muscles or to excessive loss of salt and fluids from the body through sweating. Cramp can often be relieved by stretching and massaging the affected muscle.

▶ **See also** HEAT EXHAUSTION p.203
● STITCH p.247

CRAMP IN THE FOOT

✚ YOUR AIM
● To help relieve the spasm and pain.

1 Help the casualty to stand with her weight on the front of her foot.

2 Once the first spasm has passed, massage the affected area of the foot.

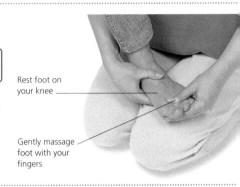

Rest foot on your knee

Gently massage foot with your fingers

CRAMP IN THE CALF

✚ YOUR AIM
● To help relieve the spasm and pain.

1 Straighten the casualty's knee and support the foot.

2 Flex the foot towards the shin to stretch the calf muscles, then massage the area.

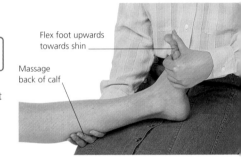

Flex foot upwards towards shin

Massage back of calf

CRAMP IN THE THIGH

✚ YOUR AIM
● To help relieve the spasm and pain.

1 Help the casualty to lie down. To ease cramp in the back of the thigh, raise the leg and straighten the knee. For cramp in the front of the thigh, bend the knee.

2 Support the leg and massage the affected thigh muscle gently but firmly with your fingers until the pain eases.

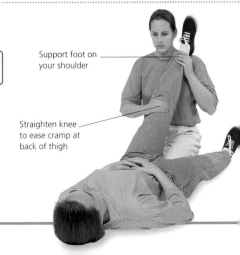

Support foot on your shoulder

Straighten knee to ease cramp at back of thigh

OVERSEAS TRAVEL HEALTH

With the increase in travel, many people are now at risk from diseases that are either not commonly encountered in their own country or pose a greater risk in other countries. Being in a hot climate can create problems such as heat exhaustion. It is important to understand any potential health risks, how they can be prevented or reduced, and how to respond to some of the medical emergencies that might arise.

PLANNING AHEAD

Many conditions can be avoided. You should consult your doctor well in advance of your planned departure – preferably at least 2 months – to allow sufficient time to arrange any immunisations that you may

need. However, do see your doctor even if you have to travel abroad at short notice – some protection may be better than none. You should tell your doctor:

- Where you are going, including any countries that you may visit en route.
- If you are or may become pregnant, as some medicines will be unsuitable for you.
- If you are taking children with you. This is especially important if any of the children have not completed their full course of childhood immunisations.

▶ See also POISONING, BITES, AND STINGS pp.217–230 ● HEAT EXHAUSTION p.203 ● HEATSTROKE p.204 ● SUNBURN p.202 ● VOMITING AND DIARRHOEA p.247

FOOD- AND WATER-BORNE INFECTIONS

Infection due to consuming contaminated food or water is one of the most common problems affecting travellers. You can reduce the risk by taking the following precautions: wash your hands after using the toilet and before eating; avoid food that has been kept

warm; do not eat raw vegetables, salads, shellfish, or ice cream; and peel all fruit. If you are in any doubt about the safety of drinking water, boil it, sterilise it with disinfectant tablets, or use bottled water supplied in sealed containers.

RECOGNISING AND TREATING FOOD- AND WATER-BORNE INFECTIONS

Disorder	Recognition	Action
Traveller's diarrhoea Spread through food and water that is contaminated with one of several disease-causing microorganisms.	● Nausea and vomiting ● Diarrhoea ● Abdominal pain	● Restore lost body fluids ● Careful hygiene to prevent spread of infection ● Seek medical advice if symptoms persist
Hepatitis A Spread through contaminated food or water. The infection may spread from person to person, especially if sanitation is poor. Protection by immunisation is available	● Abdominal pain ● Raised temperature ● Yellowing of the whites of the eyes (jaundice) and skin after several days	● Seek medical advice ● Relieve the fever, but do NOT give paracetamol ● Careful hygiene to prevent spread of infection
Cholera Spread through contaminated water, this infection can cause fatal dehydration.	● Profuse diarrhoea ● Weakness and dehydration ● Nausea and vomiting	● Seek urgent medical advice ● Restore lost body fluids ● Careful hygiene to prevent spread of infection

OVERSEAS TRAVEL HEALTH (continued)

OTHER INFECTIONS AND DISORDERS

As well as water and food-borne infections, travellers may be at risk of diseases from insects and ticks, and from unprotected sex. Simple steps should help to prevent infection.

INSECT-BORNE DISEASES

Mosquitoes are carriers of infections such as malaria and yellow fever in certain parts of the world. Protect yourself by covering arms and legs after sunset, using mosquito repellent, and sleeping under a mosquito net. Ensure that you take antimalarial medication where advised.

BLOOD-BORNE INFECTION

Abstinence from sex with a new partner is the safest way to avoid the risk of sexually transmitted infections, but you can reduce the risk by using condoms.

Any procedure in which the skin is pierced may also carry the risk of infection. Do not have a tattoo, acupuncture, or body piercing when overseas. Try to avoid having injections or surgical or dental treatment, but if you cannot, ask about sterilisation of equipment. If you need a blood transfusion, check that only screened blood is used.

RECOGNISING AND TREATING INSECT- AND BLOOD-BORNE ILLNESSES

Disorder	Recognition	Action
Hepatitis B and C Both occur worldwide. Spread through unprotected sex; sharing contaminated needles or syringes; needle-stick injury; transfusions of contaminated blood; using inadequately sterilised medical, dental, tattooing, or piercing equipment.	● May be no immediate signs ● Loss of appetite ● Abdominal discomfort ● Nausea and vomiting ● Sometimes, jaundice (yellowing of the skin/whites of the eyes)	● Seek urgent medical aid ● Restore lost body fluids ● Careful hygiene to prevent spread of infection
Lyme disease Contracted from infected ticks. No evidence of transmission from person to person.	● Stiff neck ● Fever ● Severe headache	● Seek urgent medical aid ● Relieve fever
Malaria The parasite is spread by the bites of infected mosquitoes. Antimalarial drugs must be taken as directed.	● Fever ● Headache	● Seek urgent medical aid ● Relieve fever
Rabies A serious viral infection that is transmitted via a bite from an infected dog, bat, or other animal. Immunisation is available for workers in high-risk employment.	● Headache ● Fever ● Excitability ● Fear – particularly of water ● Seizures and delirium	● Immediate, thorough cleansing of wound ● Seek urgent medical aid ● Saliva is infective: wear gloves and masks and incinerate soiled items
Yellow fever Viral disease transmitted by the bites of infected mosquitoes. Immunisation is available.	● Headache and fever ● Jaundice (yellowing of the skin/whites of the eyes) ● May progress to bleeding from nose, gums, and intestines	● Seek urgent medical aid ● Relieve fever ● Careful hygiene to prevent spread of infection

13

THIS SECTION is a quick-reference guide to first-aid measures for casualties with serious illnesses or injuries. It begins with a plan of action to help you determine how to deal with an emergency effectively. The section then describes resuscitation procedures for unconscious casualties. It is followed by first-aid treatment for casualties with serious or potentially life-threatening conditions. Observation charts are included for you to complete when monitoring a casualty.

The information in this section is also provided as a separate booklet that can be conveniently carried and used.

HOW TO USE THIS SECTION

Recognition lists help you to identify condition quickly

Cross-references direct you to extra useful information

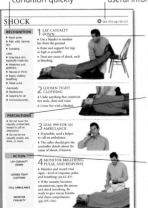

Steps and bullet points show full sequence of actions

Precautions advise you how to avoid further risks to casualty

Action points summarise first-aid measures

CONTENTS

ACTION IN AN EMERGENCY

1 ASSESS SITUATION
● Are there any risks to you or the casualty?

YES
● Put your safety first. If possible, remove the danger from the casualty or, if this is not possible, remove the casualty from danger.
● If it is unsafe, call for emergency help and wait for it to arrive.

NO

2 CHECK CASUALTY
● Is the casualty visibly conscious?

YES
● Check for other conditions (opposite) and treat as necessary.
● Summon help if needed.

NO

3 CHECK RESPONSE
● Does the casualty respond to your voice or to gentle stimulation?

YES
● Check for other conditions (opposite) and treat as necessary.
● Summon help if needed.

NO

ARE YOU ALONE?

YES
● Is the unconsciousness due to injury, drowning, or choking, or is the casualty a child or an infant?

NO

NO
● Ask a helper to call an ambulance and to pass on details of the casualty's condition.
▶ Move on to STEP 4

NO
● Call an ambulance immediately.
▶ Move on to STEP 4

YES
▶ Move on to STEP 4 Carry out the resuscitation sequence for 1 minute before calling an ambulance.

4 OPEN AIRWAY; CHECK BREATHING
● Open and, if necessary, clear the casualty's airway and check for breathing (see p.254 for an adult; p.258 for a child; p.262 for an infant).
● Is the casualty breathing?

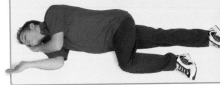

YES
● Place the casualty in the recovery position (see p.257 for an adult; p.261 for a child; p.262 for an infant).

NO

▶ Move on to STEP 5

5 BREATHE FOR CASUALTY

● Give two effective rescue breaths (see p.255 for an adult; p.259 for a child; p.263 for an infant).

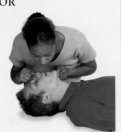

❶ WARNING

If at any stage the casualty begins breathing, place him in the recovery position (see p.257 for an adult; p.261 for a child; p.262 for an infant).

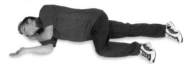

6 ASSESS FOR CIRCULATION

● Check for signs of circulation for no more than 10 seconds (see p.255 for an adult; p.259 for a child; p.263 for an infant).
● Are there any signs of circulation?

[YES]

● Continue with rescue breaths.
● Recheck for signs of circulation after every 10 breaths for an adult or 20 breaths for a child (about 1 minute).

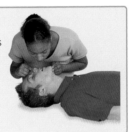

[NO]

7 COMMENCE CPR

● ADULT: Alternate 15 chest compressions with two rescue breaths (p.256); repeat as needed.
● CHILD/INFANT: Give five compressions to one rescue breath (see p.260 for a child; p.263 for an infant).

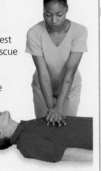

● Continue CPR, checking for signs of circulation after 1 minute and then every 3–4 minutes thereafter.

TREATMENTS FOR OTHER CONDITIONS

See the following pages for step-by-step treatments:

ASSESS THE CASUALTY

See also pp.76–77

EMERGENCY FIRST AID

1 CHECK RESPONSE

● Ask a question, such as "What's happened?", or give a command, such as "Open your eyes". Speak loudly and clearly.

● Gently shake the casualty's shoulders.

● If there is a response, leave the casualty in the position found and summon help, if needed. Treat any condition found.

● If there is no response, send a helper to CALL AN AMBULANCE then proceed to step 2.

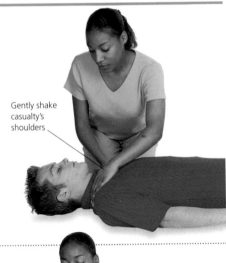

Gently shake casualty's shoulders

2 OPEN AIRWAY

● Place one hand on the casualty's forehead, and gently tilt his head back.

● Pick out any obvious obstructions from the casualty's mouth. Do not do a finger sweep.

● Place the fingertips under the point of the casualty's chin. Lift the chin.

● If you suspect a neck (spinal) injury, open the airway by gently lifting the jaw but not tilting the head (jaw thrust).

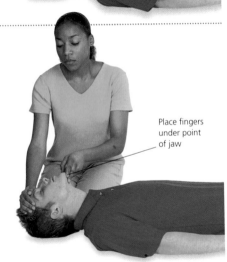

Place fingers under point of jaw

3 CHECK BREATHING

● Look for chest movement, listen for sounds of breathing, and feel for breath on your cheek. Do this for no more than 10 seconds.

● If the casualty is not breathing, begin rescue breathing (opposite).

● If he is breathing, check for life-threatening conditions such as severe bleeding. Place him in the recovery position (p.257).

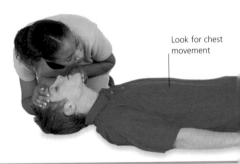

Look for chest movement

GIVE RESCUE BREATHS

▶ See also pp.78–79

1 MAKE SURE THAT AIRWAY IS STILL OPEN

● Make sure that the casualty's head remains tilted, by keeping one hand on his forehead and two fingers of the other hand under the tip of his chin.

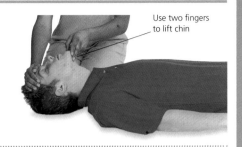

Use two fingers to lift chin

2 PINCH NOSE AND OPEN MOUTH

● Use your thumb and index finger to pinch the soft part of the casualty's nose firmly.

● Make sure that his nostrils are closed to prevent air from escaping.

● Open his mouth.

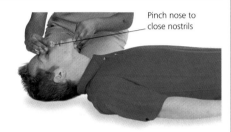

Pinch nose to close nostrils

3 GIVE RESCUE BREATHS

● Take a deep breath to fill your lungs with air. Place your lips around the casualty's lips, making sure that you form a good seal.

● Blow steadily into the mouth until the chest rises. This usually takes about 2 seconds. Maintaining head tilt and chin lift, take your mouth away and watch the chest fall. If the chest rises visibly and falls fully, you have given an effective breath.

● Give two effective breaths.

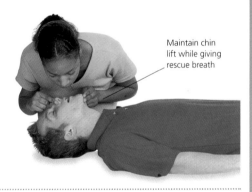

Maintain chin lift while giving rescue breath

4 ASSESS FOR SIGNS OF CIRCULATION

● Look, listen, and feel for signs of circulation, such as breathing, coughing, or movement, for no more than 10 seconds.

● If circulation is absent, perform CPR (p.256).

● If circulation is present, continue with rescue breaths. After every 10 breaths (about 1 minute), recheck for circulation.

● If the casualty starts breathing but remains unconscious, place him in the recovery position (p.257).

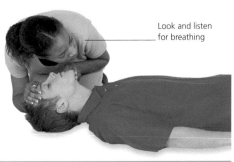

Look and listen for breathing

COMMENCE CPR

▶ See also pp.80–81

1 POSITION HANDS FOR CHEST COMPRESSIONS

● With the index and middle fingers of your lower hand, locate one of the casualty's lowermost ribs on the side nearer to you. Slide your fingertips along the rib to the point at which it meets the breastbone. Place your middle finger at this point and the index finger beside it on the breastbone.

● Place the heel of your other hand on the breastbone; slide it down to meet your index finger. This is the point at which you will apply pressure.

● Place the heel of your first hand on top of the other hand, and interlock your fingers.

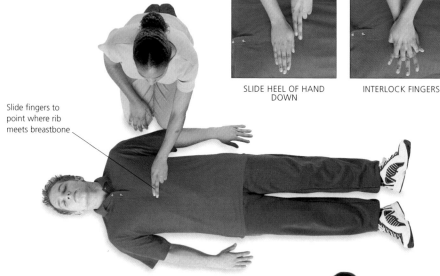

SLIDE HEEL OF HAND DOWN

INTERLOCK FINGERS

Slide fingers to point where rib meets breastbone

2 GIVE CHEST COMPRESSIONS AND RESCUE BREATHS

● Lean well over the casualty, with your arms straight. Press down vertically on the breastbone, and depress the chest by about 4–5cm (1½–2in).

● Compress the chest 15 times, at a rate of 100 compressions per minute.

● Tilt the head, lift the chin, and give two rescue breaths (p.255).

● Alternate 15 chest compressions with two rescue breaths.

● Continue CPR, checking for signs of circulation after 1 minute and then every 3–4 minutes until help arrives.

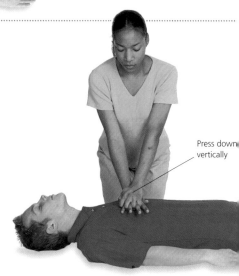

Press down vertically

RECOVERY POSITION

▶ **See also** pp.84–85

1 POSITION ARM AND STRAIGHTEN LEGS

- Kneel beside the casualty.

- Remove spectacles and any bulky objects (such as mobile phones or large bunches of keys) from the pockets. Straighten his legs.

- Place the arm nearest to you at right angles to the casualty's body, with the elbow bent and the palm facing upwards.

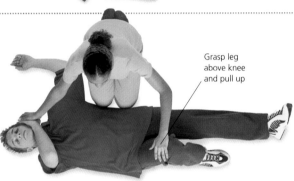

Place arm at right angles to body

2 POSITION FAR ARM, HAND, AND KNEE

- Bring the arm farthest from you across the casualty's chest and hold the back of his hand against the cheek nearest to you.

- Using your other hand, grasp the far leg just above the knee and pull it up until the foot is flat on the floor.

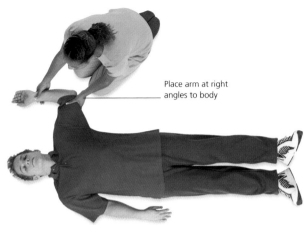

Grasp leg above knee and pull up

3 ROLL CASUALTY TOWARDS YOU

- Keeping the casualty's hand pressed against his cheek, pull on the far leg and roll him towards you and on to his side.

- Adjust the upper leg so that both the hip and knee are bent at right angles.

- Tilt the head back to ensure that the airway remains open.

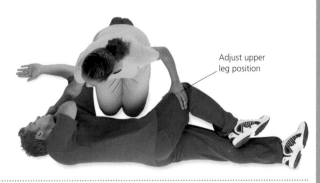

Adjust upper leg position

4 CALL AN AMBULANCE, IF NOT ALREADY DONE

- Ideally, ask a helper to make the call while you wait with the casualty.

- Monitor and record vital signs (pp.42–43) – level of response, pulse, and breathing.

UNCONSCIOUS CHILD (1–7 YEARS)
ASSESS THE CHILD

▶ See also pp.87–88

1 CHECK RESPONSE

● Ask the child a question, such as "Can you hear me?". Speak loudly and clearly.

● Gently tap her on the shoulder.

● If there is a response, leave the child in the position found and summon help, if needed. Treat any condition found.

● If there is no response, send a helper to CALL AN AMBULANCE then proceed to step 2.

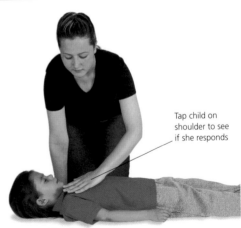

Tap child on shoulder to see if she responds

2 OPEN AIRWAY

● Place one hand on the child's forehead. Gently tilt the head back.

● Using your fingertips, pick out any obvious obstructions from the child's mouth. Do not do a finger sweep.

● Place the fingertips under the point of the child's chin. Lift the chin.

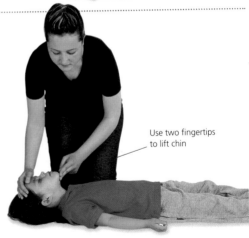

Use two fingertips to lift chin

3 CHECK BREATHING

● Look, listen, and feel for breathing: look for chest movement, listen for sounds of breathing, and feel for breath on your cheek. Do this for no more than 10 seconds.

● If the child is not breathing, begin rescue breathing (opposite).

● If she is breathing, check for life-threatening conditions such as severe bleeding. Place the child in the recovery position (p.261).

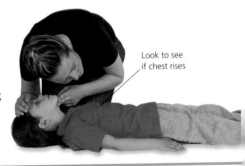

Look to see if chest rises

GIVE RESCUE BREATHS

▶ See also p.89

1 MAKE SURE THAT AIRWAY IS STILL OPEN

- Make sure that the child's head remains tilted, by keeping one hand on her forehead and two fingers of the other hand under her chin.

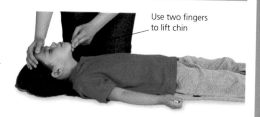

Use two fingers to lift chin

2 PINCH NOSE AND OPEN MOUTH

- Use your thumb and index finger to pinch the soft part of the child's nose firmly. Make sure that her nostrils are closed to prevent air from escaping.

- Open the child's mouth.

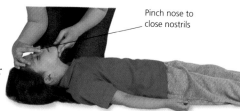

Pinch nose to close nostrils

3 GIVE RESCUE BREATHS

- Take a deep breath to fill your lungs with air. Place your lips around the child's lips, making sure that you form an airtight seal.

- Blow steadily into the mouth until the chest rises. Maintaining head tilt and chin lift, take your mouth away and watch the chest fall. If the chest rises visibly and falls fully, you have given an effective breath.

- Give two effective rescue breaths.

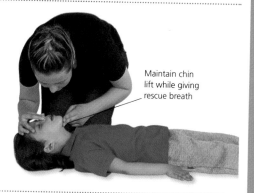

Maintain chin lift while giving rescue breath

4 ASSESS FOR SIGNS OF CIRCULATION

- Look, listen, and feel for signs of circulation, such as breathing, coughing, or movement, for no more than 10 seconds.

- If circulation is absent, perform CPR (p.260) for 1 minute, then CALL AN AMBULANCE

- If circulation is present, give 20 rescue breaths in 1 minute, then CALL AN AMBULANCE

- If the child starts breathing but remains unconscious, place her in the recovery position (p.261).

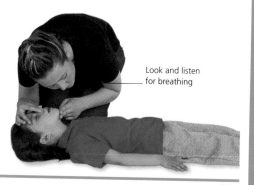

Look and listen for breathing

COMMENCE CPR

▶ See also pp.90–91

1 POSITION HANDS FOR CHEST COMPRESSIONS

• With the fingertips of your lower hand, locate one of the child's lowermost ribs on the side nearest to you. Slide your fingertips along the rib to where the lowermost ribs meet at the breastbone. Place your middle finger at this point and your index finger beside it on the lower breastbone.

• Remember where your fingers are, remove them, and place the same hand on the breastbone and slide it down until it reaches where your fingers were. This is the point at which you will apply pressure.

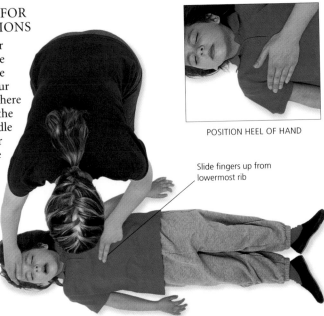

POSITION HEEL OF HAND

Slide fingers up from lowermost rib

2 GIVE CHEST COMPRESSIONS AND RESCUE BREATHS

• Use the heel of this lower hand only to apply pressure – keep your fingers raised so that you do not apply pressure to the child's ribs.

• Lean well over the child, with your arm straight. Press down vertically on the breastbone, and depress the chest by one-third of its depth. Release the pressure without removing your hand.

• Compress the chest five times, at a rate of 100 compressions per minute.

• Give one rescue breath (p.259).

• Continue to alternate five chest compressions with one rescue breath for 1 minute. Then CALL AN AMBULANCE

• Continue CPR, checking for signs of circulation after 1 minute and then every 3–4 minutes until help arrives.

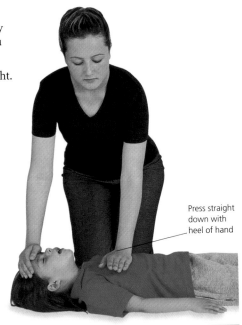

Press straight down with heel of hand

RECOVERY POSITION

See also pp.92–93

1 POSITION ARM AND STRAIGHTEN LEGS

- Kneel beside the casualty.
- Remove spectacles and any bulky objects from the pockets.
- Straighten her legs.
- Place the arm nearest to you at right angles to the child's body, with the elbow bent and the palm facing upwards.

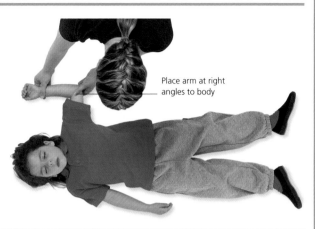

Place arm at right angles to body

2 POSITION FAR ARM, HAND, AND KNEE

- Bring the arm farthest from you across the child's chest.
- Hold the back of her hand against the cheek nearest to you.
- Using your other hand, grasp the far leg just above the knee and pull it up until the foot is flat on the floor.

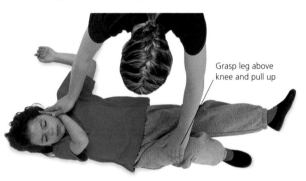

Grasp leg above knee and pull up

3 ROLL CHILD TOWARDS YOU

- Keeping the child's hand pressed against her cheek, pull on the far leg and roll her towards you and on to her side.
- Adjust the child's upper leg so that both the hip and the knee are bent at right angles.
- Tilt her head back to ensure that the airway remains open.

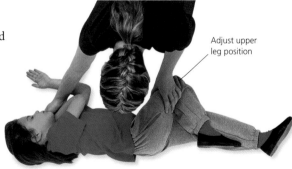

Adjust upper leg position

4 CALL AN AMBULANCE, IF NOT ALREADY DONE

- Monitor and record vital signs – level of response, pulse, and breathing (pp.42–43).

ASSESS THE INFANT

▶ See also pp.95–96

1 CHECK RESPONSE

● Gently tap or flick the sole of the infant's foot. Never shake an infant.

● If there is a response, take the baby with you to summon help if needed. If there is no response, send a helper to CALL AN AMBULANCE, then go to step 2.

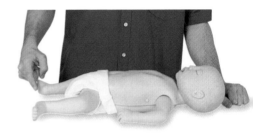

2 OPEN AIRWAY

● Place one hand on the infant's forehead, and very gently tilt the head back.

● Using your fingertips, pick out any obvious obstructions. Do not do a finger sweep.

● Place one fingertip under the point of the infant's chin. Lift the chin.

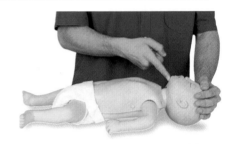

3 CHECK BREATHING

● Look for chest movement, listen for sounds of breathing, and feel for breath on your cheek. Do this for no more than 10 seconds.

● If the infant is not breathing, begin rescue breathing (opposite).

● If the infant is breathing, check for injuries and hold in the recovery position (below).

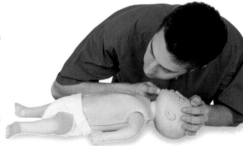

RECOVERY POSITION

▶ See also p.98

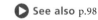

● Cradle the infant in your arms, with his head tilted downwards to prevent him from choking on his tongue or inhaling vomit.

● Monitor and record vital signs – level of response, pulse, and breathing (pp.42–43) – until medical help arrives.

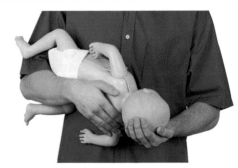

GIVE RESCUE BREATHS

▶ See also pp.96–97

1 GIVE RESCUE BREATHS

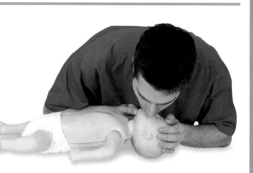

- Make sure that the airway remains open, by keeping the infant's head tilted back and the chin lifted.

- Take a deep breath. Place your lips around the infant's mouth and nose. Blow steadily until the chest rises. Take your mouth away and watch the chest fall. Give two effective breaths.

2 ASSESS FOR SIGNS OF CIRCULATION

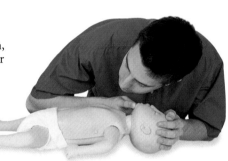

- Look, listen, and feel for signs of circulation, such as breathing, coughing, or movement, for no more than 10 seconds.

- If circulation is absent, perform CPR (below) for 1 minute, then **CALL AN AMBULANCE**

- If circulation is present, give 20 rescue breaths in 1 minute, then **CALL AN AMBULANCE**

COMMENCE CPR

▶ See also p.98

1 POSITION FINGERS FOR CHEST COMPRESSIONS

- Place three fingertips of your lower hand on the breastbone so that your index finger is in line with the nipples.

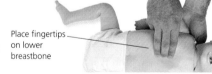

Place fingertips on lower breastbone

2 GIVE CHEST COMPRESSIONS AND RESCUE BREATHS

- Remove your index finger, then press down vertically on the chest, depressing it by one-third of its depth. Do this five times, at a rate of 100 compressions a minute.

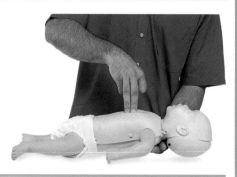

- Give one rescue breath. Alternate five chest compressions with one rescue breath. Check for signs of circulation after 1 minute and then every 3–4 minutes until help arrives.

CHOKING ADULT

▶ See also p.100

RECOGNITION

Partial obstruction
- Difficulty in speaking and breathing.
- Coughing and distress.

Complete obstruction
- Inability to speak, breathe, or cough.
- Eventual loss of consciousness.

PRECAUTIONS

- If the casualty loses consciousness, give rescue breaths and chest compressions (pp.255–256).
- Do not do a finger sweep of the mouth.

ACTION

ENCOURAGE CASUALTY TO COUGH

GIVE UP TO FIVE ABDOMINAL THRUSTS CHECK MOUTH

REPEAT SEQUENCE THREE TIMES THEN CALL AMBULANCE

REPEAT SEQUENCE UNTIL HELP ARRIVES

1 ENCOURAGE THE CASUALTY TO COUGH

- Encourage the casualty to cough to try to remove the obstruction.
- If the casualty is beginning to struggle, bend him forwards.
- Check his mouth.
- If choking persists, proceed to step 2.

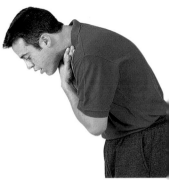

2 HOLD CASUALTY FROM BEHIND

- Stand behind the casualty.
- Put both arms around him, and put one fist between his navel and the bottom of his breastbone.

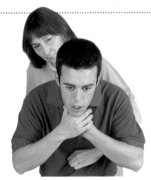

3 GIVE UP TO FIVE ABDOMINAL THRUSTS

- Grasp your fist with your other hand, and pull sharply inwards and upwards up to five times.
- Check his mouth. If the obstruction is still not cleared, recheck the mouth for any object and remove it if possible.
- If choking persists, proceed to step 4.

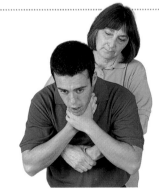

4 REPEAT ENTIRE SEQUENCE

- Repeat steps 1–3 until the obstruction clears. If after three cycles it still has not cleared, CALL AN AMBULANCE

- Continue the sequence until help arrives; the obstruction is cleared; or the casualty becomes unconscious (see PRECAUTIONS, left).

CHOKING CHILD (1–7 years)

▶ See also p.101

RECOGNITION

Partial obstruction
- Difficulty in speaking and breathing.
- Coughing and distress.

Complete obstruction
- Inability to speak, breathe, or cough.
- Eventual loss of consciousness.

PRECAUTIONS

- If the child loses consciousness, give rescue breaths and chest compressions (pp.259–260).
- Do not do a finger sweep of the mouth.

ACTION

ENCOURAGE CASUALTY TO COUGH

GIVE UP TO FIVE ABDOMINAL THRUSTS CHECK MOUTH

REPEAT SEQUENCE THREE TIMES THEN CALL AMBULANCE

REPEAT SEQUENCE UNTIL HELP ARRIVES

1 ENCOURAGE THE CHILD TO COUGH

- If the child is breathing, encourage him to cough; this may be enough to clear the obstruction.
- If he is beginning to struggle, bend him forwards.
- Check his mouth.
- If choking persists, proceed to step 2.

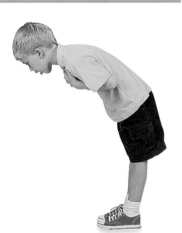

2 GIVE UP TO FIVE ABDOMINAL THRUSTS

- Stand behind the child with both arms around the upper abdomen. Make sure that he is bending well forward. Place your fist between the navel and the bottom of the breastbone.
- Grasp your fist with your hand. Pull sharply inwards and upwards up to five times.
- Check the child's mouth. Stop if the obstruction clears.
- If choking persists, proceed to step 3.

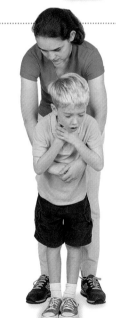

3 REPEAT ENTIRE SEQUENCE

- Repeat steps 1–2 until the obstruction clears.
- If after three cycles the obstruction still has not cleared, CALL AN AMBULANCE
- Continue the sequence until help arrives; the obstruction is cleared from the airway; or the child becomes unconscious (*see* PRECAUTIONS, left).

CHOKING INFANT (under 1 year)

▶ See also p.102

RECOGNITION

- Difficulty in breathing.
- Flushed face and neck.
- Strange noises or no sound.

Later:
- Grey–blue skin.

PRECAUTIONS

- If the infant loses consciousness, give rescue breaths and chest compressions (p.263).
- Do not do a finger sweep of the mouth.
- Do not use abdominal thrusts.

ACTION

GIVE UP TO FIVE BACK SLAPS
CHECK MOUTH

GIVE UP TO FIVE CHEST THRUSTS
CHECK MOUTH

REPEAT SEQUENCE THREE TIMES THEN CALL AMBULANCE

REPEAT SEQUENCE UNTIL HELP ARRIVES

1 GIVE UP TO FIVE BACK SLAPS

- Check the infant's mouth, but do not do a finger sweep as you may make the obstruction worse.

- Lay the infant face down along your forearm, with his head low, and supporting his body and head.

- Give up to five back slaps between the shoulder blades. If choking persists, proceed to step 2.

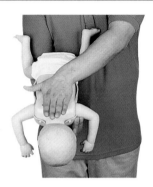

2 CHECK INFANT'S MOUTH

- Turn the infant face up along your other forearm.

- Use your fingertips to remove any obvious obstructions.

- If choking persists, proceed to step 3.

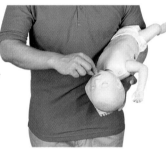

3 GIVE UP TO FIVE CHEST THRUSTS

- Place two fingertips on the lower half of the infant's breastbone, one finger's breadth below the nipples.

- Give up to five sharp thrusts inwards and towards the head at rate of one every 3 seconds.

- Check the mouth again.

- If choking persists, proceed to step 4.

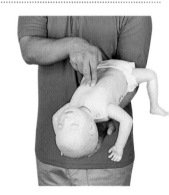

4 REPEAT ENTIRE SEQUENCE

- Repeat steps 1–3 three times.

- If the obstruction still does not clear, take the infant with you to CALL AN AMBULANCE

- Continue the sequence until help arrives; the obstruction is cleared from the airway; or the infant becomes unconscious (*see* PRECAUTIONS, left).

ASTHMA ATTACK

▶ See also p.115

RECOGNITION

- Difficulty in breathing.

There may be:
- Wheezing.
- Difficulty in speaking.
- Grey–blue skin.
- Exhaustion and possible loss of consciousness.

PRECAUTIONS

- Do not lay the casualty down.
- Do not use a preventer inhaler.
- If the attack is severe, or if the inhaler has no effect after 5 minutes, or if the casualty is getting worse **CALL AN AMBULANCE**
- If the casualty loses consciousness, open the airway and check breathing (p.252). Be prepared to give rescue breaths and chest compressions if needed.

ACTION

ALLOW CASUALTY TO USE RELIEVER INHALER

⬇

MAKE CASUALTY COMFORTABLE

⬇

ENCOURAGE CASUALTY TO BREATHE SLOWLY

1 MAKE CASUALTY COMFORTABLE

- Keep calm and reassure the casualty.

- Help her into the position that she finds most comfortable; sitting slightly forwards and supporting the upper body by leaning the arms on a firm surface is usually best.

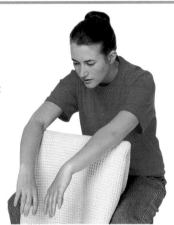

2 ALLOW CASUALTY TO USE RELIEVER INHALER

- Help the casualty to find her reliever inhaler (it is usually blue).

- Encourage the casualty to use the inhaler; it should take effect within minutes.

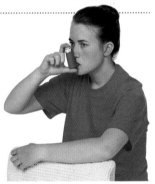

3 ENCOURAGE CASUALTY TO BREATHE SLOWLY

- If the attack does not ease within 3 minutes, encourage the casualty to take another dose from her inhaler and to breathe slowly and deeply.

- Tell the casualty to inform her doctor of the attack if it is severe or if it is her first attack.

- If the attack is severe, if the inhaler has no effect after 5 minutes, or if the casualty is getting worse, **CALL AN AMBULANCE**

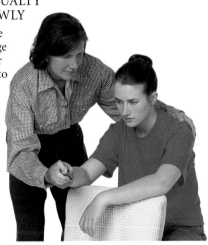

SHOCK

⏵ See also pp.120–121

RECOGNITION

- Rapid pulse.
- Pale, cold, clammy skin.
- Sweating.

Later:

- Grey–blue skin, especially inside lips.
- Weakness and giddiness.
- Nausea or thirst.
- Rapid, shallow breathing.
- Weak pulse.

Eventually:

- Restlessness.
- Gasping for air.
- Unconsciousness.

PRECAUTIONS

- Do not leave the casualty unattended, except to call an ambulance.
- Do not let the casualty smoke, eat, drink, or move.

ACTION

HELP CASUALTY
TO LIE DOWN

⬇

LOOSEN TIGHT
CLOTHING

⬇

CALL AMBULANCE

⬇

MONITOR
CASUALTY

1 HELP CASUALTY TO LIE DOWN

- Use a blanket to insulate the casualty from the ground.
- Raise and support her legs as high as possible.
- Treat any cause of shock, such as bleeding.

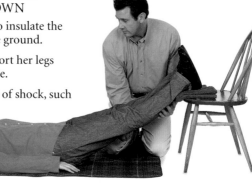

2 LOOSEN TIGHT CLOTHING

- Undo anything that constricts her neck, chest and waist.
- Cover her with a blanket.

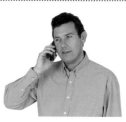

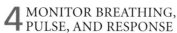

3 CALL AN AMBULANCE

- If possible, send a helper to call an ambulance.
- The caller should give the controller details about the cause of shock, if known.

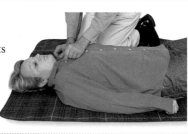

4 MONITOR BREATHING, PULSE, AND RESPONSE

- Monitor and record vital signs – level of response, pulse, and breathing (pp.42–43).
- If the casualty becomes unconscious, open the airway and check breathing (p.252). Be ready to give rescue breaths and chest compressions.

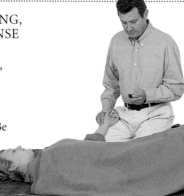

ANAPHYLACTIC SHOCK

▶ See also p.123

RECOGNITION

- Anxiety.
- Red, blotchy skin.
- Swelling of tongue and throat.
- Puffiness around eyes.
- Impaired breathing, possibly with wheezing and gasping for air.
- Signs of shock.

PRECAUTIONS

- Check to see if the casualty is carrying an auto-injector or a syringe of epinephrine (adrenaline). If necessary, assist the casualty to use it. It can save his life when given promptly.

- If the casualty loses consciousness, open the airway and check breathing (p.252). If breathing, place him in the recovery position. Be prepared to give rescue breaths and chest compressions if needed.

ACTION

CALL AMBULANCE

⬇

HELP TO RELIEVE SYMPTOMS

⬇

MONITOR CASUALTY

1 CALL AN AMBULANCE

- Pass on as much information as possible about the cause of the allergy.

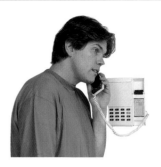

2 HELP TO RELIEVE SYMPTOMS

- Check whether the casualty is carrying a syringe or an auto-injector of epinephrine (adrenaline). Help the casualty to find and use it if necessary.

- Help the casualty to sit in a position that eases any breathing difficulties.

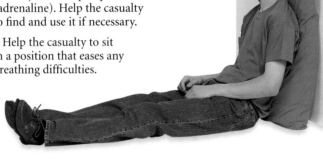

3 MONITOR CASUALTY

- Monitor and record vital signs – level of response, pulse, and breathing (pp.42–43) – until help arrives.

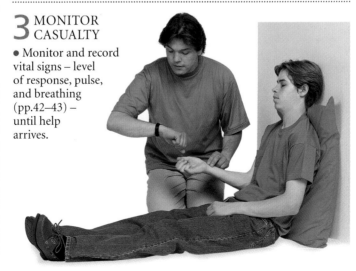

SEVERE BLEEDING

▶ See also pp.130–131

1 APPLY PRESSURE TO WOUND

- Put on gloves if available. Remove or cut any clothing over the wound.
- Place a sterile dressing or non-fluffy pad over the wound. Apply firm pressure with your fingers or the palm of your hand.

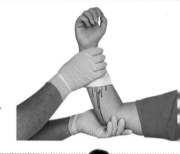

2 RAISE AND SUPPORT INJURED PART

- Raise the injured part above the level of the casualty's heart.
- Handle the injured part gently if you suspect that the injury involves a fracture.
- Help the casualty to lie down.

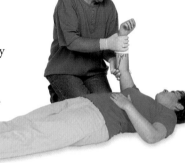

ACTION

APPLY PRESSURE TO WOUND

⬇

RAISE AND SUPPORT INJURED PART

⬇

BANDAGE WOUND

⬇

CALL AMBULANCE

⬇

TREAT FOR SHOCK AND MONITOR CASUALTY

3 BANDAGE WOUND

- Apply a sterile dressing over the pad, and bandage firmly in place.
- Bandage another pad on top if blood seeps through. If blood seeps through the second pad, remove all dressings and apply a fresh one, ensuring that it exerts pressure on the bleeding area.
- Check the circulation beyond the bandages at intervals; loosen them if necessary.

Secure bandage firmly

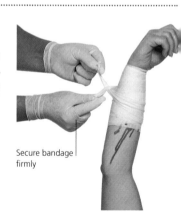

4 CALL AN AMBULANCE

- Give details of the site of the injury and the extent of the bleeding when you telephone.

5 TREAT FOR SHOCK; MONITOR CASUALTY

- Treat for shock (pp.120–121). Monitor and record vital signs – level of response, pulse, and breathing (pp.42–43).

HEART ATTACK

▶ **See also** p.125

RECOGNITION

There may be:

- Vice-like chest pain, spreading to one or both arms.
- Breathlessness.
- Discomfort, like indigestion, in upper abdomen.
- Sudden faintness.
- Sudden collapse.
- Sense of impending doom.
- Ashen skin and blueness at lips.
- Rapid, then weakening, pulse.
- Profuse sweating.

PRECAUTIONS

- Do not give fluids.
- If the casualty loses consciousness, open the airway and check breathing (p.252). Be ready to give rescue breaths and chest compressions if needed.

ACTION

MAKE CASUALTY
COMFORTABLE

⬇

CALL AMBULANCE

⬇

GIVE CASUALTY
ASPIRIN

⬇

MONITOR
CASUALTY

1 MAKE CASUALTY COMFORTABLE

- Help the casualty into a half-sitting position.
- Support his head, shoulders, and knees.
- Reassure the casualty.

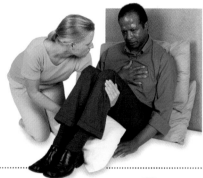

2 CALL AN AMBULANCE

- Tell the controller that you suspect a heart attack.
- Call the casualty's doctor as well, if he asks you to do so.

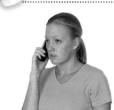

3 GIVE CASUALTY MEDICATION

- If the casualty is conscious, give one tablet of aspirin to be *chewed* slowly.
- If the casualty is carrying tablets or a puffer aerosol for angina, allow him to administer it himself. Help him if necessary.

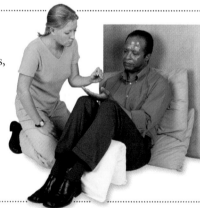

4 MONITOR CASUALTY

- Encourage the casualty to rest. Keep any bystanders at a distance.
- Monitor and record vital signs – level of response, pulse, and breathing (pp.42–43) – until help arrives.

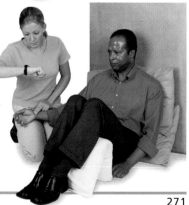

HEAD INJURY

▶ See also p.137 and p.179

RECOGNITION

There may be:
● Head wound.
● Impaired consciousness.

PRECAUTIONS

● Wear gloves, if available, to protect against infection.
● If the casualty loses consciousness, open the airway and check breathing (p.252). If she is breathing, place her in the recovery position. Be ready to give rescue breaths and chest compressions if needed.
● If the bleeding does not stop, re-apply pressure and add a second pad.
● Always suspect the possibility of a neck (spinal) injury (opposite).

ACTION

CONTROL BLEEDING
⬇
SECURE DRESSING WITH BANDAGE
⬇
HELP CASUALTY TO LIE DOWN
⬇
CALL AMBULANCE

1 CONTROL BLEEDING

● Put on disposable gloves if available.

● Replace any displaced skin flaps over the wound.

● Place a sterile dressing or a clean, non-fluffy pad over the wound and apply firm, direct pressure with your hand.

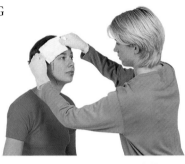

2 SECURE DRESSING WITH BANDAGE

● Secure the dressing over the wound with a roller bandage.

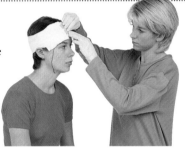

3 HELP CASUALTY TO LIE DOWN

● Ensure that her head and shoulders are slightly raised.
● Make sure that she is comfortable.

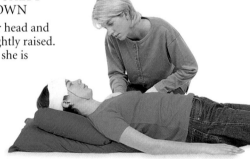

4 CALL AN AMBULANCE

● Monitor and record vital signs – level of response, pulse, and breathing (pp.42–43) – until help arrives.

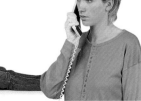

SPINAL INJURY

▶ **See also** pp.165–167

RECOGNITION

- Pain in neck or back.
- A step or twist in the curve of the spine.
- Tenderness over the spine.

There may be:
- Weakness or loss of movement in limbs.
- Loss of sensation, or abnormal sensation.
- Loss of bladder and/or bowel control.
- Difficulty breathing.

PRECAUTIONS

- Do not move the casualty unless she is in danger.
- If the casualty loses consciousness, open the airway by gently lifting the jaw but not tilting the head (*see* SPINAL INJURY, p.167), and check breathing. Put her into the recovery position only if the airway cannot be maintained. Be ready to give rescue breaths and chest compressions if needed.

ACTION

STEADY AND
SUPPORT HEAD

⬇

CALL AMBULANCE

1 STEADY AND SUPPORT HEAD

- Reassure the casualty and tell her not to move.

- Keep the head, neck, and spine aligned by placing your hands on the sides of the head to hold the head still.

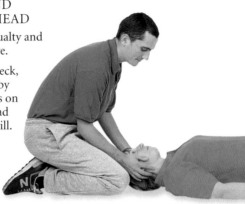

2 SUPPORT CASUALTY'S NECK

- Ask a helper to place rolled towels or other padding around the casualty's neck and shoulders.

- Keep holding her head throughout, until medical help arrives.

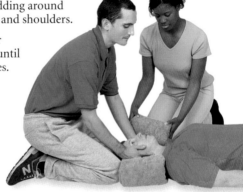

3 CALL AN AMBULANCE

- If possible, ask a helper to call an ambulance and say that a spinal injury is suspected.

- Monitor and record vital signs – level of response, pulse, and breathing (pp.42–43).

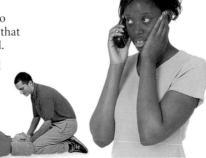

273

SEIZURES IN ADULTS

▶ See also pp.184–185

RECOGNITION

- Sudden loss of consciousness.
- Rigidity and arching of the back.
- Convulsive movements.
- Muscle relaxation.
- Regaining of consciousness.
- Grey–blue tinge to skin.

PRECAUTIONS

- Do not use force to restrain the casualty.
- If the casualty is unconscious for more than 10 minutes, is having repeated seizures, or it is her first seizure, CALL AN AMBULANCE Note the time when the seizure starts and the duration of the seizure.

ACTION

PROTECT
CASUALTY

⬇

PROTECT HEAD AND
LOOSEN TIGHT
CLOTHING

⬇

PLACE CASUALTY
IN RECOVERY
POSITION

⬇

MONITOR
CASUALTY

1 PROTECT CASUALTY

- Try to ease her fall.
- Talk to her calmly and reassuringly.
- Clear away any potentially dangerous objects to prevent injury to the casualty.
- Ask bystanders to keep clear.

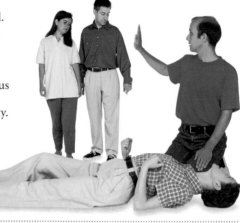

2 PROTECT HEAD AND LOOSEN TIGHT CLOTHING

- If possible, cushion the casualty's head with soft material until the seizures cease.
- Undo any tight clothing around the casualty's neck.

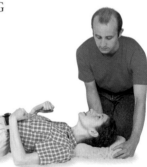

3 PLACE CASUALTY IN RECOVERY POSITION

- Once the seizures have stopped, open the airway and check breathing (p.254); then place the casualty in the recovery position (p.257).
- Monitor and record vital signs – level of response, pulse, and breathing (pp.42–43).

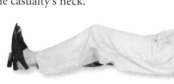

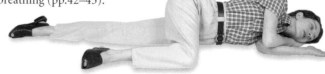

SEIZURES IN CHILDREN

▶ See also p.186

RECOGNITION

- Violent muscle twitching, clenched fists, and arched back.

There may be:
- Fever.
- Twitching of the face.
- Breath-holding.
- Drooling at the mouth.
- Loss of, or impaired, consciousness.

PRECAUTIONS

- Do not let the child become chilled.
- If the child loses consciousness, open the airway and check breathing (p.258, p.262). Be ready to give rescue breaths and chest compressions if needed (p.260, p.263).

ACTION

PROTECT CHILD
FROM INJURY

⬇

COOL CHILD

⬇

SPONGE WITH
TEPID WATER

⬇

PUT CHILD IN
RECOVERY
POSITION

⬇

CALL AMBULANCE;
MONITOR CHILD

1 PROTECT CHILD FROM INJURY

- Clear away any nearby objects.
- Surround the child with soft padding.

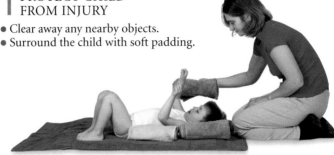

2 COOL CHILD

- Remove his clothing.
- Ensure a good supply of cool air.

3 SPONGE WITH TEPID WATER

- Start at his head and work down.

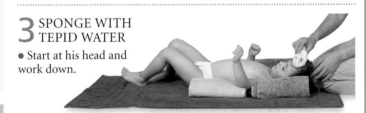

4 PUT CHILD IN RECOVERY POSITION

- Once the seizures have stopped, open the airway and check breathing (p.258, p.262), then put the child in the recovery position (p.261, p.263).

5 CALL AN AMBULANCE AND MONITOR CHILD

- Monitor and record vital signs – level of response, pulse, and breathing (pp.42–43) – until help arrives.

BROKEN BONES

▶ See also pp.150–174

RECOGNITION

- Distortion, swelling, and bruising at the injury site.
- Pain and difficulty in moving the injured part.

There may be:

- Bending, twisting, or shortening of a limb.
- A wound, possibly with bone ends protruding.

PRECAUTIONS

- Do not attempt to bandage the injury if medical assistance is on its way.
- Do not attempt to move an injured limb unnecessarily.
- Do not allow a casualty with a suspected fracture to eat, drink, or smoke.

ACTION

STEADY AND
SUPPORT INJURED
PART

⬇

PROTECT INJURY
WITH PADDING

⬇

TAKE OR SEND
CASUALTY TO
HOSPITAL

1 STEADY AND SUPPORT INJURED PART

- Help the casualty to support the affected part, above and below the injury, in the most comfortable position.

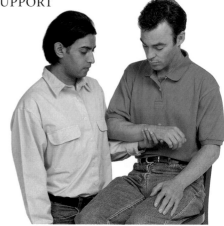

2 PROTECT INJURY WITH PADDING

- Place padding, such as towels or cushions, around the affected part, and support it in position.

- If there is an open wound, cover it with a large, sterile dressing or a clean, non-fluffy pad and bandage it in place (p.231).

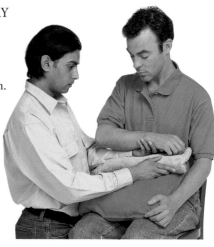

3 TAKE OR SEND CASUALTY TO HOSPITAL

- Call an ambulance if necessary.

- Treat the casualty for shock (p.268).

- Monitor and record vital signs – level of response, pulse, and breathing (pp.42–43).

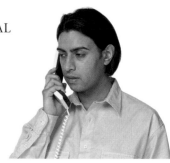

BURNS

▶ See also pp.192–201

RECOGNITION

● Reddened skin.
● Pain in the area of the burn.
● Swelling and blistering of the skin.

PRECAUTIONS

● Do not apply lotions, ointment, or fat to a burn.
● Do not touch the burn or burst any blisters.
● Do not remove anything sticking to the burn.
● If the burn is to the face, do not cover it. Keep cooling with water until help arrives.
● If the burn is caused by chemicals, cool for at least 20 minutes.

ACTION

COOL BURN

REMOVE ANY CONSTRICTIONS

COVER BURN

TAKE OR SEND CASUALTY TO HOSPITAL

1 COOL BURN

● Make the casualty comfortable.
● Pour cold liquid on the burn for at least 10 minutes.
● Watch for signs of smoke inhalation, such as difficulty breathing.

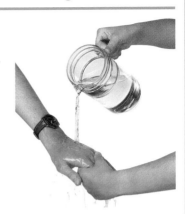

2 REMOVE ANY CONSTRICTIONS

● Put on disposable gloves if available.
● Carefully remove any clothing or jewellery from the area before it starts to swell. However, do not try to remove any clothing that is sticking to the burn.

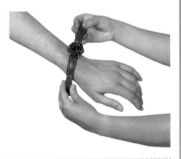

3 COVER BURN

● Cover the burn and the surrounding area with a sterile dressing, clean non-fluffy material, cling film, or a plastic bag.
● Reassure the casualty.

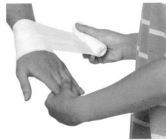

4 TAKE OR SEND CASUALTY TO HOSPITAL

● Call an ambulance if necessary.
● Treat the casualty for shock (p.268).
● Monitor and record vital signs – level of response, pulse, and breathing (pp.42–43).

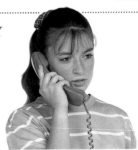

EYE INJURY

▶ **See also** p.138 and pp.200–201

1 SUPPORT CASUALTY'S HEAD

- Lay the casualty on her back, holding her head on your knees to keep it as still as possible.

- Tell the casualty to keep her "good" eye still; movement of the uninjured eye will cause the injured one to move as well, which may damage it further.

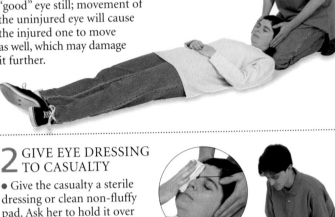

RECOGNITION

- Intense pain in the affected eye.

- Spasm of the eyelids.

There may also be:

- A visible wound.

- A bloodshot eye, even if wound is not visible.

- Partial or total loss of vision.

- Leakage of blood or clear fluid from the injured eye.

2 GIVE EYE DRESSING TO CASUALTY

- Give the casualty a sterile dressing or clean non-fluffy pad. Ask her to hold it over the injured eye and to keep her uninjured eye closed.

- Hold the casualty's head steady.

PRECAUTIONS

- Do not touch the eye or any contact lens in it, and do not allow the casualty to rub the eye.

- Do not try to remove any object embedded in the eye.

- If it will be some time before medical aid is available, bandage an eye pad in place over the injured eye.

3 TAKE OR SEND CASUALTY TO HOSPITAL

- Ensure that the casualty is transported lying down. Call an ambulance if you cannot transport her in the position in which she was treated.

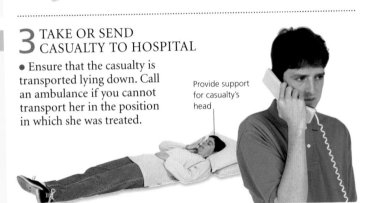

Provide support for casualty's head

ACTION

SUPPORT CASUALTY'S HEAD

⬇

GIVE EYE DRESSING TO CASUALTY

⬇

TAKE OR SEND CASUALTY TO HOSPITAL

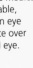

SWALLOWED POISONS

▶ See also p.220

RECOGNITION

- Vomiting that may be bloodstained.
- Impaired consciousness.
- Empty bottles and containers nearby.
- History of ingestion/exposure.
- Pain or burning sensation.

PRECAUTIONS

- Do not attempt to induce vomiting.
- If the casualty loses consciousness, make sure that there is no vomit or other matter in the mouth. Open the airway and check breathing (p.252). Be ready to give rescue breaths and chest compressions if needed.
- When giving rescue breaths, use a face shield or pocket mask for protection if there are chemicals on the casualty's mouth.

ACTION

CHECK WHAT CASUALTY HAS SWALLOWED

⬇

CALL AMBULANCE

⬇

MONITOR CASUALTY

1 CHECK WHAT CASUALTY HAS SWALLOWED

- If the casualty is conscious, ask what she has swallowed and reassure her.

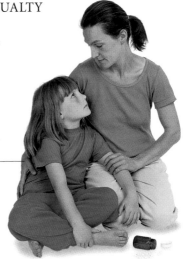

Reassure casualty as you find out what she swallowed

2 CALL AN AMBULANCE

- Give as much information as possible about the swallowed poison. This information will help doctors to give the casualty the appropriate treatment.

- Monitor and record vital signs – level of response, pulse, and breathing (pp.42–43) – until help arrives.

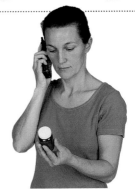

3 IF CASUALTY'S LIPS ARE BURNT

- If the swallowed substance has burnt the casualty's lips, give her frequent sips of cold water or milk.

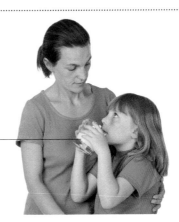

Give casualty cool, soothing drink such as milk

OBSERVATION CHARTS

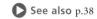 See also p.38

Fill in the following charts every time you attend to a casualty.

- On the first chart, place a dot opposite the appropriate score at each time interval.

- On the second chart, tick the appropriate pulse and breathing rates at each interval.
- The completed form should stay with the casualty when he leaves your care.

LEVEL OF RESPONSE CHART

DATE.............................CASUALTY'S NAME...

OBSERVATION	RESPONSE/SCORE	Time of observation (minutes)					
		0	10	20	30	40	50
Eyes Observe for reaction while testing other responses.	Open spontaneously 4 Open to speech 3 Open to painful stimulus 2 No response 1						
Speech When testing responses, speak clearly and directly, close to casualty's ear.	Responds sensibly to questions 5 Seems confused 4 Uses inappropriate words 3 Incomprehensible sounds 2 No response 1						
Movement Apply painful stimulus: pinch ear lobe or skin on back of hand.	Obeys commands 6 Points to pain 5 Withdraws from painful stimulus 4 Bends limbs in response to pain 3 Straightens limbs in response to pain 2 No response 1						
	TOTAL SCORE						

PULSE AND BREATHING CHECK CHART

DATE.............................CASUALTY'S NAME...

PULSE/BREATHING	RATE	Time of observation (minutes)					
		0	10	20	30	40	50
Pulse **(beats per minute)** Take pulse at wrist or at neck on adult, or at inner arm on baby (p.42). Note the rate, and whether beats are weak (w) or strong (s), regular (reg) or irregular (irreg).	Over 110						
	101–110						
	91–100						
	81–90						
	71–80						
	61–70						
	Below 61						
Breathing **(breaths per minute)** Note rate, and whether breathing is quiet (q) or noisy (n), easy (e) or difficult (diff).	Over 40						
	31–40						
	21–30						
	11–20						
	Below 11						

INDEX

285

For my parents

Acknowledgements

Huge thanks to everyone at Random House for all their work but especially to Gillian Holmes for her brilliant editing and support.

Thanks as ever to my wonderful agent Maggie Hanbury and her team. I am so glad and grateful to have you.

The life of a writer can be quite solitary, so thank you to all my friends for keeping me sane. Thank you to Alison, Nic and Tristan for giving me the idea of having a table tennis scene in this novel and reminding me of how much I love the game. But be warned I will beat you all very soon... Above all thanks to my family, my fantastic children, Joe, Amelie, Lola and to my very patient husband Julian, I couldn't do it without you. Lunch @ Bills is on me!

Chapter 1

Tor

Pregnant. Tor stared at the test in disbelief. She had been so convinced that the words **Not Pregnant** would pop up. It must be a mistake. It *had* to be a mistake. These tests weren't always right, were they? In the words of that irritatingly perky slogan that had suddenly appeared everywhere and on everything like a rash, she needed to keep calm and carry on. Even if panic and freak out seemed the more appropriate response. But she forced herself to re-read the instructions. 99 per cent accurate. She checked the tiny screen again and this time noticed the numbers 8–10. The bloody know-it-all test was even telling her how many weeks pregnant she was! She was surprised there wasn't another message pointing out the place and time of conception.

For a moment she struggled to think when that

could have been but then she remembered. It had to have been the night of her friend Spencer's annual fancy dress party – always notoriously drunken affairs, and she had got drunk. Very drunk. When she finally staggered home, minus her feather boa – she had gone as a flapper, or should that be slapper? – she had made a booty call to Ed. She had a vague recollection that a condom was not involved. But that wasn't supposed to matter as the chances of her conceiving were so remote . . . What was it that bastard doctor had told her two years ago? 'More chance of winning the lottery than getting pregnant naturally.' She had changed GP after that cruelly insensitive comment.

She wrapped the test in loo roll, and stuffed it to the bottom of the bin. Catching sight of her reflection in the mirror, she paused. She still looked the same, but felt as if she had been transported to another planet. The Planet Pregnant. Surely this could not be happening to her. She'd always had irregular periods, thanks to having polycystic ovaries, which was why the fact she hadn't had one in ages hadn't bothered her . . . until she started feeling nauseous. Very nauseous.

There was knock at the door. 'Tor, the taxi's here,' Ed called out.

Fuck! What was she going to do? She and Ed had only been seeing each other for five months. Five months – that was nothing in the scheme of things. And by 'seeing' she meant having sex. A lot of sex.

After a series of relationships that had either spectacularly crashed and burned or pathetically petered out, Tor finally thought she had got it all mapped out. She was the successful older woman, thirty-four – a cougar according to her friends, who made no attempt to hide how jealous they were of her and her twenty-four-year-old boyfriend. Not only was Ed a looker, turning heads wherever they went, he was a genuinely lovely guy. He was easily one of the nicest men Tor had ever known. They had never had a single row. He was also so laidback it was a miracle he ever managed to get anything done. He didn't have a bean to his name. He wanted to be a computer games designer, but had had no luck so far in getting a job and lived in a shared house. But that shouldn't matter because their affair was only supposed to be a bit of fun, light relief after her last relationship – three years of Horrid Harry – with a man who had systematically undermined her confidence and self-esteem. Now it seemed Mother Nature had put her foot down and decided enough was enough on the enjoyment front. *Fuck!* What was she going to do?

She and Ed were about to on their first holiday together, two weeks on a Greek island, with a group of friends as Tor was worried that it would be too intense on their own and she didn't want to put any pressure on him. She had never even spent the night at Ed's because it was too much like a student house. The one time she went round there for a

3

drink she clocked that the sink was full of washing up, it looked as if no one had cleaned the fridge *ever,* and the hallway was cluttered up with bikes. Tor did the student thing a long time ago and didn't want to do it again.

She had recently bought Ed a toothbrush for when he stayed over at her place, but every time she saw it next to hers in the bathroom she wondered if that was going a step too far . . . and now this.

Suddenly a wave of nausea rushed through her. Abandoning her position in front of the mirror, she bent over the loo and spectacularly and noisily threw up her breakfast of toast and coffee.

Please don't let Ed have heard. Though as the sound reverberated around the bathroom and he was next door in the bedroom that seemed unlikely. As if on cue he called out, 'Are you okay, Tor?'

She wiped her mouth and croaked back, 'Yes, it must have been something I ate.' She couldn't tell him the truth now. She would have to choose her moment. As they were about to drive to Gatwick airport and board a plane, this wasn't it.

Ed was sweet to her in the taxi, trying to take her mind off feeling sick and making sure she sipped mineral water. She thought of Harry, who probably wouldn't even have noticed, or if he had would have thought it incredibly inconsiderate of her to feel unwell on the first day of the holiday. *His* holiday. Ed was nothing like that.

She had asked him out for a dare. She and

her best friends Leila and Frankie had been out in Brighton, having cocktails to celebrate her birthday at the swanky Hotel du Vin. They were all dressed up and already slightly squiffy after sinking a bottle of champagne at her flat. Ed had been working behind the bar. He had been very flirtatious when he'd served her but she put that down to his barman patter, all part of the service and nothing personal.

'So where's your boyfriend taking you tonight?' he had asked, smiling and showing off perfect white teeth.

'No boyfriend. Out with the girls for my birthday. Nice teeth by the way. Like American teeth. Are they real?'

Ed laughed. 'Yep, well, that's what three years of intensive orthodontistry will do for you. You should have seen me in the brace . . . not such a good look. I like yours – that pointed eye tooth, it's cool.'

'Why, thank you,' she replied, then added cheekily, 'I sharpen it every night on the flesh of young men.' *What! Where had that comment come from?*

'Sounds promising. I'm available later. I'm Ed by the way. Happy birthday.'

Embarrassment had suddenly overtaken Tor. Just how old was he? Not young enough to be her son obviously, that really would be too weird, but she reckoned there could be ten years between them. Time to play the dignified card. She slid off the bar

5

stool, as elegantly as she could. 'I'm Tor, and I'd better get back to my friends.'

'I'll bring your drinks over,' Ed told her, treating her to another grin.

Back at their table Frankie and Leila had been blatantly checking him out. 'What were you talking to hot boy about?' Frankie demanded.

'His teeth.'

'Is that your best chat-up line? God, you're even rustier than I thought, you need an intervention.' Frankie, blunt as always.

'He was a bit flirty, wasn't he?' Leila put in, still looking over at Ed. 'Sexy forearms.' She sighed. 'I remember that was one of the first things I noticed about Tom.'

Tor wondered why her friend sounded so wistful; as far as she knew Tom was still in possession of those sexy forearms.

'I'm sure he flirts with all the ladies and selected gentlemen – it must be part of the job description. He told me he was available later. Cheeky monkey.' Tor didn't mention her own provocative comment.

'Cheeky hot-to-trot monkey! You should give him your number,' Frankie replied. Fearless Frankie, who was not afraid of any situation; teaching teenagers English in a comprehensive had given her the hide of a rhino.

Tor had been aghast. 'No way! I'm too old for him. It's tacky.'

Frankie had shrugged at this, 'So what? You only

live once. One day you'll be lying in the ground dead and the only things having their wicked way with you will be worms.'

'Ugh! Frankie, do you have to?'

'Sorry, I'm doing the Metaphysical Poets with my A-level group. All those men urging their women to jump into bed with them before the inevitable death robs them of any chance of a shag, has rubbed off on me. But seriously, Victoria.'

Tor prepared herself for the lecture to come, Frankie only ever called her Victoria when she was going to tell her what to do.

'Seriously, you should ask him out. You broke up with Harry . . . what is it? Nine months ago. You should get out there again. Not every man is like him. Thank God! Otherwise we would all be lesbians – not that there's anything wrong with that, but still. Go on, I dare you.'

'He looks really nice.' That came from Leila. She was always the voice of reason in their trio. And she was the one who seemed to have her own life sorted. Married to Tom, with a daughter, and also a fantastic career with her own radio production company specialising in dramas. When Tor grew up she wanted to be like Leila.

'Nice!' Frankie exploded. 'Tor needs someone who is going to give her the shag of a lifetime, to make up for the last three years of misery.'

'He could be nice and a good shag,' Leila persisted. 'The two things aren't mutually exclusive.'

7

Tor couldn't resist glancing over at the bar where Ed was busy mixing their drinks. He caught her eye as he was shaking the cocktail maker, and smiled. Leila was right; he did look nice. And sexy. And interested. Three things that Harry definitely hadn't been after their first year together. She smiled back.

'Anyway, it's present time. Happy birthday, you old slapper!' Frankie leant across and gave Tor a big hug before handing her a pink gift box from Agent Provocateur.

'It's from both of us,' Leila added, also giving her a hug. 'You can take it back if you don't like it.' Ever practical Leila.

'Ooh-là-là! Fancy!' Tor exclaimed, untying the black ribbon and opening the box to reveal a black satin camisole trimmed with lace, and matching briefs . . . at the exact moment that Ed arrived with the tray of drinks. Tor waited for him to make a suggestive comment but he was the model of decorum, simply placing their cocktails on the table and saying politely, 'Enjoy your drinks, ladies.'

So that was that then, Tor thought, watching him walk back to the bar, admiring his broad shoulders and feeling slightly deflated. The flirting had been part of his barman act, she was right. She shouldn't have taken it personally. But then he turned and, looking straight at her, blew her a kiss. It didn't feel as if he was leering or trying it on or that he did that to all the girls. It felt like a sweet gesture, meant just for her. At that moment she decided that she would ask him out.

And so just before they headed off to the restaurant she left the others waiting in the foyer and ran back as swiftly as her four-inch heels would allow, and handed Ed a piece of paper with her number on it and the message: *Call me if you fancy going out for a drink later Tor x*

He had rung when they were eating their desserts. By then she had convinced herself that he wasn't going to, and that she had made a complete tit of herself by propositioning him, and so she was going to have sticky toffee pudding and to hell with it. She might even order the *tiramisù* as well. It was her birthday and she would stuff her face if she wanted to. She shouldn't have run back to the bar it had looked too keen, she should have sauntered over. Or better still, not gone at all. She was never going to ask anyone out face to face ever again. She would use an online dating service if she needed to, safe behind her computer screen, in control.

'Now that's what I call a *real* dessert,' Frankie teased her once she had arranged to meet Ed and abandoned the sticky toffee pudding. 'Glad to know that the birthday lingerie will be getting an outing.'

'I'm not going to have sex with him! I've never had sex with someone on the first date. We're just having a drink,' Tor had protested. And had fully intended to stick to that resolution.

9

But within a few minutes of meeting Ed in a bar she'd realised that she absolutely didn't just want to have a drink with him. She absolutely wanted to have sex with him, as soon as she possibly could. So after they had flirted outrageously, she had asked him back to her place where they'd had the most fantastically good sex. Twice. Once without the birthday lingerie, once with . . .

She hadn't expected to see him again, thinking that it was simply an experience, something to tick off, sex with a fit twenty-four-year-old. In the morning she had woken up to find the bed next to her empty, which had confirmed her view that Ed was strictly for one night only. However, when she got up and padded into the kitchen to make herself a cup of tea as a consolation, and a poor consolation at that, she discovered that he had been out and bought provisions and was busy making scrambled egg and smoked salmon. In three years Harry had never made her breakfast, and she could probably count the numbers of cups of tea he had made her on one hand. And then Ed had asked her if she was free that night. For a split second she wondered if she should play it cool, hard to get, but there was Ed so open and warm. So yes had been the only possible reply. Since then they had pretty much seen each other every day. It was a private joke that he had been working as a waiter in a cocktail bar when she met him . . . But Tor had always secretly hoped that their relationship worked out better than the one in the song, because she really did want him.

She looked across at him in the taxi. Ed was around six foot tall, with light brown hair and dark green eyes. He still had that bloom of youth so, however knackered or hungover he was, he always looked good. He was way too young to be a dad. Men who were as young and good-looking as Ed were only ever dads in Calvin Klein adverts, photographed bare-chested on a beach, carrying their adorable offspring on their broad shoulders, while holding hands with their beautiful slender young wife, who most definitely didn't have child-bearing hips. The baby news would blow Ed's mind. It was not the right time for him to become a father. When Tor was his age all her energy was focused on building up her business and going out with her friends. She could take off to Paris or New York or anywhere at a moment's notice – the fact that she didn't wasn't the point. Anything was possible; she didn't have to answer to anyone. A baby would change everything.

Ed caught her looking at him, and smiled. 'Feeling better?'

Somehow she managed a 'yes'.

'And you're sure that I don't need to give Leila and Tom something for the villa?'

That was one of the many things she liked about him: he always tried to pay his way, even though he earned hardly anything. Harry would have been

11

thinking, *Result, free holiday,* and would have offered nothing.

She shook her head, 'Nope. We'll all share the food bills and pay towards the electricity but Leila says her parents don't want any money. They're very generous like that. I've been there several times with Frankie and Leila, and they would never accept anything.'

'Must be nice, owning a villa on a Greek island. Do Leila and Tom go there a lot?'

'Leila's been too busy to go much recently. This is the first time they've been in two years. She had to cancel their holiday last year as a project came up that she couldn't turn down.'

Ed frowned. 'That doesn't sound good on the work/life balance.'

'No, it doesn't.'

For a few minutes Tor stopped obsessing about the baby news and Ed, and thought about her friends. She knew that they were going through a bad patch in their marriage, knew it from nights spent with Leila pouring her heart out over a bottle of wine . . . knew it and wished it weren't so. She had always thought that Leila and Tom were the perfect couple, not in a smug married way, but in the way that they complemented each other, seemed so right together. If they were having problems, what hope was there for anyone else?

Chapter 2

Leila

*Have you told him yet? We can't go on like this,
Leila. I have to see you x*

Fuck! Not this. Not now. Not again. Leila hastily
deleted the text. She had already sent several
messages and left a voicemail telling Jasper in no
uncertain terms that what had happened between
them was a mistake. A one-off. That it was never
going to happen again. Ever. But he seemed
obsessed with her and wouldn't stop sending her
texts. She folded her arms, feeling as if her space
had been violated.

'Mummy, I'm hungry,' Gracie piped up from
the back seat. They'd been driving all of ten
minutes.

Leila looked over at Tom, 'Did you pack a snack
for her?'

13

He shook his head. 'I thought we could get something at the airport.'

'We'll be ages checking in and going through security . . . you know how long the queues will be! Would it have killed you to put in some rice cakes?' She knew she was snapping, even though she had promised herself that she wouldn't.

'Would it have killed you?' Tom replied evenly. 'And I thought you were going to switch your phone off? You promised. It's a holiday. It's supposed to be family time. Remember?' His tone was less even now, more than a hint of bitterness to it. This was the beginning of a well-rehearsed row. *Here we go, here we go, here we go . . .*

'I am. It's only on in case Tor or Frankie need to get hold of us. As soon as we meet up I'm switching it off, I promise.'

Tom looked sceptical. It was ironic because Leila actually wished that she could throw the wretched BlackBerry out of the window and watch it smash into smithereens on the A23. The thought of her husband stumbling across one of the texts from Jasper made her feel physically sick. She opened the window a couple of inches, needing some air.

'I'm hungry,' Gracie's voice again. The persistence of a four-and-a-half-year-old took some beating.

Leila rootled around in her handbag and came up with a half-full box of raisins which she handed to Gracie, ignoring her daughter's protests that raisins were 'Yuck'.

'I'll buy you a chocolate croissant at the airport, I promise.' *I promise* – Leila was aware that she overused that phrase.

She looked out of the window, staring blankly at the countryside. Their first family holiday in ages. Briefly she closed her eyes. *Please let everything be all right. Please let Jasper not get in touch again.* She couldn't believe how stupid she had been in getting involved with him. Stupid and selfish. She hated herself for it.

How could she have done such a thing? How could she have ended up in a hotel room with a man she now realised she didn't even particularly like. How could she?

But she forced herself to be honest. She knew why. She was worn down with feeling unhappy in her marriage, with Tom not communicating with her and being so closed off. She was worn out with feeling like the bad guy who was always nagging. She felt unloved and unwanted. It felt as if their marriage had flatlined. So when she met Jasper, who had written the drama she was directing, who was charming, entertaining and upfront about his attraction to her, it was dangerously easy to be flattered. He made her feel alive again, sexy, interesting, as if she what she had to say was worth hearing.

It should have stopped with flirtation, but one night when they were on location together it went further. It had happened over two months ago but Leila still felt raw with guilt. She had trouble sleeping as every time she closed her eyes the replay started up in her head. The anonymous expensive hotel room with its muted colours, the mocha-coloured leather headboard, the cream Egyptian cotton sheets. Jasper, his shirt unbuttoned. Slightly drunk. Too much Sauvignon Blanc. Kissing. More wine. And then on the bed in a tangle of limbs that felt wrong in spite of the wine. She didn't feel alive again, sexy and interesting. She felt cheap, in the wrong place, at the wrong time, with the wrong man. She remembered the feeling of Jasper lying on top of her, how much she'd wanted it to be over, the smell of his musky aftershave that seemed to catch in her throat, his smooth hairless chest that made her feel slightly queasy as she wondered if he waxed it. She remembered how she had waited until he was asleep before slipping back to her hotel room, running along the thickly carpeted corridor and feeling the guilt seeping out of every pore. How she had spent ages in the shower. After that night she had stopped wearing her favourite perfume, Chanel No. 5, and drinking her favourite wine. Their association with what she'd done had been too strong.

What had happened to her marriage? To her? When she had stood up in front of all her family and friends at their wedding and declared her love for Tom, she had meant it. Their relationship had seemed so strong, unbreakable. She had broken it

. . . The question she didn't yet know the answer to was whether it was beyond repair or whether she could mend it.

'Tor has offered to babysit so we can go out for dinner,' Tom's voice cut across her thoughts. 'That will be a novelty, won't it? I can't even remember the last time we went out together.'

'It was your birthday, three months ago.'

A disaster. They had gone out on their own to an expensive restaurant and Leila had felt trapped and stifled and as if she had nothing to say to him. That they were strangers. It was at the height of her flirtation with Jasper and he was all she could think of, that and knowing that she would have to have sex with Tom when they got home. Have to. And didn't want to. It didn't feel like they were ever going to get their old intimacy back, where sex was sometimes tender and passionate, sometimes erotic, a quick shag at others, but it had never mattered because of their connection. Now she wanted to get it over and done with as soon as possible and she had practically leapt on him the moment the bedroom door was shut. Which would have been funny if it hadn't felt so sad.

Afterwards Tom had simply said, 'It would have been nice to take a bit longer. I felt as if you were ticking me off your to-do list. And you didn't enjoy it, did you?'

Her denial had sounded so unconvincing. She had pretended to be tired and then, as happened

17

increasingly often, had lain awake for hours, thinking about Jasper, feeling guilty, mourning what she had lost with Tom.

Her husband changed the subject then and asked her if she had packed the laptop lead. Clearly he too remembered how grim his birthday night had been. Leila reached across and tentatively rubbed his shoulder. 'I'm so glad we're all going away together. Sorry I've been so crap with work and everything.' *Sorry I broke our marriage vows and shagged someone else. Sorry.*

'We definitely need this time. I feel as if we've been leading separate lives, and that we just happen to share a house and a daughter.'

Leila pretended to be looking for something else in her handbag and muttered, 'Yeah.' She knew perfectly well why they had not been connecting.

They were both silent for a few minutes. Leila remembered holidays in the past where they were both so excited on their way to the airport, thrilled with the prospect of all that free time stretching before them, thrilled to be together. Admittedly 'thrilled and excited' best described her reaction rather than Tom's, who'd always played his cards close to his chest and wasn't given to big displays of emotion. But she had known that he was every bit as happy as her. Now they were cautious and wary of each other.

'So have you told Frankie yet that Matt is coming?' Tom broke the silence.

18

'No, and I'm not going to until we're there. You know what she's like. More than capable of refusing to get on the plane. Anyway, it's been two and a half years since they met. Surely that's enough time for her to have got over it. Whatever it was.'

Leila still had no idea why Frankie had taken such a dislike to Tom's best friend Matt. Before the two of them met, she had been convinced that they would get on well together. Just before her wedding she had invited the pair of them round to dinner. She'd fully expected to have a lovely evening with good conversation and banter, and had a sneaky suspicion that Frankie and Matt would hit it off. But Frankie had been offhand and at times downright rude to Matt, for no apparent reason.

Tom grinned. 'Well, just to give you the heads up, I'll say it was all your idea. I know what Frankie is like when she's pissed off.'

'Coward,' Leila teased back, relieved that at least they could share this.

'Yep, and I'm not afraid to admit it where Frankie's concerned. She can be bloody terrifying! She's had all that practice bollocking teenagers, and she can do that special, withering Frankie stare that makes you feel you want to confess you've done something wrong, even when you haven't. So is she seeing anyone at the moment?'

Leila sighed. 'No, she still claims that she doesn't want a relationship, that she's too busy with work. I think she has the odd fling, but no one she ever lets into the rest of her life, and no one she ever introduces to me and Tor. She is the queen of compartmentalising. I don't think it's healthy.'

Instantly Leila felt disloyal for discussing Frankie, who was bright and witty, and spiky and sarcastic, and infuriating and generous, and just about the best friend, along with Tor, that she had ever had. They had been friends since meeting at university, nearly fourteen years ago. She just wanted Frankie to be happy. Her friend deserved to be happy after what had happened . . . deserved it more than most.

Chapter 3

Frankie

Frankie peeled off her running gear and flung it into the laundry basket. She checked her watch. Shit! She was going to be late unless she pulled her finger out. She took a shower in record time. Going for her usual four-mile run this morning hadn't been such a good idea, but she knew that she would have felt guilty if she hadn't and that would have put her on edge for the rest of the day.

She had to run every day – whether it was Christmas Day, New Year's Day, her birthday. And she ran whatever the weather. When it snowed last December she'd walked three miles to the gym, run six miles on the treadmill, and then walked three miles back. She recognised it as obsessive behaviour bordering on OCD, but she couldn't help it. She needed to run, it kept her head clear.

Out of the shower, she pulled on black denim

shorts, a black silk t-shirt, and slipped on a pair of black wedge sandals. Frankie invariably wore black. Even her nails were painted jet black. She knew that Tor would roll her eyes as soon as she saw her at the airport. Tor adored colour, the brighter the better, and had long been waging a losing battle with Frankie, trying to get her to abandon black. 'But it's me,' Frankie would tell her. 'Black is my colour.'

She didn't know if Patrick was going to be on their flight or not, but even though time was tight and it was only seven in the morning she took longer than usual on her make-up, applied a flick of black eyeliner to give her a sultry look, lashings of mascara and red lipstick, which she then rubbed off to give her lips a just-kissed appearance. Would that do? Would it be good enough to make an impact on him?

She surveyed herself critically in the mirror. Frankie always looked at herself critically. She had relentlessly dieted and worked her body into a size eight, and even though she was now in her thirties and could see the faint etching of lines under her eyes, and was well aware that the slimmer she was, the more likely she was to develop lines, she *had* to have this body. Patrick had once told her that she had a perfect body. And so the perfect size eight was how her body had to remain, all ready for when Patrick finally realised that they should be together.

Patrick. Handsome, charming, exasperating,

captivating Patrick; Patrick, with whom she had been in love for the last three years. Any other woman would have accepted defeat long ago, because although he flirted with Frankie, there was no sign that his feelings ran deeper. Besides, Patrick flirted with most women, it was a reflex action with him. But Frankie wasn't any other woman. She had been blessed, or rather cursed, with an iron will and she couldn't give up on her love for him. She was fiercely logical about everything else in her life, but not this.

She had kept her feelings secret from her friends, having a sixth sense that they would tell her that she was wasting her time; that she was too good for him; that he would never commit to anyone. Only Matt Cartwright knew, and she was hardly likely to see him again.

She had first met Patrick at Tom's thirtieth birthday. He wasn't with anyone and had just split up from his girlfriend. She hadn't had a relationship since Ross and seriously doubted that she would ever be ready for another. But she was instantly drawn to Patrick. His looks undoubtedly helped as he was half-Italian, with deep brown eyes and olive skin, outstandingly handsome with a wicked grin. It had felt all the better that he was a complete physical contrast to Ross. But it wasn't just about his appearance. Patrick was funny, irreverent, and didn't seem to care what people thought of him – again a complete contrast to Ross. Yet beneath the witty banter and the striking looks, Frankie was sure she detected a disarming vulnerability. At half-past one in the morning, when it was just the two of them left sitting at Leila's kitchen table sharing the last bottle of red wine, she found out why as he talked about his mother dying when he was ten, and how his father had remarried within a year and a half and had another child. How he'd never felt like he belonged in the new family his father had created. It was a compelling combination, the beautiful man with the broken past who needed rescuing but didn't know it. She would rescue him, put him back together again.

And then as they said goodbye they had kissed, a kiss that even three years on still had the power to stop Frankie in her tracks . . . a kiss that she thought was the beginning of something more. But Patrick had unexpectedly pulled away, had said with a wry smile that he'd promised Tom to be on his best behaviour with Leila's friends. Usually Frankie would have admired someone for keeping a promise. Not in this instance.

There had never been any repetition of the kiss and it was never mentioned between them. Instead they had become good friends, meeting in London for trips to the theatre, to film premieres, to gigs, to exhibition openings in hip places like Hoxton and Shoreditch. Patrick was a journalist on a glossy men's magazine and was always on the guest list to the latest events. He told Frankie that she was his one true female friend, the one woman he could confide in, be himself with; that it was such a relief to spend time with her, that the women he had relationships with always wanted something from him, always wanted to know what he was thinking, always wanted to own him.

'They fucking drive me mad, Frankie!' he would exclaim. 'It's like blackbirds pecking away at my head! Want, want, want! Why can't they see that I've got nothing more to give!'

I would be different, she longed to tell him. *I would just want you as you are.* But there had never seemed to be the right moment to come out with that, until now. Two whole weeks on a Greek island with no other distractions. Patrick had recently split up with his girlfriend, an incredibly beautiful, incredibly annoying model, with the incredibly annoying name of Willow – which there was no excuse for as she wasn't even American. Surely the timing was perfect. Admittedly they would be surrounded by their closest friends and a small child, but Frankie imagined the pair of them taking off together to a deserted beach, Patrick realising that all this time he had been in love with her . . . It was a fantasy that had been sustaining her for a good few months now.

She picked up her suitcase and swung her bag over her shoulder while she took one last look at her living room. When she returned, everything could be different. She could be with Patrick at last.

Chapter 4

Tor

The departure hall at Gatwick airport was heaving with people. Tor took one look at the hordes as she and Ed walked through the automatic doors and half wanted to do a runner back to the taxi, go home and back to bed. The idea of a holiday was becoming less appealing to her with every passing second. Under the unforgiving bright lights, she experienced a fresh wave of nausea and felt unpleasant prickles of sweat under her arms. It would be a miracle if she managed to board the plane without throwing up . . . most probably in the Tesco bag she had shoved in her handbag at the last minute. Needing to remind herself that she was, in spite of how she felt, a sophisticated thirty-something, she reached for her travel-size bottle of Jo Malone's Pomegranate Noir and sprayed some on her wrists. But the spicy, intense fragrance she usually adored smelt alien, as if some other woman should be wearing it.

'Bloody hell! It's rammed,' Ed commented, scanning the information screen. 'It looks like we're in Zone A.'

'Can you see any of the others?' Tor asked, trying not to think about how bad she felt.

'Yep – Tom and Leila are over there. Come on, let's join them.'

Tor trailed after him as he purposefully steered the trolley through the crowds.

Leila seemed stressed, Tor thought as soon as she saw her friend, even though she hugged both of them and said perkily, 'Happy holidays!'

'Remind me why we're going away in peak school holiday time again?' Tom asked, looking appalled by the sheer number of people surrounding them.

'Because it's the only time Frankie can come away, and because our daughter is starting school in September,' Leila explained patiently.

'She's only four, it's hardly going to prevent her from going on to university if she misses the first week of school.'

Leila raised her eyebrows at Tor as she replied, 'It will make settling in harder for her, and anyway there is no way Frankie could take time off then and I really wanted her to come. She needs a good holiday.'

'Perish the thought that the three of us might have gone away on our own,' Tom muttered quietly, but not so quietly that Tor didn't hear. She liked Tom very much, but he could have a very dry sense of humour and whereas Leila was a glass half-full type, Tom's was half-empty. Their contrasting ways of looking at the world had always complemented each other until recently – now they seemed to grate on each other.

Leila shrugged and rearranged her white pashmina around her shoulders. She was as effortlessly elegant as ever in a simple navy linen dress, and made everyone else look scruffy. She couldn't help it, she was just born that way. Leila was stunning. Her mother was Indian and her father Danish, which had given her striking blue-green eyes, fine features and silky jet black hair. She was also the most generous person Tor knew and wore her beauty lightly, always complimenting everyone else on their looks, never seeming to realise how beautiful she herself was.

'I'm hungry. When can we get the chocolate croissant?' Gracie demanded. Leila rolled her eyes and Tor guessed that this was not the first time this morning that question had been put to her parents.

'Soon,' Tom replied, as he checked through the boarding passes and passports.

'You told me that before!' she retorted.

'And when you get it, are you going to give me a bit?' Ed bent down to talk to the little girl.

'Do I have to?' Gracie replied, put out by the suggestion.

28

'Just a teeny-tiny crumb?' Ed comically scrunched up his face and looked to be on the verge of tears. 'I love chocolate croissants, they are my all-time favourites.'

'Maybe two crumbs,' Gracie conceded, while Leila looked ready to buy Ed a boxful of chocolate croissants for appeasing her daughter.

It was sweet of him to spend time with Gracie, Tor thought as she watched Ed perform some elaborate high-five ritual with the little girl that had her in fits of giggles. He was just being nice because of the free holiday. After all, what was a few minutes' banter with a tiny person if you were going to be staying in a five-star villa?

Or twenty minutes, as Ed took it on himself to be Gracie's chief entertainer as they waited in the queue, making sure that she never slipped into annoying whine mode. Not that she often did that. As young children went, Gracie was pretty chilled, though she did share Tom's unpredictable temper. Indeed, compared to all the other children Tor observed, Gracie was a shining paragon.

Several places in front of them in the queue a toddler was having a full-scale tantrum meltdown. His screams were piercing and relentless. Tor felt the onset of a blinding headache. *Please don't let him be on their flight.* But knowing her luck, he would be in the row behind and kick her seat with his chubby little legs for the entire journey. There was a fifteen-year-old boy behind her listening to his iPod, the slogan on his t-shirt reading *Your lips keep moving but all I hear is blah-blah-blah,* who looked as if he wanted to be anywhere else but here beside his family, and who, in accordance with the slogan on his t-shirt, had ignored every single comment from his harassed mum. In the parallel queue was a couple with twin boys of around six months. Both parents looked unbelievably knackered and weighed down with bags of child-related paraphernalia. It was perhaps shallow of Tor to be thinking along these lines, given that a baby was a wonderful thing, but she found herself wondering if they'd had sex since they'd had the twins. Probably not. Even if they had the inclination, they didn't look as if they would have the energy.

Was this queue trying to tell her something about parenthood? That you somehow survived the baby years and the terrible twos, though your relationship took a battering, and at the end of it all you ended up with a sullen teenager who didn't want to talk to you?

If she had this baby, would this be her this time next year? Looking totally stressed at the check-in, as if all she longed to do was collapse into bed and sleep for a month. And she would be on her own, of course. She couldn't imagine Ed staying with her and playing not-so-happy families.

He broke off from entertaining Gracie. Putting his arm around Tor, he murmured, 'This is momentous, isn't it? Our first holiday together. I never believed it was going to happen until I saw my boarding pass.'

'I thought you might have other plans with your young friends.' There was a lot of this teasing and bantering about age in their relationship – from Tor. Not from Ed, it never seemed to bother him. She was always acutely aware of the age gap, and never more so than when she met his friends. It wasn't the men who bothered her, but the terrifyingly young women. A couple of weeks ago she and Frankie had joined Ed and his friends at their local pub quiz. It wasn't exactly Tor's idea of a good night out, but she figured she should make the effort for Ed.

'Those bitches aren't even wearing make-up!' Frankie had whispered, 'Just look at their skin. It's peachy perfect. I hate them all! I hope they all get acne in middle age.' A sentiment with which Tor had to force herself not to agree. Especially when the girl sitting next to Ed, Ruby something, who he knew from university, got up and showed off an enviably flat stomach, in, of all things, a crop top. It wasn't as if Tor wanted to wear a crop top. She had always thought that they were an evil fashion invention designed to make all women feel as bad as they possibly could about their bodies. There was no way on this earth that she could ever wear one; with her curves it would be more of a flab top. Ed didn't even give Ruby of the flat stomach a second glance, but that hadn't stopped Tor from

31

vowing never to do another pub quiz with them ever again.

And then there was the brief meeting she'd had with Ed's ex-girlfriend, Anise, a leggy blonde who was German and scarily good-looking. She and Ed had been walking by the sea one Sunday morning when Anise rollerbladed by – a vision in white denim shorts and long black socks, showing off a flash of tanned, toned thigh and perfect pert bum. Tor supposed it would have been too much to ask that Ed's ex was short, fat and ugly with a massive arse and a moustache . . . or failing that someone who, although pretty, didn't look like a German supermodel. Anise had been perfectly friendly, with no hint that she still harboured feelings for him, but all the same Tor had been relieved when Ed told her that the other girl was going back to Berlin. Pity it hadn't been Australia . . . but it would have to do.

Ed kissed her. 'My friends are too broke to go abroad. Dougie and Ruby went camping in Cornwall last week and it rained every single day. Dougie thought he had developed trench foot and Ruby got a stinking cold.'

She was probably wearing the crop top, so to be fair it served her right.

'It's going to be twenty-eight in Zakynthos. No rain forecast whatsoever, until November. A kagoule will not be coming anywhere near me.' Ed continued, 'See, going out with a successful entrepreneur definitely has its advantages. I'm only with you for the villa.'

It was probably true. A non-pregnant Tor would have come back with a killer putdown, along the lines that she was only with him for his young cock. But pregnant Tor had lost her sense of humour and had nothing to say. Ed caught her grim expression, 'Oh, baby, I'm kidding!'

The baby and kidding part almost made her want to throw up. *Again.*

It was a relief when Frankie finally made an appearance, cheekily pushing into the queue as they were about to check in their luggage.

'You went running this morning, didn't you?' Tor said accusingly. 'Only you would go running on the day you were going on holiday.'

Frankie nodded. 'Yep, OCD to the last.'

'You are going to ease up when we're away aren't you? It's going to be too hot to run, you'll do yourself an injury. We'll find you at the side of the road, suffering from dehydration, hallucinating, and you know that none of us have done a first-aid course.' Tor didn't know why she was even wasting her breath as Frankie would do exactly what she wanted; she always did.

'I'll get up early. And Leila says that there is a gym with air con at one of the hotels along the coast, so I can always go there.'

'You are seriously hardcore,' Ed put in. 'A nutter.

33

And good to see that you're getting into the holiday mood with your choice of colour.'

'You know me. It has to be black.'

'Ah, and you'd look so pretty in pink.'

'You'd look better.'

He and Frankie had developed a sort of banter between them, based primarily on Frankie teasing him relentlessly. This was a good sign though as Frankie only did that when she really liked someone. The time to worry about Frankie was when she was polite.

'Anyway I have to run. I've no intention of turning into a lard arse in two weeks. You'll be lazing by the pool, drinking beer, and gorging yourself on souvlaki and chips at night.'

'Sounds good to me. But I don't think I've got anything to worry about yet.' Ed stretched his arms above his head, causing his t-shirt to ride up and give everyone a tantalising glimpse of his defined abs and the band of his black Calvin Kleins. His body was a thing of beauty, which Tor absolutely loved. She experienced a flutter of lust that was then cruelly superseded by a surge of nausea. She clamped her hand over her mouth.

'Are you okay?' Frankie asked. 'You look a bit pale.'

'Fine, I just ate something dodgy last night.' Was this going to be her mantra for the next two weeks?

Two and a half hours later they were finally on the

plane. It was easyJet, so everyone was eating their own food. Tor suddenly seemed cursed with the ability to smell everything, the Big Mac and fries three rows back, Ed's bacon sandwich, the sushi from the row in front – seriously, sushi on a plane? Surely it should be banned along with nail scissors and guns. She couldn't eat anything but managed to sip a cup of Earl Grey. Frankie had donned an eye mask and seemed to have gone to sleep, lucky thing. Tom and Leila had settled Gracie down with a film on the laptop and the long-anticipated chocolate croissant. Ed was absorbed in the latest George R. R. Martin. Tor flicked through *Vogue*, which would usually be a treat . . . but she couldn't concentrate on anything, because the *Oh my God, I'm pregnant* thought kept going round in a loop in her head, and what the hell did the sulky, skinny models wearing exquisite clothes have to do with that?

She knew that there was a twelve-week scan that she should be booked in for, that she should be taking folic acid, that she had to stop drinking and avoid seafood and was it unpasteurised cheese? *If* she was keeping the baby. She did more calculations – the baby would be due around March. *If* she was keeping the baby, what would she do about work? Tor owned and ran her own business in Brighton – a vintage clothes store that also hired out and sold fancy dress outfits. She employed Spencer – who was very high-maintenance – as manager – in fairness, that was how he would describe himself. There was also Maud, a manic depressive, who did all the alterations and didn't venture on to the shop floor, preferring the workshop at the back where she was left to her own devices and Radio 3. Tor didn't know much about Maud because she was so intensely private, but she did know that she used to be a hot shot in the City before she had a nervous breakdown. She was responsible for them all. She couldn't imagine leaving Spencer in sole charge for an extended period. He could just about cope with two weeks but she knew she would soon be getting calls from him. *I can't find the new till roll. Where are the paying in slips? Can we give a discount on such and such an item?* And so on. And while Ed might tease her and call her a successful businesswoman, the fact was that it had been bloody tough to keep the store going recently. This was going to be her first time off in ages.

Across the aisle she noticed the couple with the twins. The mum was attempting to leave her seat, but every time she got up one of the babies wailed and the dad was trying to calm down both of them and have something to eat at the same time. It looked like a fiendishly hard juggling act. Suddenly realising what was going on, Ed leant across and said, 'Here let me hold him for you.' He unfastened his seat belt and stood up. The mother looked as if she might actually fall at his feet in gratitude. 'Thanks, I'm desperate to go to the loo!'

She picked up Twin 1 and handed him to Ed. Twin 1 looked momentarily appalled and opened his mouth to release a fresh bout of bawling, but then some kind of Ed magic seemed to take over as he smiled and said, 'Okay then, fella, are you going to let your mum go for a pee? And let your dad have something to eat?' And just like that Twin 1 stopped and grabbed hold of the leather band around Ed's wrist and gurgled.

'Who are you?' Tor asked in wonder. 'The Baby Whisperer?'

Ed laughed, 'My elder sister has twins, they're five now and I've spent loads of time with them. Daisy and Milo, they're great kids.'

'I had no idea.' But that was not surprising as Tor had never met any of Ed's family. Indeed she had staunchly resisted it, fearing that they would brand her as the wicked leathery old cougar having her wicked leathery old way with their fresh-faced young son/brother.

Ed chatted away easily to the dad, who told him that it was their first holiday with the twins and that they were staying somewhere with the option of childcare.

'So you can go out with the missus?' Ed commented.

'Actually I was just thinking of going to bed. Neither of us has slept properly for six months. And as for sex . . . I can't remember. I think we might have on my birthday.' The man paused, slightly embarrassed. 'Sorry, brain too fuddled to censor my thoughts. That was too much information.'

He planted a tender kiss on Twin 2's head. 'Still, I wouldn't be without them.'

Tor had a renewed respect for Ed after this. She knew that she had a tendency to keep him in the box marked 'younger man, lover, not serious, not long-term', but there was far more to him than that. And perhaps she was wrong to dismiss the idea of Ed as a father; he was apparently brilliant with babies. How many other men would have done what he did, and done it so naturally? Most of them wouldn't even have noticed, never mind offered to help. She was actually feeling almost optimistic about her situation until they reached the baggage reclaim area in the tiny Zakynthos airport and she caught sight of two teenage girls blatantly checking him out. Oh, baby! Who was she kidding? She was too old for him. She couldn't trap him with this news. *If* she had the baby, she would be bringing up him or her on her own.

Ed hauled her suitcase off the conveyor.

'Bloody hell, Tor, what the hell have you got in here? It weighs a ton.'

She knew she had too much baggage, but she wasn't thinking about her suitcase.

Chapter 5

Leila

As she exited the plane and walked down the creaky metal steps, Leila revelled in the sensation of the sun on her face and body. It was one o'clock and burning hot. She felt like someone who had been living in a dark cave for months, only to emerge and discover that summer had arrived. What joy to be here! She loved the heat haze shimmering on the runway as if it was dissolving the tarmac, the bold blue sky, the hills surrounding the airport dotted with olive trees; she loved queuing up to go through passport control where a nonchalant Greek official with an impressively large moustache flicked through their passports but still raised a smile for Gracie who was dancing around with a scarlet *Hello Kitty* rucksack nearly as big as her strapped to her back.

She even loved walking through the automatic

doors out of the airport and breathing in the second-hand smoke from all the people hanging around outside having a sneaky cigarette. In the UK she would be mentally tutting, thinking, don't they realise how harmful it is? But here the white plumes of cigarette smoke were yet another a reminder that she was once more in Greece, back on her island, as she thought of it, which she had been coming to since she was eleven. It had always felt like a sanctuary, her special place, full of happy memories of childhood holidays, of fun weeks with Tor and Leila when they were students, of wonderful times with Tom and then with Tom and Gracie . . .

It was an hour-and-a-half's drive from the airport to the villa and some parts of the island were not so scenic, especially where the coastline had been overdeveloped with hotels, villas, tourist shops, tavernas and crazy-golf courses, scarring the island's natural beauty. But you only had to drive a little further to find stretches that hadn't been touched or that had been developed more thoughtfully, so the buildings were low-rise and you could always see the sea. It became less developed still as they drew closer to her parents' villa, and the terrain became hillier, with fiendishly winding roads that hugged the coastline. Leila drank in the vivid bursts of colours: the magenta bougainvillaea cascading over whitewashed walls, the scarlet geraniums planted in old olive-oil cans, the glittering sapphire blue of the sea. She felt as if she had been living in a black-and-white film in the UK, where it had been grey and overcast for weeks and the sun hadn't put in an appearance for far too long. Here it was a feast for the senses in full glorious Technicolor.

Gracie maintained a constant stream of chatter from the back, every now and then asking 'How many more miles?' and 'When are we there?'

Were children born with these questions already pre-programmed in their DNA? The early start and the stress that she had been under was making Leila feel frayed, impatient, and she was about to snap back at her daughter that she had just answered her when Tom said patiently, 'Last mile, Gracie. Can you remember how to spot the turning?'

Leila breathed out. Tom was a better parent than she was.

'Yes! It's the sign with the olive tree on it! Just past Jesus's house.'

Leila caught Frankie frowning in the rear-view mirror. 'She means the shrines you get at the side of the road, with a crucifix and candle. Gracie wanted to donate one of her bush-babies to keep Jesus company.'

Frankie put her arm round the child, 'That was nice of you sweetie. I'm sure he would have liked that.'

Phew! Leila had been worried there that Frankie might launch into one of her attacks on organised religion, an attack that was known to last some time,

41

even though in nearly every case she was preaching to the converted.

And then Gracie spotted the shrine and pointed out the sign. Leila's own feeling of excitement increased dramatically as Tom turned off the dusty road. Typically Gracie wanted to open the electric gates and it took her several goes to get it right with the zapper device, but then they swung open and they were going up the drive, lined with silvery-green olive trees. At the end stood the elegant villa, painted white with light blue shutters. Leila got out of the car and took in the view from here: the breathtaking expanse of sea, the olive groves, the garden with its lemon trees, scarlet hibiscus, bougainvillaea, and purple wisteria that frothed and frilled over the terrace. The cicadas were in full rasping chorus, a sound that she adored as much as any piece of music because it told her that she was back in Greece; she could smell wild thyme and jasmine. She felt as if she was home and sent up a silent prayer to this place that she had always loved: *Please,* please make everything be okay.

Almost immediately Gracie wanted to go in the pool.

Leila rifled through the suitcase trying to locate her sunsuit as her daughter danced around the bedroom like a deranged imp. Where the frig was it! And why didn't she pack it at the top? There was a knot of tension in her shoulders that wouldn't go away.

'Can't she just go in in her knickers?' Tom asked, quite reasonably.

'Of course not!' How typical of him to go for the path of least resistance. 'You'd have to slather her in sun cream, which she hates. She *must* wear the suit. Do you want her to burn and end up with skin cancer in later life!' God, she sounded like a witch. Knew it, couldn't stop it. Far too frequently this was how she spoke to Tom. She remembered hearing other women speaking to their men like this, and vowing never to be the same.

There was a resigned sigh from Tom. There seemed to have been a lot of sighs lately. A marriage built on sighs and lies and nagging.

Finally, after pulling absolutely everything out, she discovered the pink suit with the white stars on it at the very bottom of the case.

'I hate pink,' Gracie declared.

Leila was about to retort crossly, *Tough, you'll still have to wear it,* when Tom laughed and said, 'That from the girl who wanted her entire bedroom painted bright pink and wanted us to get a pink car! Come on, fickle pickle, let's get into the pool.'

He had already put on a pair of board shorts, navy with a pattern of white tropical flowers. New ones, Leila realised. He looked good in them. She should tell him, but she was so out of the habit of saying anything positive. So all she managed was, 'Those shorts are an improvement on your porno ones.' She was referring to a pair of black Speedos, worn thin and see-through by long exposure to chlorine and leaving little to the imagination.

'Yep, better than porno shorts, though I like to think the ladies and certain selected men of the Prince Regent Pool are going to miss their twice-weekly outing. I'm imagining there will be speculation about their disappearance on Twitter: #have you seen porno shorts? Possibly even a reward offered for them.' He grinned, 'And won't you miss them?'

'Not really.' Leila knew she should come back with a witty, provocative comment, something that showed that she was still interested in him, but she couldn't. That side of her seemed to have been put into cold storage since *that* night.

'Will Ed come in too?' Gracie asked.

'Yeah, when the lucky bas—' Tom checked himself. 'When the lucky thing's had a beer.'

As Gracie stripped off her clothes and put on the accursed pink suit, Tom slid his arm around Leila's waist. Resting his chin on her shoulder, he whispered, 'Do you remember our very first holiday here?'

She tried not to flinch at the physical contact. She did remember. It was just the two of them, when just the two of them meant something to be treasured and not something to be avoided. They spent the mornings on the beach swimming and sunbathing, then, when the sun got too hot, they returned to the villa for long afternoons of making love, their bodies golden in the light filtering through the wooden shutters. In the evenings they'd take off on a moped, her arms wrapped tightly round his waist, for dinner at Nikos's taverna. She remembered how intensely connected she'd felt to Tom back then; felt as if she had found her soulmate. She didn't think they had ever been closer. It seemed like another era to Leila; to have happened to another woman, and another man. She couldn't imagine feeling like that now.

There was no time for further conversation as Gracie grabbed Tom's hand, shouting, 'Come on, Daddy!'

'Bring me that beer when you get chance,' Tom said ruefully, allowing himself to be dragged away to the pool.

Feeling exhausted, Leila sank back on the bed. Her phone beeped with a text. Oh, God, surely not him again? Reluctantly she pulled it out of her bag. The message was from her mum, telling her to have a great holiday and not to think about work. Relief. But only for a few minutes. Just as she was changing into her bikini her phone beeped again.

I must talk to you, Leila, there are things I have to tell you. I know you said that you didn't want to see me, but I don't believe you. We need to work this out so that we can be together. Call me. I can't stop thinking of that night, the feel of your skin, the taste of you x

In spite of the heat, she felt herself go cold. She deleted the message and switched off the phone, wishing that she could erase Jasper from her life as easily. The idea that they should be together was insane. He barely knew her. He was talking about what had happened as if it was the start of an incredible love affair instead of a drunken shag, and not even a very memorable one, certainly not a good one. What was she going to do? She contemplated replying, telling him to leave her alone, but rejected the idea. It hadn't worked so far. Silence was the best policy. Surely even Jasper would give up if she didn't respond.

Suddenly she couldn't bear to be on her own with her thoughts for another second. Opening the drawer in the bedside table, she shoved her phone under a novel she was planning to read. She quickly put on a long white t-shirt over her bikini, and tied her hair back into a ponytail. She grabbed her sunglasses and practically ran out of the room and down the wide terracotta-tiled staircase. The living-room doors had been folded back to reveal the infinity pool set in the terrace, beautifully designed by her architect dad so that the water seemed to blend into the Ionian Sea beyond, making a breathtaking expanse of blue.

Tom was in the pool, encouraging Gracie to jump in. Leila looked at the pair of them. They seemed so joyful and carefree, so innocent. How could she ever have threatened the life she had with her family?

'Oi! Where's my beer?' Tom called over to her. 'I'm a desperate man.'

'Coming right up!' she replied, forcing herself to smile, to slam the door shut on thoughts of Jasper. She padded back through the large open-plan living room, enjoying the feel of the cool limestone floor beneath her bare feet, and into the designer kitchen with its glossy white units and azure glass tiles. It was considerably nicer than her own kitchen at home, which was in urgent need of an upgrade. Tom kept nagging her about it, but she could never find time to think about what she actually wanted. It was a bloody metaphor for her life.

She pulled open the door of the sleek fridge-freezer. Her mum had asked Alexa, a local woman who oversaw the villa, to stock up with food and drink. Leila appreciated the gesture, she couldn't face going round a supermarket today. She reached for two bottles of Stella. She never drank beer back home, but here she liked nothing more than an ice-cold beer in the afternoon. It said, relax, you're on holiday.

'Is there another one of those going?' It was Frankie.

''Course,' she replied, grabbing a third from the fridge.

'It is so gorgeous here, Leila. You are so lucky. I'd come here all the time if I had a place like this.'

'I know, I'm really lucky.' She really didn't feel

47

lucky. But Leila smiled as she flipped the lid off the bottle of beer and handed it to Frankie.

'Cheers!' The two women clinked their bottles together.

'I must get this one out to Tom,' Leila said, after taking a glug of beer. She looked at Frankie, who was wearing a bikini top, black of course, and a pair of tiny denim shorts that Leila probably couldn't pull over her knees.

'Looking good, Frankie. I reckon you could crack walnuts with your thighs, they look so toned. In a good way, not as if you've been taking performance-enhancing drugs,' she added hastily, knowing how ultra-sensitive Frankie could be about her body.

Immediately her friend frowned. 'I thought I'd put on a bit of weight actually. I'll have to watch it this holiday.' She held up the beer. 'Not too many of these. Do you know how many calories there are in a bottle of beer?'

Leila ignored that question; she made a point of ignoring any calorie-counting comments from Frankie. 'There's no way you've put on weight – in fact, you could do with putting more on, if for no other reason than to make me feel better about my flabby stomach and cellulite thighs. It's your duty as one of my best friends.'

'Rubbish! You've lost weight. I was going to ask if you'd been on a diet.'

Leila had been so anxious about the whole Jasper thing that she had hardly been eating. She should market her secret – the cheat-on-your-husband-and-the-weight-falls-off-you-diet. She might be on the fast track to getting divorced, but at least she would be thin. The truth was, though, she would rather have her old life and her old body back.

She couldn't tell Frankie this. 'Nope, and even if you think I look thinner, the truth is I'm flabby and un-toned.'

'Oh, shut up! Girl you're beautiful!' Frankie sang *à la* Christina Aguilera, using the beer bottle as a microphone.

'"Who cares what they say",' Tor joined in as she walked into the kitchen. She had showered and changed into a green maxi dress.

'And you've got a beautiful child.' Now Frankie reverted to an American accent. Not a very good one.

'A beautiful child who has wrecked my pelvic floor.'

'Did having Gracie wreck your pelvic floor?' Tor asked. An unexpected question from her as she tended not to talk about childbirth and babies since she'd found out that she probably would not be able to have children.

'It's just about all in working order, but I should do my exercises more often than I do, which is never . . . God, d'you remember when I asked Tom to buy some pads after I'd got home from the hospital with Gracie and he bought Tena incontinence pads by mistake? I said, I'm not quite there yet, thanks!

And when I sent him out again he came back with pant liners – like *they* were going to do anything.'

'I can just imagine him rushing into the shop and grabbing the first thing, being too embarrassed to check what he was actually buying. It was sweet of him to try,' Tor put in.

'I threw them at his head. I was so awash with hormones that I couldn't laugh about it, and then he had to go out again, by which time I was about to abandon all hope and rip up sheets like they used to in the olden days.'

Even talking about this funny incident depressed Leila because it was a reminder of how distant she and Tom had become and how very far away they were from the couple they had been when Gracie was born. She remembered the two of them lying on the bed when Gracie was a few days old – in between them their tiny daughter with her rosebud mouth – and at that moment Leila had felt like the happiest, luckiest person in the world.

'D'you want a beer, Tor?'

'Actually I'm still feeling a bit dodgy, I'll have water.'

Both Leila and Frankie did a double take. Tor really must be under the weather – she was not known for refusing alcohol.

Outside the three women settled themselves on the loungers surrounding the pool. Leila opened up the large white parasol, mindful of Frankie who had very pale skin and never lay out in the sun, and was strict to the point of obsession about wearing factor fifty and hats. In fairness, it wasn't because she was worried about getting wrinkles and aging prematurely, it was because she only had to be in the sun for a few minutes before she burned.

Ed strolled out of the villa in a pair of red swimming shorts, waved at them and dived straight into the pool. It was hard not to stare at his body as he cut through the water with an energetic front crawl that displayed his broad shoulders and lean hips.

'Nice view,' Frankie commented, smirking as she sipped her beer.

Tor pursed her lips. 'Bet you won't be saying that when you see me in my bikini looking like Miss Porky Pig of the universe. In fact, I don't even know if I'm going to wear one. It'll be a burqini for me.'

Leila looked at her; it was also not like Tor to be so down on herself, she had always accepted that she had curves – curves that were the envy of many women and that all men seemed to adore. At a voluptuous size 12, she was not quite in the Christina Hendricks category, but she had an hourglass figure. Leila wondered if everything was okay with her friend.

'Don't be mad, you know you've got the ideal bikini body – not like me with my flat-as-a-pancake chest.' Frankie glanced disparagingly at her own bikini top.

51

'What is this? A body dysmorphia support group!' Leila declared. 'Ladies, we are on holiday. We are going to eat, drink and be merry. We are going to wear our bikinis with pride . . . and no hang-ups.'

Tom hauled himself out of the pool. 'At last I can have that beer. I'm gasping.'

Leila handed him a towel and the longed-for bottle and they watched as Ed and Gracie messed about in the water, with Ed pretending to be a shark and chasing Gracie, to her huge delight. Leila felt a tiny loosening of tension. Perhaps everything would be fine . . .

'So what's the plan?' Frankie asked. She was renowned for finding it incredibly hard to relax and had to know exactly what she was doing at all times. Serendipity was most definitely not her middle name.

Tom glanced over at Leila, and she knew that he was sharing her thoughts as he said, 'Well, we're going to chill by the pool for the next couple of hours. And chill, Ms Harper, means not doing anything. Nothing at all. *Nada. Rien.* And then –' he checked his watch and adopted the brisk tone of a sergeant major '– at nineteen hundred hours I suggest showers; twenty hundred hours a pre-dinner drink, a dry white wine perhaps, accompanied by pistachios, olives and crisps; twenty hundred and thirty hours sit down for dinner on the terrace and . . .

'Okay, okay, very funny, I get the picture,' Frankie

interrupted. 'You know I can't help it. But I will relax.'

She said it as if it was a command to herself.

'And what time is Patrick arriving tomorrow?' she continued.

Leila avoided meeting her gaze. 'I think the flight gets in just after lunch,' she said vaguely. This probably was the moment to mention that Matt would also be joining them, but she couldn't bear it if Frankie got into a strop. By tomorrow she would be more relaxed. Well, relaxed by her standards. Leila would make sure she plied her friend with alcohol tonight . . . a hangover might blunt Frankie's capacity for outrage. And maybe she wouldn't have a problem with Matt any more and would hit it off with him this time, in the way Leila had hoped they would. She would keep her fingers and toes crossed on that one.

53

Chapter 6

Frankie

By half-past two the following day Frankie had worked herself up into a complete state about seeing Patrick again. She had missed him so much. Their last meeting six weeks ago had been a bitter disappointment to her. She had dashed up to London, even though it was his turn to come down to Brighton and she was up to her ears in writing end-of-term reports. She had been anticipating a leisurely dinner, wine, chat and flirtation. And there was always that tantalising possibility that she might finally be able to tell him how she felt, and the tantalising possibility that he might feel the same. It was only when she met him in a crowded pub in Covent Garden that he told her that he had double booked and could only meet her for a drink after all. And even then, as they sat drinking white wine at a table sticky with spilt beer, he had been

54

distracted and kept checking his phone.

She remembered travelling back on the train, downing a gin and tonic that she bought from the station because she needed something, *anything*, to make her feel numb. It didn't work, she had felt like the saddest, loneliest person in the world . . .

This morning she had forced herself to go for a five-mile run, in spite of having drunk far too much the night before. It had only been half-past seven but already blisteringly hot. The ancient farmer with his wrinkled walnut-brown face who had driven past her in his tractor, pulling a trailer loaded with watermelons, had looked at her as if she was stark raving bonkers as she pounded along the side of the road, sweat pouring down her back.

She had failed to make any progress with the book she was reading – a thriller that was supposed to be unputdownable but which she was finding very putdownable. She had checked her appearance about twenty times, tied her hair back, taken it down. Now she was sitting in the shade of the wide terrace with its prime view of the tree-lined driveway. Tor and Ed were in their bedroom having a siesta; Leila was glued to her novel, Tom was lying by the pool and Gracie was watching *Toy Story 3* on DVD. Leila had already warned her that it was Gracie's current favourite and that by the end of the holiday Frankie would be word perfect in it. It could have been worse. Earlier in the year

Gracie was apparently obsessed with *Alvin and the Chipmunks: The Squeakquel*, a film so sadistically annoying it almost drove both Leila and Tom to take up smoking again. 'Crack,' Leila had told her, only half joking.

Frankie stood up. 'D'you want a drink?'

'No, thanks,' Leila murmured, not looking up from her book.

Frankie wandered back inside and into the kitchen where she poured herself a large glass of water and ticked off what she had eaten so far today. She had overindulged last night – with alcohol rather than food – two beers and three glasses of wine, and she would have to ease up otherwise she would end up bloated. Not a good look in her bikini, not the look to impress Patrick. She half wondered if she had time to do some sit-ups, a quick fifty might ease some of the guilt she felt for having drunk so much.

Suddenly the doorbell rang, and she nearly dropped the glass. *He was here!*

'Can you buzz them in?' Leila called out.

Frankie was too hyped up to wonder why Leila had said 'them'.

'Hey,' she said into the receiver, pressing the door release. Her heart was pounding as if she had completed a 10K in record time.

'Hey, yourself.' Patrick's familiar drawling tones sent mini shockwaves of anticipation through Frankie. She ran out to the terrace and felt like a child racing downstairs to see what presents Santa had left under the tree . . . Two whole weeks with Patrick all to herself! She felt like hopping around with excitement, just like Gracie when she knew that she was in for a treat.

She watched the silver Peugeot drive slowly towards the villa. Its black-tinted windows made it impossible to see inside, but Patrick opened his and stuck out his arm to wave at her. Frankie self-consciously smoothed down her hair and fiddled with the bracelet on her arm. The fragile string broke and the turquoise beads cascaded on to the terrace, scattering everywhere.

'Oh, no!' she exclaimed. It was her most treasured piece of jewellery, a present from Ross. She always wore it. She knelt down and frantically attempted to gather up the beads, assisted by Leila. She heard the car door open, the crunch of Patrick's footsteps on the gravel drive. She looked up, and caught her breath. Patrick looked as handsome as ever in faded blue jeans and a white shirt. She could look at him all day long – she would be able to look at him all day long! But he was not alone. There was another man who seemed very familiar. Horribly familiar. The man she never let herself think about. But surely it couldn't be him? No way. Why would it be? Oh, fuck! It was him. Matt Cartwright. She loathed Matt and he couldn't stand her either. Why had no one told her he was invited? She never would have come if she had known.

'What's *he* doing here?' she muttered through clenched teeth.

'Tom asked him. It's not a problem, is it?' Leila looked guilty as hell. She was the world's worst liar.

'You should have told me! You know we don't get on.'

'Shush!' Leila ordered, then said, 'Who the hell's that?'

They both watched a young woman getting out of the car. You couldn't miss her as she was wearing a bright red playsuit patterned with black love hearts, staggeringly high red sandals that must have been torture to walk in, full-on make-up including fake lashes, and to complete the glamour-girl look her long hair was dyed a deep red. It was a colour Frankie knew only too well as so many girls at her school had gone through a craze of dying their hair that shade in homage to Rihanna – even though it did none of them any favours. She must be Matt's girlfriend, though she didn't exactly look like the kind of girl that serious businessman Matt would date. Dinner parties with his stuck-up friends and their stuck-up partners must be interesting . . . Or perhaps she wasn't allowed to go to them.

'Frankie! Darling! I know you're pleased to see me, but you didn't have to kneel.' Patrick bounded on to the terrace and, reaching for her arms, pulled her up and folded her into a tight embrace, kissing her on the lips. His body felt unbelievably good against hers. He hadn't been a figment of her imagination. He was here. At last. She got a hit of his familiar aftershave that she adored – Tom Ford's Extreme – and breathed in sandalwood, cedarwood and Parma violet. She had even bought a bottle and sometimes sprayed the scent on her pillow, fooling herself that Patrick was close by . . . She always had to remember to put it back in the drawer in case any of her friends saw it.

She wished she could lose herself in this embrace, but she was all too aware of Matt and the girl walking up the steps. The redhead stumbled in her ridiculous heels and Matt reached out to steady her.

Patrick broke away, 'And this is Candy.' He gestured to the girl in red. He paused. 'My girlfriend.'

What the fuck!

Candy stepped forward shyly, holding out her hand. 'Hiya, pleased to meet you.'

She was very pretty in spite of the heavy make-up. Very pretty and very young. Somehow Frankie reached out and shook her hand, noting the long fake nails, also red. She'd had absolutely no idea that Patrick had a girlfriend. He certainly didn't mention Candy when they'd met for a drink. She would have remembered that piece of information.

'I hope it's okay with you, Leila? I know there's plenty of space here, and Candy's very easygoing. A total sweetheart, you'll love her,' he said smoothly.

'Of course. It's lovely to meet you, Candy, I'll show you your room.' Leila always had impeccable manners, even if she had been taken by complete surprise.

Candy looked uncertain. 'Oh, I'm sorry, didn't Patrick tell you that he had invited me?' She had a husky voice and quite a strong Brighton accent that sounded even more noticeable against Leila's perfect RP.

'Not exactly, but it's no problem, I promise.' Leila did her accomplished hostess thing. The words would have choked Frankie had she been in her place.

'I'll grab the bags,' Patrick said, keen to avoid any further awkward questions, 'And I've got presents for the ladies.' He winked at Frankie as he ran back to the car.

Matt moved to stand in front of her. 'Hello, Frankie.'

He was much bigger than she remembered, taller, with wide shoulders and a powerful athletic build – a total contrast to Patrick who was lean and lithe. He was also better-looking than she had remembered, with intensely blue eyes. His dark blond hair had been longer then, now it was cut short against his head. It suited him. But his good looks didn't cut any ice with her. She was willing to bet that he was still a total wage slave, only caring about money and success and status.

She had an unpleasant flashback to Tom and Leila's wedding, and what would go down as the worst night of her life. That was the last time she had seen Matt – a bastard in a black morning suit and peacock blue waistcoat to co-ordinate with the bridesmaids' dresses. She had very, *very* much hoped that she would never have to set eyes on him again . . .

'Hello, Matt,' she said coolly. 'How are you?'

'Very good, thanks. Looking forward to two weeks off.'

She folded her arms across her chest. 'I bet you're going to do some work though, aren't you?' She shouldn't needle him; she should try and keep things civilised. But she had been knocked sideways by the arrival of Candy, and channelling her dislike of Matt seemed a better option than crying in her bedroom.

'I might have to,' he admitted. 'The odd email, maybe a conference call.'

'Your work is so important, isn't it? I imagine the world would stop turning if Matt Cartwright didn't reply to one email.' Frankie knew how rude she must sound. Knew it, couldn't stop it.

He didn't rise to her bait. 'Probably not. Do you know which is my room?'

Frankie guessed it must be the one next to hers, 'Yep, I'll show you.' She smiled a not-very-nice smile at him. 'Just so long as you're not planning on bringing anyone back as it only has a single bed.'

Matt shrugged. 'I could always go to their place, I suppose, if that situation arises. Although a single bed will take me right back to my student days and

61

it suited my purposes just fine then. I hope the walls aren't as thin as my halls of residence though – for your sake.' He grinned at her.

The smile vanished from Frankie's face. She didn't want to imagine Matt in bed with anyone, least of all in the room next to hers.

Patrick returned from the car carrying one suitcase and wheeling a hot pink number – no prizes for guessing who owned that item. He abandoned his own suitcase at the steps leading up to the terrace and lugged the pink one up, groaning with the effort.

'I don't know what she's got in here. I mean, how much stuff do you need for two weeks? She'll be wearing a bikini most of the time.'

'A shedload of make-up, I imagine, judging by how much she's wearing,' Frankie said acidly. 'You'd better warn her that it will slide off in this heat. And that's *so* not a good look.'

Patrick waved a finger at her. 'Now, now Frankie, that's not very sisterly of you.'

'So how long have you been seeing her?'

Patrick looked sheepish. 'Don't tell Leila because she'll go all moral high ground on me and probably make us sleep in the barn, and I do appreciate the fine Eyptian cotton sheets she has in the guest rooms, and the en suite bathrooms.'

He was trying to fob her off. It wasn't going to work.

'Well?'

'It's just been a month.'

He went away with this girl after a month! A measly four weeks!

'And where did you meet her? Your local lap-dancing club?' Frankie was struggling to keep her emotions under control. This had been the biggest slap in the face. Ever.

'Tut tut, Ms Judgmental. I only went to that lap-dancing club to research an article. And just because Candy looks a little bit like a girl you might pay to have sex with, it doesn't mean she *is* that sort of girl. She's adorable and funny and bright.'

'You mean, she lets you do whatever you want,' Frankie retorted.

Patrick laughed. 'You know me too well, Frankie.'

'You haven't answered my question,' she persisted. God only knew why. It wouldn't make her feel any better and would possibly make her feel a whole lot worse.

'If you must know, Candy was one of the shots girls at some tedious gig I went to. The vision of her dressed as an Indian squaw in a suede tasselled mini dress and knee-high boots, coming at me with a bottle of tequila, was an arresting one. She's a beautician when she's not doing that kind of thing. Brighton girl. She could have gone to your school. You might even have taught her. Be nice and maybe she could give you some treatments. She's good. She's already waxed my back.' He winced. 'Bloody painful, but very professional results.'

63

'I don't need anything waxed,' Frankie snapped back. 'And just how old is she?'

'Sweet twenty-two. And before you give me a lecture about being a lecher, remember, you never give Tor a hard time about her toy boy. Equal opportunities and all.'

'You're going out with someone who was born in the 1990s?'

'It always was my favourite decade,' he replied, grinning. 'All that girl power, all that zig ah zig ah.'

'Well, Candy was six when "Wannabe" came out,' Frankie muttered. She didn't usually remember pop trivia, but had recently been in a pub quiz where the date of the Spice Girls' first hit came up.

Patrick shook his head. 'You won't make me feel bad about this, Frankie so you can stop with your judgmental act. What are you going to do, miss? Put me in detention?' He flashed her his extra-naughty-boy smile. 'Seriously, if you'd been my teacher, I would happily have had detention every day. You are way too sexy to be a teacher.'

Why her and not me? Frankie wanted to say. Why? Why? Why? But sensing that the interrogation was over, Patrick swiftly wheeled the pink suitcase inside.

While this exchange had been going on Matt had been quietly gathering up more beads from Frankie's bracelet. He seemed to have located nearly all of them. 'Here you go,' he said, carefully handing them to her.

'Thanks,' she muttered, shoving them into the pocket of her shorts and not sounding nearly as grateful as she should, but she was trying not to let on how upset she was. 'I'll show you your cell . . . sorry, room . . . as Leila must be giving Candy the grand tour.' She turned on her flip-flopped heel and marched through the living room. She was about to go upstairs when Gracie, noticing Matt, tore herself away from *Toy Story* and hurtled towards him.

'Mattie Matt Matt!'

'Gracie!' Matt picked her up and swung her round.

You traitor, Gracie, Frankie thought, conveniently forgetting that the little girl was only four.

Matt looked over at her, 'Lead the way to my palatial room then. I can't wait to see it.'

Frankie stomped upstairs while Gracie chattered away, telling Matt all about the lizards she had spotted in the garden. Leila and Tom had the master bedroom, with an en suite bathroom and a balcony with stunning views across the Ionian Sea; Gracie was next-door to them, and further along a cool terracotta-tiled corridor and up a small flight of steps was Frankie's room, also a double with its own balcony. Beside it was a luxurious shower room, with floor-to-ceiling marble tiles, and then Matt's room. It was the smallest, least luxurious room in the house. Leila had christened it 'the nun's room' and had hung over the bed a kitsch picture of the

Virgin Mary with eyes that lit up, which her dad kept threatening to take down as it was not exactly in keeping with the elegant style of the rest of the villa. If it was anyone else being put in here Frankie might have felt some sympathy, but it was Matt so she didn't.

'Knock yourself out,' she said sarcastically, but once again he refused to be riled. Ignoring her tone he threw his suitcase on the bed and opened the shutters to take in the glorious view, the silvery-green of the olive trees and the blue promise of the sea. Gracie dashed off to find one of her toys to show him, while Frankie leaned against the doorframe.

'Perfect,' he said, then turned to face her. He gave her a considering look. 'I got your number from Leila and I did call you a couple of times, but you never called me back.'

Of course she hadn't called him back! Why the hell would she?

'Oh, yeah, busy with teaching probably. It can be very full on.' She looked straight at him, daring him to challenge her.

'Sure. I understand. I had tickets for a play I thought you might have liked.'

'Oh, right. Sorry.' She wasn't.

'So how have you been, Frankie?'

'Good, thanks. Glad it's the holidays.' She was not going to open up to Matt of all people.

'Really? You seemed pretty rattled just then.' He

paused. 'I thought you'd be over Patrick by now.'

Fuck! She was convinced that Matt would have forgotten; she had prayed Matt would have forgotten. She played dumb. 'I'm sorry, I don't know what you're talking about.'

'He's not worth it. Believe me, there is so much less to Patrick than meets the eye.'

'I thought you were supposed to be his friend!'

'I am, and I like him – in small doses – but I'd never want to have a relationship with him. Patrick is incapable of having a relationship with anyone other than himself. He's entertaining, charming – if you like that kind of thing – and easily one of the most selfish people I've ever met. You're one of his closest friends, and you didn't even know that he had a new girlfriend, did you?'

Frankie was momentarily speechless.

'Yep, thought not. Anyway, that's all I have to say on the subject. I'm going to get changed and hit the pool.'

When Frankie didn't move – she was still in shock – Matt grinned and said, 'You're welcome to watch if you like.'

Like she ever would! Frankie stormed out. She locked herself in the bathroom and looked at herself in the mirror. Her face was shiny with sun cream, her hair had gone limp in the heat, she looked ugly and pale. No wonder Patrick preferred Candy, even if she did look like a stripper. Scrap that, no doubt he preferred her precisely because she looked like a stripper. She turned on the shower then collapsed on to the marble floor, pressing her hands over her eyes as tears of humiliation and hurt spilt out.

Chapter 7

Tor

Tor stood in front of the full-length mirror brushing her hair. She felt unbelievably uncomfortable in her skin, wished that she could unzip it, get another one. Nothing she wore made her feel good, and usually she could rely on the right outfit to boost her confidence. If only her clothes weren't so bright and attention-seeking. She longed for an unassuming black number. She should borrow something from Frankie, though nothing would fit her. What she required was a black tent – a large one. But she didn't do black and she didn't do unassuming, so instead it was the red-and-white polka-dot swimsuit which showed far more cleavage than she would have liked. But she couldn't help that, her boobs were swollen, and felt as if they were bursting out of her top. This was eight weeks? At this rate they'd soon be the size of bazookas.

Did they actually make bras big or strong enough to contain them?

It wasn't her body that was her main concern, though. She was still reeling from the news. She was desperate for advice, longed to confide in her friends, but it would be wrong to speak to Leila and Frankie without telling Ed first. The trouble was, she couldn't imagine telling Ed. They had never really talked about where their relationship was going. There had been no discussion about babies, and no mention of love. Did she love Ed? She loved being with him, that was certain. She couldn't imagine not being with him. It had been a wonderful, joyous release after Harry.

It had seemed to her that both of them had been content to live in the moment. Though to be fair, there had been times when Ed had tried to discuss the future. For instance, he had wanted her to meet his family, but Tor had always been quick to say that she wasn't ready for that, she wanted to enjoy what they had and not worry about anyone or anything else. But the pregnancy was something she couldn't brush away.

For so long she had believed that she would never have a baby, and had carried that knowledge with her, a twist of pain in her heart, always there in the background, even when she was really happy. And now she was pregnant, she had confounded that horrible doctor; she had won the lottery. She should be over the moon, but she couldn't stop thinking that it was the wrong time. But was there ever a right one? She couldn't imagine what her life would be like raising a child on her own, but then again she couldn't imagine ending this pregnancy. This might be her one and only chance to have a baby. Her head was so full of contradictions and questions. She didn't know what the answers were.

Ed emerged from the en suite bathroom. He was naked, and even after just a few hours in the sun his skin was already turning golden brown. He had a beautiful body – a body she had revelled in touching and kissing and fucking . . . All that seemed strange to her now. He came up behind her and put his arms around her waist.

Don't touch my boobs! She almost flinched as he ran his hands over her shoulders. Great. So now on top of having the world's most immense boobs, she had become frigid.

Ed kissed her neck. 'You look gorgeous.' She could feel his hard cock pressing against her and usually she would want nothing more than to tumble on to the bed with him. She adored the fact that he loved sex as much as she did. Harry had barely showed any interest in it for the last year of their relationship. She could still remember what it felt like when he rejected her, making yet another excuse about being too tired or too stressed. After a while she had stopped suggesting it and retreated to her side of the bed, wrapped up in the duvet, feeling like a leper. But Ed was never too tired, he was always up for it and so was she, until now . . . He unfastened her costume and murmured, 'Any chance of a quickie?'

'Do you mind if we don't? I still don't feel great.'

'Sorry, I thought you were okay.' He kissed her forehead. 'Yeah, you do still look a bit pale.'

'I'm sure I'll be fine tomorrow.' Tor had no idea how she would feel tomorrow, but she had to say something. She refastened her costume.

There was a knock at the door and Ed barely had time to reach for a towel before Frankie steamed in, oblivious his near-nakedness.

'Don't mind me,' he commented, grabbing his trunks and retreating into the bathroom for some privacy.

'Can you fucking believe it!' she exclaimed, coming to a halt in front of Tor, hands on hips, dark eyes blazing. 'Not only do I have to put up with wanker-banker Matt for two weeks, but there's also that girl! This is supposed to be a holiday! Not a fucking endurance test!' She grimaced. 'I mean, Candy. What the fuck kind of name is that? It's the name of a lap-dancer. What's her second name? Floss? She looks like she's straight out of *TOWIE* – not that I've ever seen it. Did you see her nails? Gross. And all that make-up? What is Patrick thinking of? She's far too young for him. What can they possibly have in common or talk about?'

Tor was tempted to reply that she didn't think Patrick was with Candy for her conversation, but didn't. And she wanted to point out that there was nothing wrong with having an age gap in a relationship. But Frankie didn't seem to want an answer anyway, just to vent. 'I hate the way she looks . . . everything fake . . . everything out there . . . everything about sex. I see young girls dressed like that and it does my head in. It's like feminism never happened! Pandering to this idea that we should all look like lap-dancers, and that women are objects with no brain, no ambitions, beyond looking like Barbies or those hideous Bratz!'

Oh, lordy! Frankie was well and truly off on one. Tor didn't know why she was so riled by Candy. Usually Frankie was supportive of all women, especially those who were younger than her, and especially someone like Candy. She'd taught girls who turned out just like that, and was usually full of compassion and hope for them, never judging them.

Frankie paused momentarily to draw breath and Tor seized the opportunity to speak up. If she didn't it would be another king-sized rant.

'Don't get so wound up, Frankie, Matt's a decent bloke and he's not a wanker-banker, he's a partner in a law firm. Candy seems sweet. She might not have gone to university, and she wears too much make-up and has overdone the fake tan but that doesn't make her a bad person. She's probably really nervous. We're all older than her and it's not easy meeting a bunch of strangers.' *Especially judgmental scary ones like you.* She kept the last thought quiet.

It didn't go down well. 'Hah! I'd like to hear you sounding so reasonable when she's got her fake nails into Ed, batting her fake lashes at him and thrusting her twenty-something tits in his face . . . which are probably fake too.'

'Candy's not my type,' Ed said calmly as he walked out of the bathroom, in his trunks, 'so Tor doesn't have any worries on that score. Or on any other score.' He put his arm around her. She smiled at him. Even after five months it was still a novelty to hear someone be so complimentary to her. In the early weeks Tor would think that Ed was taking the piss, as she had been so used to Harry routinely putting her down.

Frankie was less impressed. 'Are you for real?' she demanded. 'Please don't come out with my all-time least-favourite quote from a man about his woman.'

Ed looked blank. Tor interpreted, 'It's Paul Newman on why his marriage lasted. "Why fool around with hamburger when you have steak at home?"' She put her hand up to her mouth then, feeling queasy again at the mention of food. Ugh! When was this feeling going to go?

'I don't suppose Ed even knows who Paul Newman was,' Frankie commented. 'I loved that actor, but comparing women to pieces of meat? Outrageous! Unforgivable! And I'm too pissed off to think of another word for outrageous. Fucking outrageous!'

Ed rolled his eyes, 'And you an English teacher, Frankie . . . I'm not stupid. Of course I know who Paul Newman was. *Butch Cassidy and the Sundance Kid* is one of my dad's favourite films, I've watched it about ten times. And Tor's right, Matt and Candy are okay. You're on holiday. Chill.'

Frankie was so far from looking as if she was going to take his advice that Tor almost laughed, but knew it would only make matters worse if she did.

'I bet you'll hardly see either of them. I heard Matt say he wants to explore the island and stay a couple of days somewhere in the north with some friends who are already out here, and Patrick and Candy . . .' She was about to say they would be spending most of their time together, when Ed interrupted.

'Patrick and Candy will be exploring each other.'

'Thanks, I feel so much better now,' Frankie replied in a tone so sarcastic Tor was surprised it hadn't withered the clematis growing round the window.

Tor barely had time to roll her eyes at Ed after Frankie had stomped off before Leila and Tom knocked at the door. Leila seemed as wound up as Frankie. 'I could strangle him!' she hissed.

There was no need for Tor to ask who she meant.

'So he hadn't given you any idea that he was bringing her?'

'None at all!' Leila glared at Tom. 'He didn't tell you, did he? And you forgot to pass it on.'

Tom sighed, 'No, he didn't bother to tell me either. And if he had, even I would have remembered that he was bringing someone called Candy.'

'Knowing him, he probably got pissed one night and suggested it to her – and she jumped at the chance of a free holiday. And Patrick didn't even stop to think about whether she would fit in or not. This is meant to be a relaxing holiday for close friends. She looked as if she was dressed to go clubbing when she arrived here. God knows what she'll wear if she actually goes out clubbing. Hot pants and nipple tassels!'

Tor hoped that Candy was well out of earshot.

'Let's hope she does,' Tom attempted to joke, but no one smiled.

'She seemed okay,' Tor said cautiously. 'Knowing Patrick, he didn't tell her that he hadn't bothered to let you know.'

'I just don't need this,' Leila groaned, sitting on the bed and putting her head in her hands.

'Don't get so wound up, Leila, it isn't a big deal. We've got plenty of room and she seems perfectly nice. She actually stopped to talk to Gracie, which is more than Patrick did after he'd shoved that new teddy bear at her.' Tom sounded more irritated with his wife.

At this point Tor was sure that Ed must be wondering why exactly he had agreed to go on holiday with her and her friends, who gave new meaning to the word uptight . . .

After Tom had managed to persuade Leila to go and have a swim and calm down, Ed exclaimed, 'Your friends are tense, aren't they? They won't be like that all holiday, will they?'

He probably wished he had gone camping in Cornwall, in spite of the rain.

'God, I hope not,' Tor replied, then instantly felt disloyal. 'I can understand why Leila is so annoyed, but she'll be okay. And Frankie will relax soon.'

'You know what she needs,' Ed continued, grinning, 'a holiday shag. We'll have to go out clubbing and fix her up with a fit Greek.'

'I'd like to see you suggest that to her,' Tor replied, thinking that there was absolutely no way she was going to a club. She didn't especially like going clubbing when she was on top form and able to have a few drinks, never mind feeling like an elephant in a maxi dress with boobs the size of WMDs.

Clubbing and festivals were two areas where she had put her foot down with Ed. He had wanted her to go to Glastonbury with him and six of his friends back in June, expecting her to jump at the chance. But Tor had never been a festival chick. Every summer when the magazines published pictures of slender girls rocking a tiny pair of shorts that flaunted most of their bum cheeks, a vest, and Hunter wellies, her heart sank. Tor was about fifties dresses, fitted shirts and pencil skirts. Heels. Glamour. Make-up. A blowdryer. Access to hot and cold running water.

'I don't do camping,' she had told him. 'I might consider glamping, in the VIP area in a camper van – no, hang on! Not big enough. A Winnebago with a double bed . . . a proper one, not a fold-down excuse . . . and its own shower and loo. Can you promise me that?'

'I've got a two-man tent, a blow-up mattress and a really good torch,' Ed had said hopefully. 'We can zip our sleeping bags together – it'll be cosy. You don't need to have a shower, you can use baby wipes, and the chemical loos are much better than the holes in the ground they used to have. Go on, Tor, it'll be fun.'

Fun and the words 'two-man tent', 'no showers' and 'chemical loos' to Tor did not compute. She had resisted. And felt fully vindicated when it rained the entire weekend, and turned the fields into gigantic mud baths. Ed's tent had collapsed under the sheer weight of water and he'd had to share with his friends. Because their tent wasn't big enough, they'd had to sleep in shifts. He got bitten by a horse fly and his arm turned black, he developed a stye in his right eye and someone nicked his phone. Ha-ha-ha. Fun indeed.

When she had met him at Brighton station she

had hardly recognised him as he was so filthy, crusted in mud from head to toe as if he had been rolling in it. At the time she had laughed but now that memory made her feel blue, as it was a reminder of how very different her life was from his. That was his idea of a good time. If on the rarest of chances he wanted to be involved in their baby's life, he would want them to go camping. It would be baby wipes all round . . .

Chapter 8

Candy

Leila had been perfectly polite to her, giving her a guided tour of the villa and introducing her to all her friends, who had been equally polite, but Candy was no fool. She could tell that her hostess had been taken aback by her arrival and was most likely mightily pissed off with Patrick. Candy was feeling pissed off with him herself as he had promised her that he had told his friends – she could clearly remember him saying, 'Oh, yeah, Leila says she can't wait to meet you. She loves a full house. She's the hostess with the mostest. The more the merrier.' It was bollocks! He hadn't got round to telling her. But Patrick was flaky and unreliable. Candy knew this after just four weeks. And now she was going to have to face the consequences with these women she was pretty sure she had zero in common with . . .

'I'll leave you to get unpacked. There are fresh towels on the shelf in the bathroom, and then do come and have a drink by the pool,' Leila had said as she showed Candy the guest bedroom.

It was about five times the size of her own pokey bedroom in the council flat she shared with her two younger sisters. Everything here looked expensive and well made: the elegant wrought-iron headboard, painted white, the mother-of-pearl inlaid bedside tables, the matching dressing table, the elegant white wardrobe – and this was the guest bedroom! The whole villa was stunning, furnished in what Candy thought was called a shabby chic French style in the bedrooms with expensive, distressed furniture, cool pastel-coloured walls and delicate silk curtains, while the bathrooms, living room and kitchen were all ultra-modern and minimalist. She had run out of adjectives to praise everything and there were only so many times she could say 'Wow'.

She wondered what Leila would make of her tiny flat, where everything had come from charity shops and car boot sales, where the door on the fridge was a bugger to close, there was a damp patch in the lounge that was getting bigger, and no shower but for one of those annoying rubber attachments that you put over the taps, but which always managed to spring loose when you were halfway through washing your hair, spraying the floor with water.

She wanted to call her sisters, Keira and Mollie,

to check they were okay, but Patrick walked in, dragging her case with one hand and clutching a bottle of beer in the other.

He kicked the door shut behind him, handed her the beer and began unzipping her playsuit. 'So what d'you reckon? Two weeks of sun, sex and more sex.'

Candy put her hand over his, to stop him. 'Someone might come in.'

'No one will.' He manoeuvred her back on to the bed, silencing her with a kiss.

Oh, well, Candy reflected as Patrick fumbled with her knickers, he never took that long. And indeed, some five minutes later it was all over.

'You didn't come,' he said reproachfully as Candy rolled out of his hot embrace.

She didn't care. All she could think about was getting outside in the sun. This was only her second time abroad. Well, the first time didn't exactly count as it was a school camping trip to the Isle of Wight where it poured with rain the entire week. She wanted to experience something new, not lie in bed with Patrick, who had seemed so promising when she met him, but who was becoming a disappointment on so many fronts.

'Yeah, well, later.' Knowing that there probably wouldn't be a later as Patrick would have drunk too much by then. 'I'm going to have a shower.'

'We could have one together,' he murmured. 'You know I'm very good with my hands.'

Really the moment had passed for her. 'Like I said, babe, later.'

When she'd met Patrick she'd thought he was one of the most handsome men she had ever seen, and fit, and charming, and funny. He seemed to belong to a world where anything was possible, where if you wanted something it was easy to get it, there was nothing to hold you back. And she still thought that he was handsome and all the other things, but she also thought that Patrick had a drink problem – not that he would admit this for a second. But Candy's uncle was an alcoholic and she knew all the signs, all the denials, all the lies, all the 'I can stop any time I want', all the bullshit.

She was categorically not in love with him, but he was good company and she fancied him, and when he'd suggested coming away she thought, why not? Yes! Why not? She never did anything impulsive – she never could as she was responsible for her sisters. But they were older now and she was owed loads of holiday from the salon, and Carly, her aunt, no longer married to the alkie uncle, had offered to look after the girls. And it was the anniversary of her mum's death in August and Candy felt she had to do something different, experience something different. Her mum would have approved, especially as it was Greece. She had gone to Corfu with Candy's dad when they first got together and had loved it, always longing to

83

go again and take Candy and her sisters. But they could never afford to go. The closest any of them got to Greece was looking at the photograph her mum had hung over the kitchen sink of a deserted beach in Corfu, where the water was an astonishing vivid green.

Yes, she needed a holiday. But now she was here, in this luxurious villa, she was having second thoughts. She had noticed the way the other women looked at her . . . especially that pale-faced Frankie. If looks could kill, Candy had a feeling she would be toast. Burnt toast. She shouldn't have worn so much make-up, but she'd had no idea what to expect and had decided to go all out for glamour. Wrongly as it turned out. She would tone it down. In fact, it would be a relief not to put on so much make-up. Claudia, who owned the salon where she worked, expected all the girls to wear full make-up all the time, and Candy was sick of getting up an extra half an hour earlier than she needed to in order to pile on the slap.

She spent ages in the shower, enjoying the sensation of the powerful jets of water cascading on to her skin. She used Patrick's delicious-smelling and no doubt expensive Molton Brown Blissful Templetree bodywash (whatever that was), knowing that he wouldn't mind. He was very generous with his things and his money, one of his better qualities. But then he'd probably never known what it was like to be scrabbling around in your purse for enough coins to buy tea for your two sisters and yourself; always to go to the cheapest supermarkets and at the times when they reduced foods that had reached their sell-by dates; sometimes only to have enough money for the girls to share a bag of chips, even though you knew, and didn't need Jamie Oliver to tell you, that they should eat healthy food, five portions of fruit and vegetables a day. He'd probably never had to turn off the heating and huddle under duvets, all three of them together in front of the TV, because even though it was freezing they were too worried about paying the bill to have it on . . . No, there was no way that Patrick would know about any of this. His very comfortable world revolved around him and no one else.

Candy's friend Madison thought her romance with Patrick was like the plot of *Pretty Woman*, her all-time favourite film. And she had forced Candy to watch it with her. Candy loathed rom-coms. She was all for fantasy – *Game of Thrones*, *True Blood* – things with a bit of bite. She considered *Pretty Woman* the most ridiculous film ever. Like, who would seriously believe that the sensationally beautiful Julia Roberts was a prostitute! She would have been instantly snapped up on *America's Next Top Model*! And she wasn't even a high-class escort, operating out of a penthouse suite with champagne in the fridge and a Jacuzzi, but a prostitute who hung out on street corners. A prostitute with a heart of gold, though, who was only waiting for her prince in a white limo to rescue her so she could go and get her high-school diploma. Madison told her off for going on Facebook during one of the romantic scenes. No, Patrick was not Edward Lewis/Richard Gere and she didn't need anyone to rescue her, thank you very much. Candy was perfectly capable of doing that herself.

When she returned to the bedroom, wrapped up in a large white fluffy bath towel, Patrick was not there. It was a bit of a relief. She unzipped her suitcase and tried to decide which bikini to wear – the leopard print had seemed a good idea when she bought it from Primark, but now she worried that it was too tarty. She could just imagine the look that Frankie would give her if she wore it. She went for her pink one, with the gold rings at the side of the briefs, put on some pink lip gloss, a pair of sparkly flip-flops then made her way outside.

The infinity pool with the sea beyond almost took her breath away, it was so perfect. The impressively big pool was lined with shimmering turquoise mosaic tiles and the water sparkled invitingly in the sunlight. It definitely didn't look like the kind of pool where you'd find revolting old plasters or hairbands covered in hair lurking in the depths or where you'd end up with a verruca the instant you dipped your foot in the water. Expensive-looking loungers were arranged around the wide paved area along with two huge white parasols. It was straight out of the pages of a glossy magazine – your perfect getaway. Candy had never ever been anywhere like this before. The wealth and opulence were almost overwhelming. As she walked over to one of the loungers she tried to act as if she belonged there, rather than feeling like an intruder who had stumbled into the wrong place and was about to be found out.

Patrick was floating on a lilo in the centre of the pool, a bottle of beer in his hand; Gracie was in the shallow end with her dad, practising handstands in the water. Tom seemed like a really nice bloke. He could do with a shave, though – his two- or three-day old beard made him a look a bit of a scruff. Hunky Ed with the abs was sunbathing next to Tor. Candy admired Tor's good looks. She had fantastic bone structure, a knock-out figure and highlighted blonde hair, cut in a stylish shoulder-length bob. Candy had dyed her hair peroxide blonde once – she had gone through practically every colour – but it had turned ginger and she'd had to fork out a fortune at the hairdresser's to correct it. She stuck to darker colours now.

Frankie was lying under one of the parasols. If she wasn't looking quite so sulky she would be exceptionally pretty, with shiny dark brown hair that was obviously natural, beautiful dark brown eyes, well-shaped eyebrows and a wide, sensual mouth. She was pale, so pale she almost glowed. She could definitely do with slapping on a bit of fake tan. Candy considered offering to lend her some, but couldn't quite see Frankie and her getting girly and pally and swapping beauty tips. Leila was lying next to her. Her skin was a gorgeous brown that Candy doubted was fake. She looked elegant, sophisticated. As if she entirely belonged.

Candy wondered where Matt was. From the moment she'd met him at the airport Matt had been lovely to her, a real gentleman, old-school style. If he was surprised to see her with Patrick, he certainly hadn't shown it. He had put her at her ease, chatted to her about Brighton, which he knew well, about *Game of Thrones*, which it turned out he was a fan of too, about her sisters and his nieces, while Patrick flicked through *GQ* and bitched about the features and the journalists who had written them and downed a double vodka and tonic before they even got on the plane. It had only been half-past seven in the morning, but he'd claimed it was one of his rituals before flying. She and Matt each had a latte from Pret.

'Come in the pool, Candy, there's room on the lilo for two,' Patrick called out.

'No, thanks,' she replied. In spite of living by the sea in Brighton she couldn't swim and never liked to be out of her depth.

She sat down on one of the loungers and attempted to adjust it so she could sit up. It was five in the afternoon and the sun was still burning hot. Candy loved the feel of it on her skin. All those hours and hours she spent inside the salon:

massaging, squeezing, plucking, exfoliating, spray tanning, waxing other women and the occasional male – only ever a back wax, mind you. She drew the line at back, sac and crack. Compared to that this was sheer paradise. Compared to anything this would be paradise!

'Is everything okay with the room, Candy?' Leila asked.

'Great, thanks. Everything's lovely here. It's like a hotel,' she gushed, then stopped. 'I mean a luxury hotel, of course. Like a boutique one, I imagine. I've never stayed in one.'

Leila smiled. 'Thanks. My dad designed it and spent ages agonising over every single fitting.'

'It's not a hotel though. We do have to do our own cooking and clearing up.' That from Frankie, said not especially warmly, which made Candy wonder if she knew what she and Patrick had been up to for all of five minutes . . .

'Oh, yeah, of course,' Candy replied. She was still attempting to adjust the lounger and not having any luck – at this rate she would snap one of her nails and she doubted that any of these women would know where the nearest nail bar was.

'Are you going to have some kind of rota?'

Patrick snorted with laughter, and nearly fell off the lilo. 'Rota, my arse! This is what will happen. Leila nags Tom, who does all the shopping and most of the cooking; Tor sets the table, and stacks and empties the dishwasher; I'm in charge of booze, purchasing of, opening of and drinking most of. Frankie does fuck all, but interrogates Tom about what he's going to cook to make sure it's not too calorific for her. I'm not sure about Ed yet – he's most likely going to be eye candy – no pun intended – for the ladies. But maybe he can clear the table and be the pool boy too.'

Not surprisingly there were mutters of outrage from all the women, and Ed didn't exactly look thrilled.

'That is not true, Patrick!' Leila was the first to retaliate. 'We all pull our weight.'

There was a pause when everyone was looking at Patrick and he seemed to register that he had overstepped the mark.

'Sorry, just teasing. It was all a lie except for the part about me and Tom. Oh, by the way did you like the perfume, Leila? You wear Chanel No. 5, don't you?'

She managed a smile and a lie, 'Yes, thanks, Patrick. Very generous of you.'

'It was the least I could do to thank you for having us,' he replied.

He could actually be quite sweet when he put his mind to it, Candy reflected. He had spent a small fortune in duty free buying perfume for Leila, Tor and Frankie, a teddy bear and a watch for Gracie. He had bought her a pair of Chanel sunglasses, perfume and an iPod. It was like there were two sides to him – good Patrick and bad Patrick. She was about to give up wrestling with the lounger when Ed noticed her struggling, came over and easily slotted the top part into the correct groove.

'Thanks,' Candy said gratefully.

'No problem,' he replied.

He smelt deliciously of sun cream, was even better-looking close up, with a cute smattering of freckles on his nose, and those abs were quite something . . . If he wasn't already with Tor, Candy would definitely enjoy having a bit of a flirt with him. But he was out of bounds. She was aware of Tor looking at her now.

Take a chill pill, sweetheart, she felt like saying, *I'm not after your man.* But she knew it wouldn't go down well, so instead she went for flattery. 'I love your costume,' she told Tor, which was partly to get her on her side, and partly true as she did like the red-and-white polka-dot number. 'It's very retro.'

'Thanks. I'm feeling a bit too lardy to wear a bikini. And retro is my thing. I own a boutique in the Laines, you'll have to come in sometime.'

'Thanks, I will. And I know what you mean about the costume. I have days like that when I feel really fat.'

Tor cracked a smile. Phew, job done. It would be nice to know that at least one of the women there didn't think Candy was a slag in a Primark bikini who had no right to be here.

Ed and Tom were looking at the pair of them in bewilderment.

'I don't know what you're talking about,' Ed commented. 'Words are coming out of your mouth but they make no sense at all. None of you are fat, what are you on about?'

''Course you don't understand, you're a bloke,' Candy said, rolling her eyes at Tor and Leila. Then added, 'Where's Matt by the way? He was so nice to me on the flight. It was the first time I'd been on a plane and I was dead nervous.'

'It was so sweet. She actually wanted to watch the air steward's safety demonstration, can you believe it?' Patrick drawled. 'I told her we wouldn't need to know any of it because if the plane crashed we'd all be dead. Putting on a life jacket or oxygen mask and knowing where the emergency exits are would be bugger-all use.'

'I imagine that was an immense comfort to Candy,' Leila replied sarcastically.

'It really was.' Candy was equally sarcastic. 'And then he fell asleep for the entire flight. Matt was the one who held my hand when we hit some turbulence. I had no idea what it was and I was freaking out, thinking that we were going to crash.'

That got Patrick's attention. 'Did he now? I hope that's all he held.'

'He was a real gentleman actually,' Candy replied.

'Hmm, don't be deceived. I'm sure Matt has it in him to be a dirty dog,' Patrick drawled. 'Filthy, in fact. Those posh, clean-cut, ex-public-school types are always the worst.'

'Not everyone is like you,' Leila exclaimed, then quickly added, 'Sorry, Candy. I've known Patrick a long time.'

'It's okay,' she replied cheerfully, 'I haven't known him long at all, but I already know what he's like.'

'Hey!' Patrick called out. 'Stop talking about me as if I'm not here.'

'You should hear what they say when you're really not here, mate. And they don't even know the half of it.' That from Tom, who had been quiet up to now.

Patrick looked slightly pissed off. He flipped over on to his stomach and paddled the lilo to the side of the pool where he left his beer bottle (empty by now) and then slid off the lilo and swam underwater. Candy was sure that it was so he could avoid hearing any more negative comments about his character. He was very good at dishing it out, not at all good at taking it. She closed her eyes. Ah, well, she was sure she could handle him. Two weeks wasn't long, and she really did need this holiday . . .

Chapter 9

Leila

Leila glanced surreptitiously in Candy's direction. It was hard not to stare at her. The young woman was wearing a teeny-weeny pink bikini, the bottoms of which were so small Leila was convinced they would fit Gracie. The halterneck top was struggling to contain her assets. But thankfully she was still wearing it. She might look a bit tarty but she was sexy with a capital S. She was already tanned to a glorious deep rich brown, fake or natural, Leila couldn't tell, but her money was on fake. Leila couldn't help feeling a little middle-aged by comparison, rather drab, a little too Miss Goody Two Shoes in her turquoise bikini, which she had bought because of the generously cut briefs which offered 'full rear coverage' according to the website blurb. She wondered how Candy's tiny pair had been described. Cheek baring? Arse flashing? Bootilicious briefs? Mind you, if Leila's bum looked as pert as Candy's she might have been tempted to go for them . . . She wondered what the men – specifically Tom – made of Candy, and then decided she would rather not go there.

'How come you're so tanned, Candy? Have you been away already this summer?' Frankie asked. 'Or is it from going on sunbeds?' There was a definite judgmental edge to her voice. Leila would have to mention it to her in private; she couldn't bear being surrounded by tension. It was bad enough Patrick landing the surprise guest on her without Frankie adding to the mix.

'No way! I'd never fry myself on one of those . . . far too bad for your skin. I don't want to end up a wrinkled old bag with skin cancer.' She gave a throaty, sexy laugh. 'No, I got a spray tan yesterday – Fake Bake. It's good, isn't it? They do a range for fair skin as well.' Candy seemed to be trying her best to be friendly but Frankie was still looking at her as if she was something she had found on the bottom of her flip-flop.

'Thanks, but I prefer being pale.' Frankie paused. 'I always think that fake tan looks so, well – fake. And it always smells so vile. It must be all those chemicals.'

'Meow! Saucer of milk for Frankie!' Patrick called out. He was back on the lilo, sprawled out in his tight black trunks that showed off his impressive physique. He had defined abs that a man ten years younger would be proud of. And didn't he know it.

Frankie was renowned for being direct and outspoken and Leila had always liked her for those qualities, but not at this precise moment. At this moment she wanted her friend to be polite and easygoing. She might as well wish for the moon on a stick.

She waited for Candy quite rightly to take offence, but to her surprise the girl laughed it off. 'Actually it smells okay, and as you can see I like a bit of fake. I've got fake nails, fake lashes and dyed hair. In fact, I've forgotten what my natural hair colour is, I've been dying it for so long. A boring mouse-brown, I think.'

And just as Leila was thinking that was it, Frankie started up again. 'And did you make-up your name, Candy?'

Bloody hell! Couldn't she give it a rest?

'No, my mum loved that Jackson 5 song "Candy Girl". And I like it. It's different.'

'It suits you,' Frankie replied in a neutral tone, but Leila knew what a depth of disapproval was lurking underneath.

'And what about you – is Frankie your real name?' Candy asked.

Hah! That served Frankie right. She absolutely hated her real name, never used it.

'No, my real name is Francine, but I've been Frankie all my life. My mum thought Francine was really stylish and sophisticated, but from the moment she saw me she realised I had to be Frankie.'

'It suits you,' Candy replied in as neutral a tone as Frankie had used.

Clearly Candy was no bimbo, in spite of her best efforts to look like one, and Leila liked the way she could answer Frankie back and put Patrick in his place – God knows he needed it. And she seemed to have grasped that she needed to win the women over as she had complimented Tor, which had gone down well. Thankfully. They could all do without Tor being jealous of Candy as well.

Leila knew how insecure Tor felt about younger women around Ed, though she had no reason to, as he so clearly adored her. Leila thought that he was one of the best things ever to happen to her friend. She'd had her doubts when they first got together, mainly because Tor had an unfortunate knack of picking total bastards, as if it was her special gift only to go out with men who started out charming but all too quickly became charmless. But from the word go Ed had been nothing but lovely to her. Leila had registered the way he always listened to her, clearly respected her, and looked as if he believed he was the luckiest man in the world to be with her. He had looked after her when she had 'flu, he always made an effort with her friends, and seemed to strike just the right balance between wanting to be with her, and giving her space to do her own thing.

If Leila were being really picky she would say that perhaps Ed was too lovely and too easygoing, that he didn't have the edge that someone like, say, Tom did. But that really was being picky because surely nice was better than a man with such an edge he ended up making you feel bad about yourself? Secretly Leila harboured a wish that Tor and Ed would move in together, not that she had dared mention this to Tor, who was always downplaying the seriousness of the relationship, saying that it was casual, easy come, easy go, and she was massively hung up on the age gap.

'God, I fucking love the sun!' Patrick declared, hauling himself out of the pool and flopping down on the lounger next to Candy's. Then he caught sight of Leila's frown. 'Shit! I mean, sorry! I keep forgetting there are little ears present, I'm so unused to being around kids. I will do better, I promise.'

Luckily Gracie chose that moment to duck underwater. Leila had lost count of the number of times she had asked Patrick not to swear in front of her daughter. At this rate Gracie would return home swearing like a trouper, all thanks to him.

'It's absolutely wonderful here, Leila,' he continued, 'Thanks so much for having us. You and Tom are complete stars.' He reached for his cigarettes and lit one. That was something else she would have to ask him not to do around Gracie. Leila hated being cast as the killjoy nag. She waited for Frankie to say something as she knew her friend loathed people smoking near her, but for some reason she didn't.

'You're welcome,' she replied, trying not to sound too tight-lipped and not at all sure she succeeded.

'So how's your work going?' Tom had left Gracie to her own devices in the pool and had joined them. Patrick was a features writer on a glossy men's magazine. He was always jetting off to glamorous locations to interview actors, musicians, models. She wondered if Tom envied him, and hoped not. The two men had met seven years ago when Tom's own career as a journalist was on the rise, like Patrick's. There had been lots of bonding during drinking sessions at the pub that ended with Tom staggering back to Brighton on the last train and waking up with a raging hangover and vowing never to do it again – until the next time. Leila had always found Patrick entertaining company in moderation. It was Tom who had persuaded her to ask him to the villa, and as she had asked two of her friends, it had seemed only fair.

Patrick shrugged. 'Same old, same old. I'm getting tired of interviewing actors. They're all so cagey these days, I could write the bloody piece without ever meeting them – it's all so tightly controlled by their PRs. No one is ever honest about anything any more. They all want to come across as whiter than white. No drugs, no sex, no carbs. No fun. It's so fucking tedious. I'm thinking of writing a novel, I've got enough source material.'

'Sounds good, what would it be about?'

Leila admired the way that Tom could sound interested. Patrick had been talking about writing a novel for as long as they had known him. He had zero self-discipline and could only work when he had pressing deadlines. He was never going to write one.

'Contemporary. A crime slash love story. Parts set in London, parts in Hong Kong, parts in Sydney. I've got so many ideas,' Patrick said airily. 'So what about you, mate?'

'Well, I'm only doing two days a week at the sports desk because Leila's been so full on with her production company. There is a possibility of ghost writing an autobiography, but nothing concrete. The rest of the time I'm looking after Gracie.'

'Good for you.' Patrick said, sounding as if it was very much rather you than me . . . 'D'you get to hang out with MILFs and hot nannies in cafés? I bet they're all desperate for a bit of male attention.'

Typical of Patrick to drag this conversation down to his level.

Tom gave rather a strained laugh. 'It's not like that, Patrick. It's a lot of going to the park, and to different groups – art, dance, gymnastics, that kind of thing. And there are quite a few other dads. And I look after my daughter because I want to. We're not stuck in a time warp when men go out to work and women stay at home. It's called the twenty-first century, Patrick.'

'But we are going to look at work schedules,' Leila put in. 'So Tom can work more. It's only fair.'

But by then Patrick had closed his eyes as if the conversation was just too boring, and was busy blowing a perfect smoke ring.

She smiled at Tom to show that she was on his side and that she appreciated everything he did. The smile wasn't enough. Patrick's comments had hit a raw nerve. Tom didn't acknowledge Leila. Instead he got up and dived into the pool. She looked back at Patrick. God, he could be insensitive! He was too cool for school, incredibly good-looking, but he had never done anything for Leila – probably because she knew him far too well, and was aware of his appalling track record with women. Besides, his looks were more pretty boy and she preferred her men rugged. She definitely wouldn't want a man who was slimmer than her, which was why she hadn't minded that Tom had put on a bit of weight over the last year, though it was fair to say that he'd looked more toned recently, with no sign of the slight paunch he had been developing.

While she had been feeling so on edge, Tom seemed to be in full holiday mode. He had been brilliant with Gracie today, playing endless games with her in the pool. He calmly made lunch for everybody and didn't even get wound up by Frankie hovering at his shoulder checking how much olive oil he was putting in the salad dressing – Patrick had got that bit right. But then Tom wasn't riddled with guilt, he didn't dread switching on his phone for fear of what he might find. In fact, Leila hadn't switched on her phone at all today – and if she had her way she wouldn't switch it on for the entire holiday. Tom didn't feel like the worst person in the world. He wasn't the worst person in the world. She was. She was amazed no one else could see it . . .

Matt strolled out on to the terrace and Frankie immediately made an excuse about being too hot and practically jogged inside. It was glaringly obvious that she was avoiding him, but thankfully he didn't comment on it.

'I'm sorry you've ended up with the smallest room,' Leila told him. 'I had intended to toss a coin between you and Patrick, but—'

'I turned up,' Candy interrupted, sounding upset. 'I'm really sorry.' She sat up and hugged her knees, suddenly seeming very uncomfortable. Leila felt a flash of sympathy for her. She was so young and it wasn't her fault that Patrick hadn't checked before bringing her.

'It's no problem at all, Candy,' Matt replied easily. 'I don't intend to spend much time in my bedroom.'

Leila smiled at him gratefully. Thank God for Matt being so easygoing. Just as well as he was going to be spending two weeks with Frankie, the human antithesis of easygoing. Matt was one of Tom's oldest friends, he had been his best man and Leila had always got on well with him. But Matt's hectic work schedule and the fact that he lived in London meant that Tom had hardly seen him lately. It was a pity as Leila could imagine him confiding in Matt whereas she couldn't imagine him doing the same with Patrick.

Chapter 10

Frankie

She had already had a beer today and had decided that one was her limit, but when Frankie opened the fridge intending to get out a bottle of water she reached for a beer instead. Christ knows she needed something to take the edge off. A double vodka would hit the spot better, but beer would have to do. At this rate she would be flying home a bloated functioning alcoholic . . . or maybe not so functioning.

It had taken a monumental effort to pick herself up off the bathroom floor and saunter downstairs as if she didn't have a care in the world. All she could think about was Patrick having a girlfriend. Her entire, carefully constructed fantasy about finally getting together with him lay in ruins, demolished by a girl with too much make-up and the name of a porn star.

She flipped off the lid and took a long swig, and was rather inelegantly wiping her mouth with the back of her hand when Matt walked in. He was wearing a pair of black swim shorts and a blue shirt, unbuttoned. There seemed to be so much of him. He was all broad shoulders, muscular chest and long legs. She almost didn't know where to look and felt awkward and self-conscious in her bikini.

Was there going to be no escaping him? Couldn't he take a hint? What else could she do? Wear a badge saying 'I can't stand you, Matt Cartwright, bugger off'? She was all set to make an escape upstairs when he unexpectedly said, 'Do you fancy a game of table tennis? I need to do something active after the flight.'

She wanted to say, *WTF! Why would I want to play table tennis with you after what happened at Leila and Tom's wedding? We could be the only two survivors after a nuclear war, just us plus a table tennis table, two bats and a ball, which inexplicably haven't melted, and I still wouldn't want to play with you!*

The fact that Frankie had a very competitive streak and adored table tennis, and actually ran the table tennis club at school, was irrelevant here. She absolutely couldn't stomach the idea of spending any time alone with him. Was he taking the piss? Deliberately trying to provoke her?

The blue eyes looked sincere so maybe not, or maybe he was skilled at deception. Yep, must be the latter. She couldn't believe he would actively want to spend time with her.

'Actually I was going to have a lie down in my room.' She knew she sounded abrupt. Rude was her default setting with Matt. 'But I'm sure one of the others will play with you.'

'Okay, but I was kind of hoping it would break the ice between us. You clearly didn't know that I was going to be here and I'm sorry about that. But I'm here now so how about we make the best of it?'

He was being so grown up and reasonable, Frankie should be able to follow his lead. But she couldn't forget what had happened in the past. She had thought she would be over it by now, but two and half years on, confronted by him, she found the humiliation as searing now as it had been back then.

'Yep, I agree, but I really am tired.' A pause. 'It's not that I have a problem with you.'

Matt looked as unconvinced as she sounded.

'Another time then. We've got two whole weeks, after all,' he replied.

Like she needed to be reminded of that fact . . .

Upstairs she flopped on the bed and stared up at the ceiling. Of all in the people in all the world, why, oh why, did it have to be Matt Cartwright sharing the villa? She had first met him at Leila and Tom's pre-wedding dinner party – a chance for Tom's best friends to meet Leila's best friends. It should have been a perfectly friendly relaxed night, but Frankie arrived in a terrible state. She had met Patrick for a quick drink early that evening, and he had revealed that he was now living with Willow. He had gazed at her, all starry-eyed, and said, 'Maybe she's my "one".'

'You hardly know her!' Frankie had exclaimed, knocked sideways by the news.

He had shrugged. 'I just feel this connection to her that I can't explain.' He paused. 'I know you're going to say it's too soon, but I'm thinking of asking her to marry me. I've asked my dad to look out my mum's engagement ring. It was my grandmother's before her. What do you reckon, Frankie – a diamond from Tiffany's or the vintage?'

Somehow she had managed to come out with a reply. 'If it were me, I would want the vintage. But Willow's not into that kind of thing, is she?' Subtext she was a shallow, money-grabbing bitch compared to Frankie, who had integrity and appreciated the past. It was too subtle for Patrick.

'You're right. I'd better start saving – the bigger the better I think. Cheers, Frankie, I knew you'd know what to do. I should have you as my best woman, if Willow says yes.'

She should have cancelled dinner; she was in no state to see anyone after that, but she had forced herself to go. Somehow it had felt like a less painful option than staying in. Matt was already there, and because everyone else was coupled up she'd assumed that this was another of Leila's set-ups. He was good-looking – admittedly he was blond and Frankie tended to be attracted to dark-haired men, just like Patrick – and he was broad-shouldered and tall where Patrick was slender and only a little taller than she was. But Matt's looks made no difference. He could have been George Clooney's *doppelgänger*, she wasn't interested. She felt as if someone had taken a sledgehammer to her heart and then trampled over the pieces. It was made even more exquisitely painful by the fact that Patrick and Willow had also been invited, and spent the entire meal looking sickeningly loved up.

Frankie was bruised, hurt and vulnerable, but she wasn't going to show it. So instead she was feisty, opinionated Frankie. She took issue with Matt's job – he was partner in a law firm, specialising in commercial work, therefore she decided he had no social conscience – and with his politics, or rather with what she had decided were his politics. He was a City boy Tory in her head, and so was fair game. Matt had been perfectly polite, hadn't risen to any of her scathing comments. And all the time Frankie was aware of Patrick and Willow, who were so wrapped up in themselves they barely took any part in the conversation.

At one point Leila had cornered her in the kitchen. 'Why are you being so horrible to Matt! He's a lovely guy, what is your problem?'

Frankie had shrugged. 'I told you I didn't want

you to set me up with any more men. I'm perfectly happy being single.'

'I don't believe you, and that doesn't explain why you're being so rude to him. He's going to be Tom's best man so you'd better snap out of it. I'm not having any tension on my wedding day. I'll bloody turn into Bridezilla and make you wear a disgusting bridesmaid's dress in peach taffeta, with an empire line that will make even you look the size of a bungalow. One with really bad double glazing and pebbledash and some gnomes in the front garden – not in an ironic way!'

'You wouldn't.' But you could never tell with brides to be. Every woman, even the most rational ones like Leila, went a bit loopy as the big day drew near . . .

'I might, so promise me you won't be like this on my wedding day?'

Leila was standing near the knife block at the time, so it seemed sensible to make that promise.

But things only got worse when Patrick and Willow left the dinner party early as she had a shoot the next day. Pre-Willow Patrick would have stayed on, but now he trailed after her like a love-sick puppy.

'So finally Patrick has found someone he loves even more than himself,' Matt commented after they'd gone. 'Luckily Willow is just as self-obsessed so it's a perfect match. I'm sure they'll be very happy together.'

109

To hear him voice that criticism was like a red rag to a bull.

'Why are you so down on him? Especially when he's not here to defend himself?' Frankie retaliated.

Matt had shrugged. 'I'm not down on him. I haven't seen him for a while and I'd forgotten how immense his ego is, that's all. It's always the world according to Patrick, isn't it?'

Tom nodded. 'Yep, I don't think I heard him ask anyone else about their work. He just held forth about all the brilliant articles he's writing, in between gazing at Willow.' He grinned at Leila. 'D'you know, he actually fed her some of the dessert from his spoon. I thought you said that was unforgivable in public?'

'Probably the first time she'd had a taste of cheesecake in a decade,' Leila replied. 'Mind you, she is absolutely beautiful.'

'Stunning,' Tom agreed.

'Too thin,' Matt replied. 'And terribly dull. But like I said, perfect match for Patrick.'

To hear her friends discussing Patrick and Willow like this made Frankie reach for the wine. She entirely blamed Matt for bringing up the subject. By the end of the night she had drunk far too much, but instead of making her mellow, she felt strung out, tense, as if she could carry on drinking all night and it wouldn't even touch the pain. She ordered a taxi, and just as she was putting on her coat Matt asked her if he could share it back to his hotel. She could hardly say no. But she was resolutely silent on the journey, staring out of the window at Saturday night Brighton out on the lash, gangs of girls giggling as they tottered along in short skirts and high heels, their hair whipped up by the wind, lads in t-shirts, showing off their tattoo sleeves, and low-rise jeans showing off their underwear.

It was only when the taxi pulled up outside Matt's boutique hotel that he spoke to her. 'I'll get this.' He pulled out his wallet and went to hand her twenty pounds.

'It's okay, I'll pay.'

'Don't be silly, you're a teacher and I'm a wicked lawyer who worships money.'

Frankie hadn't said that in so many words . . . but clearly he'd got the gist. 'No, I want to.'

'How about we go halves?'

Of course that's what she should have agreed to.

'No I'll get it,' she insisted.

'We could have an arm wrestle to settle it,' he had suggested. 'But I think I'd win.'

'That's so childish. I told you: I'll pay.'

Thinking about it now, she could feel her herself blushing. She had been absolutely vile to him.

Matt had looked at her closely, 'I would suggest that you came back for coffee, but I think you'd probably kill me. Goodbye, Frankie. I think underneath it all you must be a nice person – you'd have to be for Leila to have you as her best friend. She's

111

one of my all-time favourite people. I hope you can sort out whatever is troubling you. And maybe you shouldn't go on any dates for the foreseeable future.' He was calm and polite when no doubt she had just caused him to endure one of the worst evenings of his life. He'd be dining out on 'my blind-date from hell' experience for a while.

She should have left it right there. Should. Didn't. 'Nothing's troubling me other than the fact that my best friend thinks I might have anything common with someone like you.'

Matt had shaken his head at this. 'I don't think tonight had anything to do with me.' And before Frankie could come out with another scathing putdown, he had opened the taxi door and got out.

That night would have been bad enough. But what happened at Tom and Leila's wedding made that look like a picnic in the park. Frankie never allowed herself to go there – she was usually adept at compartmentalising her feelings. But now she was stuck at this villa with Matt, she couldn't bring the shutters down and, as she lay on her bed, she relived the experience in full colour and surround sound.

There had been no avoiding Matt at the wedding as she and Tor were Leila's maids-of-honour – though maid-of-dishonour would have best described her, Frankie always thought afterwards. She behaved impeccably during the ceremony, smiling politely at Matt, warmly at everyone else, delivering a heart-felt reading of the Maya Angelou poem 'Come, and Be My Baby'.

It was at the reception, held in the grounds of a hotel in the heart of the Sussex countryside, that things went pear-shaped. Willow had arrived halfway through the wedding breakfast, a vision in a gold-sequined 1920s-style dress and matching headband that made her resemble a character from *The Great Gatsby*. Frankie hadn't realised that she was coming as Patrick had said that that they'd had a massive row and Frankie was secretly hoping that was it. However, they made up with a full-on snog and afterwards Willow had remained glued to Patrick's side.

'Not so much willow, more like bindweed,' Frankie had commented to Tor. 'And don't you think she's far too skinny? It looks as if you could snap one of her twig-like legs with your bare hands.' She had hoped it didn't sound too much like she wanted to do just that . . .

Tor had shrugged. 'There's no such thing as too skinny if you're a model, is there?' Then she had done a double take. 'Oh, my God! Check out the size of that rock. Did you know they were getting engaged?'

As if in the grip of a nightmare Frankie had taken in the diamond ring on Willow's slender finger. Its cold, hard, expensive glitter signalled the end of her dream. The song had got it all wrong –

113

diamonds were only ever a girl's best friend when you were the girl who was wearing them. It had taken Frankie every ounce of self-control to reply, 'Oh, yeah. I thought I'd told you.'

'Good luck to her then,' Tor replied. 'She'll need it with Patrick.'

Somehow Frankie switched to autopilot and got through her best woman's speech with Tor, and applauded politely at the end of Matt's best man's speech. A good one, she would give him that, with just the right balance of humour and feeling and no inappropriate sexual references that would have made parents and in-laws squirm. But after that she proceeded to hit the champagne. From then on she could only recall fragments of what happened, but those fragments were branded into her memory as if they'd happened yesterday.

Once the music started she was up on the dance floor, dancing alone or with anyone she could persuade to dance with her. She even managed to drag Matt up and could remember dancing to Prince's 'Kiss' with him, strutting around as if the night of the dinner party had never happened. She recalled shimmying up to him and wiggling her hips provocatively. The shame! Take the shame. He had been a surprisingly good dancer for someone she had down as an uptight Tory, and she remembered thinking he looked pretty good in a suit. Not as good as Patrick, but not bad. They had both thrown themselves into a succession of songs including 'Dancing Queen', 'Stayin' Alive' and 'Don't Leave Me This Way' – Leila loved her disco music – until Matt pleaded exhaustion and sat down. Frankie lasted for a couple more numbers then she grabbed a bottle of white wine and joined him, where she gabbled an apology.

'I'm really sorry about that night at Leila and Tom's. I was very rude. It was work . . . stress, you know. And I'd probably drunk too much. Sorry. I'm not usually that rude and I don't usually drink that much.' That wasn't strictly true, but he wasn't to know.

It was quite hard for her to focus. Matt's face kept going fuzzy. But fuzzy was good; it stopped her thinking about Patrick and Willow. The glittering diamond ring. Fuzzy was good. Fuzzy was what she wanted.

'No problem, Frankie, consider it forgotten.'

'And who knew Tories could dance so well? You're inspired on the dance floor, Matt. Great hip movement. Impressive performance. You've got the moves like Jagger and everything.'

He had shrugged. 'I'm not a Tory. And you're not a bad mover yourself.'

Details were even more hazy after that. She had decided, in spite of the blond hair and his job, that she quite fancied him. She had flirted with him and she thought he must have flirted back – she couldn't really remember any specifics but she remembered Matt's intense blue-eyed gaze that seemed to lock on to her and made her feel as if they were the only two people there; she liked the fact that he had undone his waistcoat, the top buttons of his shirt and loosened his tie, and she had an urge to undo all the buttons. Surely she would not have been flirting with him if there hadn't been some interest on his part? It was hard to be objective because of how the night ended. This was the moment when Frankie wished that she was living in a future where it was possible to have certain parts of her memory erased. She would have paid anything for that to happen. *Anything.*

'How about we raid the mini-bar in my room?' she had suggested, after Leila and Tom had retired to their honeymoon suite. By now she was in that state of drunkenness when she didn't want to be alone, didn't want to watch Patrick and Willow slow dancing to 'The Look of Love', didn't want to think about how the next wedding she came to might well be theirs. She wanted, needed, to be with someone. She'd had nights like these before, when she'd slept with men she wouldn't have if she'd been sober or not feeling so alone. It was precisely why she had promised herself not to get this drunk again . . .

Looking back she wondered why Matt had agreed. Revenge for her childish behaviour the first night they met? Because he was as drunk as she was? She had no way of knowing. All she did know was that once they were in her hotel room she had kicked off her shoes, put her arms round Matt's neck and kissed him. He had kissed her back. A good kiss, she remembered that much, a sexy kiss, a promising kiss. His body had felt gratifyingly solid against hers. She began unbuttoning his shirt, touching his skin, wanting to see and feel what he was made of, and she was all set to pull him on to the four-poster bed with her. There seemed no point in any further conversation, they both knew why they were here. There was no need for any beating around the bush, unless it was hers – at least she hadn't come out with that comment, a very small mercy in the big merciless scheme of things.

But suddenly Matt had stopped with the sexy kisses, let go of her and stepped back. She had managed to undo all the buttons, had glimpsed flat, hard abs.

'Sorry, this is all wrong. I'm drunk, you're very drunk and in love with someone else and I don't do this kind of thing any more.' He'd sounded regretful but that didn't take the sting out of his words. They pierced through Frankie's alcohol daze to where it hurt.

'What are you talking about?' She regretted kicking off her heels as he towered over her.

'Frankie, you know exactly what I'm talking about. I've seen the way you look at Patrick. You don't need to pretend with me. And right now, a meaningless fuck is not on my list of things to do. I'm sure it would be good, but in the morning

117

we'd probably both feel like shit and regret it. Do yourself a favour, have a glass of water, go to bed and we don't need to talk about this again. Sorry Frankie, we shouldn't have got into this situation.'

She was so stunned that she couldn't even come up with a reply. Instead she had stood there, in her fifties-style peacock blue bridesmaid's dress, which had been designed by Tor, and watched him walk out of the door. Then she had done the only possible thing in the circumstances: she had raided the mini-bar and downed two brandies, a Bacardi and a ready-mixed mojito, desperate to get the fuzzy feeling back and block out what had just happened. She contemplated knocking on Tor's door and confessing everything but thankfully couldn't find her key card. Anyway by now the room was spinning round and round as if she was riding a carousel from hell, and she had to lie down and close her eyes. At some point she thought she heard a knock at her door but she ignored it. She eventually passed out in bed fully clothed. In the morning Matt had already left and Frankie never wanted to set eyes on him or the peacock blue bridesmaid's dress ever again.

She had never told Leila and Tor about the night of shame and could only hope that Matt had been as discreet. And now here he was. For two whole weeks. The man who knew her secret. She didn't see his behaviour as that of a gentleman. To her it was rejection, pure and simple. To Frankie it was so very much worse than if they'd gone ahead with that 'meaningless fuck'. She drained her bottle of beer. How the hell was she going to get through this holiday?

Chapter 11

Tor

'At eight weeks old your baby is the size of a kidney bean, and is constantly moving. His fingers are slightly webbed.' Tor was hunched over her laptop avidly reading about fetal development. She looked at the accompanying picture in wonder. Something the size of a kidney bean was taking over her body and her life. It was amazing, incredible, and absolutely terrifying. She read on. 'The nerve cells in your baby's brain are branching out to connect with one another, forming primitive neural pathways.' The kidney bean's brain was developing! It was mind-blowing.

She heard the door open behind her and quickly closed down the page on her laptop. Ed stepped on to the terrace. Damn, she'd thought he was playing table tennis with Tom. She was desperate to do some pregnancy research but there never seemed to be a moment when she could be alone.

'Were you working?' he asked.

'No, no, just checking the news.'

'So what's been going on?'

Her mind was still full of baby facts, of translucent eyelids and newly formed earlobes. She stared at him blankly.

'What do you mean?'

'In the news, you said you were reading it. What are the big stories?'

'Oh, the wi-fi was so slow I gave up. I thought you were playing table tennis.'

'Matt and Tom are still at it – they seem to have rediscovered their childhood passion. I thought I'd leave them to it.'

Instantly Tor wondered if he felt left out because he was the youngest man there. Tom had always been friendly to Ed and, though she didn't know Matt as well, she had the feeling that he would always be pleasant. But maybe they were just humouring Ed, and thinking, *Must be nice to Tor's boy toy.* No, no, she had to stop thinking like that; it was so insidious.

'So are you okay? Not bored? You wouldn't rather be jet skiing or bungee jumping?'

He sat down. 'It's hard to go jet skiing and not look like a total wanker who is disturbing the peace and quiet of everyone on the beach, and no doubt every living creature in the sea. And as for bungee jumping . . . you know I suffer from vertigo. Believe it or not, it's fantastic being here with you, Tor.' He looked out at the view then turned to her and smiled, his gorgeous warm Ed smile.

'Better than being in Cornwall in a tent, with rain lashing against the canvas? Eating a tin of cold baked beans because it's too wet to light a fire to cook anything?' she bantered back.

'Most tents are made of polyester with a breathable coating now, Tor – I worked at Halfords one summer, I know my tents. As for food . . . we'd eat at the pub. And as for where I'd rather be, it's great here but I wouldn't mind wherever we were. And one day I will persuade you to try out camping, and I bet you'll love it.'

He had failed to see that this was not a challenge Tor was ever going to rise to.

'Nope, it's not my thing. *Really*. I'm allergic to tents – even more so now that I know they're made of polyester. I hyperventilate in confined spaces, and as for sleeping bags . . .' She gave a mock shudder. 'I haven't been camping since I was at school and even then I hated it. Getting into a damp sleeping bag at night and staying freezing cold. And then Darren Andrews, the naughtiest boy in our class, snuck into our tent and farted, so we had to evacuate in our PJs. *And* I've never ever seen a stylish kagoule for a grown woman. And, yes, I am shallow, Ed. I thought you would have realised that by now.'

He narrowed his eyes, 'We could take a duvet.

And a bigger tent. You shouldn't be so set in your ways, Tor, you should be open to new experiences.'

If only he knew – she and the kidney bean were having a new experience to end all new experiences.

She hesitated. Since she'd found out about his sister having twins, she had been itching to ask him more. She was wondering if she would be able to gauge his attitude towards children without having to come out with a direct question, which seemed too blatant, too out there.

'So have you ever been away with your sister and her twins?' It was holiday-related and therefore safe territory, a perfectly reasonable question to ask.

'Yeah, it was crazy, but fun. When they were six months old my parents rented a big house in Devon in the middle of nowhere, and I went, along with Libby, her husband, the twins and my youngest sister. We all took it in turns with the babies. I think the case of wine my dad took along helped us get through it, except for my sis who was breastfeeding and kept pointing out how many units we were having.'

'It must have been really hard work when the twins were little?'

Ed didn't need to stop and think about it. 'Totally knackering. You remember that couple on the plane? My sis and her husband looked exactly like that. They were like sleep-deprived zombies who could barely string a sentence together, and when they did manage to talk it was all about feeding, and sleeping, and whose turn it was to change the nappies. It put a massive strain on their marriage as his job was under threat, so he felt that he couldn't take too much time off and she felt she had to do everything. But they're cool now. They got through the baby years and they're really happy. And, like I said, the twins are great.'

Tor was trying to focus on the positive but all she had really taken on board was *knackering, zombies* and *massive strain*.

'You'll have to meet them when we get back. My mum's been nagging me to fix it up ever since she saw a picture of you.'

Tor didn't like to imagine what his mother's reaction had been. Typically she made light of it. 'And I'm sure she said, "Get your hands off my fresh-faced son, you raddled old witch. Pick on someone from your own decade." I bet she loved Anise.' Anise of the natural blonde hair and glowing skin. Anise who has not trapped her precious only son by getting pregnant . . .

An eye roll from Ed. 'She liked Anise, but I think she was glad when we split as Mum thought she was too bossy. And she *was* bossy. And a neat freak. I could never leave anything lying around. Ever. It did my head in.'

Ah, so Anise of the natural blonde hair and glowing skin was not perfect. And Ed, for all his many attributes, was annoyingly messy. Tor was not usually given to *schadenfreude* but there was a brief moment when she revelled in the thought of the stunning Anise doing her stunning nut when she picked up yet another pile of Ed's magazines, papers and pants.

'And Mum said you looked beautiful.'

'It must have been a flattering photograph, she can't have seen the lines.'

And now there was a sigh of exasperation from him. 'For once take the compliment, Tor! You know, I sometimes wish I'd lied about my age when I met you. If I'd told you I was thirty, you never would have made an issue of it. It's only a number. And it's all in your head.'

'Sorry, I can't help it. I don't know why.' She knew why. She was insecure enough about being older than him, and now there was the kidney bean to consider. She was convinced that Ed's family would think she'd deliberately set out to get pregnant, like one of those women she'd read about in magazines who were so desperate for a baby that they opted for DIY insemination by stealing their boyfriend's sperm from used condoms. The fact that she had never even contemplated this wouldn't convince them . . .

Ed smiled and reaching out to stroke her hair. 'You worry too much about things that don't matter.'

He was so lovely. She leant her head on his shoulder and was almost feeling reassured until Patrick sauntered by with his arm around Candy, who had put a sheer pink kaftan over the revealing bikini.

'Nothing like a bit of young flesh, is there?' He winked at Tor. 'You'll never want to see someone your own age afterwards.'

A comment that was wrong on so many levels.

He laughed when he registered the stony expression on everyone else's faces.

'Lighten up, people! It was only a joke! I'm with Candy for her mind. The fact that she has a killer body is just a bonus. I didn't even notice it when we met. We were too busy discussing Nietzsche.'

Candy thumped him on the arm.

'Ouch! That hurt!'

'Good. It was meant to.' She broke free from him and marched into the villa.

Patrick rolled his eyes at Tor. 'It really was only a joke. You know I have great respect for women.'

He didn't wait for her answer, which was just as well because she wasn't about to agree with him.

When he was inside, no doubt trying to make-up with Candy – good luck with that – Ed said under his breath, 'I really like most of your friends, but I have a problem with him. He can be a real dickhead.'

Tor sighed. 'I know what you mean. I haven't seen Patrick for ages and he seems to have gone a bit off the rails since he broke up with his fiancée; he never used to be like this. He used to be great company, always entertaining. But now it's like he doesn't censor what comes out of his mouth.'

'Total crap comes out of his mouth,' Ed muttered. 'I feel really sorry for Candy. She's too good for him. *Anyone* would be too good for him.'

'I'm sure she can take care of herself. She probably knew what she was getting into – with Patrick, what you see is what you get.'

They were quiet for a few minutes after that and it was a silence that felt comfortable, Tor realised. With Harry she would have been wondering what he was thinking, if he was okay just sitting there, or if he would rather have been doing something else, and should she suggest it? Everything was always about him. However tough things were going to be in the months ahead, at least she was no longer with Harry.

'What are you thinking?' Ed asked her. And that was something Harry had never done.

'Just that I'm happy to be here. With you.' She really meant it.

Chapter 12

Leila

Leila picked up her bag from the bed, all set to go out for dinner, when a squeaking sound made her pause.

'Tom, can you hear that? Is it the air con playing up? Can you take a look at it? There's no way I'll be able to sleep with it making that noise.'

'D'you really not know what it is?' he replied, sounding amused. Then he frowned as he added, 'Though I'm not surprised, it's been so long. Lucky Patrick, getting into the holiday spirit.'

And Leila realised that the rhythmic, squeaking noise was not a malfunction of the air conditioning but was in fact the sound of Patrick and Candy having sex – energetic sex – in their bedroom. It should have made her laugh, as the creaks and squeaks were like something out of a *Carry On* film. Instead it made her feel even more uptight.

'Oh, for Godsake! He could have shut the window! That's so typical of Patrick, only ever thinking of himself.'

As if in reply to her Patrick let out a strangled 'Oh, Candy' and the creaking abruptly stopped.

'Well, at least he remembered her name,' Tom muttered, walking towards the door. 'And don't look so pained, it is a perfectly natural thing to do. We used to do it, I seem to remember. You used to want to. You used to enjoy it. It didn't used to feel as if you were doing me a favour.'

Ouch! She wanted to protest but Gracie waltzed in then wanting to know when they were going as she was starving, and could she have a vanilla ice cream with chocolate sauce for pudding? And she had counted seven lizards that day, which made a total of twenty, and where do lizards sleep? And do they lay eggs or have babies? And could she take one home as a pet? And by the time Leila had dealt with all her questions, Tom had left the room. Once again she felt as if they were leading parallel lives. But he had been right about sex, the lack of it.

Last night when they were in bed he had put his arms around her and Leila knew he wanted to have sex. And even though she knew that if she went along with it, it might help break the tension between them and bring them closer, she couldn't because of what had happened with Jasper.

'I'm sorry,' she had said, 'I'm too tired.' Hating

129

herself for the lie, another one on top of all the others.

'Sure,' Tom had muttered, withdrawing his arms and turning over when she longed for him to hold her. She had lain awake for hours after that. Again. When she lived in North London, in her twenties, every morning when she walked to Finsbury Park tube station she would look up at the same piece of graffiti sprayed across a railway bridge that seemed perfectly to sum up her life now: *Situation normal, all fucked up.* She didn't want this situation to be normal any more.

There were many tavernas on the island, but for Leila there was only one place worth going to and that was Nikos's. It was a couple of miles away from the villa, set on a hill surrounded by pine trees and overlooking the sea. It was a stunning location and the food was fantastic, but the real draw were the friendly owners, Nikos and his English wife Ellie, whom Leila had known since she was a child.

Now as Leila and Gracie walked into the restaurant, followed by the rest of the gang, Ellie and Nikos rushed over to greet them.

'You look tired, Leila! You're working too hard!' Ellie scolded, hugging her and enveloping her in the familiar scent of sandalwood. When she wasn't helping out in the restaurant Ellie was a masseuse and taught yoga. At fifty-nine she had the body of someone at least twenty years younger – she was a great advert for yoga. She was always trying to get her husband to take it up, but he had always resisted as his ample stomach attested.

If Ellie knew the real reason why Leila looked so washed out, would her greeting have been quite so warm? Leila doubted it. She couldn't imagine Ellie ever doing anything so deceitful as having an affair.

'Yes, but I'm here now, and I can relax.'

Ellie gently kneaded her shoulders. 'And have a massage, you're full of tension.' Spot on there.

Nikos made a huge fuss of them, kissing the women, shaking hands with the men, and picking up Gracie and swinging her around. 'The best table for my friends,' he declared, showing them to one overlooking the sea. He clicked his fingers to summon one of his waiters to come and take the drinks order straight away. It was the closest Leila ever got to feeling like a VIP in a restaurant.

There was nothing fancy about the taverna, but she loved everything about it. She loved the fairy lights decorating the olive trees, the vines trailing over the whitewashed walls. She loved the cats prowling around for food – thankfully Ellie was a cat lover so these were not the skinny strays you saw in other tavernas, but well fed and looked after. She loved the blue-and-white checked paper tablecloths, the baskets of crusty white bread and bottles of olive oil, which was made on the island. She even loved the wine, which packed a punch and was considerably rougher than the wine she drank at home.

She remembered coming here with Tom on their first holiday together, ten years ago. They would sit and talk for hours over thick garlicky *tzatziki* and aubergine dip, Greek salad with salty feta cheese, and crispy calamari. Everything had seemed so hopeful and exciting, their future stretching out before them, golden with possibilities. She had loved him so much. Leila sipped the slightly acidic white wine and willed Tom to remember those happier times, but he was deep in conversation with Matt and didn't look at her. She tried to imagine what her twenty-three-year-old self would have thought of her now. Nothing good that was for sure.

She turned to Tor, who surprisingly was still on the mineral water, and then to Ed.

'This place is great,' he told her. 'The villa, the island, everything. Thanks so much for inviting us, Leila.'

'It's a pleasure. I've been wanting to come here with a group of friends again for ages.'

'And a complete stranger,' Tor said quietly, glancing over at Candy who was sitting at the end of the table.

'I don't mind,' Leila replied. 'I know I sounded like a total cow when I first met her, but to be honest I infinitely prefer her to Willow. God, she was so high-maintenance, do you remember? She had a hissy fit at my wedding because there was only vegetarian and not vegan food, and she hadn't even told me that she had become a vegan. She wouldn't eat the vegetables because they'd been cooked in butter, and when I suggested she have some bread, she said she didn't eat wheat either. Apparently she made Patrick get rid of his leather sofas because she couldn't bring herself to sit on them.'

'I suppose we should be grateful that it's Candy here and not Willow, though at least she got him to bin the leather trousers too,' Tor replied. 'He used to strut around in them like he was God's gift, and I would just think, eew! Sweaty crotch!'

'Can any man get away with leather trousers?' Leila mused.

'Yes, but they have to be under thirty and called Johnny Depp.' Tor again.

'So does that mean I have to get rid of mine?' Ed asked, grinning.

'I reckon you could get away with them, Ed,' Leila said. 'What do you think Tor?'

'Two words, sweaty crotch.'

They were all still laughing when Gracie said, 'Mummy, will you push me on the swings?'

There was a small children's play area nearby which was naturally a magnet for Gracie, but Leila just wanted five more minutes with her friends,

'Why don't you whizz down the slide and I'll there in a minute?' she replied. 'I promise.'

'No, come now, *please!*'

She was about to stand up but Candy beat her to it. 'I'll push you on the swing Gracie.'

'Are you sure?' Leila asked. Candy wasn't exactly dressed for a children's play area. She was rocking a pair of tiny black shorts, a low-cut white vest embellished with silver sequins, and pair of six-inch pink wedges, plus her fake lashes, as if she was all set for a night clubbing.

'Yep, no problem.' She turned to Patrick. 'Can you order me something veggie? I don't mind what.' Then she took Gracie's hand and walked, or rather tottered, over to the swings.

'I didn't have Candy down as a vegetarian,' Frankie commented.

'She is, won't even eat fish. But she's not averse to a bit of prime sausage.'

Patrick winked at Frankie as the whole table chorused, '*Patrick!*'

Leila picked up some bread. Breaking off a piece, she dipped it in the dish of olive oil. Patrick had often regaled them with stories of his many conquests and it had never bothered her before. He could always be relied on for a hilarious anecdote, but lately she felt that he was becoming crude, a bit of a bore. Maybe she was getting older and less tolerant; maybe it was to do with his drinking. They'd barely sat down and he'd already drained one glass of wine and was on to his second. She was sure his drinking had got worse. He never used to drink so heavily when he was with Willow. She should mention it to Tom, see if he could have a quiet word with him. Life suddenly seemed so much more complicated for all of them.

Ellie came over to take their order, accompanied by a handsome Greek lad in his early twenties. He was tall, with soulful brown eyes, and his long black hair was tied back in a ponytail. Ellie introduced him as her nephew, Dimitri who was working there for the summer before returning to university in Athens. He was holding a bottle of mineral water, poised to pour out glasses for the diners, but was riveted by the sight of Candy, who had kicked off her ridiculous shoes and was pushing Gracie on the swing and chatting away to her.

He rattled something off in Greek to Ellie, who laughed and said quietly to Leila, 'He wants to know if the beautiful girl over there has a boyfriend.'

'I'm afraid so, she's with Patrick,' Leila replied discreetly. A frown creased Dimitri's handsome young face and he muttered something under his breath.

'I think it's best if I don't translate that,' Ellie said wryly. 'He was rather hoping that she might go to one of the clubs with him later.'

Dimitri progressed along the table filling glasses, but every now and then Leila noticed that he couldn't resist sneaking another look at Candy. Oblivious to the fact that she was the object of his attention, she was now teaching Gracie how to cartwheel and flashing her hot pink bra as she demonstrated the moves.

'Oh, to be young,' Tom said, raising his wine glass and clinking it against Leila's. She was grateful for the gesture, hoped that it meant he had forgiven her for last night's rebuff.

'He'll get over it,' Frankie said, joining in their conversation. 'He's bound to have a girlfriend back home, that sort always does. Most likely he wants a quick summer fling with an English girl.'

'So you don't believe in love at first sight?' Matt commented.

Leila fully expected her friend to come back with one of her cynical putdowns, but she was confounded when Frankie replied, 'I do actually. I don't think it ever works out though. What about you?'

'I think I need to get to know the person first.'

And just when Leila was thinking that maybe Matt and Frankie were going to be friends after all, Frankie came back with, 'Yeah, I bet you need to know that they earn enough to be worth it, and that they vote the way you do.'

Or maybe not.

'I don't know why you think you know how I vote.'

Frankie curled her lip. 'Oh, what? You're going to tell me that Matt Cartwright, corporate lawyer, is a Socialist! Isn't that, like, a contradiction?'

Leila shot Frankie at WTF look. Her friend could

be so, like, obnoxious! She didn't know anything about Matt – who was definitely not a Tory, and who outside office hours mentored children from his local school in London and gave them work experience opportunities. It was down to Tor to rescue Matt, asking him about his plans to explore the island. At this rate the poor guy would leave the villa and never come back. It was supposed to be a holiday for him, not a perpetual inquisition from Rottweiler Frankie.

A resounding cry of 'Bollocks!' from Candy brought the conversation to a standstill as the whole table, and most of the other diners, looked over to where she was sitting on the swing, clutching her right foot.

'Candy's cut herself,' Gracie called out.

'Poor baby, I'll be right over.' It actually looked as if Patrick was going to tear himself away from his wine glass, but then he said to Leila, 'Actually, can you go? I hate the sight of blood and you're a mum, you're used to that kind of thing.'

She scrabbled in her bag for some antiseptic wipes, but was beaten to the scene by Dimitri, who abandoned the table he was serving and sprinted over to Candy, where he fell to his knees and gently wiped away the blood from the heel of her foot with a napkin. Clearly he was not the squeamish type. 'I don't think there is any glass in there,' he said, carefully examining the injury. Feeling rather superfluous, Leila handed him the wipes.

'Trust me to step on it,' Candy replied, adding, 'I'm sorry I swore in front of Gracie, Leila.'

'Don't worry, she's heard far worse.' She turned to her daughter. 'Go and see Daddy, he's got some breadsticks for you.' Once the child was out of earshot she continued, 'Last time she and Tom went swimming at the pool in Brighton, she jumped into the water and shouted out, "This water's bloody freezing, Daddy!' Tom was mortified.'

Candy smiled, then looking at Dimitri, who was still on his knees, said, 'Thanks for helping me.'

'You are welcome. I'm Dimitri, Ellie and Nikos's nephew. I'm working here for the summer – at the taverna and also at the turtle conservation project over at Gerakas beach. You should come and see what we do. And one of my friends is running a club. I can get you –' he paused '– and your friends free tickets.'

Had he actually drawn breath once? He was a quick worker!

'I'm Candy.' She stared back at him, seeming to register that this wasn't any old waiter tending her foot but a drop-dead gorgeous Greek God!

Leila smiled to herself. Patrick definitely had some competition here. It would serve him right for being such a big baby about a little blood.

'That's a pretty name. It suits you very well,' Dimitri was saying.

'How come you speak such good English?' Candy asked. 'It's better than mine!'

138

'My mum got a job in England for a couple of years when I was fourteen so I guess I picked it up then. And I should get a plaster for that cut.' Dimitri glanced at the abandoned pink shoes. 'And I will ask my aunt if she has some flip-flops you can borrow.'

What a total sweetheart, Leila thought as she and Candy watched him run back inside the taverna.

'He's a very good-looking boy, isn't he?'

'Is he? I hadn't noticed. Long hair, not my thing.' Candy replied, and self-consciously fiddled with one of the straps of her top. 'Nice of Patrick to shift his arse,' she added.

'Hates the sight of blood apparently.'

'What a wimp.'

Oh, dear, it hadn't taken long for Candy to realise what he was like. Leila wondered if their romance would even survive the holiday.

'So do you think you guys would be up for going to a club?' Candy asked, trying to sound casual. 'I wouldn't mind going – with Patrick,' she quickly added.

'I could pimp up my Zimmer frame,' Leila teased. 'We're not that old!'

'I didn't mean it to sound like that. I meant I didn't know if clubs were your sort of thing.'

'Well, I haven't been to one for a while, but we used to go every now and then. A lot when Tom and I first met in our twenties. He's a really good dancer and I can bust some moves myself, after a

139

few cocktails. I bet you go all the time in Brighton, don't you?'

She imagined Candy out on a Saturday night with her girlfriends, all dressed in revealing clothes, with way too much make-up on, tottering down West Street to one of the many clubs that were close to the seafront. Whenever Leila saw those gangs of girls she was always tempted to shout out, 'Aren't you freezing? Put a cardigan on! And don't drink too much!' But maybe that was because she was getting older.

Candy shook her head. 'Only on special occasions – it's too expensive and I never really got into it because I couldn't leave my sisters when they were little.'

'Oh? Did your parents always work at the weekend?'

Her reply was totally unexpected. 'No, my dad left when I was ten and my mum died when I was seventeen. She had breast cancer.'

How terrible to lose your mum at such a young age. Leila felt awful. She had been busy writing Candy off as a fun-loving girl who didn't have a care in the world. How little she knew. She reached out and lightly touched her shoulder. 'I'm so sorry, Candy.'

She was looking away but Leila could see the tears welling up in her eyes. 'It's okay. I mean, it's not really. I still miss her. Every day.' She waved her hands in front of her eyes. 'Oh, God, I can't cry with my false lashes on, they'll fall off.' She took a deep breath. 'Mum would have been so pleased to know that I was here in Greece. She came once and fell in love with it. She always wanted to come back.'

'How old are your sisters?'

'Mollie is fifteen and Keira's seventeen.'

'So they were really little when your mum died. Who looked after you all?'

Candy shrugged. 'There was just me. I knew there was no point trying to get hold of my dad, he'd had nothing to do with us for years. My aunt helped out a bit, but her husband was an alkie and her hands were full with him.'

She sounded so matter-of-fact.

'So you had to bring up your sisters on your own, when you were only seventeen? That must have been very hard.' Leila couldn't imagine having that responsibility at such a young age. She found it challenging enough sometimes being the mother of one, with a husband, supportive parents and in-laws and a reasonable income.

'It was, but we're okay. Mollie is doing her A-levels at college and Keira is getting her GCSE results in a couple of weeks. They should be good, and then she's going to do A-levels as well.'

'I am in awe of you, Candy. When I was seventeen I was completely self-obsessed, too caught up with having a good time with my friends and fitting in my A-levels to think about anything else. I don't think I could even boil an egg, never mind run a home and look after my siblings. We'd all have ended up in care.'

Leila had meant it as a light-hearted comment but a shadow seemed to fall over Candy's face as she said quietly, 'There was no way I was going to let that happen. I knew we'd be separated.'

'You must be a very strong person,' Leila replied, feeling humbled by Candy's example. She wondered if Patrick had any idea about his girlfriend's past. Probably not. Most likely he had her down as a good-time girl. Less complicated for him that way.

'I just wanted to do my best for them.'

Dimitri dashed back with a pair of purple flip-flops incongruously clutched in one hand. He looked so noble and manly, with his fine profile and athletic body, as if he should be holding the Olympic torch. Leila glanced at Candy and saw that the young woman was gazing at Dimitri with frank admiration. She hadn't looked at Patrick that way. Dimitri quickly got to work, carefully applied a plaster to the cut, then slipped the flip-flops on for her.

'You have beautiful feet,' he told her. 'Very elegant.'

He really must like her if he was complimenting her feet!

'I feel like Cinderella,' Candy joked.

'Darling! I've poured you a glass of wine,' Patrick called out. 'You've been so brave.'

'Is he your prince then?' Dimitri asked.

'I wouldn't go as far as that,' Candy muttered as she stood up. Instantly she winced as her injured foot touched the ground, and Dimitri sprang up to help her, 'If you lean on me, I'll take you back to the table.'

Leila considered offering to help too, but decided it would spoil the moment for the two of them. She was amused to observe that Patrick had finally clocked that Dimitri had more than an eye on his girlfriend and had jogged over to the couple.

'This is better than a soap opera,' Tor commented.

'A soap opera crossed with *Romeo and Juliet*,' Leila replied. 'You should have seen the way they were gazing at each other, like star-crossed lovers. It was very romantic. He even liked her feet.'

'Perhaps he's a foot fetishist,' Tom joked.

'Don't spoil it, it was so sweet.'

'And now for the stand-off,' Tor murmured.

'You've done more than enough, mate,' Patrick told Dimitri as the two men stood facing each other. 'You can leave my girlfriend with me now. I'm sure you've got some tables to serve, haven't you? Can't keep the customers waiting for their moussaka and chips.'

Dimitri looked as if he'd like to tell Patrick exactly where he could stick that moussaka. Leila didn't blame him, Patrick sounded *so* patronising.

'I hope they're not going to have a fight over her,' Tom whispered to Leila, 'I don't rate Patrick's chances. Though it would be entertaining. Less *Fight Club*, more *Diary of a Wimpy Kid*.'

'It's no problem,' Dimitri replied, defiantly maintaining his hold on Candy's waist. But clearly Patrick had decided that action was called for. To the amusement of Leila and her friends, he stepped forward and slid one arm around Candy's waist, dislodging Dimitri's, and with his other arm around her neck he managed to swing her into his arms. There was nothing chivalrous about the move as it looked as if he was lugging a sack of coal. Candy screwed up her face in embarrassment as Patrick staggered back to the table, where he dumped her unceremoniously on to a chair. Nonetheless the whole restaurant erupted into applause and Patrick took a bow. Dimitri stomped back into the kitchen.

'My back's killing me now, Candy, I'll need an extra good massage from you later,' Patrick commented, taking a long slug of wine. It didn't exactly scream Prince Charming to his Princess – more like the Ugly Sister bossing Cinders around. But Candy wasn't listening; she was looking wistfully in the direction of the kitchen.

The rest of the meal passed without incident, though Leila was still aware of Frankie's antagonism towards Matt – she didn't seem to miss an opportunity to disagree with anything he said, whatever the subject, even picking an argument over which series of *Mad Men* was the best when Leila knew for a fact that Frankie had loved all of them. Dimitri recovered his composure sufficiently to hand out free tickets for his friend's club to everyone – including Patrick.

'Blue Oasis? Sounds like a lap-dancing club,' he commented, throwing the ticket on the table.

'Should be right up your street then,' Tom said wryly.

Patrick was topping up his glass and didn't hear him.

But even surrounded by her closest friends Leila couldn't shake off the negative thoughts, the nagging feeling that she didn't deserve to be happy, because of what she'd done. A moment of madness, a moment of dissatisfaction, where she was thinking only about herself . . . How would she feel if Tom had been unfaithful to her? It would hurt, even though they weren't getting on. It would hurt like hell.

Nikos and Ellie joined them for coffee and sticky-sweet baklava at the end of the night. Tom was now on Gracie duty in the play area. They had hardly spoken to each other during dinner; Leila missed the banter they used to share.

'Your daughter is adorable! She looks exactly like you!' Ellie exclaimed, watching the little girl zoom down the slide with her long black hair flying out behind her. 'How old is she now?'

'Four and a half.'

'It would be a good age gap, wouldn't it?' Ellie went on. Leila was used to her being so direct.

145

But right now she wasn't in the mood for such a conversation; she wanted the spotlight away from her life, which didn't bear inspection.

'I guess,' she replied, sounding non-committal.

'I had a six-year gap between Theo and Otis,' Ellie continued, on a mission now. 'And when I look back, I wish I hadn't left it so long before I had Otis. They never really played together when they were little.'

Leila knew she wouldn't get away with saying nothing.

'I do want another baby but the timing is all wrong with my work. I'm so busy, and Tom and I barely get any time on our own as it is.' Leila sighed, 'I wish we lived here, life would be so much easier.' *No Jasper for a start.*

'Don't leave it too long, is my advice,' Ellie replied. 'You're a wonderful mother.'

Leila felt her eyes unexpectedly fill with tears; she wasn't worthy of Ellie's praise and good opinion. 'I don't think I am, and I'm a bad wife. Work is the only thing I'm good at.'

Ellie looked at her searchingly, and was about to speak when Tom and Gracie returned.

It was only when the party came to leave that Ellie hugged Leila and said quietly, 'Come and see me any time.' Leila nodded, but she couldn't imagine confiding in Ellie about her sordid affair.

Chapter 13

Frankie

'I've hardly spoken to you, Frankie, how's it going? Any men in your life that I should know about it?' Patrick was in the kitchen with her, opening yet another bottle of wine. Finally they were alone together. All day Frankie had been waiting for this. Patrick was close enough for her to smell his aftershave, and as she breathed in the familiar scent she experienced a pang of longing so intense that she almost couldn't bear it. This was the moment she could tell him. Come right out and tell him that there was no one except him, and there never would be. She couldn't keep up the pretence any longer.

Patrick gave her his sexy smile. 'Come on, Frankie, don't spare me any details. I want full disclosure. I always tell you everything and you know that I'm completely unshockable. So give it up, Ms Harper.'

Actually he didn't tell her everything. He certainly hadn't mentioned Candy, she would have remembered that, but Frankie wasn't going to be sidetracked. She took a deep breath. This was her chance. Now. Do it now. Seize the moment.

Or not, as Matt wandered into the kitchen and said, 'Is anyone up for a game of poker with Tom and me?'

Talk about bad timing. Frankie glared at him. *Wanker!* Christ! Had she said that out loud? She knew how obnoxious she had been to him at dinner, and Leila had read the Riot Act to her in the Ladies'.

'But he doesn't like me!' Frankie had protested. She hated being told off; knew exactly how her students felt when they were on the receiving end of a bollocking. It made her want to rebel even more.

'Rubbish, he's perfectly civil to you. You're the one who is constantly jumping down his throat.'

There was no way that Frankie could bear to say, 'Actually he *really* doesn't like me. He turned me down on your wedding night and humiliated me more than any other man ever has.' Though that would get Leila's attention. Instead she mumbled something about finding him smug. It didn't pacify her friend.

'You have to promise me that you'll be nice to him. It's ruining my holiday, seeing you constantly antagonise him. I don't need this, Frankie. This is the first time Tom and I have been away in ages.'

Leila was on the verge of tears. Frankie instantly gave in. 'Okay, okay, I promise.'

Now as she looked at Matt she realised it was going to be a very hard promise to keep.

He looked straight back at her. 'You've a very odd expression on your face. Have you got indigestion, Frankie? Perhaps it was the stuffed vine leaves? Or the calamari? Or the baklava?'

Who was he? The food police? Jesus! Was he now keeping tabs on everything she ate?

'I didn't have any baklava.'

'You should have – it was delicious.' He grinned. 'Not that you're not sweet enough already.'

Leila should be here to witness him deliberately provoking her! Frankie just looked at him as if making an actual reply was beneath her. Something she had perfected in the classroom. She had a variety of looks and stares in her repertoire.

'I'll play if we're using real money,' Patrick declared. 'There's got to be something at stake to make it interesting.'

'I'm sure just having the lovely Frankie join us will make the game interesting enough.'

It really was going to be tough keeping that promise to Leila . . . She doubted that Matt wanted her to join them and she was hardly in the mood for a game of cards, but the alternative was to go to her room and brood and she didn't want to do that either. She would take up Matt's offer and ruin his night by winning, it would serve him right for ruining hers.

Or not. Three rounds in and she was losing badly.

'You're too impulsive,' Matt told her as he won yet again. 'And I know exactly what kind of hand you've got every time. It's funny because I thought you would be good at hiding your feelings, but you're no good at it at all.'

Was that a dig about her and Patrick?

Tom eyed her nervously. 'I think Matt's only trying to be helpful.'

Frankie was all set to say that, yeah, he was extremely fucking *trying*, but managed not to.

'Frankie baby, you need a good poker face like Matt's,' Patrick put in, and then proceeded to give an appalling rendition of Lady Gaga's 'Poker Face'. He was slurring his words now after guzzling most of the bottle of wine and well over a bottle at the taverna, and there had been all those beers during the day. Frankie felt embarrassed on his behalf and couldn't look at Matt or Tom. No one else had drunk anything like as much as Patrick.

'Don't let Candy hear you singing or she'll definitely go off with that good-looking Greek boy,' Matt joked. 'That was more like Lady Gaga's "Shit-faced".'

Patrick slammed his hand on the table, nearly knocking over one of the citronella candles they had lit to keep away the mosquitoes. 'I don't have anything to fear from Stavros, trust me. A waiter compared to an award-winning journalist, for fuck's sake! I bet he still lives at home with his mama and dreams of opening his own taverna. Yeah, aim high, Stavros, you'll always be a loser in a waiter's uniform.'

There was an awkward pause before Frankie muttered, 'He's called Dimitri and he's a Psychology student.' Much as she loved Patrick, she wasn't going to let him get away with a comment like that. And the award-winning journalist bit made her cringe. He had won that award five years ago, far too long ago to be bringing it up now.

'Whatever, he's no threat to me. Candy won't even remember his name by the morning, I guarantee it,' he replied, getting up from the table and throwing his cards into the middle. 'I'm done for the night.'

'Another hand?' Matt asked, expertly shuffling the cards as Patrick walked slightly unsteadily back into the villa. There was no point in her going after him now and trying to have that conversation. He was far too drunk. And if Frankie was really honest with herself, she hadn't especially liked the way he'd been tonight. The snide comments about Dimitri, his excessive drinking. That wasn't the Patrick she thought she knew, the Patrick she wanted.

Frankie shook her head. She would be bound to lose again and there were only so many times her ego could take that with Matt. She felt a familiar

151

bleakness overwhelm her, knew that she wouldn't be able to sleep for hours and hours.

'Or how about that game of table tennis?' he continued. 'Though prepare to be beaten. I am King of Ping.'

'It must have been all those hours you played at boarding school in between wanking over a biscuit, or whatever you posh boys got up to when Matron wasn't looking. Or perhaps she *was* looking. Public schools are full of perverts, aren't they?'

'I didn't go to one. But thanks for that delightful image. You really do have a mind like a sewer, Ms Harper. Do they call you that in school or is it just miss?'

Frankie folded her arms and gave him her best 'you don't impress me at all' look, honed by many hours of deploying it on naughty fifteen-year-old boys. 'You did go to private school though, didn't you?'

It was like they were playing a game of conversational table tennis. When Frankie came out with yet another barbed comment – wham! – Matt deflected it – *bam*! 'I did, but I don't think that makes me a bad person. A lot of complete bastards come out of comprehensives too. Private schools don't have the monopoly.'

Of course Frankie knew that, but she wouldn't admit it.

'So are you going to play or are you too scared of being beaten at this as well?'

She hesitated. It would mean spending time alone with him, but maybe it would help clear the air, and she couldn't avoid him for two weeks. It was surely better than lying in her room and not being able to sleep in any case.

'You're on.'

Tom looked at each of them in turn. 'I'm going to bed. Try not to kill each other. Or if you must, do it quietly. I don't want to be woken up.'

Ten minutes later they were both sweating profusely as they battled it out over the table tennis table in the converted barn at the far end of the garden. It was just as well that they were some distance from the house as they had both been swearing as they played with intense concentration. Matt had matched Frankie word for word. She liked him better when he swore. And she liked him even more now she was beating him. She'd had an easy victory for the first two games, taking Matt by surprise with her mean serve that barely bounced at all and her killer backhands. He fought back in the third with some nifty volleys that wrong-footed Frankie, but it wasn't enough to defeat her and she took that game as well. She slung her bat on the table. Yes! She had beaten the bastard. Job done. And, as the added bonus of keeping her promise to Leila, she had actually been nice to Matt. Well, maybe that was pushing it. 'Jammy bastard' and 'twat face' had been uttered in the heat of the moment during the game and so didn't count – though she had enjoyed coming out with them.

'You've played before then,' he said, running his hand through his hair. 'Did you go to boarding school?' He grinned. 'So that's where you got all your kinky ideas about what goes on in one. Personal experience.'

'Ha-ha, very funny. I did not. We had a table in the garage when I was growing up, and I got back into the game a couple of years ago. Thanks for playing.' She was trying not to sound too gleeful, though she wanted to punch the air.

'Where are you going?' he said. 'We haven't finished yet.'

'Best of five, wasn't it?'

'Let's do best of seven,' he replied, with steely determination. 'I'm just warming up.'

'Is that what you call it? I say sweating it out like a loser.'

'That was tough! Don't act like it was a breeze.'

She paused as she heard the whine of an approaching mosquito. Damn, she hadn't put any bug spray on; she'd be eaten alive.

It definitely hadn't been a breeze, but she was not going to let on. 'Okay, I'll get some water. You probably need to conserve your energy for the game.'

'Not so cocky, Harper, I've been observing your style. I know exactly where your weaknesses are.'

'It won't be enough, I'll still whop your arse!' she

shouted over her shoulder as she jogged back to the villa. By now it was close to one a.m. but she was feeling energised and realised that she had been playing table tennis with Matt for over half an hour without remembering anything about their history. Perhaps this would be the way forward for the rest of the holiday – they would be fine as long as they played table tennis and didn't have to talk.

She returned with a bottle of mineral water, glasses, two beers and the bug spray.

'Cheers,' she said, raising the bottle to her lips.

'Cheers,' replied Matt, then after a quick sip put his bottle down and said decisively, 'Come on. Let's get on with it. I'm itching for revenge.'

'Hang on, I just need to put some of this on or I'll be itching. This barn is Mosquito Central.' She waved the bottle of insecticide and began spraying it on to her arms and legs. It smelt disgusting.

'D'you want some?' she asked. Really she should be recording this for evidence for Leila. The caring sharing Frankie. This would definitely win her a stack of brownie points.

'Yeah, thanks, and shall I do your back?'

'Sure. Thanks.' She stood still while he aimed the nozzle at her skin.

'Thanks,' she repeated when she thought he must have finished. But he reached out and began rubbing the liquid in with firm, assured strokes that reminded her that she hadn't been touched in a while. It felt good, too good, and it also reminded

155

her that the last time Matt had touched her had been in a hotel room, just before he'd upped and left. She could feel her face burning at the recollection.

'You've got beautiful skin, Frankie.'

That wasn't going to help the burning face situation, and just as she was wondering what would make a suitable reply, he said briskly, 'There, all bug-proof. Ready?'

She turned round, hoping that she didn't look as unsettled as she felt. 'Yep, if you're sure. Three-nil doesn't sound too bad. Five-nil? Not so good.'

But Matt had been observing her and took the next two games. Now Frankie's lead was under threat. He was matching her killer serve for killer serve, slice for slice. That beautiful skin comment had distracted her. But with some cunningly angled forehands she managed to clinch the next game, making her the overall winner. Matt was far more gracious in defeat than she would have been in his place. He actually shook her hand.

'You're a demon player, Frankie. See how I resist calling you a jammy bastard?'

These ex-public-school types had jolly good manners, she had to concede.

'We'll have to have a return match tomorrow. You play a mean game.'

'You're not too bad yourself.'

Matt gave a mock double-take. 'Did you just say something that was very nearly a compliment by your standards?' He reached out and touched her forehead as if to check whether she had a fever. 'Are you feeling okay?'

Another touch that unsettled her. 'Just a statement of fact actually.'

It was strange walking back to the villa together, she was more used to marching away from him. Without the distraction of table tennis they were both quiet. For the first time since she'd seen him again Frankie wondered what he was thinking. Had he known that she was going to be at the villa? Would he have come if he had? Did he dislike her as much as she was convinced he must? Though dislike was too strong a word. He had been okay to her during their game, more than okay. She had been so wrapped up in her own feelings she hadn't even considered his.

'D'you want a brandy?' Matt asked once they were inside. 'We can toast your victory over me. You should make the most of it because it will be your only one.'

For a moment she was almost tempted. But what would they talk about? Discussing their mutual passion for table tennis wouldn't take long, and once they'd covered that, what else was there? There were no pleasant strolls down Memory Lane for them. 'Oh, yeah, do you remember the time I was so drunk that I tried to seduce you in a hotel room and you turned me down because you didn't want a meaningless fuck? Hilarious wasn't it?

157

How I laughed into my pillow after you'd left . . .'
Nor did she want him to mention her feelings for
Patrick again. No, it was best to avoid being alone
with him. They'd played table tennis; it had been
civilised (swearing apart), and it had broken the
ice. From now on she would be able to be in the
same room as Matt without wanting to insult him
or escape. That had to be enough. Anything more
would be pushing it. Though there had been that
moment when he'd touched her . . . but it was
probably best not to dwell on that. She would put
it down to the late night, and to the wine. It hadn't
meant anything.

'Thanks, but I'm knackered. Goodnight.'

But Frankie couldn't sleep. The day had been an
unrelenting emotional rollercoaster. It had begun
in such anticipation and excitement, only to have
those feelings smashed by Patrick's arrival with
Candy as well as Matt's unexpected appearance.
She would try and keep her promise to Leila and
be nice to him. After this holiday she would never
have to see him again.

But Patrick. What to do about Patrick? Seeing
him with Candy had been pure torture. For added
salt in the wound, Tom had joked about overhearing
them in the afternoon . . . at least Frankie had
been spared that. She knew Patrick well enough to
realise that Candy was just a fling. He wasn't in love
with her. So why was he with her?

She had believed, when he finally split up with

Willow, that it would be her big chance. That prospect seemed to be fading fast. Maybe she should book a flight home. It would take some explaining away to Leila and Tor . . . and it would be miserable returning home with nothing changed between her and Patrick. But wasn't that better than seeing him every day with Candy? Or should she find a way of telling Patrick how she felt, whatever the consequences?

Frankie turned over. She always had a plan, but in this instance she hadn't a clue. From next door she heard the creak of Matt's single bed. Perhaps he couldn't sleep either. She found it strangely comforting to think of him lying awake as well, but doubted that he was tormented by pangs of unrequited love. He was probably worrying about work.

Chapter 14

Tor

Tor padded into the bedroom after her shower, wrapped in a white bath towel. It had been a good day on the sickness front; she'd only felt nauseous once. She had even pretended to drink a bottle of beer, knowing that her friends would certainly comment if she carried on refraining from alcohol, and then when no one was looking had poured it away in the garden. She hoped it wouldn't kill the geraniums.

Ed was already dressed for dinner in a pair of long black cargo-style shorts and a white t-shirt. He had to be one of the few men who still looked sexy in shorts and not like a boy scout about to go on a camping trip. He was lying on the bed reading. If she hadn't had the baby news rattling around in her head, she might have thought that it was brilliant spending all this time with him; that they got on incredibly well, so much better than she could ever have believed. As it was, she hardly dared to allow herself to think that. It was only setting herself up for a massive fall. Ed put down his book and watched her as she opened the wardrobe.

'Have you got any shorts?'

She spun round. 'I only ever wear dresses and skirts, you know that! I don't think they make shorts large enough to cover my arse.'

He sprang off the bed. 'I won't have a word said against your derrière. I love it, it's perfect.' He put his arms round her and hugged her. 'I'm only asking because I'm taking you out for dinner tonight and we need to go on the moped as I'm not insured to drive the car. So don't wear a long dress.'

'God! I haven't been on a moped for at least ten years. When I did my boyfriend of the time drove straight into the wall of a tunnel and then blamed me because I hadn't reminded him to take his sunglasses off. He spent the rest of the week sulking about his grazed knee. You're not going to be like that are you? I'm strictly a passenger and not a co-driver.'

She knew he wouldn't be without even asking. One of the many things she liked about Ed was that he never sulked or gave her the silent treatment.

'Nope, and I'm sure you'll be good at getting your leg over – the bike,' Ed teased her. Clearly he was still feeling frisky from the brief encounter they'd just had in the shower once Tor could be persuaded that no one could possibly hear them. Patrick might not give a fig about anyone overhearing his antics, but Tor would be mortified. She had actually enjoyed the experience, to her surprise and Ed hadn't seemed to notice that her boobs had doubled in size.

She flicked through her dresses, and settled on a pretty knee-length blue-and-white checked sundress. 'This is the shortest dress I've got.'

'You'll have to tuck it in your knickers, we can't have it catching in the spokes, causing us to veer off the road and die tragically young.'

'Tragically youngish in my case. And anyway,' she replied, momentarily feeling back to her old self, 'who said I'd be wearing any knickers?'

'Really?' Ed was definitely still feeling frisky.

She punched him lightly on the shoulder, 'Of course I'll be wearing knickers! Ugh! So unhygienic. Who knows who's been on that seat before?'

'Pity. What if I bought a brand new moped that no one had ever sat on before, would you consider it then?'

'And end up on YouTube? Knickerlesspassenger. org. No, thanks. #Pervert.'

'It was worth asking. #Hopeful.'

In the event Tor managed to tuck her skirt under her bum. She had a brief run-in with Ed when she said she wasn't going to wear a helmet as it would wreck her hair, and he put his foot down and refused to go unless she did.

'You're very sensible,' Tor teased him as she wrapped her arms around his waist. She had an urge to hum Bruce Springstein's 'Born to Run' as he turned the key in the ignition and kickstarted the bike. She resisted.

'Yeah, well,' he shouted over the sound of the engine, 'I don't want you to have an accident and end up with brain damage just because you didn't wear a helmet. Not on my watch.'

Suddenly she felt one of those flashes of optimism about a future that just might involve Ed the dad. She imagined him being strict with their son about wearing a helmet when he scooted along the seafront or cycled to the park, and saying, 'No helmet, no play.'

The kidney bean was definitely a boy, she had decided. A boy who would have Ed's green eyes, brown hair, cheeky grin and easygoing nature.

Ed had chosen a taverna in Zakynthos Town as recommended by Leila. It was set on a hill and had views over the picturesque harbour, where expensive-looking yachts were moored alongside fishing boats. The sea was silky calm and lights from the town shimmered on its smooth surface.

'This is very nice,' Tor commented as they sat down at a candlelit table. 'And unexpected.'

'Yeah, I thought it would be good if we had a

night on our own. I mean, I really like being with everyone, but I want to spend time with you as well.'

He smiled at her, showing off those perfect teeth, and Tor smiled back. Maybe she should seize this opportunity to tell him her big news. Their big news. The waiter came over to take their order and Ed chatted to him about where he was from, and where he would recommend they visit on the island. It was typical of Ed, who always got talking to people.

The feeling of optimism continued to gain momentum, especially when he pointed out how cute a little Greek girl looked, tucking into an ice cream that was practically the size of her head.

Tor smiled when really she wanted to exclaim, *Oh my God! You notice children!* She couldn't remember any of her other boyfriends ever doing that. Harry had been godfather to his best friend's daughter and had shown zero interest in the baby. Tor was the one who had bought the Christening present, wrapped it up and exclaimed over the newborn. During the service she'd had to whisper to Harry to stop checking his phone and yawning. Mind you the baby girl got her revenge by being sick all over his Prada jacket when the parents insisted he hold her for a photograph.

And Ed had been really sweet with Gracie, and always played with her whenever she asked. Tor didn't think he could be putting on an act – maybe the first time, but not after three days. In contrast

Harry had been appalling with Gracie. He would look at her as if she were some kind of inferior being, not worthy of his attention. It had been embarrassing.

Right from the start of their ill-fated relationship, Harry had told her that he wasn't sure if he wanted children. Although he had made a show of being sympathetic when she had revealed that she might have trouble conceiving naturally, Tor was sure that he was secretly relieved.

The waiter arrived with their main courses and for the first time since she had found out she was pregnant, she actually felt hungry. She tucked into the stuffed tomatoes and aubergines with relish. Maybe they really could make this work – her and Ed. Okay, it wasn't ideal, he was much younger, but other men became fathers in their twenties. He had yet to embark on his proper career, but maybe he could be a house-husband like Tom, at least for a while. She tried not to think about how Tom being a house-husband seemed not to be going so well. That must be down to Leila working too hard. Tor was sure it was about balance. Maybe she could reduce her hours at the boutique and employ someone else part-time. It would be a stretch financially, and quite a challenge to find someone who could deal with high-maintenance Spencer and antisocial Maud, but surely not impossible. And it would mean that she could be at home more.

'You look thoughtful,' Ed commented as the

waiter cleared away their plates. 'I hope you're not worrying about the store, I'm sure they're getting on fine without you. You deserve this holiday.'

After the baby news, everything else had paled into insignificance and so far Tor had only spoken to Spencer twice to check everything was okay and even then had hardly taken in what he'd said. 'No, I'm not, for once. It all seems to be going smoothly. Spencer hasn't had any meltdowns – he's back with his boyfriend Federico who is good at keeping him calm. And apparently Maud has got a dog – a rescue greyhound – which seems to have brought her out of herself.'

'That's great. So you can really relax. And maybe next year we could go away for longer.'

He was talking about the future, their future, that was positive. Of course, he didn't know that next year there would be three of them . . . She couldn't wait any longer, now was definitely the time to come out with it. She clenched her hands together under the table.

Ed waved at the waiter, who to Tor's surprise brought over two glasses of what looked like champagne. 'What's this for?' she asked. He couldn't already know, could he? She'd thought that she had been so careful. But if he did know then surely the champagne was a good sign, a brilliant sign. And one sip wouldn't hurt the kidney bean, would it?

'I've got some news.' Ed leant forward and

reached for her hand. 'You've been so good about me not having any money, but starting from September it's all going to change.'

Hang on, he didn't know, so what was the champagne for?

'Don't look so worried, Tor. It's nothing bad. It's the opposite. I've got a job. My dream job! I'm going to be working at Sony. I found out the day before we came away on holiday. I've been dying to tell you, but I wanted to do something special to celebrate. My treat, for a change.'

The fantasy of Ed the dad and Ed the house-husband disintegrated before her eyes. She had been an idiot ever to imagine it was a possibility. Somehow she managed to say, 'That is amazing news, Ed!' She made herself pick up the champagne glass and clinked it against his. 'Well done.'

She raised the glass to her lips and took the smallest of sips. The champagne tasted acidic, she had to force herself to swallow it.

He beamed at her. 'I bet you thought I'd never get my act together, that I'd be working as a barman for ever.'

''Course not! I know how tough it is getting a job at the moment.'

'The only downside is that I'll be working in London. I figured commuting is going to be way too expensive, so I'll stay with my sister in the week, and then at the weekends either stay with friends – there might be a chance that Dougie and Ruby have a spare room – or . . .' He paused and looked at her expectantly.

He wasn't going to be living in Brighton any more was all Tor had heard. He had the job of his dreams; he would be working all the time. There was going to be no Ed the dad. *If* she kept the baby it was going to be Tor the single mum. *If*. She was back to the world of ifs.

'Or,' he repeated, 'I wondered if I could stay with you at the weekend – I mean, move in. I know we haven't been seeing each other that long, but it doesn't seem that way. We get on so well. I love being with you.'

There was a pause. She knew that she was supposed to say something positive here, but she didn't, she couldn't, her mind was in a complete scramble. Ed carried on, 'And you work Saturdays anyway, so I swear I won't invade your space. I won't leave my stuff lying around, I promise. What do you reckon?'

He looked so happy, so full of optimism and excitement, thinking about his brilliant new life. She couldn't see that there would be any room in that life for a baby.

'I think it's great, Ed,' she said quietly. 'Really great. You totally deserve that job and you'll be fantastic at it. But,' she paused, 'I'm not so sure about the weekend thing. Can we see how it goes with staying with Dougie? We have only been seeing each other for five months. Every weekend is a big commitment.' *Not as big as having a baby. Obviously.*

'Oh.' Ed was taken aback; it was clearly not the answer he'd been expecting. 'It's just, I know how much I'm going to miss you. We've spent practically every night together for the last five months. Maybe I could come down one night in the week? Or you could come up and see me? I know you're busy, but it doesn't take long on the train. It's only forty-nine minutes on a fast one. It will take an effort on both our parts, but it's worth it. You do believe that, don't you?'

'Sure. And we can always Skype.' Tor knew she sounded cool and offhand, like she barely cared, but she was struggling to keep it together. She couldn't tell him about the baby now; it wasn't fair on him.

Ed frowned, registering the tone.

'Oh, I get it, Tor. You're doing your, "I'm the older woman, I'm the one in control, stay in your place, little boy." It's really boring and insulting. Do I ever mention the age difference? I don't give a flying fuck that you're seven or eight years older than me, I don't even remember. It doesn't mean anything to me. It's just a number. I don't know why you're so hung up on it. Or is it a convenient way of keeping me out? I'm only for fucking, is that it? You won't be serious about me because I'm younger than you. I know your last boyfriend really fucked you up, but I'm not like that.'

She had hurt him and she hadn't intended to.

There were so many things she wanted to say in reply, and so many things she couldn't. 'I know you're nothing like Harry. And I know I go on about the age gap, but I do feel it. It is an issue for me.'

'I'm not a teenage boy, Tor. Give it a rest!'

She could see other diners turning and looking over at them, at his raised voice. The waiter approached to refill their glasses but Ed shook his head and he retreated. The night was ruined and she didn't know how to make amends. Suddenly she felt overwhelmed with nausea. The kidney bean certainly knew when to pick his moments. She quickly got up, knocking over the glass of champagne in her haste, and rushed to the loo where she promptly threw up.

She was gone so long that Ed came to find her, knocking on the door to check that she was okay. She dragged herself over to the sink where she washed her hands and face. She caught sight of her reflection in the mirror and winced. Under the bright fluorescent light she looked pale, her mascara had run and her lipstick had smudged. The crash helmet had flattened her hair to her head, making her look as if she'd had a 1970s feather cut. It was not her best look. She couldn't summon up the energy to care. She opened the door.

'I've been sick. Maybe I've had too much sun or I haven't got over what I had before. I'm really sorry to mess up your celebration.'

'Oh, baby, I'm sorry for having a go at you. I know it's a lot to take in. Come on, I'll get you home.' Ed put his arms round her and held her tight. She could do without the 'oh, baby', but the hug felt good.

They were both subdued on the drive back, there were no jokes about knickers or lack of. At the villa Tor went straight to bed with a cup of peppermint tea. Ed wanted to stay with her but she told him she needed to sleep and that he should play poker with the boys and Frankie, that she was better being left alone. It would be good practice, after all.

And then it was just her in the darkness, feeling sick and very, very alone. For the first time she lightly touched her stomach, in the place where she imagined the tiny kidney-bean baby was.

'Oh, baby,' she said out loud. 'It's just you and me, kid.' And she admitted what she had known all along: that there was not going to be any *if* she kept the baby, she was going to keep the baby. But there would be no more fantasies about Ed the dad. She would do this on her own. She was not the first single mother in the world . . . she would cope, somehow. She had to.

Chapter 15

Leila

'Can you pass me the honey please?' Tom asked as they sat on the terrace having breakfast, barely glancing up from the iPad, on which he was reading the *Guardian* online. It was practically the only thing he had said to Leila all morning, but then they hadn't had a meaningful conversation since coming on holiday. It was all about Gracie or to Gracie or they were making small talk: *How did you sleep? How's your book? What shall we have for lunch?* There had been no sex – Tom wouldn't suggest it again after she had rebuffed him, and Leila couldn't imagine bridging the gulf in their bed to attempt it. They didn't even hold each other any more when they went to sleep, and Tom always used to sleep with his arm around her, his body tucked into hers. They were strangers sleeping side by side, fifty shades of we don't have sex any more. All their energy seemed to be directed towards ignoring the big fat elephant in the room that was their crumbling marriage.

Leila felt like one of those couples in restaurants who managed to have entire meals without saying a single word to each other. Those were the couples she and Tom used to laugh about in the past, unable to comprehend that a relationship could become that dried up, little imagining that they would one day morph into that relationship. It made her want to shout out, *What are we doing! What's wrong with us! This isn't what I want!* Instead she passed the honey.

It was a relief when Candy limped outside on to the terrace. She had stopped wearing the fake lashes and was wearing hardly any make-up. She looked ravishingly pretty.

'How's the foot doing?' Leila asked.

'It feels much better today than it did yesterday, thanks.'

'It must be the healing hands of Dimitri,' Leila teased, but Candy didn't rise to it. She quickly replied, 'It wasn't a very big cut.'

Tom immediately offered to make her breakfast and disappeared into the kitchen. Leila sensed that he was glad to be doing something, so he didn't have to be confronted with the sight of her talking far more easily to Candy than she ever did to him.

'I can do it,' the girl protested, 'I don't expect to be waited on.'

Clearly she remembered Frankie's barbed comment that this wasn't a hotel.

173

'I know you don't. You've been brilliant at playing with Gracie, you always tidy up, and anyway Tom likes cooking.' Leila wanted to reassure her, make her feel that she belonged here.

'I don't think Patrick knows what his oven's for. We either go out for dinner or he orders a takeaway. So does Tom do a lot of cooking?'

'He makes supper in the week and I'm in charge at the weekends.' That wasn't strictly true; more often than not Leila was too knackered and resorted to takeaways herself.

'Lucky you. It's my fantasy to come back from work and find my dinner's been made – something healthy and delicious. My sisters and I take it in turns. My youngest, Mollie, isn't bad, and does a mean *penne arrabbiata*, but Keira's bloody useless. She can only do jacket potatoes, beans and cheese, and she either incinerates the potato or it's uncooked in the middle. Like, how difficult can it be! There is nothing more depressing than an underdone jacket potato after a long day at work.'

Leila smiled sympathetically and thought about what it had been like for her returning home from work recently. The silences, the feeling that their relationship wasn't working, the guilt. She had taken to suggesting they ate the supper in front of whatever box set they were watching. Anything to avoid making conversation. Thrillers or black comedy worked. Romance was definitely out, it was too upsetting to be reminded of what they didn't have any more. So it was *The Sopranos* with Jamie Oliver's lasagne, *The Killing* with Nigel Slater's baked red mullet with saffron and mint, *Breaking Bad* with Nigella's spaghetti with prawns and chilli. Tom was a great cook but lately she felt as if she couldn't taste what he'd made – everything tasted the same.

Tom returned with a plate of poached eggs, toast, grilled tomatoes, and wild mushrooms, home-made guacamole, and a bowl of fruit salad.

'Thanks, Tom, that looks amazing,' Candy exclaimed. 'Usually I have Rice Krispies.'

'Is Patrick still in bed?' he asked, sitting back down.

The answer was bound to be yes as Patrick hadn't been getting up before midday. Candy rolled her eyes. 'Yep, he's snoring away. I'm surprised we can't hear him, it's so loud.'

'Sleeping it off then,' Tom commented. 'He hit the brandy last night. We played poker and then, fresh from her triumph over Matt the night before, Frankie challenged us all to table tennis. God, that woman is so competitive!'

'I bet that went down well with Patrick,' Leila put in, remembering from past experience what a bad loser he could be. It was one of his least-attractive qualities.

'What do you think? He actually threw his bat on the floor and stamped on one of the ping pong balls.'

175

'OMG! That is so shameful and childish!' Candy exclaimed. 'I'm glad I wasn't there.'

'Yep, it was. I thought Frankie would read him the Riot Act, but she was the one who calmed him down and managed to persuade him to go to bed.'

Candy's phone beeped with a text message. Leila noticed her wistful expression as she read it.

'Message from home?'

'Yeah, from my sister Mollie. I asked her to text me every day so I know that she and Keira have got up in time. They're both working at Asda for the summer and staying at my aunt's, but she's a bit flaky and isn't exactly a morning person.'

'How many brothers and sisters have you got?' Gracie asked.

'I've got two sisters. Mollie's fifteen and Keira's seventeen.'

'You're so lucky, I wish I had a sister or a brother.' It was Gracie's turn to look wistful.

Leila's heart sank. Gracie hadn't mentioned her lack of siblings for a while and she had been secretly hoping that her daughter had dropped this particular obsession. It had been a nightmare when she'd started nursery and become aware that all her friends had siblings, and every week seemed to bring news that one of them was soon going to have a baby brother or sister. Sometimes Leila felt like the only mother there who didn't have an enormous baby bump or a newborn in a sling. She was aware of Tom's gaze on her – the will they, won't they have a second child discussion had become one of the no go areas. Plus, of course, you had to have sex first and there had been precious little of that. And you had to know that your marriage was going to work out . . .

Candy seemed to pick up that this was a bone of contention as she said diplomatically, 'Well, it's great having your mum and dad all to yourself, isn't it? Babies take up loads of time.'

'And Mummy's always working,' Gracie replied in a matter-of-fact voice. And before Leila could defend herself, her daughter had slipped off her chair and sprinted to the sunny part of the terrace, back on the lizard hunt again.

'Yep, Mummy is always working,' Tom said pointedly, 'which is probably why Gracie doesn't have a sister or a brother. Or maybe there is another reason that Mummy hasn't shared with me yet.' He picked up his coffee cup. 'Is it okay if you have Gracie this morning? I'm going into town with Matt.'

Tears sprang into Leila's eyes and she lowered her head so neither he or Candy would see. She preferred it when they only made small talk. This was too much like washing their dirty linen in public.

'No problem.'

Tom went inside and Leila said quietly, 'I'm not always working actually. If I were a man no one would comment on my working hours, but because I'm a woman I'm supposed to be the one who can

177

juggle everything. I hate it.' Oh, God, she had said too much, and in front of Candy whom she barely knew.

'I guess it's hard getting the work/life balance right when you have a family.' Candy was quite the diplomat. It must be all those hours of listening to her clients offloading their problems on her. Therapy with the wax, facial or whatever. 'So would you like more children?'

Leila hesitated. 'Yes, I think I would, but things are quite difficult at the moment.' She was saved from having to elaborate further by the arrival of Frankie and Tor.

'So what's the plan for this morning?' Frankie asked, picking up a slice of watermelon and typically steering clear of the chocolate croissants. She'd probably last eaten one ten years ago. She had the strongest willpower of anyone Tor knew.

'I don't know, I'll have to check the itinerary,' Leila teased her. Four days into the holiday Frankie still hadn't got the hang of relaxing. She could just about manage to read for half-hour bursts before getting up and energetically swimming lengths. Mind you, Leila didn't exactly feel relaxed either. She still hadn't been able to bring herself to check her phone, which had remained in her bedside drawer, and the problem of what to do about Jasper was never far from her thoughts.

'How about going to the beach before it gets too hot?' she suggested.

'Good idea, I could cycle there,' Frankie replied.

'Bloody hell!' Candy put in. 'It's boiling already.'

Frankie shrugged. 'I need to do something, and I don't know if I'm up to running – I drank too much brandy last night.' She pulled a face. 'I never drink brandy, I don't know what got into me.'

'Yeah, we heard about your table tennis contest and Patrick's queeny fit,' Leila said. She was expecting Frankie to revel in her victory, especially over Matt, but her response was altogether different.

'I'd forgotten that Patrick finds it difficult to lose.'

'What?' Leila couldn't hide the exasperation in her voice. She thought it was pathetic that he was such a bad loser. She wouldn't tolerate such behaviour from her daughter.

'It brings back memories of his dad criticising him for not being good enough at sport. He always felt like such an outsider anyway, and the fact that the rest of the family were so sporty made it even worse.'

'That doesn't excuse his being such a bad loser, he is thirty-four! I thought he might have addressed those issues by now.'

'All right, Leila. Sometimes you need to cut people some slack. We can't all be perfect like you.'

Where did that come from? 'I don't think I'm perfect, Frankie. Far from it.' She was stung by her friend's comment.

Frankie put her head in her hands, 'Okay, okay, I'm sorry. This hangover is vicious. I'm going to have to skip the beach and go back to bed.' She picked up her cup of coffee and went back inside the villa.

'We can still go to the beach,' Leila said, trying not to show how much Frankie's words had got to her. 'And Ed as well. I reckon we could all squeeze in one car.'

Tor shook her head. 'I think Ed's going to hang out at the villa.'

'Do you think I should stay here until Patrick wakes up?' Candy asked. 'I don't want him to think that I'm abandoning him.'

'He'll be asleep for hours, and by the time he surfaces it will be too hot to go to the beach. Anyway, he abandoned you to get pissed.' Leila absolutely didn't feel like defending Patrick.

'So how was your dinner out last night?' Candy asked Tor.

'Oh, yes, was the taverna okay?' Leila had been so wrapped up in herself that she'd completely forgotten Tor and Ed had gone out. He had hinted that he had something important to tell Tor.

'It was fine, thanks.'

Tor seemed unusually subdued. As far as Leila could remember the taverna was lovely, with delicious food, and she would have expected more than *fine* in response to her question.

'So what was the big news?'

Tor swirled her spoon round a bowl of Greek yoghurt and said quietly, 'He's got a new job in London, working as a games designer. It's what he's always wanted to do.'

'Wow, Tor that's fantastic!' Leila knew it must have been tough on her invariably being the one to pay when they went out, even though she had never once complained. And maybe she would stop obsessing about the age gap now Ed was starting his career.

'I know, it is really good news.' She didn't sound like she thought it was, though.

'So is he going to be moving to London?' Perhaps this explained why Tor was so subdued.

'During the week, yes.' She paused. 'Actually we had a bit of a row about that. Ed suggested that he spend every weekend in Brighton with me.'

'And?' Leila thought it was a really good idea. 'It won't be such a big commitment as living together all the time. You'll have the best of both worlds, as you'll have the weekdays to yourself.' There, she was brilliant at solving everyone else's dilemmas, absolutely appalling at addressing her own.

Now Tor looked at her. 'I don't know, Leila. I don't want to rush into things. And every weekend might be too much.'

Leila didn't understand why Tor was being down-beat. She got on so well with Ed. And surely enough time had gone by since her disastrous relationship with Harry?

181

Candy got up from the table and picked up her plate. 'I'll just get my stuff together for the beach.'

Poor girl, she must be wondering why she hadn't gone on holiday to Ibiza with her mates, she was surrounded by so much thirty-something angst.

'Is that all it is?' Leila asked gently, instinctively feeling that there had to be something else going on.

'Well, weekends are still a big commitment. I messed up by moving in with Harry too soon, and you know what a nightmare it was when we split up. I don't want to repeat the same mistake.'

'It was a nightmare *before* you split up! You were practically decorating the street with bunting when you actually left him. We all were.'

Tor managed a smile. 'I felt like decorating the whole of Brighton with bunting, having a firework display and burning an effigy of him.' The smile faded. 'But the whole living together thing . . . I just don't know if it's for me. What if it goes wrong? Don't you remember what it was like dividing all my things up with Harry when we split?'

'I remember what a complete and utter shit he was about it, and how he kept the TV and computer that you had bought together and didn't give you any money. And how he held on to the sofa even though he had moaned non-stop about you choosing a pink velvet one because it was too feminine.'

'It was pure spite because he knew how much I

loved that sofa. The bastard! I hope every time he sits on it he feels his dick shrivel. His new girlfriend will need the Hubble telescope to find it as he was never exactly blessed in that department!'

That was more like it, Tor.

'You were unlucky with Harry, but Ed is nothing like him. He would never behave like Harry if things went wrong – for a start, it's your flat and everything belongs to you. But I don't think it would go wrong. You're really well suited.'

'Well, we'll see.'

Somehow Leila got the feeling that Tor had already made up her mind.

The beach was a three-mile drive away, through a small village, past several tavernas and along a fiendishly bumpy track, that always made Leila fearful for her tyres. On the drive over she told Candy about the island being one of the main nesting sites for the loggerhead turtle, *Caretta caretta*, which returned year after year to the island to lay its eggs on the same beaches, and about how there was a growing conservation movement to protect the turtles and their nesting sites.

'I'd love to help out at something like that, something worthwhile,' Candy replied, gazing out of the window. 'It would make a change from giving someone a Brazilian. I can't say they give me a great deal of job satisfaction.'

'What's a Brazilian?' Gracie asked.

Yikes! Leila did not want to explain to her four-year-old daughter about intimate hair removal.

'It's just a boring beauty treatment I have to do,' Candy said quickly.

'Balding more like,' Tor said under her breath.

'So have you ever seen any turtles, Gracie?' Candy asked, in a welcome change of subject.

'Yes, and I've adopted one. I've got a certificate with her name on it and some pictures. She's called Hera and she's two years old.' Gracie chatted away to Candy and thankfully seemed to have forgotten about Brazilians. But knowing Leila's luck it would be one the thing she remembered on her first day back at school, and she'd ask the teacher. Still, it could have been worse, Candy could have said vajazzle.

'Oh, look,' Tor commented as they approached the beach, 'isn't that Dimitri over there?' It was indeed Dimitri and a young woman in her early-twenties, who had dyed blue hair and a nose ring. They were sitting at a table under a bright orange parasol and handing out information about the rules for going on the beach.

Dimitri smiled warmly at Candy. His long hair was still tied back and he was wearing a white t-shirt advertising the turtle conservation project. He looked young, clear-eyed and very handsome.

'I don't imagine Patrick looks that good this morning, after the night he had,' Tor whispered to Leila. 'I could hear him snoring when I walked past his bedroom. I bet the room reeks of alcohol.'

'So is your boyfriend with you?' Dimitri asked. Leila could lay money on him hoping that Patrick wasn't.

'No, he's still asleep. It's just us girls.'

'And me!' Gracie piped up.

Dimitri waved at the little girl. 'Who could forget you, Gracie? Would you like a sticker with a turtle on it?'

He was very cute, and by the way Blue Hair Girl was looking at him, she thought so too.

'And your foot is okay?'

So kind and considerate . . . what wasn't to like?

'Fine, thanks,' Candy assured him.

A small queue of tourists had formed behind them, and Blue Hair Girl muttered something in Greek.

'I'll come and see you on the beach when I have my break,' Dimitri said, without once taking his eyes off Candy, which provoked Blue Hair to glare at her and say, 'And, remember, no parasols except in the designated areas, and no disturbing the turtles' nests. It is most important.'

Her terse 'Enjoy your visit' didn't exactly sound sincere. She probably hoped that Candy would fall into a turtle's nest and then she could be banned from the beach.

'She's obviously got her eye on the lovely Dimitri,' Tor whispered as they headed for the beach. 'But I reckon he prefers Candy.'

185

'I don't blame him,' Leila whispered back. 'She looks stunning without all that make-up on, doesn't she?'

'She does, but she is only twenty-two. We all looked that good when we were that age.' She sighed, 'Except, of course, that I was fatter than her. But still a lot slimmer than I am now.'

Not the age/weight comment again. Leila hoped that Tor hadn't been talking like this in front of Ed. She had it on good authority from Tom that there was no greater turn-off than a woman obsessing about her appearance.

She and Tor settled on sun loungers under a parasol and read while Candy paddled in the sea with Gracie. This had always been Leila's favourite beach. It was idyllic. A wide sandy bay with crystal-clear waters and no development to mar its natural beauty. It was wonderfully peaceful too as all water sports were banned to protect the turtles. After some ten minutes of uninterrupted reading, which seemed more like an hour to her as it was such a rare treat, she felt guilty about leaving Candy playing with Gracie and went over to relieve her. The water felt deliciously cold against her legs.

'Mummy!' Gracie exclaimed, and instantly rushed over and took her hand. 'We've been counting fish. I've seen seven.'

'That's brilliant, sweet pea! Feel free to have a swim,' she said to Candy.

For some reason Candy looked embarrassed.

She checked that Gracie wasn't listening and said quietly, 'I'm rubbish at swimming. It's one of those things I never got round to doing properly. I was hopeless in the lessons we had at school and ended up bunking off for most of them.'

'Oh. Well, you could have lessons now, couldn't you?' And then Leila thought of Candy having to juggle work as well as run the home for her two sisters, and regretted her comment.

'Yeah, I guess,' the girl said slowly.

'Or I could get Tom to teach you. He taught Gracie. He's a really good teacher.'

'Maybe. It is supposed to be his holiday. You go for a swim if you want, I'll stay with Gracie.'

Then, when Leila hesitated, Candy repeated, 'Go on, you're not taking advantage of me. I'm happy playing with her.'

'Thanks, I won't be long.' Leila swam out to sea, relishing the sense of space and freedom. Then she lay on her back looking up at the blue cloudless sky. This was bliss, sheer bliss. Surely here on her island she and Tom could sort their problems out . . . and she did want them to. She didn't want to be a single parent. She wanted to make their marriage work. She remembered hearing other couples talking about working at their relationships and had never understood it. Until now, her relationship with Tom had always felt so easy. Now everything seemed hard. How did they bridge the gulf that had developed between them? And then there was

Jasper. Part of Leila wanted to tell Tom everything, to wipe the slate clean, start again . . . but that was more about her, not about him. She wanted him to forgive her, which was hardly fair when she didn't forgive herself.

By the time she swam back to shore Gracie and Candy were hard at work making sandcastles, decorating them with shells, stones and strands of seaweed. Candy seemed perfectly happy to be covered in wet sand. She had tied her long red hair into a messy ponytail and seemed very different from the girl who'd arrived with her full face of make-up.

'Stop any time you want and I'll take over,' Leila told her.

'Honestly, Leila, I'm having a great time. I'd tell you if I wasn't. It's so lovely being outside. I spend so much time inside when I'm at work, and the treatment rooms have no windows. It's like being in prison.'

Leila was about to grab her towel when she noticed Dimitri coming on to the beach. He must have escaped the clutches of Blue Hair for his break. She probably had a telescope trained on him, or maybe she had him electronically tagged . . .

'Well, you might want to stop now. I think you've got a visitor.'

He was certainly very easy on the eye, thought Leila, watching him stride towards them.

Candy hastily stood up and attempted to brush away the sand coating her legs.

'I was just thinking I needed to exfoliate,' she tried to joke, but she was blushing and looked flustered.

'You look great, like a surfer chick – and I mean that as a compliment,' Leila told her as Candy wrapped a purple sarong around her waist.

Dimitri chatted politely about the conservation work he was doing, which included night patrols of the beach to ensure the nesting turtles remained undisturbed and that once their eggs had hatched the baby turtles made it safely to the sea. But all the time Leila was certain that he would so much rather be alone with Candy.

'You could come and help out,' he told the girl. 'You and your boyfriend.'

Well done, he had managed to say the word without choking. 'We're always looking for volunteers.'

Candy smiled. 'I can't exactly see Patrick patrolling the beach at night unless you provide alcohol. And then he'd only get pissed and end up falling in one of the nests and crushing the eggs. But I'd like to get involved.'

She was rewarded with a dazzling smile from Dimitri that could probably have been seen from the next island.

'I have twenty more minutes left of my break and I wondered if you wanted to go for a walk along the beach?' he asked, attempting to sound casual though hope was radiating off him.

'Can I come?' Gracie piped up.

Leila quickly intervened, 'Let's have a competition to see who can build the biggest sandcastle, and the winner can choose whatever ice cream they want.'

'Anything? Can I get a Nobbly Bobbly? A white chocolate Magnum? A Feast? A Fruit Pastel lolly? A Mini-milk . . . but only if they have the strawberry one.'

Should she be worried that her daughter knew the names of so many ice creams? Leila wondered if she could name as many vegetables.

'Anything.'

Gracie picked up her spade and began energetically filling her bucket with sand, conveniently forgetting about the walk. Bribery worked every time.

For a few minutes Leila watched Candy and Dimitri as they strolled by the shore. They were deep in conversation and kept looking at each other. She remembered walking on this same beach hand in hand with Tom before Gracie was conceived, and then when she was pregnant. Could they ever get back to that? She had to hope they could.

Chapter 16

Candy

Candy had been thinking about Dimitri a lot since their encounter. Especially when Patrick had been snoring away next to her, preventing her from going to sleep. She had been thinking about chocolate-brown eyes and gentle, strong hands, broad shoulders and a very sexy smile. About someone who had gazed at her as if she was special. Not leered at, not grinned at suggestively. Not looked at her tits . . . or if he had, he'd done it discreetly. No, he had gazed at her. She felt a touch of guilt, but only a touch because Patrick had been so intensely annoying since they'd arrived. All he wanted to do was drink, and he would do that until he was completely pissed, said stupid things, and then passed out. He hadn't been like this before the holiday – if he had, she certainly wouldn't have come. God, no way! And yet, if she hadn't come she never would have met Dimitri . . . and just seeing him again was making her heart beat faster, giving her butterflies that she had never got with Patrick. Sometimes life was a complete bugger.

'So where is your boyfriend now?' Dimitri was bound to ask, she supposed. They had talked about what she'd done the day before, where she was from, where he was from . . . enough for Candy to know that she liked him, and really, really fancied him. Did that make her sound a complete slut? Possibly. It was only four weeks ago that she'd really fancied Patrick . . . It had been hard to remember why when she'd slipped out of bed this morning and he let out a particularly loud snore.

She shrugged. 'Still asleep probably – he stayed up late drinking.' *No change there then.*

Dimitri stopped walking, 'I don't understand why you are with him. You're so young, and he is—'

'He's not that old! If that's what you were going to say,' Candy exclaimed. 'And he is funny and good company. Most of the time.'

Some of the time. Rarely since we've been here. And he drinks way too much, and I don't like the way he treats me as his plaything. These were the things that she could have said . . . but didn't. There was no point.

She sat down on the sand and gazed out to sea. She wasn't comfortable talking about Patrick. She couldn't help feeling that Dimitri was judging her for being his girlfriend. He sat down next

192

to her. Reaching inside his rucksack, he handed her an ice-cold bottle of water. There was an instant when their fingers touched that felt more significant than when she had kissed Patrick for the first time.

'I'm sorry, I just don't get why a girl like you is with someone like him,' Dimitri persisted.

'I like Patrick. Okay, he's not the great love of my life, we're not going to get married, I'm not going to have his babies . . .'

She was trying to keep it light but Dimitri interrupted her.

'So why are you with him? You're worth more. So much more.'

The questions were making her feel uneasy. She turned to face him. 'What is this? Judgement Day? I met Patrick when I was doing some crappy job trying to earn a bit of extra money, and he was nice to me, lovely in fact. We'd been seeing each other a month, and when he asked me to come on holiday, I thought, why not? I've always wanted to come to Greece.' She was aware that last part made her sound as if she was a bit of a freeloader . . . maybe she was a bit of a freeloader.

'I'm just jealous of him. I'm sorry,' Dimitri said, shamefaced.

'Why are you jealous of him?'

He looked down and said quietly, 'Because he's with you.'

It stopped her in her tracks. *I wish I wasn't, you*

193

have no idea how much, she wanted to tell him. But what good would that do?

'Do you really think a beautician who lives in a council flat is such a great catch?'

Dimitri probably didn't even know what a council flat was. Now as well as coming across as a bit of a slut, she sounded as if she had a massive chip on her shoulder.

He turned to look at her, but she couldn't see his eyes behind his sunglasses. 'I think you are beautiful and kind. It doesn't matter to me what you do, or where you live. You are not defined by those things.'

Wow! This was the kind of conversation people had in books or films – the kinds of rom-coms her friend Madison adored – not in life. Patrick's opening line had been, 'You're the sexiest woman here, tell me you haven't got a boyfriend.' It was so close to 'Get your coat, you've pulled' that she had burst out laughing. She had gone to bed with him a week later, still laughing then. It was fair to say that he hadn't made her laugh much since they had been here.

No man had ever said anything as romantic as Dimitri on first meeting her. Candy wanted to hoard the words, treasure them, for when she got home, back to reality. She would replay them at the salon when the endless appointments were getting her down, when she felt as if her life was slipping through her fingers without ever really getting started. But then her naturally cynical, streetwise side kicked in.

'Yeah, right, I bet you say that to all the pretty girls. There'll be someone else who catches your eye soon, I expect. There must be loads of them on the island, all looking for a good time with someone like you. English girls are probably your best bet. We all know what people think about English girls abroad. And what would your girlfriend in Athens think of that?'

Dimitri shook his head. 'I don't have a girlfriend in Athens and I'm not interested in any other girls. Only you. Maybe we shouldn't talk about this.' He scuffed at the sand with his foot.

Instantly Candy regretted her outburst. It sounded as if he was being perfectly sincere. She hadn't meant to hurt his feelings.

'So what are you a studying at uni?'

'Psychology. I'd like to become a child psychologist one day.'

'That's impressive.'

'Not really, it's just what I'm interested in. And did you always want to be a beautician?'

'Yeah, it's my lifelong ambition. Waxing is my dream. Bring it on!' She couldn't help being sarcastic and feeling envious of someone who could go to university and pursue whatever they wanted to do. It had never been an option open to her. Dimitri looked slightly taken aback by her tone. It wasn't his fault that her life had turned out the way it had, and she didn't want to offend him, so she added, 'Actually I wanted to train to be a midwife, but I had to drop out of college when my mum died. I had to earn money, and being a beautician meant I could learn on the job and get paid.'

She hated talking about this – tried to avoid it wherever possible. It reopened too many wounds, too many what might have beens, too many if onlys.

'It sounds like you had a tough time.'

Candy thought of the endless struggles to pay the bills, of worrying about her sisters, of the time Mollie truanted from school and Candy became paranoid that she and Keira would be taken away from her and put into care, of never being able to go out with her mates except on the rarest of occasions, of having to give up her ambition to be a midwife. Tough didn't exactly cover it.

'But, you know, you could still do it. You're so young,' Dimitri insisted, optimistic for her chances. 'And I think you would be very good at it. You're a real people person.'

'Maybe.' She thought about how Patrick never asked her any personal questions and had no idea that she wanted to be a midwife. He would have made a joke about it. Patrick made a joke about everything.

Dimitri looked at his watch and sighed, 'I'll have to get back in a minute or Naida will be annoyed and will sulk for the rest of the afternoon. And that's even worse than when she tries to flirt with me! Let's go for a swim first.' He stood up and peeled off his t-shirt. His skin was a beautiful rich brown, so smooth that it made her want to reach out and touch it.

He held out his hand to help Candy up, but she remained sitting where she was. 'I can't swim.'

He did a double take. 'Really? I could teach you. I've been swimming since I was a baby. You should let me, and by the end of the holiday you'll be swimming as if you've been doing it all your life.'

She shook her head. 'No, thanks.' She was starting to feel insecure – as if she was Dimitri's little project for the summer: teach the poor little English girl all about turtles, and how to swim. Big tick for being such an all round good guy and maybe even get a shag in the process.

He remained where he was, obviously not used to being turned down. 'Are you sure?'

'I am. Thanks.' She paused. 'And anyway, I don't know what Patrick would think about you teaching me. It would probably dent his male pride. He had to pick me up the other night, don't you remember? I don't think I can take any more of that. I don't think his back could either.'

Dimitri frowned as if the mention of the other man had pained him. 'Your boyfriend, of course. I forgot about him. So if you won't come for a swim, how about coming to the club? I don't care what you say, Candy, I have to see you again. There is something between us – a connection. You can't deny it.'

And before she could fob him off, he raced into the sea and dived straight into the water. She watched him swim out with an effortless front crawl. Then he stopped, turned to look at her and blew her a kiss. 'I will see see you again, Candy. That's a promise.'

He sounded so determined that she couldn't stop a smile from spreading across her face.

'Maybe,' she called out.

'For certain,' Dimitri shouted back.

She was still smiling when she rejoined Leila and Tor.

Chapter 17

Frankie

Day five of the holiday from hell, Frankie thought as she hauled herself out of bed, determined to go for a run. She hadn't gone the day before, which was unheard of for her. A hangover had had her in its evil grip all morning and it was far too hot by the time she recovered, so she *had* to go this morning.

That she was not enjoying the holiday was an understatement. She had not had a moment alone with Patrick. Either he was asleep or he was with Candy or he was too drunk. She couldn't go on like this. She would have to do something, *say* something.

She had been running for ten minutes and was already sweating in the early-morning sun when she was aware of someone running behind her and then drawing level. She was all set to nod and say 'hi' as she would back home, when she saw it was

Matt. No, no, no! Not on her run. She could handle being with him when they played table tennis or were in a group, but not here, not during the one opportunity she had to clear her head.

'Hi, I thought it was you,' he said, barely out of breath at all, adding, 'I didn't know anyone else who would be mad enough to run in this heat.' He was in a white running vest and black shorts. He looked good. If she didn't know him, she would think he looked fit. In both senses of the word. And for a second Frankie had a flashback to the wedding, to how that fit body had felt when they had embraced. And just as quickly she remembered him rejecting her . . . the gut-wrenching humiliation. She wanted to tell him to go away, leave her alone. They had discovered that they had table tennis in common, couldn't he just leave it at that?

But she had promised Leila, and so she tried to sound pleasant as she turned down the music on her iPod – she had been listening to 'The One That Got Away' – Katy Perry was her guilty pleasure for running to. 'I didn't know you were into running.'

'I didn't know you were into Katy Perry. I'd have had you down as listening to something moody like New Order or Arctic Monkeys.'

Tits! He'd heard her music! 'I like Katy Perry,' she mumbled. Correction – she *loved* Katy Perry. Thank God she hadn't been singing along when he'd caught up with her, which she liked to do. It

200

wouldn't exactly have fitted her kickass image. She had even gone to see Katy Perry's film, *Part of Me*, on her own because none of her friends wanted to see it, and had the mortifying experience of being spotted by about ten of her Year Nine pupils when the house lights came up.

'And, yes, I run at least three times a week,' said Matt. 'Good for releasing those endorphins and relieving stress. How about you?'

'I run every day usually.' *Now shut up.*

'So, d'you mind if I run with you?'

Bollocks!

'It's okay,' he added, as if reading her thoughts. 'We don't have to talk if you don't want.'

'No problem,' she replied and turned her music back up as if to emphasise that she certainly wouldn't be talking.

Usually Frankie hated running with anyone, preferring to set her own pace, and she definitely didn't want to talk. All day, every day when she was teaching she was talking, talking, talking; she had to be across everything in the class and everyone. It was stimulating, interesting, important work – and absolutely bloody knackering. Running was how she recharged, got some headspace and perspective, nothing ever seemed quite so overwhelming after a run. But, and this was a big surprise, she didn't find it annoying having Matt by her side. It actually encouraged her to push herself to go that bit faster. She couldn't quite believe that she was thinking this, but he was a lovely runner, with a completely natural and smooth action. They fell into pace together.

She was the first to break the silence. 'You're a really good runner.'

'Thanks, so are you.' He glanced at her. 'D'you know, that's the second nice thing you've said to me? And, yes, I am counting. Are you mellowing in the sun? Are you sure you don't want to add, "a really good runner for a capitalist"?'

'Nope, I promised Leila I would play nice from now on. She had me pinned against the hand dryer in the Ladies'. You might not think it to look at her but she can be bloody scary.'

'Pity.' Matt grinned. 'I quite like our little disagreements. Can't you say something insulting? Otherwise I won't know how to be around you. Go on, you know you want to really.'

Was it her imagination or was there a flirtatious edge to his voice? It was impossible to tell with him. Where Matt was concerned, she knew nothing. Less than nothing.

'Definitely not, Leila will kill me.'

Another grin. 'I'm sure it won't be long before I do something that annoys you and you'll break that promise.'

'Probably, but I'm not going to let on. I'm going to "Zip it, lock it, put it in your pocket" – as my friend who is a primary school teacher says to her class of seven-year-olds. You can still say things when they're that age. Something happens to them when they reach secondary. If I came out with that, I'd just get WTF looks.'

'So do you still enjoy teaching?'

'Yeah, I know you think that I'm a cynical cow but—'

'I did before I knew you liked Katy Perry. Now I don't know what to think. Sorry, carry on.'

'I love working with young people . . . their energy and enthusiasm and their humour. Even the ones who are bolshie and difficult, it can be so rewarding helping them find something they are good at, something they can be proud of.' Frankie gave a wry smile. 'You're going to think that this sounds really wanky, but I want to make an impact on their lives.' She was getting out of breath; she was not used to talking so much when she was running.

'I don't think it sounds wanky at all. I think it sounds inspired, and I bet you're great teacher.'

'I do my best.' They were silent for a few minutes after that. Frankie had always been terrible at accepting compliments, and least of all from someone she was wary of. The road twisted and turned along the coast, with the constant vivid blue of the sea beside them. They ran past whitewashed houses, with shutters and doors painted green or blue, past orange trees and fig trees. Being out here felt like a shot of happiness . . . it almost made her forget about Patrick. Almost.

But then Matt had to ruin it all by talking again. 'Is it tough seeing Patrick with Candy?'

This was not a conversation Frankie wanted to have, and definitely not with Matt. She tried to keep her tone neutral as she replied, 'I just think she's far too young for him.'

'That's not what I meant. Don't you think it would help to talk about it?'

Her promise to be nice went out of the window as the old defensive, spiky Frankie responded, 'I didn't realise you'd become a therapist as well as a lawyer – good for you, Matt, multi-tasking. I didn't think men could do that, but apparently you can. But this is none of your business!' And then she couldn't stop herself from going further and blurting out, 'I don't want to talk about it with anyone, least of all you. Let's drop the pretence. I know what you think of me – you made that obvious at the wedding.'

And to underline her point she picked up her pace and pulled ahead of him. Her legs and lungs were protesting, and she was getting a stitch, but she wouldn't give in and she practically sprinted round a corner, thinking that even thick-skinned Matt would get the message that she wanted to be alone.

A few metres ahead of her she noticed what she thought was a bag of rubbish dumped at the side of the road, but as she got closer she realised, with a sickening feeling, that it was the body of a cat. The poor thing must have been hit by a car. She stopped, and forced herself to check that the cat was dead. It was. She hoped that it had died instantly. For all her cynical, hard exterior, Frankie couldn't bear to think of anything suffering – she even rescued spiders from the bath, and had been the designated spider-catcher when she'd shared a flat with Tor and Leila as students. A slight movement in the ditch close by caught her attention and she noticed two tiny kittens mewing piteously. They must only be a few weeks old and would not survive without their mother. One was a tortoiseshell, one jet black with a white patch on its chin. She couldn't just leave them there. She bent down and tried to coax them over. Matt came to a halt beside her.

The tortoiseshell seemed to make-up its mind that Frankie was not going to hurt it and walked unsteadily over to her. She scooped it up. It was only a little bit bigger than her hand and she could feel its tiny heart beating away frantically.

'What are we going to do?' She put on hold her feelings for Matt, in fact she was grateful to have him here with her. They were at least four miles away from the villa and could hardly run back with the kittens, and if they left them the chances were they would meet the same fate as their mother.

'I'll phone Leila and get Ellie's number. She adores cats. She's bound to know what to do.'

'Oh, yes, of course!'

Frankie listened as Matt made the calls. He was calm and efficient. Within a few minutes he had described their location and arranged for Ellie to come and pick them up. She found herself thinking about Patrick and imagining what he would do in this situation. She forced herself to be clear-sighted and concluded that he wouldn't have wanted to help, that it would all have been too much effort for him. She could almost hear him saying, 'Come on, Frankie, they're only bloody cats. I'm dying for a beer.'

'Thanks,' she said as Matt finished the call.

'No problem,' he replied. Bending down, he managed to pick up the black kitten. 'Did you think I wouldn't care?'

'Of course not.' She hesitated. 'And sorry that I was rude to you yet again. You were right, it wasn't long before I broke my promise. Don't tell Leila.'

'And I'm sorry too. I know that Patrick is a sensitive subject. I won't say anything more about him.' Now Matt hesitated. 'But I'll say this one last time . . . he really isn't worth it, Frankie.'

She glared at him. 'I thought you were going to stop!'

'That's it, I promise.' He paused. 'And about what happened at the wedding. We were both drunk. We should forget it. And I could tell you that—' he broke off and shook his head.

'Tell me what?' Her curiosity was piqued.

'Nothing. I just wanted to say, let's call a truce.'

With an effort she replied, 'Truce.' And then, because it was ridiculous to be glaring at a man in sportswear who was holding a cute kitten, while clutching a kitten herself, she added, 'Anyway my kitten is cuter than yours.'

Matt shook his head. 'No way. You've got the runt of the litter.'

Frankie stuck her out tongue.

They both sat down by the side of the road to wait for Ellie. To deflect any questions about herself, Frankie turned her attention to Matt, almost pretending that she didn't know him, as if they were meeting for the first time. That way she wouldn't get wound up and she could fool herself that the encounter at Leila's wedding never actually happened. And in that ten minutes she discovered things that she'd never known about Matt. He lived alone in Islington. He had split up with his long-term girlfriend not long before Leila and Tom's wedding.

'Why did you break up?' Frankie asked, never afraid of a direct question when they weren't being directed at her.

He shrugged. 'She wanted more commitment, and I didn't. It wasn't fair to carry on. It was very comfortable but also unchallenging, and that's not what I want in a relationship.'

Frankie raised an eyebrow, thinking, Typical commitment-phobe.

Matt saw the look. 'I do want to settle down and have kids, before you dismiss me as another guy who can't commit, but it wasn't right with Sinead.'

'And since her?'

'A few casual flings, I guess. Nothing more serious.'

Frankie imagined that Matt was seen by many women as extremely eligible. Good job (if you liked that kind of thing), okay personality (if you liked that kind of thing) and good-looking (again, if you liked that kind of thing). Frankie always judged other men against Patrick's brooding dark good looks and it was hard for anyone to compete with him, but even she had to admit that Matt was a looker.

She smiled. 'Well, if you get lucky on a night out, you can always have my double bed.' She wanted to make amends for being so foul when he first arrived. She was back on track with her promise to Leila to be nice.

He looked at her, and gave a wickedly cheeky grin. 'Is that an offer of a threesome, Frankie?'

Frankie who had always prided herself on having an answer to everything – she had to as a teacher – found herself blushing, and stuttered, 'I only meant that you could have my bed and I would have yours.'

Matt was still giving her that grin. 'Pity. Thought it might be something I could tick off my bucket list.'

The arrival of Ellie in a battered white Fiat saved

Frankie from coming up with a reply, which was lucky as she didn't have one.

'The kitten saviours!' Ellie declared as she got out of the car in a waft of sandalwood and swirl of her long purple skirt. She had brought along a cat basket and they carefully placed the kittens inside. 'I'm going to get them checked out by my local vet, and then Leila's agreed that they can stay at the villa while you are here as two of my rescue cats have just had litters and we're rather kittened out. And I'll have to do some sweet talking to Nikos as I had promised him there would be no more cats.'

'I bet you always get your own way, don't you, Ellie?' That from Matt.

She laughed. 'Naturally! So are you running back or d'you want a lift?'

Frankie hesitated; she really should run back. She'd only run about four miles, but it was much hotter now and all she wanted to do was have a shower and swim in the pool.

'I'll have a lift, thanks,' she replied, fully expecting Matt to do the same.

'And I'm going to run back.' He turned to Frankie. 'Lightweight – I'll see you later.' Again there was the bantering tone.

He set off at speed. *Nice bum*, she found herself unexpectedly thinking, watching him go.

'That is one good-looking man,' Ellie commented, her thoughts clearly running along the same lines as Frankie's.

'D'you think?' she replied. 'I've never been into blond men. They're too healthy and hearty-looking for me, I like my men dark and mysterious.' She truly hoped that she wasn't blushing after saying this, though she could always blame it on the run.

Ellie gave her a sideways glance. 'Hmm, I think blond men can be very sexy. And he's single, and so are you. Ideal holiday romance, I'd say, or maybe something more. This is the island where I met Nikos when I was island hopping and I thought it was only going to last the summer. And here we are, thirty years and two children later.'

Frankie shook her head. 'I really don't think so, Ellie, we don't especially like each other. I doubt we'll see each other again after the holiday.'

She looked sceptical. 'You seemed to be getting on very well just then. There was more than a whiff of flirtation – trust me, I'm practically an oracle in these matters.'

'Yeah, well, the whiff was probably sweat and the rest was the influence of the kittens, honestly. And I promised Leila that I would be nice to him.'

But that was only half the truth because Frankie had been surprised by how well she'd got on with Matt and by how much she had enjoyed talking to him – apart from the comments about Patrick and the wedding. It would be good if they could salvage some kind of friendship after their rocky start.

Chapter 18

Tor

Tor and Ed were sitting on the terrace having a late breakfast. Or rather Ed was having breakfast, Tor was sipping peppermint tea; she couldn't face eating anything. She had already thrown up twice already. The morning sickness seemed to be going up a gear. So much for thinking it had been getting better . . .

'So have you thought any more about what I said the other night?' Ed asked.

Tor had thought of nothing else and still didn't know what to do. If she told him she was pregnant, would he run a mile? Or would he feel that he had to stay, but feel trapped and resentful?

'I need time to think about it, Ed.'

He frowned. 'How much time? Because if you don't want me to move in, just tell me. I'd much rather you were honest with me.' He had never sounded this pissed off with her before.

'Just a week or something, Ed.' She knew how annoyingly vague that must sound.

A shrug from him. 'I still don't get what the big deal is. I feel as if we've been coming at this relationship from two different angles. I thought we were going somewhere, but you're acting like we're not. I want this – us – to mean something, to matter, because it matters to me.'

What was she doing? At this rate she wouldn't have a relationship. She put her arm tentatively around his shoulders, 'I'm sorry if I'm giving you that impression. I do think our relationship matters. I really do.' She hesitated. 'I might have started out thinking that it was going to be casual but that was more of a defence mechanism. It's not how I feel now. It hasn't been for a long while.'

She wanted to say more, but at that moment her phone rang. It was Spencer. Shit, talk about bad timing! 'Sorry, it's Spencer, I'd better take it in case it's urgent. He might have frozen the card machine or got locked out. You know what he's like.'

A resigned sigh from Ed. 'Yeah, whatever.'

'Hi, Spencer, how are you?' said Tor, trying to sound cheerful, like someone who was having the time of their life on holiday, as she headed for the privacy of their bedroom.

'*Ciao, bella*! Sorry I don't know any Greek apart from *Kalispera* and *Efharisto*. But "good evening" and "thank you" were enough to get me a shag with a hot Greek barman last time I went to Mykonos on holiday – oh, happy times. Do you know, it's pissing down with rain here? It's so dreary, every single day and Federico says he can't take any time off this summer. I think I'm developing SAD and vitamin D deficiency. I need colour, Tor! Come on, cheer me up.'

It was clearly not urgent.

She sat down on the bed with the feeling she was not going to be able to lift his spirits. Her own were weighing her down too badly.

'It's lovely here, Spencer. Idyllic. Hot. Relaxing. Blue skies, beautiful beaches.' A relationship that was teetering on the edge, a kidney bean that was taking over her life.

'Lucky, lucky, lucky you! I don't think I can remember what blue looks like any more. So how's it going with Ed? Your first holiday together. A relationship milestone.'

Spencer adored Ed. Not only did he fancy him like crazy, but Ed had achieved hero status in his eyes for repairing his laptop and for not being Harry. Spencer loathed Harry.

'It's good, really good.'

But Spencer knew her too well and instantly picked up that it was not really good at all. And so Tor found herself telling him about Ed's job and the idea of him moving in.

'But that sounds like the perfect arrangement! And it's fantastic about Ed's job. Why are you sounding so downbeat, you crazy, mad, insane lady! Do you think there are lots of Eds out there? Honey, I've looked high and low, in every nook and cranny, and there are none. You have the only one. He's a keeper.'

She couldn't tell him about the baby. It was tempting. Very tempting. But he would be off-the-scale hysterical, and she needed calm.

'I don't know. Maybe Ed and I are only supposed to be a fling and it's past its sell-by date.' Tor didn't believe this and didn't know why she even said it. It was as if she was protecting herself against future hurt.

'You are kidding me! That man is the best thing to have happened to you in such a long time. Such a very, very long time. Do I need to remind you what it was like BE? Before Ed. You were with *Harry*. The time of low self-esteem and no sex and never looking forward to going home. Not ever, because you never wanted to spend any time with Harry.

'Ed adores you. And you adore him, I know. The pair of you are so good together. It *would* be sickening and I *would* hate you, except for the fact I love you both. Obviously you more than him,' he quickly added. 'But don't make me choose. I need to have Ed's abs and technical ability in my life.'

Tor managed a smile. Spencer could infuriate her when she worked with him every day, but she loved him too. He had a heart of pure gold. He had always looked out for her and after her, from the moment she'd employed him eight years ago. Her brother from another mother, he often teased her.

'I've really pissed him off by not saying yes straight away. I don't know what to do.'

'Just tell him that of course you want him to move in! You're making a problem where there isn't one. It's because of Harry, but you mustn't let the experience of living with him taint what you have with Ed. You can forget the past, Tor. You have to let it go. Oh my God, I sound so sensible and together, what's happening to me? Hurry up and come back, I need to be trivial and shallow again!'

'You'll always be trivial and shallow, Spencer. Those qualities run through you like stripes of colour in a stick of Brighton rock.'

'Thank you, I take it as a compliment.'

'Good, it was meant as one.' And then, because she couldn't bear to have the spotlight on her any longer, Tor asked about the store and Federico and Maud.

Everything and everyone was fine. Maybe they could get by without her. Maybe she did need to let go and trust. Maybe. By the time she went back outside all the friends had congregated on the terrace and were transfixed by the arrival of two kittens, rescued apparently by Frankie and Matt.

Ed and Gracie were playing with a cute tortoiseshell, waving a piece of string in front of it while it batted away at it with its paw. She wanted to go up to Ed and wrap her arms around him, tell him how much he meant to her. But when he looked across at her, he still looked subdued and so she didn't.

Chapter 19

Leila

Between two and five the sun was far too intense for them to do anything much at all, apart from laze around the pool and occasionally dive in to cool off. Leila always loved this time of day on the island. Back in the UK she would be charging around, organising everyone if she was at work, and if she was at home she would be doing the same, but with fewer people who listened to her less. Now as she lay on a lounger under the parasol, with her eyes closed, she felt the heat envelop her, giving her permission finally to relax, to let go. Gracie was inevitably watching *Toy Story* and playing with the kittens; Tom was reading. For this small window of time no one wanted anything of her. She could just be. There was no breeze and no sound apart from the cicadas in full chorus.

She allowed her mind to wander, fantasising that

she and Tom and Gracie lived out here; that life was simple, that they were happy, back to the way they were. She imagined directing two or maybe three dramas a year; Tom writing more; imagined that she never snapped at him; that they talked more; that they were having another baby; that she hadn't slept with another man. The fantasy came to an abrupt halt. She opened her eyes, sighing, and reached for her book, needing to escape into another reality. She had barely read two pages before she was interrupted by Frankie.

Her friend flopped down on the lounger next to hers. In a navy-and-white striped bikini she was as pale as ever, though her face had the faintest sun-kissed glow about it and she looked better than she had in ages. Perhaps finally she was relaxing.

'Do you think you're going to get a tan at all?' Leila enquired.

'You know I don't get tanned. I burn, turn the colour of a tomato, and then it all peels off, which makes me look as if I've got radiation poisoning. An attractive look, I think you'll agree. So no, I'm sticking with lily white. Okay with you?'

'I don't mind what you do, sweetie, so long as you're having a good time.' Leila paused. Until now Frankie hadn't looked as if she was fully into holiday mode, though she seemed to have cheered up with the arrival of the kittens.

'Yep, and I've been nice to Matt *and* I rescued two kittens. Can't you see my halo shining?' She gave a cheeky grin. 'You'll have to set up one of those roadside shrines to me – Saint Frankie. It has a good ring to it. I expect fresh flowers – none of your artificial crap – wine – none of your cheap stuff – and money. In fact, gold. Less chance of it losing its value.'

'Don't push it.'

'And what about you? Are you having a good time? Or is it tough being the hostess, even though you always seem to do it so easily?'

Without hesitation Leila replied, 'It goes without saying. My favourite place with my favourite people. I'm having a brilliant time.' What an accomplished liar she had become.

She had always told Frankie everything, but she couldn't confide in her about Jasper, she was too bitterly ashamed. She judged herself harshly enough over what had happened. She couldn't handle anyone else's bad opinon of her. Nor did she want to burden Frankie with her toxic secret. Tom was her friend as well. It wouldn't be fair. As a result Leila felt that there was a distance between them. It might only have been in her own mind, but she hoped Frankie hadn't picked up on it.

'We should have a girls' night out tonight, don't you think? Have a good gossip over some cheeky cocktails. The boys can go out another night and talk about whatever boys talk about when they're alone.'

Frankie curled her lip. 'Does that mean Candy

would have to come? There's only so much time I like to spend discussing – oh, I don't know – the latest craze in fake lashes or fake tans. Or,' and at this point Frankie thrust her chest out and put on a simpering voice, 'how lovely my tits are. Bet you'd like to touch them, boys.'

So much for thinking that she seemed more relaxed. 'It's up to Candy, and she probably won't want to if you're being like that!' Leila pointed out. 'She's not stupid, Frankie, I'm sure she knows exactly what you think of her.'

'What, me? When I'm always so good at disguising my feelings? I am Ms Inscrutable. Really I should work in espionage, I'm wasted in front of all those teenagers.'

'Hah! I can read you like a book – like an easy-to-read book with enormous print, for people who can't see.'

Leila had no scuples about being rude to Frankie, knowing full well that her friend always gave as good as she got. 'I like Candy – I didn't think I would when I first met her, but I do,' she went on. 'And she's had a bloody tough life. Did you know that she brought up her two sisters on her own after their mum died? She was only seventeen. That can't have been easy. And apparently her dad buggered off when she was little, so it was all down to her.' Leila was piling it on thick, aiming to make Frankie feel guilty.

It worked like a dream as her friend appeared to

be genuinely mortified and said quietly, 'I had no idea. Poor girl. God, I really am such a bitch. Don't let me be horrible to her ever again.'

Leila smiled to herself. 'I'll hold you to that. So now there's two people you've got to be extra nice to – Matt and Candy.'

'Bloody hell, I really will deserve a sainthood,' Frankie muttered. But she wasn't subdued for long as she shot Leila an accusing look. 'So why didn't you tell me you were asking Matt here? It wasn't a last-minute thing, was it? You planned it all along.'

That was a no-brainer. 'Because I knew you wouldn't come if I told you. I know how stubborn you are.'

'I hope you weren't trying to set me up with him?'

'God, you are an egomaniac! We asked Matt because he's Tom's best friend, we weren't thinking about you! But Matt's a really decent bloke, if only you'd give him a chance.'

Leila was fully prepared for one of Frankie's acid putdowns, but instead she replied, 'Yeah, he is. I had no idea. I'm sorry I was so obnoxious to him before.'

'Oh my God! Have you had some kind of per-sonality transplant?' Leila teased. 'I never thought you would say that!'

Frankie refused to be provoked. 'I am capable of changing my mind about people, Leila.'

She was temporarily speechless. She had never

known Frankie change her opinion about anyone. She knew that her friend was incredibly fair and patient in the classroom, but the price she paid for that meant that she often displayed zero tolerance outside school.

Leila watched as Frankie dived into the water. Her friend was a brilliant swimmer and glided the length of the pool in a smooth breast stroke, even performing the nifty tumble turn at the side that Leila had always wanted to be able to do and had never managed.

She looked over to the villa as Matt wandered out with a towel slung over his shoulder. She would be able to observe at first hand whether Frankie could stick to her resolution, she realised. Matt stopped when he saw that Frankie was already in the pool, but she called out, 'Come in, Matt, it's great after a run.'

She really had had a personality transplant . . . Frankie was usually the kind of swimmer who got pool rage if anyone dared to swim in the fast lane when they weren't as speedy as she was, and was quite capable of telling that person to shift lanes.

Matt was obviously as surprised as Leila by the invitation, 'Are you sure? I don't want to interrupt your swim. I know how you like your own space.'

He glanced over at Leila, 'I've already ruined her run this morning by joining her.'

'No, no, Frankie said how much she enjoyed

your company, and that she's hoping to go running with you every day. She loves exercising with other people. Can't get enough of it.' Leila would suffer for this, but couldn't resist it.

'Really?'

Leila ignored the filthy look Frankie shot her.

'Yeah, that would be good,' her friend managed to reply, halo still intact, just about. 'Come on then, I'll race you.'

'You're on,' Matt replied, throwing his towel on a lounger and diving in. When he surfaced he called to Leila, 'You be the judge, I don't trust this one not to cheat and play mean.'

'Cheek!' Frankie glared at him, smoothing her hair back and adjusting her goggles.

'And I bet you're a really bad loser.'

'Well, you won't get to see that. Prepare to be beaten, motherfucker!'

Leila was absolutely certain that Frankie would not admit this, but she and Matt were flirting. Frankie only ever swore like that with someone she really liked. Could Leila be witnessing the start of a beautiful something? The conviction grew stronger in her as she watched the pair of them race up and down the pool, and Matt just pipped Frankie to win.

'That was too easy,' he declared. 'To be honest, I wasn't even trying.'

'Pah! I let you win,' Frankie retorted. 'I didn't want to dent your male pride. I know it doesn't take much to wither a man, especially after I annihilated you at table tennis.'

'Re-match then.'

'No, I'm done,' she replied. But as she began climbing the steps Matt grabbed her round the waist and pulled her back in and under the water. The moment an outraged Frankie surfaced, she pushed him down. This was textbook flirtation, Leila thought gleefully as she watched them mess around together.

'Best of three then,' Matt spluttered when he surfaced. 'And then I'm going to have to head off.'

'Oh?'

'Yeah, I'm meeting my friends in the north of the island and it's a two-hour drive.'

'Are you staying there then?'

Leila was convinced that Frankie actually sounded wistful, as if she was going to miss Matt.

'Yep, so if you don't beat me now, you'll have to wait three days to do it again. And I doubt that even you, with your iron determination, can improve in that short space of time.'

'You know I said that Matt was okay?' Frankie drew Leila into the conversation. 'Well I was lying.'

'Don't listen to her, she's just bitter and twisted about losing. Do you know she propositioned me on our run?'

Now this really was interesting.

'I did not!'

'She can deny it now, but she implied that she would be up for a threesome.'

He was clearly pulling Frankie's leg but the flirting tone was very much in evidence.

Frankie rolled her eyes. 'I'm *so* going to make your kitten prefer me while you're away.' She swam over to the side of the pool, 'Now get in position . . .' She caught Matt giving her a cheeky grin. 'I meant for the race!'

He was still laughing when Leila shouted 'Go!' and as a result Frankie won. But he pulled himself together for the final race and beat her.

'You know, usually I'm not that competitive, but there's something about you that brings it out in me,' he told Frankie as he hauled himself out of the pool. 'Keep practising and you may have a small chance of beating me again when I get back. Provided I give you a head start – say half a length.'

With true Frankie charm she gave him the finger.

Matt laughed. 'I knew it wouldn't be long before you were rude to me again.'

'I was provoked!' she exclaimed.

Leila was bursting to say something, but managed to contain herself until he was safely out of earshot. 'You two really *are* getting on better.'

Frankie shrugged and tried to act nonchalant. 'Like I said, he's okay.' And as if to prevent any further questions from Leila, she dived off the stone steps and swam the entire length of the pool underwater.

Humming the tune to 'It's a Thin Line Between Love and Hate', Leila wandered back inside where she found Tom lying on the sofa reading with the black kitten fast asleep on his lap. Gracie had named both kittens after her favourite characters in *Toy Story* – the black one was Jessie and the tortoiseshell was called Buzz. He glanced up. 'You look cheerful.'

She perched on the arm of the sofa. 'I think I might just have witnessed something extraordinary.' She lowered her voice so that her daughter, who had the hearing of a bat, wouldn't overhear and then repeat it to the world: 'Frankie and Matt were actually flirting.'

'That *is* extraordinary. Are you sure you haven't had too much sun? One too many beers? Your eyes need testing?'

Leila smiled and shook her head, feeling in a better mood than she had for ages, and told him about Frankie and Matt competing against each other and the way they had messed about in the water.

'By the way,' Tom said as she was about to get Gracie a drink, 'Candy has offered to babysit so you and I can out for dinner tonight. Just the two of us.'

Dinner for two. There were so many times in the past that Leila would have loved nothing more than that. Now the idea struck dread into her as she worried that she wouldn't have anything to say to him, that the fault lines in their marriage would be exposed.

'Oh, Tom, I'm sorry but I've promised the girls that we'll have a night out tonight. Can we make it tomorrow instead?'

He looked disappointed. 'Okay, whatever you say.' Then muttered, 'As usual.'

The happy mood vanished. 'That's not true – stop making me out to be such a bad person. I don't need any help from you on that score, if you must know.'

Tom didn't get chance to reply as Gracie butted in, wanting to know if they could take the kittens home. It was the question that Leila had been steeling herself for since the arrival of the strays, but now she welcomed it. *Anything* was better than bickering with her husband.

'I'm sorry, darling, they'll have to stay here, but we'll be able to see them whenever we come on holiday. And I'm sure Ellie will send us pictures of them.'

Naturally that wasn't the answer Gracie wanted and so there was a long drawn out discussion . . . well, discussion was probably the wrong word . . . as Gracie kept asking *why* on a loop, with her usual tenacity, until Leila changed tactic and said, 'How about we get a kitten when we get home? In fact, why don't we get two and they can be company for each other?'

That provoked a disbelieving look from Tom. He had been saying for ages that it would be good for Gracie to have a pet, subtext because she was an only child. But Leila had always resisted, thinking that it would be too much hassle – even though, in fairness, Tom would be the one looking after the animal.

'Can we really!' Gracie exclaimed. 'I want one exactly like Buzz.' She scooped up the little tortoiseshell and stroked him. 'But I promise I won't forget you, Buzz.'

'Are you sure about this?' Tom said quietly. 'There'll be no going back on it now. She won't forget.'

'Absolutely, so long as you clean out the litter tray.'

Leila said it half jokingly but Tom shot back with, 'I clean everything else so I wouldn't expect it to be otherwise.'

Leila wanted to say that she knew this and that she was sorry, that she would try and work less and help out more, but Patrick and the others returned at that moment laden down with shopping – in Patrick's case laden down with beer and wine – and she had to help them unpack. And then Gracie wanted to go in the pool so Leila had to coax her into her sunsuit, make sure she had sunscreen on her face and spent the next few hours either swimming with her daughter or watching her, so there was no time to make things up with Tom.

Chapter 20

Frankie

They had chosen a quiet bar overlooking a pretty little cove for their girls' night out. It was the perfect location to watch an impressive sunset turn the sky brilliant shades of orange and red, tinged with pink. Frankie wondered if Matt had met up with his friends by now and if they were out having dinner. She also found herself wondering if there was someone there who was more than a friend to him. And then stopped herself. No. She and Matt were friends, or rather nearly friends. Nothing more. And yet there had been that bantering between them today, that had felt more than friendly. She had enjoyed being with him, she hadn't bantered with anyone like that since – well, for a very long time.

She had also been slightly apprehensive about coming out with Candy, but she was definitely warming towards her and it wasn't just the effect of the two cocktails she'd had. Candy was easy to talk to, and friendly, and funny and it didn't feel like an effort to be with her at all. It helped that Patrick wasn't there, talking about *his* Candy, coming out with suggestive comments, putting his arm round her possessively.

'So did you always want to be a beautician?' Tor asked her.

Candy rolled her eyes, 'Yeah, it was always my lifelong ambition to give women Brazilians, and back, sac and crack waxes to men – or BSCs as we in the trade call them.'

'Eeow!' Tor and Leila exclaimed in unison while Frankie smiled. She found she appreciated Candy's dry sense of humour.

'It's so intimate! How can you do it?' Leila wrinkled her nose. 'Princess Leila' Frankie sometimes secretly called her, because she liked everything to be perfect.

'And I'd hate it if a man had everything whipped off down there! What woman cares if a man has hairy balls. It's not like the scrotum is a thing of unparalleled beauty!' Tor exclaimed. 'Keep it covered!'

'Actually teabagging is better with less hair,' Candy replied, shooting a cheeky grin at Frankie who shook her head, knowing that Leila wouldn't have clue what this particular sexual practice involved.

Sure enough she wanted to know, and when

Frankie explained, she exclaimed, 'I could cheerfully have lived all my life without knowing that and been perfectly happy! And Tom had better not get any ideas . . . I'm not going to go there.'

'You did ask. So do you have to do the BSCs, Candy?'

'I draw the line somewhere and I draw it there. I leave all that to Olga, who claims to enjoy it. She's got a sadistic streak and issues since she found out that her boyfriend, who had led her to believe that he was going to propose to her, was in fact a married man with a wife and two kids he had no intention of leaving. And as for Brazilians . . . I've done so many now that I'm on automatic pilot. I don't even think about it. I'm less keen on doing the Hollywoods – that's everything off,' she explained to Leila, who was looking blank again.

At this point Frankie could have said that she didn't think women should remove all their pubic hair; that the fashion – if you could call it that – had come directly from the porn industry. And that pubic hair was perfectly natural, not the devil's work, and men should bloody accept it! But she didn't. Having an argument over pubes, or lack of, seemed rather silly. And after all Candy was only doing her job, she could hardly refuse to give someone a Hollywood as a matter of principle . . . she would be fired.

Instead Frankie asked her what she would rather do. She'd fully expected her to come up with the immortal line, '*I'd like to be a model.*' She had heard it so many times from her students, along with the other line, '*Miss, I just want to be famous.*' Their lack of ambition and originality drove her mad and sometimes she felt as if she was waging a one-woman battle against reality TV shows that held out the promise of instant fame along with instant infamy. She would cheerfully have taken up picketing the *X Factor* auditions and telling all those wannabes to go and do something more worthwhile, like one of those fanatics with a sandwich board declaring that the end of the world was nigh, except she would end up on YouTube.

'Don't laugh, but I've always wanted to be a . . .'

She paused and Frankie was convinced that Candy's mouth was forming an 'm' – for model. Bloody bollockingly typical. Sometimes she hated being right.

'A midwife.'

Candy's answer was so entirely unexpected that for a second Frankie wondered if she'd heard correctly, then she burst out with, 'Brilliant! You should do it!'

'I couldn't do the training after my mum died as I needed to earn money right away and had to drop out of college. A friend of my mum's owned the beauty salon and offered me training on the job, so I took it.'

Frankie thought of the huge sacrifice Candy had made for her sisters. She herself had always done exactly what she wanted. She had never felt that opportunities were being closed off from her. She'd wanted to go to university and she did; she'd wanted to take a year off to travel and she did. She'd always had the support of her parents. She felt very lucky and rather spoilt by comparison to Candy. And humble. And ashamed of her earlier judgmental attitude.

Candy glanced at Frankie, a challenging look in her blue eyes. 'I bet you weren't expecting me to say that, were you?'

'No.' She decided that honesty was the best policy. She was pretty sure that Candy would see through any lies. 'You're right. I thought you'd say something like model.'

'You can't judge a book, et cetera,' Candy replied, but she didn't say it nastily. If only she hadn't been Patrick's girlfriend there was a real chance that they might have become friends.

'It's never too late to go to college,' Frankie replied.

'I'm hoping to go once my youngest sister has done her A-levels.'

'I bet you'll be a fantastic midwife,' Tor put in.

'Might have to ditch the false nails though,' Frankie teased. 'If I were in labour I wouldn't want those anywhere near me – especially down the business end.'

'Pity,' Candy replied, considering her perfect red nails. 'My real ones are shit.'

Leila ordered them all more cocktails except for Tor who was drinking Diet Coke, claiming that her stomach was still upset after the bug. 'I think it's the longest time I haven't had a drink in years,' she joked. 'My liver must have completely regenerated.'

'Well, I need this,' Leila declared, taking a large sip of her mojito.

'So what are the boys doing tonight?' Candy asked, 'Please tell me they're not going to let Patrick get drunk again. He snores really loudly when he's had a skinful and I can't wake him up.'

'And they say romance is dead,' Tor commented.

'Does he always drink this much?' Candy continued.

Frankie looked down at the table; she didn't want to be part of this conversation.

'I don't think so. I've suggested that Tom should have a word with him about it, but I'm not sure if he has. I think Tom feels it's yet another instance of me telling him what to do.' Leila suddenly sounded flat, as if all her natural spark had deserted her.

'I'm sure he doesn't think that,' Tor replied – ever the peace-maker.

'Don't you believe it. I'm already the Wicked Witch of Brighton, and now it seems of Zakynthos as well. And he's right, it's official. I've become a nag. It's what I'm best at. I hear the way I speak to him sometimes and it's awful, it's everything I never wanted to be.' She looked at Candy. 'Sorry,

234

I'll cheer up. This was supposed to be a fun night out, not me moaning.'

'Has something happened?' Frankie asked quietly.

Leila didn't meet her eye. 'No, nothing at all.' She paused. 'I suppose it's coming back to this island. It's where we came on our first holiday together, and I remember what it felt like to be so in love with him. Such a very long time ago.'

'You still are in love with him, aren't you?' Tor said anxiously. Frankie knew exactly how she felt. She and Tor had fallen in and out of love and had their share of heartbreak, but Tom and Leila had always been there – a constant in their lives, a reassuring reminder that relationships did work out, that you could find your soulmate and be happy. She knew that Tom and Leila had been through a bit of a rough patch, but she hadn't realised that it was serious.

'Of course, but it's different from when we first met. There's not that intensity any more. We bicker more often than not. Sometimes I think we take each other for granted. He doesn't know what I'm thinking and I've no idea what he's thinking. We spend more time watching box sets together than talking – thank God for box sets! The patron saints of marriage.' She was trying to sound light-hearted, but Frankie wasn't convinced.

'That's what happens to all couples, isn't it?' Candy put in. 'Children and life change a relationship. But

235

isn't that a good thing? Could you really go around with that crazy in love butterfly feeling all the time? It would be bloody knackering. You'd never get anything done.'

Frankie wondered if Candy was crazy in love with Patrick. On the balance of evidence, probably not.

'You're right,' Leila conceded. 'How did you get to be so sussed out at the age of twenty-two?'

Candy shrugged. 'I don't know. My mum always said that I had an old head on my shoulders.'

They sipped their drinks for a few minutes and looked towards the beach. The sun had disappeared now, the sky was still tinged with pink and the sea was silver and silky calm, tiny waves gently lapping at the shore.

'Hey, isn't that Dimitri over there?' Tor said, gesturing over at the bar. They all looked in the direction she was pointing to where a group of young men stood chatting and drinking beer straight from bottles.

'No, it's not him,' Candy said. 'He'll be working anyway, on the beach.'

'Oh, yes – do you think you might help out one night?' Leila asked. 'He really wanted you to go along, didn't he?'

Candy rolled her eyes. 'Yeah, and the week before I'm sure he wanted some other gullible English girl to go. But I have a boyfriend, remember.'

How could she forget? Frankie felt a stab of longing for what she couldn't have . . . This was exactly the kind of beach where she had imagined being one day with Patrick. But whereas before the holiday that fantasy ran very smoothly in her head, with Patrick declaring his love for her, now all she could see was the pair of them sitting there in silence. He would be drinking – of course. But she couldn't imagine what he would say, unless it was to order another bottle of wine. Could she really hear him saying that he loved her? That he had wasted so much time apart from her? That they belonged together? She didn't know if she could any more.

'I think you're in there!' Tor nudged Frankie as one of the lads in the group stared directly at her. A definite checking her out gaze.

He was pleasant enough looking with short brown hair and a cheeky grin, but far too young. 'Really not my type,' Frankie replied, sipping her cocktail, which just happened to be called Sex on the Beach. Well, not with him, that was for sure.

'So who is your type?' Candy asked. 'No, hang on, let me guess – it would have to be someone really intelligent and good-looking, but not in an obvious way. A quirky Indie boy, I reckon.'

For a second Frankie wondered what would happen if she replied that Candy knew exactly who her type was as she was going out with him . . . but she would never say that. She might have been tempted when she'd first met Candy, but not any more. She wouldn't want to hurt her.

So instead she went for an approximation of the

truth. 'I haven't had a boyfriend for ages, to be honest, I just haven't met anyone I was interested in.' She hoped Candy left it at that. Frankie really didn't want to answer any questions about this. She *never* liked to answer questions about this.

But Candy was on a mission. She was halfway through her third cocktail, pleasantly tipsy, and probably hadn't picked up the signs that Frankie was reluctant to open up. It was meant to be a girls' night out, a bit of fun, so why would she?

'No way! You need to get out there, lady!' Candy persisted. 'You're so attractive. You could do with a bit of fake tan – no offence – and you can be a bit scary – no offence – but I bet you have loads of men after you. And what about Matt? He's gorgeous and single.'

'And we have absolutely nothing in common. Oh, apart from table tennis and running.' Brutal honesty was the best approach to ending this conversation. 'I have sex with a man every now and then, I'm not living like a nun, it's just I never feel the need for it to go any further. I like my own space too much.'

She caught Tor and Leila giving her their concerned looks. 'What?' she challenged. 'There's nothing wrong with that. Men do it all the time. It's not a big deal. It's just sex.' She knew that her friends wished she was settled, that they worried about her. Maybe she should be worried about herself . . .

'Yes, but you don't want to be living like that when you're forty,' Tor put in. Forty was now Tor's big number by which time things i.e. life had to be sorted. It had been thirty, but Frankie realised that none of the friends had sorted anything out, except perhaps Leila.

'Thanks, Tor! I am only thirty-three; I've got some way to go. I know you're obsessed with age, but I'm not. It's only a number.'

Shit! She shouldn't have said that. Tor instantly looked hurt.

'So have you never had a long-term relationship?' Candy again. Frankie had to hand it to her for getting to the heart of the matter. Now Tor and Leila looked anxious. Even after six years the subject of Ross was still a painful one.

She took a deep breath. She had to get this over and done with, like ripping off a plaster. It was the only way. Procrastinating would make it worse. 'I did, in my twenties. I was actually engaged. I was going to get married – hard to believe, I know – in a country church, in a white dress, with three cute bridesmaids. He wanted to have the traditional wedding with me the cynical atheist. And yes, in answer to your question, he was really intelligent, and good-looking, but not in an obvious way.'

'So what happened?'

Candy must be imagining some dramatic tale of her jilting her fiancé at the altar and sprinting out of the church with her big white dress and veil flowing cinematically behind her, dropping her bouquet in her flight. Or maybe of him cheating on her with one of her friends, and of her walking in and discovering them in bed together. *If only.*

She shredded the garish paper umbrella that adorned her cocktail and scattered the purple paper on the table, like confetti. Funny what you remember – the vicar telling them when they met him to book the church that they couldn't have confetti, it was hellish to clear up. Actually he probably hadn't said hellish. Frankie was going to use pink and white rose petals instead. The vicar didn't have a problem with those.

'He died,' she explained. 'He was suffering from really bad headaches, I kept nagging him to go to the doctor, but you know what men are like. When he finally went and was referred for tests they discovered he had a brain tumour. It was inoperable but they tried radiotherapy. It didn't work. He died five months later. Two months before we were supposed to be getting married. I wanted us to get married anyway, ditch the white wedding and have a small ceremony in a register office. I wanted him to know how much I loved him; I wanted everyone to know how much I loved him. But he wouldn't. He didn't think it was fair on me.'

There was a pause during which she could hear the soothing sound of the waves breaking and swishing on to the shore. She imagined the water smoothing the sand, erasing out all imperfections, leaving a perfectly smooth surface behind. She wished she could lie there and let the water wash over her, take away the pain; erase the memories. *And this too will pass*, she said to herself, her mantra from the bad years. She forced herself to meet the anguished eyes of Candy.

'Frankie, I'm so, so sorry. I had no idea.' She sounded as upset as she looked. Poor girl, it wasn't her fault that she had ventured into the emotional landmine-strewn site of Frankie's life. Really she should carry a health warning. Get too close to me and you'll feel like shit.

Frankie took pity on her, and reached out to touch her hand as if Candy was the one who had lost her fiancé and needed comforting. 'It's okay, why would you know? It's not something I ever talk about. I've hardly mentioned it to Patrick. He didn't know Ross.'

'But it's tragic. He must have been so young.' Candy actually had tears in her eyes. Frankie had no more left to cry over Ross. Cry me a river? She already had.

'It is. He was. But you know what it's like to lose someone you love. You have to carry on because it's what they would have wanted.' Even though you didn't, you absolutely didn't, because the weight of your grief felt as if it was crushing the life out of you and all you wanted to do was lie down and give in to it. 'Anyway, let's talk about something else. *Please.* And I'm okay now. Really.' She shouldn't have added the 'really', it never convinced anyone.

But as she had suspected this had killed the light-hearted conversation stone dead, as dead as her sweet Ross. There could be no more jokes about one-night stands and waxing, of course there couldn't. She looked at the fragments of paper again. In the end there were no pink and white rose petals raining down over her and Ross as they made their joyous exit from the church, only the white roses that she along with his mother and sister had laid on his coffin. She didn't believe in life after death, but when Ross died she clung on to the idea that a part of him lived on, in his friends, in the people whose lives he had touched. There was some comfort in that. *And this too will pass.*

They finished their drinks and Tor drove them back to the villa. They were all quiet in the car. There was none of the earlier banter. Frankie knew that Tor and Leila would be thinking about Ross, who had been a close friend of theirs too, so his death was their loss as well, and his parents', and his sister's. She couldn't just hoard it to herself. And she suspected that her friends would be worrying about her. Again.

Back at the villa Candy's prediction had come true as a drunken Patrick lurched on to the terrace and demanded to know who they had flirted with. No one was in the mood for that. Frankie grabbed a bottle of mineral water and said a hasty 'Goodnight', anxious to avoid an '*Are you all right?*'

conversation with Tor and Leila. She was not up to that. Not by a long way. And she was not all right. Not by a long way.

Upstairs she willed herself not to think about Ross, but the images from the past were crowding into her head and they were persistent.

She had met him in their first week at Sussex University at the Student Union bar – though met was probably not the right word. He had collided with her and managed to pour his entire pint of Guinness over her fake-fur leopard print jacket.

'You wanker!' had been the very first words Frankie had uttered to him, outraged at the ruination of her favourite vintage coat. Ignoring his apology, she had stormed to the Ladies' to dry it off.

When she emerged with the coat bundled up under her arm, still damp and smelling of wet dog, Ross had been waiting for her.

'I'm really sorry about your coat. I'll pay for it to be dry cleaned. Or I could get you another one. Of course I won't be able to eat for a few weeks or have the heating on, so I'll probably get hypothermia and that will be my promising academic career over and . . .'

Suddenly Frankie had registered that while Ross was undoubtedly annoyingly clumsy and he had undoubtedly ruined her coat, he was also undoubtedly the best-looking boy she had

243

seen since arriving at uni. Auburn hair, gorgeous hazelnut eyes, razor-sharp cheekbones. He was tall, angular, artistic-looking as if he played in a band. Just the kind of look she liked. Actually just the kind of look she loved.

'It's okay, you can get me a drink,' she conceded. 'Vodka and tonic. A double. We'll call it quits.'

One drink became four and conversation lasted long into the early hours. They saw each other every night for a week, talking, flirting, teasing, until finally tumbling into Frankie's single bed in her hall of residence. She was studying English, he was studying Physics and Astronomy. Right from the start they both said that this wasn't going to be serious, and joked about how they had nothing in common, though that wasn't strictly true as he was almost as well read as she was and they were both into Britpop – Pulp, Blur, Suede performed the soundtrack to their romance – and they both loved films, going at least twice a week to the cinema. At the weekend while Frankie would lie in bed, or mooch round the vintage clothes shops, or spend hours over one cup of coffee with Tor and Leila at their favourite café, Ross would be out cycling across the Downs, or playing football, or surfing. But right from the start they both knew it was more than a fling. They were together for the next nine years. She loved him; he loved her. They planned to spend the rest of their lives together. And then he died. Actually she had lost him a month before his death, when the effect of the tumour pressing on his brain meant that he didn't know her or anyone else any more.

She opened the drawer to the bedside table and took out her sleeping tablets, reserved for very special occasions. Like now, for instance, when the pain was cutting through her like a shard of glass and she felt as if she couldn't breathe.

She found herself wishing that Matt was next door, that she could hear the familiar sounds of him getting ready for bed, the creak of the single bed as he turned over, the light being switched off. Just for someone to be there.

Chapter 21

Tor

Tor knocked softly on the door of Frankie's bedroom. Her friend hadn't left her room since last night and it was now midday. She was worried about her, knowing how much it would have shaken her up to talk about Ross. 'It's Tor, can I come in?'

A muffled, 'No, I'm fine,' didn't convince her. Choosing to ignore it, Tor quietly opened the door and walked in. The shutters were still closed and Frankie lay curled up on the bed. It broke Tor's heart to see her friend looking so desolate, just like she used to after Ross died.

She sat down on the edge of the bed. 'Can I get you anything? Some toast?' She didn't know why she mentioned that, Frankie never ate bread, not the evil carbs. 'A cup of tea?'

Frankie lifted her head off the pillow; she looked as if she hadn't slept at all, there were shadows under her eyes and creases from the pillow criss-crossed her cheeks.

'A cup of tea would be good, thanks.' She uncurled her hand and Tor saw that she was holding several turquoise beads. She had been holding them so tightly that they had left a red welt across her palm. Tor had been with Ross when he'd bought Frankie the bracelet for her birthday. She had insisted on going with him after he had let slip that he wasn't sure what to buy Frankie, and was considering some scented candles.

'And I'll tell you what she'll do with those candles if you get them and it won't be pretty,' Tor had told him. 'Candles are what you buy your mum or your gran.'

But in the end Ross had chosen the bracelet without any help from her, and Frankie had loved it. She had been going to wear it on her wedding day – her something blue.

'How about you have a shower and come downstairs? Everyone's gone out so we have the place to ourselves.' Tor was convinced that Frankie's staying up in her room was not healthy. She remembered how she and Leila would try and coax her out of her flat after Ross had died, encouraging her to come for a walk with them by the sea. At first she would only ever come when it was dull and overcast, ideally raining. It took two months before she'd agreed to go out when the sun was shining, and then she had sobbed all the way along the seafront, telling them

247

that she couldn't bear to feel the sunshine on her face, knowing that Ross couldn't . . .

'Ed as well?'

'Yes, he wanted to go windsurfing, and he's gone to some water sports centre with Tom and Leila.'

'Didn't you want to go?'

'Not really my thing, Frankie.' But while that was true, the real reason she hadn't gone was that she'd wanted to keep an eye on Frankie, and had also thought that she and Ed might benefit from some time out from each other. She'd hoped that she would have the chance to think further about what she wanted to do but she was no closer to getting any clarity.

Frankie managed a smile. 'No, Tor, I can't exactly see you windsurfing.'

'I might be unexpectedly good at it, you never know,' Tor bantered back. 'I might have a hidden talent for it and take it up when we get back to Brighton. I'll be out all weathers in my wetsuit. A windsurfing ninja.' The idea was insane, she would never in a million years wear a wetsuit. Did they even make maternity ones?

'I think we do know, Tor,' Frankie sighed. 'Okay, give me ten minutes and I'll come downstairs.'

Tor used the time to check out the pregnancy website. She had been desperate to do so for the last two days and this was the first chance she'd had. By the time she went back to Brighton the kidney bean would be 5.4 centimetres long and able to curl his fingers, and his reflexes would be more honed – if she prodded her tummy he would squirm, though she wouldn't be able to feel it yet. She lightly patted her stomach, and whispered, 'Did you feel that, kidney bean?'

Then she reached for her pen and started making a list of all the things she needed to do on her return. Lists usually made Tor feel more in control.

1. See doctor and midwife
2. Book scan. (Hang on, did she book it or do they? She had no idea. She was sure Leila would have told her what happened with Gracie, but it would have gone in one ear and out the other. She wished she had paid more attention now . . . but when you weren't pregnant yourself, it didn't seem so relevant. And when you had thought you couldn't have children, it hadn't seemed relevant at all.)
3. Work out what to do about the boutique and her hours. Part-time? Full-time but reduced hours?
4. Nanny or childminder? Nursery?
5. Tell Ed.

It was number 5 that was causing her most anxiety. She was still worried that he would feel trapped. She needed to have sorted herself out before she came out with the great revelation. She

249

needed to demonstrate that she had everything under control, and that while his help would be appreciated, it wasn't essential. But the list was an exercise in self-denial. She didn't feel as if she had anything under control.

She looked up. Frankie had managed to drag herself downstairs. She was ethereally pale, but at least she had showered and got dressed. Tor tried not to appear furtive as she closed her notebook.

'I'll get you that tea, you sit down.'

She was pleased to be doing something for Frankie, however small. Her friend was notoriously independent and resistant to asking for help. Tor wished she could rustle up a delicious wholesome snack, but knew that Frankie wouldn't eat it. In the end she made do with an offering of tea, and a Greek yoghurt with honey and banana.

'Thanks, Tor.' Frankie clasped her hands around the mug as if it was a chilly day rather than being close to thirty degrees.

'Where would we be without tea? It was the only thing I could drink after Ross died. I didn't drink coffee for about two years, it reminded me too much of him. He always loved that first cup of coffee in the morning. He claimed not to be able to function without it. He made such a performance of making his coffee in that silver espresso coffee pot that he bought when we went to Italy, was convinced that it tasted better that way than in a cafetière. Do you remember?'

Tor did remember. She remembered going round to Frankie and Ross's tiny flat for breakfast after a big night out, and the smell of freshly made coffee while he cooked them all a fry-up. They'd sat round the kitchen table, which always wobbled, gossiping and laughing. She remembered the sheer happiness that radiated from Frankie when she was with him. Tor hadn't seen her like that since – well, since before they found out about Ross's illness. She remembered how she would look at the two of them together and think that was the kind of relationship she wanted for herself.

She remembered how brave Ross had been when he told her and Leila about his diagnosis, far more concerned about them being upset than he had been about himself. He wouldn't let them cling on to false hope, but laid out the facts as if it was one of his physics lectures. There was no cure. He was going to die. He wanted them both to have fantastic lives and to look after Frankie.

'And then when he became ill he stopped wanting to drink it, he couldn't smell it. He couldn't smell anything. I couldn't bear to drink coffee after that,' Frankie was saying.

She looked at Tor. 'Do you think we'd still be together if he hadn't died?' Her dark brown eyes were pools of loss. Ross had always called her his 'brown-eyed girl', after the Van Morrison song.

How was Tor to answer this? As far as she knew Ross was the love of Frankie's life and she of his. Of

251

course they would still have been together. They were meant to be together. They would have got married and most likely would have had children. She desperately wanted to protect Frankie, to say something that wouldn't make her feel even worse, but lying was out of the question. Frankie would know instantly.

'I do,' she said quietly.

'I agree,' Frankie replied, and looked down. 'He drove me mad sometimes, though. Do you remember when he was training for the marathon and banned me from having any alcohol in the house? I felt like an old wino coming round to yours to get my fix. And how he always saw the good in everyone? He would never let me bitch about anyone! I used to have to save it all up for when I saw you and Leila and let it all out.' She sighed. 'I was a better person when I was with him. I've become such a horrible, cynical old bag. Ross wouldn't even like me if we met now.'

'That's not true.'

Frankie shook her head, not convinced. 'Let's not talk about it any more. I'll be okay soon, I promise. It just takes a while, you know, to process it all, to put it all back.'

She took a sip of her tea. 'So what about you? Have you decided what to do about Ed staying weekends with you?'

It was Tor's turn to shake her head.

'I'm in no position to give anyone any relationship

advice, but I have such a good feeling about Ed. You should go for it, Tor. Life is too short not to.'

If it was anyone else Tor would bat away the comment. But it was Frankie so she didn't. Frankie knew what she was talking about. Frankie knew what it was like to be planning what music you wanted at your wedding one moment, and the next to be planning what songs to play at the funeral of the man you loved. Tor still couldn't listen to Nina Simone singing 'My Baby Just Cares For Me', which was played at the funeral, without crying, and she imagined Frankie couldn't either. Frankie knew what she was talking about.

Chapter 22

Leila

For four whole days Leila hadn't switched on her phone. It had remained in her bedside drawer, out of sight, unfortunately not out of mind. She knew that Tom was pleased that for once she hadn't been glued to her phone, he obviously thought that she was finally showing that she could achieve some kind of work/life balance. How ironic was that?

But as she was getting ready for their dinner for two Leila remembered that she would have to take her phone with her as Tom's didn't work abroad, and what if Candy who was babysitting Gracie needed to get hold of them urgently? Reluctantly she opened the drawer and picked up the novel that had been covering it. The purple BlackBerry seemed to have taken on a malevolent quality. She imagined it like a spider, crouching there in the darkness, pulsating with messages that she didn't want to hear or read. *Oh, for God's sake!* she told herself, reaching for it and switching it on. *It was just a phone.* But she almost held her breath as she waited to get a signal. For a minute or so it looked as if she didn't have any messages. He'd realised it was over. Giving him the silent treatment had worked. But then the signal strengthened and the texts and emails started registering on the screen. Fuck! She had fifteen texts and twenty emails.

She checked the email folder first – nothing from Jasper – but then he always texted. All except two of the texts were from him. She read them with a sickening feeling in the pit of her stomach. The words swam before her eyes in a blur . . . *miss you, want you. Why haven't you been in touch? I can't live without you, Leila. I love you.* What! He loved her? The man was crazy – he hardly knew her. How could he say he loved her? What had she unleashed by getting involved with him? Leila felt frightened by the intensity of this obsession, because that's what it was. She would have to see him when she got home, tell him to leave her alone, make him understand that this had to end. She couldn't have this hanging over her life. What if he took it a step further and came round to the house? How would she explain that to Tom?

And she had to find a way of blocking his number, she couldn't bear to read any more of his messages, though she had absolutely no idea how and could hardly ask Tom who usually sorted out her phone.

He opened the bedroom door, startling her. 'Are we ever going to get going? At this rate we'll be in time for breakfast tomorrow morning.'

'Sorry, I've been faffing about, I couldn't decide what to wear but I'm ready now. Do I look okay?' Her voice sounded falsely bright and upbeat. Tom would surely pick up on it.

He didn't. 'You look lovely,' he said, taking in the white halterneck dress. 'Have you lost weight?'

'Um, a little, I think. I could do with losing more.' She didn't deserve compliments from her husband.

'No, don't lose any more, you're in great shape.' He ducked down and kissed her on the cheek.

'Thanks.' She reached out and tentatively touched his flat stomach. 'So are you. I meant to say before.'

And she noticed that he had shaved for the first time all holiday, giving him a clean, fresh look that she would take over stubble any day.

'Yep, well, I have been making an effort to exercise more and eat less crap. I was getting chubby. Too many cupcakes in the park after nursery with Gracie. And finishing up her tea. Polly, one of the mums says that she puts any leftovers straight in the bin and then squirts them with Dettox. I was seriously thinking of doing it myself.'

Polly? She vaguely remembered seeing a slender young woman with long blonde hair at the nursery. Leila had been dropping off Gracie in a mad rush to get to work, as usual. Polly had been sitting with her daughter India at one of the art tables, looking as if she had all the time in the world to make a necklace with pieces of dried pasta. When Gracie had been upset that Leila had to go, Polly had been the one to comfort her.

'That's a bit extreme, isn't it? Has she got some kind of eating disorder? She is very thin.' And young and very pretty, definitely one of Patrick's MILFs.

'I don't think so, it's just to stop any temptation.'

If only other temptations could be so easily Dettoxed away.

Discovering the texts from Jasper had been the worst possible start to her 'date' night with Tom. Leila was distracted and on edge on the drive to the taverna. She kept having to ask him to repeat what he'd said.

'You're very quiet, are you okay?'

She thought of the desperate messages on her phone, of the hotel room, of how much she wished it hadn't happened.

'Oh, sorry, I was miles away.'

'Hope you weren't thinking about work,' Tom said grimly. 'You give enough of your time to the company as it is, without it eating into your holiday.'

If only she had been thinking about work . . . how innocent and easy to explain that would be.

'No, I wasn't, I was thinking about Frankie.' What

was one little lie compared to the big betrayal? 'I'm worried about her. She had to tell Candy about Ross last night. It really upset her but she wouldn't talk about it.'

Actually this wasn't a lie. Leila had been concerned about her friend. Frankie had been subdued afterwards and had spent much of the day shut away in her room.

'It's a pity Matt went away when he did, I think she was finally warming to him.'

'He'll be back soon.'

'Yes, but then the moment might have passed. You know what she's like.'

The conversation about their friend lasted for the rest of the journey. With any luck, they could spend most of dinner discussing Tor, Ed, Patrick, and their daughter, and avoid any analysis of their marriage, which was being held together by sticky tape and thin air.

And initially that's exactly what happened, until halfway through his swordfish Tom pushed his plate to the side, leant across the table and said, 'We really need to talk, Leila.'

She forced herself to meet his eyes. This was exactly why she hadn't wanted to come out to dinner. She didn't want to talk, she was far too afraid of what might come out. When she didn't reply Tom continued speaking.

'We need to talk about us, about our marriage. It's not working, is it? We never spend any time together, and on the rare occasion that we do, we either bicker, or we talk about other people, or watch a fucking box set.'

Part of her was relieved that he obviously didn't know about Jasper, the other part terrified that he was talking like this. For the past year Leila had thought she was doing a good job of pretending that everything was okay; that all marriages went through difficult patches; that they could get through this. She had never actually managed to convince herself. And apparently she hadn't convinced Tom either.

A small group of musicians had wandered into the taverna and was doing the rounds, playing a selection of traditional Greek tunes, with great gusto. The lead singer had an enormous pot belly and was inexplicably wearing a gigantic black sombrero with gold tassels that bobbed crazily up and down. At any other time that would have made Leila smile. Now she thought the possible end of her marriage was being played out against the theme to *Zorba the Greek* and there was nothing funny about it.

'I love you, Leila, and I want our marriage to work. I know I can be difficult, and hard to live with, that I can be crap at letting you know how I feel, and I intend to change that, I promise. Do you want our marriage to work?'

For ages she had told herself that it was all Tom's fault. That he was dissatisfied with his role of house-husband. That he was closed off and impossible to communicate with. It was Tom's inability to express his emotion that had driven her to have the affair. Her get out of jail card free for being unfaithful had been that she felt so lonely in her marriage. But it wasn't the cold, remote Tom sitting in front of her now. This was the old Tom, the Tom she'd fallen in love with. This man was passionate, strong, and not afraid to show his feelings. She felt a sudden rush of love for him. 'Yes. Yes, of course I do.'

'Well, we both need to make changes. You have got to treat me as an equal, not as someone you start bossing around the moment you step through the front door. I know I don't always keep the house exactly how you want it, but you can't have everything.' He hesitated. 'And I need to know that you still want me, that you still find me desirable. I don't want sex to be an afterthought, something you do because you feel you have to, to keep me happy. That's not enough for me, and I don't think it should be for you either.'

He was so right, and oh, how Leila wished they could have had this conversation before. Way before that night one month ago when she didn't think about her marriage vows, about her family, when she only thought about herself. Her eyes blurred with tears as she replied, 'I want things to change as well, and I will make those changes. I know I've been selfish.' But even as she made this declaration she could feel the guilt burning away inside her.

She had always seen herself as a decent person; the one-night stand had destroyed that belief.

Tom reached out for her hand. 'We can do it, I know. I love you, Leila.'

She laced her fingers through his. 'I love you too.'

And then the small band of musicians reached their table and switched from the jaunty *Zorba the Greek* theme to something altogether more plaintive. Leila had no idea what they were singing about, but it sounded like a love song.

'Did you pay them to do this?' she whispered to Tom.

'No, if I had, I'd have asked them to play the first song we had at our wedding reception.'

Leila smiled at the memory of the two of them dancing to 'Can't Take My Eyes Off You'.

After dinner they walked by the harbour and stopped off at a bar for a brandy – a Metaxa twelve-star, the only brandy Leila had ever liked. They drank a toast to a new start, and kissed. It was as if they had found each other again. Everything was going to be all right.

'That was nice. More than nice,' Tom kissed the top of Leila's head. They had just made love for the first time in what seemed like ages. And for the first time in what seemed like ages, it had felt good; it had felt right. She hadn't gone to bed with him because she felt she had to, she had done it because

261

she wanted to; she wanted him. Now, as she lay with her head on his chest, she felt as if she was back to where she belonged. Everything was going to be all right . . . She would not think about the phone just a few feet away from her, she would not think about Jasper. Everything was going to be all right. It had to be.

Chapter 23

Frankie

It was eight o'clock and already the sky was a relentless cheerful blue that screamed, 'Get up and seize the day'. *Give me a break . . .* Frankie paused at her window. Grey would be more fitting to her mood. A washed out, miserable, dirty grey. Clouds. Some rain even. Proper rain that was, not a weedy drizzle that made you feel listless and lethargic, but a downpour that drenched you, made you feel as if you had experienced something outside of yourself. That was not going to happen here, it was too bloody idyllic for words. She sighed, sat down on the bed and tied the laces on her trainers, feeling as if she hardly had the energy to do that – never mind run four miles. That was the thing about grief. It took everything else away, all your spirit, zest for life, and left only the greyness and the pain.

Yesterday she had done nothing and seen no one except Tor. She had lain in bed, brooding over the past. She couldn't face any of the others, especially not Candy. She couldn't bear to see the sympathy in the girl's eyes. She had to put herself in quarantine. Solitary confinement for the misfit. But she couldn't allow herself to have another day like that. She'd had far too many days like that in the past. And she had promised herself no more.

She forced herself to begin her stretching routine, telling herself that she would feel better after the run. Those perky endorphins would do their job and a new and improved Frankie would return to the villa – okay, maybe that was pushing it. She would return to the villa and actually be able to talk to her friends. Her phone beeped with a message, an email, probably spam. She accessed her mailbox without any curiosity, but it got her attention as it was from matt.cartwright13@gmail. com. Surprisingly she felt something emerge from the greyness, something bright and vibrant.

Hey, Frankie, no one's being mean to me here – I'm not used to it. I almost miss it. Yes, I do have a masochistic streak – hangover from private school, you probably think, and maybe you're right. Prepare yourself as I have been playing table tennis! Hours of the stuff and, though I say so myself, my improvement is exponential. Just tell yourself that it's not the winning that counts, it's the taking part, as I wipe the floor with you. You'll be begging me for mercy

*(clearly a sadist also as I like that image . . .) and for tips
on how to improve.*
Matt

Even though she felt like hell she smiled. It was an
email to pull her out of herself, a reminder that
life went on. And there was that hint of flirtation
again. A hint that awakened something in her. She
quickly typed back:

*Hey, loser! There is no way you'll beat me. I was only
playing at a quarter of my capacity and I had my eyes
closed for some of the shots. Begging you for mercy, my
a***! Your kitten now loves me more than you and who
can blame him? I let him sleep on my bed. So it's game
over for you on all fronts.*

She paused for a second. To sign off with an x or
not? It was how she signed nearly all her messages
to her friends. But Matt didn't so nor did she.

She was almost out of the door when her phone
beeped again. She should get on with her run;
she had to be back in time for the boat trip Leila
had organised. Should do, but instead she was
irresistibly drawn to her phone.

*Loser yourself! Who beat you at swimming? Who nearly
beat you at TT? And Buzz will forget all about you
the minute I return, he's only humouring you. He's a
discerning kitten. Back in two days' time – an extra day*

as forgot it's my friend's birthday. It's a shame as am itching to beat you. Don't get big-headed but no one here is as good as you. It's also a bit of a drag as am surrounded by couples. I feel like a bit of a spare part. Do you know that feeling? Or have you copped off with someone? Am I going to be the only single on the island?
Matt

Frankie had no intention of copping off with anyone and suddenly she realised that she hadn't been obsessing over Patrick at all for, oh, at least the last three days. He had knocked on her door last night and asked her if she wanted a glass of wine – that would, of course, be his answer to everything. Still sad about your dead fiancé? Have a drink. Hasn't worked? You still feel bad? Have another one. And another. And so on. He had no idea. After Ross's death she had actually stopped drinking for over a year. She hadn't wanted to feel numb and out of it; she had wanted to hold on to the pain, the grief and the loss. It had been the one thing that still connected her to Ross. She couldn't imagine explaining that to Patrick, he wouldn't get it. And so instead of welcoming the chance to spend some time alone with him, as she certainly would have done at the beginning of the holiday and at any other time during the last three years, she had said no. He didn't attempt to persuade her but returned downstairs to his bottle of wine, probably very relieved to be let off the hook. She knew him well enough to realise that he didn't handle displays of emotion from other people very well.

I have not copped off with anyone, though a pretty young thing gave me the eye in a bar the other night and I was tempted, until I realised how young he was.

She hadn't been but the pretence was fun.

Even I draw the line at eighteen . . . But we're all going clubbing, so who knows? When you return I might be shacked up with a German called Jonas, who is a yoga teacher . . . and even though I am rubbish at yoga (hamstrings too tight from running) maybe I will be prepared to over look that because of his incredible flexibility and stamina. The positions that man can get into! Phew – he is one hot yogi! If only he would stop wearing sweatpants! Can't stand them! They are an aberration! Whatever my gay hairdresser says.

In the meantime we're going on a boat trip. Maybe there will be a Greek able seaman I can ogle before I meet the German yogi. I'm thinking a strong silent type who won't annoy me, mainly because he will rarely speak, hardly knows English and he'll be away at sea a lot. Let's call him Hector. He'll have exceptionally muscular forearms and shoulders and a tattoo of a swordfish on his back. In fact I'm thinking that I have could have both of them on the go at the same time. I live in hope.

She pressed send, did a couple more stretches, paced up and down. She really should get going but she couldn't resist seeing if he replied.

Another message from Matt pinged back.

Do you like younger men then? I wouldn't have thought you did. Not nearly enough of a challenge for you. You could have them for breakfast . . . Hmm, may have to revise my opinion of you. And Jonas won't last; you'll be rude to him, and he won't be able to take it. It will interfere with his chakras. And even though he wanted to bring you to the path of enlightenment, loosen your hamstrings, and he fancied you bad, he will be forced to dump you. Kindly, of course. He'll say it was more him than you. He'll say a little prayer for you every time he performs his sun salutation – in his sweatpants. And he will always wonder about the woman with the beautiful dark brown eyes and too-tight hamstrings . . . I can't see Hector working out either, he'll be passive aggressive, talk about needing his own space and smell of fish, however many times he showers. Even though he thought you were a great catch! ☺

Cheek! I predict that I'll dump him! Frankie quickly typed back.

Once I've had my wicked non-yogic way with him. Hector will smell of the ocean, thank you very much, and lend me his lovely chunky navy blue cable-knit sweater that will look adorable on me. I take your point on the passive

268

aggression though. Can't abide that. So I will dump him and keep the sweater.

PS: Ha-ha re catch pun, and am sure he will reason that there are plenty more fish in the sea.

PPS: Never use emoticons with me. It's instant detention for any students who put those in their work. What next? Love hearts over your 'i's??? Are you a man or a teenage girl???

She was smiling as she typed, enjoying the flirt, the tease, the something bright and vibrant, the not being drowned in grey.

'The sweater would suit you. Good to wear something other than black, Ms Harper, you really should branch out sartorially. Red would also be good on you. Bad news about the emoticons. Do you know, I can do one in the shape of a kitten? Do you want to see it? I am imagining the expression on your face. It's the classic Ms Harper stare. It has teenage boys running for the hills, scared out of their hormonal wits, and makes Medusa's look a bit limp. But I am not a teenage boy and I am not afraid.

*FYI my stare works on everyone – except my mum. And what the f***!!! A kitten!!! Keep that quiet amongst your corporate cheeses or they'll think you've gone soft and you'll never work in business again. You'll no longer be able to say things like 'ball-breaking contract' and 'Let's seal the deal with vintage Bolly', or 'Wake up and smell the coffee'. And now I feel nauseous for coming out with* *those wanky phrases. Oh, and not all my clothes are black.*

Is wanky a word, Ms Harper, English teacher? Your mum must be formidable if she can resist the stare . . . My nine-year-old niece taught me the kitten thing – come on, admit that it's cute. I'll share it with you on my return, you'll be doing it to sign off your emails before you know it :D
PS: I'm guessing you don't wear black underwear, maybe?

I refer you to my previous answer, what the f***!!! Never, ever, ever will I use an emoticon. And now I must go for my run – got to keep myself looking good for Jonas and Hector.
   Stop speculating about the colour of my knickers, you pervert!

But the phone was still in her hand when he sent another reply.

And enjoy your dancing at the club. I'm jealous, I love a good dance and you're a great dancer, I seem to remember. Have fun, and happy ogling. Jonas and Hector won't know what's hit them. Mx
PS: Pink. And I'm not a pervert.

All the fizz and sparkle, the teasing and the banter, went out of Frankie at the mention of dancing. In its place came a flashback of hitting the dance floor with Matt at the wedding. The dance of

270

shame, followed by the hotel room of shame; Matt walking out; the taste of brandy and bitterness in her mouth. The soul-searing feeling of rejection. She barely registered that he had complimented her and signed off with a kiss. The greyness was creeping back in along with something that wanted to lash out. Without pausing to think, she typed back:

Well, I imagine they'll be good for a dance and a meaningless fuck. But sometimes that's what you need.

She pressed send and instantly regretted it. She slung her phone on the bed and slammed the door. Why had she done that? Sabotaged whatever it was that they had going on between them? Sabotaged something that had made her feel better. She was an idiot.

Not even Katy Perry could cheer her up on her run, but Frankie pushed herself and completed the four miles. She could do that at least.

As soon as she returned the first thing she did was check her messages. Matt had replied:

This is hard to do by email, but sorry. Only meant to say that you're a good dancer, not trigger any bad memories. There is no subtext. We're okay, aren't we, Frankie? x

It was very good of him to reply. She knew that in a similar situation she wouldn't have. God, never mind Hector, perhaps she was the passive aggressive one . . . or maybe just aggressive.

Yep. We are. And I'm sorry too. I'll let you know how it goes with Jonas and Hector. x

And just as she thought that would be it, she received a response:

Good, look forward to hearing all about it. xx
PS: I challenge you not to wear black on your night out.

272

Chapter 24

Candy

It was only midday but already Patrick had downed three beers. Candy was not impressed. She had been looking forward to this afternoon as Leila had organised a boat trip around the island. Yesterday she had spent the entire day at the villa with Patrick while everyone else went out, and he had driven her mad by drinking non-stop. He had been so tedious to be around, bitching about people at work, whom she had never met, moaning about having to go to his dad's sixty-fifth birthday party when he got back to the UK, and about his stepbrother and sister. The only good thing had been that he was too pissed for sex. He had suggested it, late-afternoon, after a bottle of wine on top of all the beers, and when Candy said that she would meet him in the bedroom, she had left it a good half an hour before joining him, knowing he would fall asleep first. Sure enough, when she tiptoed into the bedroom to check he was out for the count.

Now looking at Patrick as he attempted to do up the buttons on his shirt and then gave up as it required too much coordination, she wondered if she had better suggest that they stay behind again.

'Are you sure you want to go?'

'Yeah, I love a boat trip, especially with you draped over one of the seats in that sexy little bikini.' He slipped his hand down the back of Candy's bikini bottoms.

She sighed and removed the hand; she was beginning to wonder why she'd ever found him attractive. Right now she thought that he was an epic fail – the drink, the smutty comments, the passing out . . . it just wasn't cool.

'But you've drunk all that beer. You've been drinking far too much.'

'And? I'm on holiday! I can drink beer for breakfast if I want. Stop fussing. It's boring and it doesn't suit you. I don't want a nag as a girlfriend.'

She thought back to being on the beach with Dimitri, to the way he had made her feel so special, so interesting . . . she wished she hadn't been so chippy with him. She'd probably blown it; he wouldn't want to talk to her again.

Outside Tor was already in the driver's seat so there was no question of Patrick driving, thankfully – as no doubt he would have claimed to be fine . . . right up until he crashed the car.

'How's Frankie?' she asked quietly while Patrick was talking to Ed. She had felt so guilty for making Frankie talk about Ross. Had wanted to go up to her room and tell her how sorry she was. But even after knowing her for such a brief time, Candy guessed that the other woman wouldn't welcome the intrusion. When someone like Frankie said that they wanted to be alone – they meant it.

'She's much better today. She's gone ahead with Leila and Tom.'

'I feel so bad. I never would have asked those questions if I'd known.'

'But you didn't and Frankie doesn't blame you at all. So forget it. Honestly.'

'You worry too much,' Patrick put in. 'Frankie sounded fine when I spoke to her last night. It was all a long time ago.'

'You wouldn't say that if you had known Ross,' Tor said, sounding upset. Ed put his hand on her shoulder. At least one man in the car had some empathy. Patrick seemed to have used his up, or maybe he didn't possess any in the first place. Most likely he was too awash with alcohol to realise how insensitive he was being.

'So are we going to take it in turns to skipper the boat?' he asked, oblivious to any upset he had caused. 'I'll take the first slot. It's been years since I drove a motorboat but you never forget that kind of thing. It's like riding a bike.'

'A very big powerful bike,' Ed muttered.

275

'Actually Dimitri is going to be skippering the boat,' Tor replied, smiling at Candy in the rear-view mirror. 'I don't think you would be insured, Patrick.'

Candy tried to keep her voice neutral as she replied, 'Is he? I thought he'd be working.'

'It's his day off.'

The motorboat was moored at a small fishing harbour. She spotted Dimitri as soon as she got out of the car and again felt that tell-tale flicker of anticipation. She reckoned she could even overlook the long hair . . .

'Shouldn't he be in uniform?' Patrick commented as they approached the boat.

'Yeah, I bet he'd look even better in a white sailor's uniform, tight white trousers, fitted jacket, nothing underneath,' Tor teased. 'Very Jean-Paul Gaultier perfume ad. Is that what you had in mind, Patrick? Maybe you should suggest it.'

Candy swallowed a grin. Patrick looked disgusted.

They were last to board the boat. The butterflies went into overdrive as Dimitri smiled warmly at Candy, and said, 'Hi, how are you?' He looked so young and handsome in a pair of cut-off jeans and a white t-shirt that showed off his tanned arms.

'I'm good, thanks,' she replied, aware of Patrick behind her who was no doubt giving Dimitri the evil eye – that was, if he was still able to focus . . .

Dimitri reached for her hand. His grip was firm

as he helped her on to the deck. He then offered his hand to Patrick, who shook his head dismissively and nearly lost his balance. Dimitri shrugged and looked at Candy as if to say, *What are you doing with him?*

What indeed.

She took a seat next to Gracie who was wildly excited about being on the boat and the possibility of spotting some turtles. Patrick sat behind, next to Frankie, and cracked open a beer. He asked if anyone else wanted one. No one did.

'What is this? An AA meeting?' he attempted to joke. He raised his bottle, 'Well, cheers anyway.'

The powerful roar of the engine made conversation difficult, and it was a relief not to hear any more of Patrick's comments. Candy gazed out to sea. Every now and then she sneaked a glance at Dimitri. Not only did he have an exceptionally handsome face, he also had a gorgeous body. She was just admiring his broad shoulders and lovely pert bum when he turned round. For a moment they stared at each other and Candy could only hope that he didn't realise she had been blatantly checking him out . . .

'Do you want to have a go at steering the boat, Gracie?' Dimitri called out.

'Are you sure that'll be okay?' Candy put in, looking over at Leila and Tom, but they both nodded and Leila said, 'It's fine, Dimitri knows what he's doing.'

277

As she was sitting next to Gracie it made sense for Candy to take her to the bow of the boat.

'Just keep your hands like this.' Dimitri gently placed Gracie's hands on the wheel. Gracie looked solemnly in front of her as if taking her responsibilities very seriously. Candy was standing so close to Dimitri that for the first time she noticed that his brown eyes were flecked with gold and that he had a small scar just below his right eyebrow. He smelt fresh and clean with hint of citrus aftershave. She thought of Patrick breathing his beer fumes all over her, sweating out the alcohol at night.

'Very good, Gracie, you make an excellent sailor,' Dimitri told her after Tom had snapped away with his camera for a few minutes. 'Will you let Candy have a go now that you've shown her how it's done?

'No crazy turns, now Candy,' he teased as she took over the wheel.

Candy laughed. She suddenly felt an immense sense of freedom and exhilaration as the boat sped through the glittering blue expanse stretching out in front of them. She felt herself shedding those persistent worries about her sisters, the routines that pinned her down, the fact that she wasn't doing what she wanted to. She imagined cutting through all those negative thoughts as easily and cleanly as the boat through the waves, and leaving them far behind.

'Turn the wheel slightly to the right,' Dimitri told her, and it was a thrill to feel the vessel respond.

Ahead of them she spotted a motorboat speeding towards them and it seemed to her that they were on a direct collision course. 'I can't do it!' she panicked. 'We're going to hit that other boat.'

But Dimitri simply leant over and slightly adjusted the wheel. 'Of course you can do it. I'm here.'

For a few minutes they stood side by side. Candy wished that they could stay like this for the rest of the afternoon, wished that there were just the two of them on the boat. Usually she felt completely in control around men, flirting had always been a bit of a game to her, a game that she was in charge of. She didn't feel like that with Dimitri. It was exciting. If only there wasn't Patrick . . .

'I hope I didn't offend you the other day on the beach,' Dimitri said quietly. 'I think I may have sounded arrogant. I didn't mean to.'

'No, it was me. It must have seemed like I had a massive chip on my shoulder.'

Dimitri frowned; his English was good, but not that good.

'I meant, I was defensive.'

'So no hard feelings?'

'None at all.' Oh, God, absolutely none at all.

He smiled at her and she couldn't take her eyes off him. So much for playing it cool.

'And you will come to the club with me?'

'Yes – but everyone else has to as well. I won't be able to come otherwise.'

Dimitri frowned. 'That wasn't exactly what I had in mind.'

'That's the way it has to be.'

'You will dance with me though?'

'Yeah, I don't think Patrick's into that.' He would most likely be propping up the bar. Candy didn't say that, it would sound too disloyal.

Dimitri reached out and put his hand over hers. 'So it's a deal then?'

'Deal.'

Candy would happily have stayed like that, but Ed suddenly called out that Tor felt sick and could they please slow down?

Instantly Dimitri took over at the wheel. Candy returned to her seat. Tor was leaning over the side of the boat; she looked wretched. Ed was rubbing her back. He was so considerate. Candy tried and failed to imagine Patrick doing that for her. He wimped out at the sight of blood so he was bound to be completely useless around anyone feeling ill. He would probably have to lie down himself to recover.

'Sorry,' Tor mumbled, 'I thought I'd grown out of being seasick.'

Candy recalled the last four mornings when she'd heard Tor sprint to the bathroom, and throw up. It wasn't seasickness she was suffering from.

Chapter 25

Tor

Boats and morning sickness definitely did not make for a good combination, Tor reflected bitterly, as she gripped the side of the boat and leant over, willing herself not to throw up. The trip – to explore the famous blue caves of the island, then have a picnic on a deserted beach – had sounded like the perfect excursion. Yep, perfect if you weren't suffering from morning sickness. Pure bloody torture if you were.

'Okay now?' Ed asked her as she sat back on her seat.

'I'll be fine,' she replied.

She was feeling too rough to talk and instead watched her friends, hoping that she didn't look as ill as she felt. Patrick was lounging at the back of the boat, clasping the inevitable bottle of beer. They had all noticed how much he had been drinking, discussed it, and worried about what they could do. Tom finally had a word with him the other day, in the brief window of time that he was actually sober. Apparently Patrick laughed off his concern, told him he was on holiday and relaxing, that he had everything under control and that he'd cut back as soon as he went back to work. Tor was not so sure. Patrick had always been a big drinker, but there was something different about the way he had been drinking lately, as if he was seeking oblivion, trying to hide from something. He'd always been funny and charming after a few drinks in the past, the life and soul of any party, but there had been little evidence of that here. Instead he had displayed a hard mean streak, as if he wanted to wound with his words.

Frankie was sitting next to him, as usual fully covered up from the fierce sun in a large white sun hat, a long-sleeved shirt and sunglasses. She had been laughing and joking with Patrick and appeared not to have a care in the world. She had even been saying how much she was looking forward to going clubbing. But you could never tell with Frankie. She was the past master of putting on a brave face, and Tor knew how much it would have hurt her to talk about Ross.

Leila and Tom seemed much happier together. For the first time in ages Tor noticed that they were being affectionate to each other in public. Tom had his arm round her now and she was smiling at something he'd said. At least there was someone Tor didn't have to worry about.

And then there was Candy. Leila had told her about Candy bringing up her two sisters on her own, with no help and very little money, and Tor had felt inspired by her story. If Candy could do it, then surely she could . . .

But she still didn't feel able to tell Ed. Nor did she have an answer for him about the weekends. They hadn't argued. Instead they had been polite, tiptoeing round each other, which somehow made it worse.

She looked towards the bow where Candy had returned to Dimitri's side and was taking turns with him to steer the motorboat, though Tor was certain that Dimitri was always in control. Patrick would be furious with her for saying this but Candy and Dimitri looked good together, and it was obvious that they were drawn to each other. She had seen the glances they exchanged when they thought no one else was looking. That Candy would be attracted to Dimitri was a no-brainer. Not only was he handsome, he was also interested in her, kind and considerate. Patrick hardly seemed to notice that she was there, unless it was to make a suggestive comment or gesture.

Dimitri took over the wheel as they approached the dramatic Blue Caves, carved out of the cliffs by the sea. He steered the boat into one of them where it was blissfully cool in the shade, like being in a cathedral with the rocks shaped into natural arches. Tor thought about the caves existing for thousands of years in the past and for centuries to come and had one of her flashes of optimism and hope. What was a baby in that space of time?

She tuned back into Dimitri who was giving them some background. 'These caves are one of Zakynthos's best-loved tourist spots. They were discovered in 1897 and the most striking thing about them is the way their white walls reflect the colour of the sea – you can see an incredible range of blues.'

'I didn't know Stavros was a tour guide as well as a waiter,' Patrick commented snidely to Frankie. 'Is there no end to his talents?'

'For God's sake, Patrick, he's not called Stavros. And he's a student!' Frankie hissed back. Even she seemed to be losing patience with him, Tor noticed, and Frankie wouldn't usually say a word against Patrick.

'Whatever. So long as he keeps his hands off my Candy,' he replied.

'She's not yours, Patrick. You don't own her.' Tor couldn't bear the way he treated Candy as if she were his personal plaything. She had never seen him like this before. It must be the alcohol.

'I know, Tor,' he said, suddenly sounding weary, 'I was just making a joke.'

'It wasn't funny.'

'No, I agree. Bad boy Patrick. Must try harder.

Must not upset Frankie and Tor.' His voice was thick with sarcasm.

Frankie shook her head as if despairing of him. Patrick plucked a cherry from paper bag, ate it, then spat the stone over the side of the boat as if he couldn't care less. What was wrong with him?

Fortunately neither Dimitri nor Candy had heard this exchange and they motored on to a deserted cove, a gem of a beach with what looked like pure white sand. It was surrounded by sheer cliffs and was only accessible by sea. The plan was for the strong swimmers to swim ashore and for the others to get there by dinghy, and then they'd all picnic on the beach. Frankly at this point, however unspoilt the location, all Tor wanted to do was go back to villa and crawl into bed.

'Are you going to swim?' Ed asked her. He had barely said a word on the trip, which wasn't like him at all. He had been glued to his iPhone – no doubt texting his friends back in Brighton to let them know what a cow his girlfriend was. A big fat cow.

'I'm not. But you swim if you want.'

'Do you really care what I do?' he said quietly.

Oh, no, not now. She glanced round the boat, hoping that they hadn't been overheard.

'Of course I do, Ed.' She lowered her voice. 'I said I would think about you moving in, please can we leave it at that for now?'

'Yeah, right.' He stood up and pulled off his t-shirt.

She turned away, trying not to let on how upset she was. Frankie was already in her bikini and slathered in factor-50. She had an amazing body, with the flattest stomach, but she could also do with putting on a bit of weight. Patrick stripped off his shirt. She wondered if she should say something about whether swimming after so much beer was a good idea, but knowing Patrick he wouldn't take a blind bit of notice and would just tell her to stop fussing.

'Come on, Candy Girl, let's beat these suckers to the beach!' Patrick declared. He seemed to want to come across as extra-macho when he was around Dimitri. Tor was only surprised that he didn't beat his chest and come out with the Tarzan cry. She found it rather pathetic and was pretty sure that Candy wasn't impressed.

'I'm going in the dinghy,' she replied, carefully walking over to him as the boat gently bobbed up and down. 'I'll meet you there.'

'Don't be so boring! I bet you're only worrying about your hair. It'll be fine. Honestly, the hours this girl spends straightening her hair you wouldn't believe. It's the first thing she does when she wakes up every morning.' He sounded so patronising. He never used to speak to Willow like this. He wouldn't have dared.

'I'm not bothered about it actually, Patrick,' Candy shot back. 'And you wouldn't know what I do in the morning. You're always asleep.'

Tor rolled her eyes at Leila. When she glanced back Patrick was doing his he-man act and had picked Candy up.

'Come on, baby! You're on holiday. You need to live a little.'

'No, Patrick, please don't!' Candy exclaimed, as he swung her round.

Tor would be livid if he did that to her. He was behaving like a dickhead teenager. The boat listed violently from side to side.

'What's that Buzz Lightyear geezer always saying, Gracie? "To infinity and beyond!" And forget about your hair!'

'Put me down!' Candy shouted, sounding genuinely scared. But with a grunt of effort Patrick flung her over the side of the boat.

Candy screamed and there was an almighty splash as she hit the water. She briefly surfaced, arms flailing, but seemed to be struggling to stay afloat. What was she doing! Why wasn't she swimming? She lost the battle to keep her head above water and went under. She looked as if she was drowning. Oh my God! Tor realised in absolute horror. She *was* drowning!

'Patrick!' Leila yelled. 'Candy can't swim!' Gracie burst into tears.

'What!' Patrick looked stunned, but before he could act Dimitri grabbed the life belt, sprinted the length of the boat and dived into the water, closely followed by Ed.

There was a terrifying wait, which probably only lasted a minute, as the two men struggled to bring Candy to the surface. Dimitri towed her to the side of the boat where Tom and Patrick reached down and pulled her up. They laid her on the deck where she spluttered and retched. Tor and Frankie knelt down next to her and wrapped her up in a beach towel. The poor girl was shivering uncontrollably and coughing.

Patrick looked ashen-faced. 'I had no idea that you couldn't swim, Candy. Why the fuck didn't you tell me?'

Even now he was trying to pass the buck as if it was her fault that he had nearly drowned her.

'For God's sake, Patrick! Leave it now,' Frankie bit back at him. 'She's had a massive shock.'

'All right, all right, I'm sorry, okay? I fucked up, and I'm sorry. But I never would have done if I'd known, what do you take me for?'

He went to comfort Candy but she turned away from him and muttered, 'Go away.'

Patrick slumped down on one of the seats and reached for his cigarettes and lighter. His hand was shaking so much that it took several attempts before he was successful in lighting one. No one offered to help him.

By now Dimitri was out of the water and by Candy's side. He reached for her hand and held it tightly. 'You're okay now, Candy, I promise.'

'Thank you,' she murmured, gazing at him. 'You

saved me.'

It was game over for Patrick, Tor thought.

No one felt like a picnic after that. They cut the boat trip short.

'So would you rescue me?' Tor asked when she and Ed were alone in the bedroom. She intended it to be a light-hearted comment; she desperately wanted them to get back to where they had been. She missed that and she missed him. She wanted him to put his arms around her now and rescue her; she felt as if she was drowning on dry land.

Ed paused in fastening the buttons on his shirt – he was about to go out for dinner with Tom, Frankie and Patrick. Everyone thought it best if Patrick spent some time away from Candy.

'I'm sure you'd never put yourself in a position where you'd need to be rescued. You'd make some comment about how I was too young and you could do it yourself. Or that you would let me know in a few months' time – you know, when I've passed whatever test it is you've set for me.'

'That's not fair, Ed.'

'Isn't it? I don't know where I stand with you, Tor. I thought that you inviting me on holiday was a step forward in our relationship. But I'm not at all sure it is. Maybe Patrick was right when he said I was here to provide the eye candy. You really don't take our relationship seriously, do you?'

Tor couldn't believe how angry and hurt he

sounded.

'Of course I do, Ed!' And she wanted to tell him that being with him had made her happier than she had ever been. That she felt she could be herself with him . . . but something stopped her, and it wasn't just the baby, it was her. The legacy of her dysfunctional relationship with Harry was that she now doubted herself, afraid of giving too much away, afraid of admitting how deep her feelings were for him, in case she got hurt all over again. And this time it would really hurt.

'I want to believe you,' Ed told her, 'but I just don't know. I heard from Anise today. She's back in Brighton and says that I can rent a room in her house, no problem. So I won't get in your way. Maybe we can see each other every other Saturday – if you're not too busy.' Hurt had turned to sarcasm.

The ex-girlfriend? 'I thought she had moved back to Berlin.' Tor suddenly felt nervous and very, very insecure. Her legs turned to jelly and she had to sit down on the bed. She had never been good at confrontation, at arguing her corner.

'Yep, she did, but she missed Brighton too much. I can move in the weekend we get back. So you don't have to worry about anything any more. Everything can carry on as usual. Minimal disruption to your life, Tor.'

Missed Brighton or missed Ed? 'But I thought you said that she was a neat freak? Won't that drive you mad?'

'At least she wants me there, which is more apparently than you do.'

Ed would be living with his ex? The beautiful, non-pregnant Anise? The thought was like a grenade exploding over and over in Tor's head. Ed was already walking out of the door. 'See you later,' he called out. He left without giving her a kiss.

Tor picked up the t-shirt he had just taken off and pressed it against her face, breathing in his aftershave and unique Ed scent. She had to do something or she was going to lose him.

Chapter 26

Leila

Candy was still shaken when they got her back to the villa, but as she'd just had a near-death experience it was entirely understandable. Poor girl, Leila thought. This was definitely not the holiday she had signed up for. She knocked on the bedroom door and Candy called out a tentative, 'Come in,' adding a less tentative, 'so long as you're not Patrick.'

Leila found her curled up on the bed. In spite of the heat Candy was wrapped up in a white fluffy bathrobe Leila had lent her and she was still shivering.

'I've brought you a brandy,' Leila told her. 'For the shock.'

'Thanks, but I hate brandy.'

'Try it, I'm sure it will help.' She handed her the glass and Candy reluctantly took a sip. She coughed and pulled a face, but took another sip.

'And we've made some food – it's just pasta and salad.'

'I'm really not hungry.'

'I think it would be good if you had something – you didn't have any lunch.' Leila couldn't help feeling responsible for Candy. 'And I'm really sorry about what happened. Patrick was a complete idiot.'

'A complete wanker!' Candy said with feeling. 'I'm sorry, I know he's your friend, but I'm really pissed off with him.'

'You don't have to apologise. He was a complete wanker; he's been a complete wanker all holiday, I don't know what the matter is with him. He is very sorry about what he did, though.'

'Yeah, I bet he's showing how sorry he is by sinking another drink.'

Of that Leila was certain.

'Anyway, we're on the terrace, so please come and have something to eat and then maybe we can watch a film. It's just me, Tor and Gracie.'

'No Frankie?'

'She's gone out with all the men. I think she's hoping to have a talk to Patrick, to try and find out what's going on with him. There's a chance he might open up to her.'

'He's an alcoholic, that's what's going on with him.'

Leila frowned, slightly taken aback by Candy's certainty. 'Do you think? I know he drinks a lot but

I've never thought of him that way. He's got a good job, seems to be able to hold it together.'

'He's a functioning alcoholic, that's the term they use. Just because he's not downing cans of Special Brew at seven in the morning, and passing out in the street, it doesn't mean he's okay. He's got a serious problem, Leila. I didn't realise it before we came away, probably because I hadn't spent that much time with him. But now I think about it, every time I saw him he was drinking.'

'That's so awful, he's messing up his life. What can we do?'

A shrug from Candy. '*You* can't do anything. It's what *he* needs to do. Sorry, I probably sound harsh, but my uncle is an alkie and I've seen what it does to families. There is no one more selfish than an addict. And he's never going to stop until he wants to, no matter what anyone else says to him.'

'I see,' Leila said quietly, feeling lost. She wished Tom were here so she could talk to him about it, and get his perspective. She realised that she hadn't had that thought in a very long while.

She went out to the terrace where Tor was sitting with Gracie, who was absorbed in drawing a picture of a cat. Well, Leila guessed it was a cat, though without the extravagantly long whiskers it would be hard to tell what the purple squiggles were. Thankfully her daughter seemed to have recovered from seeing Candy nearly drown, but

Leila was steeling herself for the nightmares that were bound to happen.

'How is she?' Tor asked.

'As well as can be expected. Shocked and very, very angry with Patrick. I doubt she'll ever forgive him. I wouldn't in her place.' She lowered her voice. 'She thinks he's an alcoholic. What do you reckon?'

She'd expected Tor to look surprised, but instead heard the calm reply, 'I've been wondering that myself.'

'God, really?' Leila had been so preoccupied with her own problems, she felt as if she'd been oblivious to everyone else's.

'His drinking seemed to get much worse after he split up with Willow. I've barely seen him sober since then. I reckon she was the love of his life, not that he would admit it. He's still in love with her, I'm sure.'

'Are you talking about Patrick?' Candy had walked on to the terrace without either Leila or Tor realising. She had tied her hair back into a ponytail and put on a pair of shorts and a t-shirt.

Shit! Could things get any worse?

'It's okay,' Candy went on, sitting down, 'I wondered if he might be on the rebound from someone.' She looked at Leila and Tor, and smiled. 'You don't have to look so worried. I'm a big girl, I can take care of myself. And I can't exactly say that Patrick is the love of my life.'

That was just as well, Leila reflected. It would be a nightmare having him as the love of your life. So unpredictable and flaky. And selfish. She thought of Tom and felt a sense of calm. She had him back at the centre of her life now. It felt right. She felt restored. She was never going to take him for granted, dismiss him, undervalue him, again. Or she would try her very best not to. They could have a good marriage, a strong marriage. She could be who she wanted to be with Tom. She suddenly remembered that she hadn't checked her phone or blocked Jasper's number. If there was anything from him, she would delete it without reading it.

Candy sighed, 'What a mess. I'm sorry to be so negative about Patrick. I really had no idea he hadn't asked you about bringing me. And I know you probably don't want me here.' She paused. 'Believe me, if I could afford to pay for my flight home, I would go right now.'

'Don't be silly! I admit it was a surprise when you arrived, but it's been lovely having you here. I really mean that,' Leila was quick to reply.

'And Frankie likes you, and you know what a tough act she is,' Tor added.

'I know someone who really, really likes you,' Gracie piped up.

Damn! Leila hadn't realised that her daughter was listening.

'Dimitri!' she said triumphantly. 'He helped you

when you cut your foot, and he dived into the sea. In his clothes and his shoes.'

'I think Gracie has a point,' Tor said, smiling. 'It was pretty spectacular. I swear, I have never seen anyone move so fast in my life. It was like witnessing a hero in action. Daniel Craig, eat your heart out.'

Candy was blushing. 'He just felt responsible because he was in charge of the boat.'

No one was buying her attempt to underplay the rescue.

'It was more than that,' Leila said knowingly.

She was only teasing but Candy looked awkward and sounded serious as she replied, 'I've got a boyfriend, remember? Or I did have until this afternoon. I know you think I dress like a slapper, but I'm not one. And anyway, even if I was single, Dimitri is so far out of my league. He could have anyone. He's at uni studying to be a psychologist – he wants to be a child psychologist. His father is a leading psychologist in Athens. Mine is an AWOL loser.'

Leila was mortified. Instead of cheering her up, they had made Candy feel more insecure. 'I don't think he is out of your league in any way. But we won't go on about it. Now will you please have something to eat?'

She was relieved when Candy agreed to have a small bowl of pasta.

'And then will you watch *Toy Story?*' Gracie put

in. It was very cunning of her daughter to target someone when they were at a low ebb.

Leila was all set to say no when Candy replied, 'You're on, Gracie.'

'Really?'

'Definitely. That's all I'm up to at the moment.'

After supper Candy offered to clear up, but Leila wouldn't hear of it. When she took them each a bowl of chocolate ice cream, her daughter and Candy were spread out on the sofa with the kittens.

She poured herself another glass of wine and went back outside. She loved her daughter more than life itself, but if she had to hear another line from *Toy Story* – much as she loved that too – she would be forced to break the DVD to preserve her sanity.

'Actually, Leila, I'm going to go to bed,' Tor told her. 'Sorry to be so boring. I'm still feeling wiped out after that bug, and the seasickness today didn't help.'

'D'you want me to bring you anything?'

'No, I'll be fine.' She hesitated. 'It's good to see you and Tom getting on better, you seem much more relaxed around each other.'

'Yes, we finally talked when we went out for dinner and said all the things that had been bothering us. It cleared the air. I feel we can move on.'

'I'm so glad, I've been worried about you. And, selfishly, I couldn't bear it if you split – you've always been my ideal couple. It would be like my mum and dad splitting up again.'

Leila smiled ruefully. 'I'm going to cut down my hours when we go back, so that he has more opportunity to work. I just wish . . .' She paused, realising with a jolt that she was about to tell Tor about Jasper, and she absolutely didn't want to burden anyone with that poisonous information.

Tor looked at her. 'You wish what?'

Leila shook her head. 'Nothing. Just that you don't realise what you've got sometimes until you nearly lose it. I know that sounds like such a cliché, but it's true.'

Leila remained on the terrace sipping her wine after Tor had gone to bed, enjoying the peace and the sunset. The whole thing with Jasper felt like a bad dream. But its intensity was fading. She was going to put it all behind her.

She wondered how Tom was getting on with Patrick. She was looking forward to seeing him and talking about what had happened. She had felt locked up in herself for so long that she almost wanted to shout, laugh, sing in relief, now that it was over. She loved him, she always had. This holiday would wipe the slate clean for them. They could start again. She felt a dizzying rush of happiness as she realised what this meant. When he got back, she would tell him that they should try for another baby.

The door buzzer startled her from her reverie.

She hoped it was the others back from the taverna. She couldn't wait to tell Tom. Instead it was the hero of the hour on his moped – though really he should be on a white charger. She buzzed in Dimitri and told Candy that she had a visitor. The effect on her was immediate. She dashed into her bedroom to check her appearance. So much for saying that she wasn't interested . . .

'You're a hero!' Leila exclaimed, greeting Dimitri on the terrace.

'Not at all – I did what anyone would have done.' He kissed her politely on the cheek but she was aware of him looking around. No prizes for guessing who he was looking for.

'She'll be out in a minute, can I get you a beer?'

'Thank you.'

Candy stepped outside. She'd put on a bit of mascara and lip gloss but still looked pretty and fresh-faced. Immediately Dimitri stood up.

Nice manners, Leila thought approvingly. She felt protective of Candy after what had happened, and the more she had got to know her, the more she liked the girl. She deserved someone who would treat her well . . . someone like Dimitri. Leila didn't feel disloyal thinking this about Patrick's girlfriend. He definitely didn't deserve Candy.

'I had to see that you were all right after your ordeal,' Dimitri was saying.

'I am, thanks to you,' she replied shyly, sitting down.

'It was nothing,' he said, sitting down next to her. 'It was like a reflex when I saw what happened. I spent last summer as a lifeguard, so I remembered my training.' He smiled. 'You are much prettier than the last guy I saved – a drunk Englishman who fell off his pedalo and then realised he couldn't swim. Fortunately I did not have to give him the kiss of life.'

Leila was feeling very much like a gooseberry. She nipped inside for the beers and hoped that she could leave them to it. But when she returned with the drinks Candy insisted that she join them.

'I should really give Gracie her bath . . .'

'There's still another hour left of *Toy Story*,' Candy replied. Then mouthed '*Please stay*' when Dimitri wasn't looking. Okay, so Leila was their chaperone. She was the nurse to their Romeo and Juliet. She just hoped that Candy and Dimitri's story had a happier ending.

'Where's Patrick?' Dimitri asked. 'I thought he'd be here looking after you.'

'Leila sent him off to the taverna, he's not exactly my favourite person.'

'Mine either,' Dimitri replied. 'Sorry,' he added, not sounding sorry at all. He smiled at Candy. 'Does this mean you're going to dump him?'

Wow! Full marks to Dimitri for being direct.

'He didn't know I couldn't swim, so I guess it wasn't his fault.'

301

The smile instantly went from Dimitri's face. 'Please don't defend him. There is no excuse for what happened.'

Candy looked upset and Leila quickly intervened. 'Maybe it's best if we don't talk about Patrick or the accident.'

'Yes, of course, I'm sorry.'

So they talked about other things. Conversation was easy with Dimitri, he was interested in everything Candy and Leila had to say. He told them about his family – his two younger brothers, his mother who was a children's author, his grandmother who was an actress and lived with his family. It sounded such a wonderful vibrant home. The kind of home Leila wanted to create for her own daughter.

'You're so lucky,' Candy said with feeling. 'I've only got my aunt and my two sisters. It must be amazing to be part of such a big family.'

They both gazed at each other and Leila got the gooseberry feeling all over again. Fortunately at that moment Gracie wandered out. 'The film's finished, Mummy, can you read me a story?'

'Of course I can, sweet pea, I'll be right in.'

Dimitri had gone by the time the others returned, which was just as well as it was entirely possible that he would have punched Patrick if he'd come face to face with him.

Leila was sitting up in bed reading when Tom

walked into the room. Immediately she put her book down. 'Okay?'

'Yeah, a bit pissed but okay.'

'Too pissed for a shag?'

Tom did a double take. 'Never too pissed for that.'

He quickly moved over to the bed and Leila put her arms around his neck and pulled him down on top of her, where she kissed him deeply.

'That's nice,' he murmured.

'Now take off all your clothes,' she ordered, undoing his belt. She couldn't believe there was a time when she'd thought she didn't desire him. Now all she could think of was how much she wanted him.

Tom, naked and ready for action, reached over and foraged in the the bedside drawer for a condom.

'We don't need one,' she whispered.

She waited for him to question her but he was so lost in his desire for her that he didn't. It was only afterwards that he asked why.

She trailed her fingertips across his shoulders, suddenly anxious that he wouldn't want the same thing, that she was springing this on him, that it was another example of her control freakery. But she had to tell him, 'Because I'd really like us to have another baby.' She paused. 'But only if you would.' She held her breath.

He looked as if he couldn't quite believe what

he'd heard, but then he exclaimed, 'God, yes!' He drew her towards him and kissed her, sealing the deal.

Chapter 27

Frankie

Leila's usually sophisticated, stylish bedroom had been turned into a tip. Clothes were strewn all over the bed and armchair, high-heeled shoes covered the floor, turning it into an obstacle course; pots and tubes of make-up cluttered the elegant dressing table. The air was heady with the scent of hair spray competing with Acqua di Parma (Leila), Pomegranate Noir (Tor) and Agent Provocateur Maitresse (Candy). Black Eyed Peas 'I Gotta Feeling' was blasting out of the speakers, and Leila was singing along and dancing. Candy was making final adjustments to Tor's make-up. She'd clearly been hard at work giving Leila and Tor makeovers.

'Blimey! Here come the girls!' Frankie exclaimed, surveying the scene.

Tor was in false lashes and considerably more make-up than usual, and her blonde hair had been straightened into a sleek bob. She looked gorgeous, sensual, a real come-up-and-see-me-sometime girl, showcasing her curves in a pillar-box red dress and heels. Leila, who usually made do with the barest minimum of make-up, had upped the ante in false lashes and metallic bronze eye shadow that made her green eyes smoulder.

Frankie had said no to a makeover, figuring that she didn't want to end up looking like a drag queen or mutton or both, but in fact her friends looked like sexy confident women, supremely comfortable in their own skins, out to have a good time. She suddenly felt plain by comparison, the ugly duckling to their swans, Cinders before the arrival of the Fairy Godmother. She tried to jolly herself out of it by putting on a sleazy foreign accent and adopting a swagger. 'Hey, sexy ladies! D'you wanna dance with me?'

'Only if you buy me a very big cocktail,' Leila bantered back, pouting her lips suggestively and batting her eyelashes. Then she snapped out of it to ask slightly anxiously, 'Is this dress too short?'

She was wearing a backless green dress that Frankie hadn't seen before. It wasn't the kind of thing Leila usually wore on a night out – she was more of a tea dress sort of girl. This dress was a show-off number, a flaunt it if you've got it, and Leila had it.

'You've got the legs for it, babes, go for it.'

'Candy lent it to me, she said my floral dress was too square.'

'It was. You looked like you were going to some posh drinks do or a garden party.' Candy put on a deliberately plummy accent. 'Who are you? Kate middle-aged Middleton? You've got to be able to shake your booty. You can't shake it in a frumpy dress!'

'Cheeky girl!' Leila declared, but she smiled. 'I bet you don't talk like that to any of your clients.'

'None of my clients would ever dream of wanting to look middle-aged, they're all forty going on twenty. They would be making that short green dress even shorter, wanting longer fake lashes, and slapping on even more make-up.'

'Now the only question is what to do about you.' Tor dragged herself away from checking out her new look in the mirror, to consider Frankie. She wrinkled her nose, unimpressed by what she saw.

'What do you mean?' Frankie said, a little defensively.

Typically she had gone for black. She hadn't risen to Matt's challenge, principally because she didn't possess clothes of any other colour except for her red knickers, but she was hardly going to be showing those off, so it was black shorts, black halterneck, black wedge sandals. A little more eye-liner than usual, an extra layer of mascara, but that was it.

'You're wearing black to go to what is bound to

be a tacky club. We are never going to see anyone from there ever again. Live a little, wear some colour, slap on some more slap!'

Frankie sat down on the bed and poured herself a generous glass of white wine from the bottle the others had already made inroads into. 'Okay, then, do something with me, I'm in your hands.'

'Yay!' Candy declared with a glint in her eyes. 'I've been wanting to do this for ages.'

Fifteen minutes later Frankie hardly recognised herself in the mirror. Gone was the understated lip gloss, in its place a daring red; her eyes were expertly made up with shimmering gold shadow; her usually pale skin had been given a glow with bronzer, but more dramatic was the long fringe that Candy had cut into her dark brown hair that instantly highlighted Frankie's eyes and cheekbones and gave her an exotic, sexy look.

'What do you think?' Candy said, sounding slightly nervous. 'The fringe will grow out really quickly if you don't like it.'

Frankie had worn her hair in the same style for years: shoulder-length, straight-ish, with a side parting. 'I love it! I never thought I would, but I do.'

'And now for the outfit. How about this?' Tor held up a gold sequined t-shirt dress.

'What is this? *Strictly Come Dancing*? You'll be giving me a spray tan next.'

Tor threw the dress at her, 'Go on, I dare you.'

It was way out of Frankie's comfort zone but she figured, what the hell? She went into the bathroom and slipped out of the black clothes and into the dress – though she was not sure that dress was the right description. It was not quite in knicker-flashing territory, but it wasn't far off. She walked out to wolf whistles from the girls.

'I'm proud of you, ladies,' Candy told them. 'You are ready for clubbing!'

Frankie held out her phone. 'Will you take a picture of me – this may well be the one and only time I ever wear this much make-up. I should record it for posterity.'

That led to all of them taking pictures of each other, and group shots, posing and pouting outrageously for the camera.

'Promise me that you won't post these on Facebook?' Frankie asked Candy. 'Just on the slightest chance any of my kids at school should somehow find them and I'll end up on the front page of the local paper – "Teacher moonlights as prostitute".'

'Are you insulting my makeover?' Candy arched a perfectly shaped brow.

'You know what I mean. I don't usually wear this much slap is all. And I meant high-class escort.'

As they clattered down the stairs in their heels, Frankie decided that there was someone she would like to send the photograph to. Matt. They had been in regular email contact with more teasing, bantering, and, yes, some flirting. It didn't mean anything, she was sure, but it did give her that vibrant, bright feeling that she wanted to hold on to. She paused to type a quick message to accompany the photo.

Just been given a Candy makeover b4 clubbing. No black, see, I can wear something different. I am not stuck in style rut. Do you think Jonas will like it? Alas, there was no Hector for me to ogle at on the boat, and I so wanted that navy blue jumper . . . damn him. You were probably right, he would stink of fish and smoke roll-ups and have a yellow index finger. How are you? x

She pressed send and wondered what Matt would think of her new look.

The men's jaws didn't quite hit the floor when they saw the women, but they weren't far off.

'Bloody hell! You all look amazing!' Tom spoke first. 'Are we going to have to watch out that you don't get whisked away from us?'

'No chance of that,' Patrick said with his usual confidence, though when he went to kiss Candy she abruptly turned her head away. He looked thoroughly pissed off. Candy had yet to forgive him. Frankie doubted that she ever would. He was banned from the bedroom and had to sleep on the sofa, claiming that Matt's single bed had hurt his back too much when he had tried it out.

Only a few days ago she would have been

delighted at such a rift between the couple and seen it as her chance. But that was before the subject of Ross came up, and before she realised Patrick was drinking so much, and before she had started to feel closer to Matt. And now, even when Patrick kissed her on the cheek and told her how beautiful she looked, she felt none of that old pull towards him.

Everyone was in the mood for kicking back when they arrived at the club. It was a huge cavernous place, playing pumping dance anthems that they all vaguely knew and channelling a kitsch vibe with vast rotating glitterballs that cast silver discs over the walls. Classy it most definitely was not but that was all for the good, it added to the holiday mood. Tom and Leila hit the dance floor straight away. Gracie was staying with Ellie and Nikos and they were keen to make the most of their freedom. Tor seemed to have left her inhibitions back at the villa and was dancing enthusiastically with Ed, and somewhere in the middle of the throng was Candy. Frankie was all set to join them when Patrick took one look at the packed dance floor, put his arm round her and said, 'How ghastly. Come on, let's go and get a drink.'

He led her to a black leather booth and immediately signalled to the waitress. How ironic that it took Patrick's nearly drowning his girlfriend for them finally to spend some time together alone

. . . ironic too that after all these years of yearning Frankie wasn't sure of her feelings for him any more. While Patrick ordered the drinks she sneaked a look at her phone. There was no reply from Matt. She was surprised to find that she was disappointed.

She glanced over the dance floor and noticed that Dimitri had joined Candy. They weren't even attempting to play it cool but were staring at each other as they danced closely together, directing all their moves at each other, in a world of their own. Luckily Patrick had his back to them and was too lost in his own thoughts to wonder what his supposed girlfriend was up to.

He seemed unusually subdued. He'd been subdued since the accident. 'My life is such a fuck-up,' he declared gloomily as he took a slug of his vodka martini. Frankie couldn't help noticing that he had chosen the strongest possible cocktail on top of God knows how much he'd already had back at the villa. Here we go. She'd had all this from him last night when they'd taken him out for dinner, where Patrick had lamb souvlaki, a bottle and a half of wine, and a large helping of self-pity.

'Your life isn't a fuck-up. You made a mistake and you've apologised. Candy will forgive you.' Frankie wasn't convinced that last part was true, though.

'Haven't you noticed? Candy's not speaking to me. I slept in the living room last night. Jesus, this holiday was supposed to be fun. It's a fucking nightmare – the nine circles of hell would be a picnic compared to this. '

God, Patrick was such a drama queen! 'She *will* forgive you, just give her some space.'

'I don't even know if I care either way. To be honest, I've got more important things to worry about.' He paused and took another gulp of his drink. 'I haven't told anyone else but I've been sacked from the magazine.'

'What!'

'They said I was pissed when I interviewed some bloody C-list actor, who made a stink to his PR who then complained to the mag . . . and the upshot was they kicked me out. Two days before we came away. Ten fucking years I've slogged my guts out for them.'

Frankie didn't know what to say. She doubted that he'd been sacked for that one misdemeanor – no doubt there was a long list of other incidents. She decided to be positive. 'Well, you did say that you wanted to write your novel, and there are lots of other magazines out there. You're a very talented writer, Patrick, you could do whatever you wanted.' *If you put your mind to it and stopped drinking.*

'Yeah, you're right. I should have told you earlier, it would have saved me stewing over it all on my own.' He reached out and put his hand on hers and gazed at her, giving her the intense Patrick stare she had only ever seen him deploy on Willow before.

313

'Where would I be without my Frankie?'

'I'm always here for you,' she replied. Even though he was upset, more than a little drunk and close up she could see that his hairline was slightly receding, and that he had lines under his eyes, he was still the most beautiful man she had ever seen. But she felt it objectively . . . there was none of the longing she used to feel for him.

'Thanks. I don't know why you are, though. I don't know why anyone likes me any more. *I* certainly don't.' He was wallowing in self-pity, and suddenly she realised that he hadn't even asked her how she was after the other night when she had been so upset about Ross. And now she came to think of it, she couldn't remember when he'd ever asked her how she was, it was always all about him.

He drained his martini glass and signalled to the waitress for another. Catching Frankie looking at him, he said defensively, 'Don't start on the drinking either. I know I'm having too much and I'm going to cut right back when I'm home. I can deal with it. I've done it before. I can knock it on the head any time I want, no problem.'

Frankie had heard that one, but she simply nodded.

'It started to get bad when Willow left me for that musician.' He gave a snort of derision. 'I mean, he calls himself a musician, but he's barely scraping a living with his band. He has to teach guitar to kids.

314

It's not exactly the rock and roll lifestyle, is it?'

This was news to Frankie. Patrick had always made out he broke up with Willow. She couldn't remember the reason he'd given. She stayed silent as he continued, 'I told her that there would be no more trips to Paris or New York or to that exclusive yoga retreat in Bali, no weekends at Babington House, no more designer clothes, no more dinners at Nobu, no more shopping at the Conran Shop for furniture. And she said she didn't care about any of that; that she was in love with Andy.'

He paused, looking disgusted. 'She doesn't love him! She can't. Andy – what kind of name is that for a musician? She lives with him in a poky studio flat in Shepherd's Bush. How fucking ironic is that? She was for ever moaning that my three-bed roomed fucking massive apartment was too claustrophobic!'

'She always did seem a little spoilt,' Frankie said quietly. She glanced over at the dance floor, wishing she could join her friends. Patrick was dragging her down.

'I begged her to come back to me, but she wouldn't even consider it. Said she couldn't be with anyone who was unfaithful.'

He begged? He was unfaithful? This was also news to Frankie.

'You had an affair?'

A shrug as if it was nothing. 'It was a one-off with some girl I met in New York when I was over there doing an interview. It was a stupid mistake. I got pissed. She was there. It was no big deal. But Willow read some of the texts this girl sent me and freaked. I don't know why I slept with the woman. I can't even remember her name. It's like I've got a self-destruct button.'

'And then you met Candy.' She was piecing together Patrick's recent life and it wasn't pretty.

'Yeah. Then I met Candy. You know how shit I am at being on my own, and there she was . . . sweet, available, young.' He paused. 'I don't love her and I know for sure she doesn't love me. She loathes me. Poor girl. I'm not the man she thought I was. Jesus, that sounds like the lyrics for a really sappy song. I should send them to Andy.'

He sighed. 'I need someone strong to keep me in check, someone who doesn't put up with any of my shit, an equal.' He looked at her as if seeing her for the first time. 'Someone like you, Frankie. I would be good with you.'

Now? He told her now? In this tacky nightclub where a euro pop anthem was blasting out (something about tonight being the night) and the lights kept switching to ultraviolet, which made Patrick's teeth (and no doubt her own) go a funny luminous white and there was dry ice swirling on the dance floor. She wanted to laugh. This had been the moment she had been waiting for, longing for, praying for, except it wasn't any more.

'Actually, Patrick, I don't know if you would. And

you're just saying that because you're drunk. We're friends, good friends.'

He seemed to slump. 'No one wants me. I've got no job. Nothing.' He drained his glass and went to signal the waitress for another, but Frankie reached out for his hand.

'Come on, why don't we go back to the villa and talk properly?' She was afraid of him making a scene if they stayed there any longer.

Somehow she managed to manoeuvre him out of the club. There was no chance to tell any of the others what she was doing and she didn't want Patrick to run into Candy and Dimitri. Patrick passed out in the taxi, his head lolling against her shoulder. She checked her phone and there was still nothing from Matt. And she had been so sure that he would reply, that there had been something between them . . . She sighed and sent Leila a text telling her she'd left the club.

Patrick woke up as they arrived at the front gate and was able to stagger up the drive, leaning against Frankie. It was after one a.m., a beautiful night, with a full moon and the stars out in force in a velvety black sky. She wished she could sit outside on the terrace on her own. Once they reached the villa he went inside to get a bottle of brandy, ignoring Frankie's comment that she didn't want any. She lit the citronella candles in the hurricane lamps and sat on the sofa, steeling herself for his return. She found herself wondering what Matt was doing, wishing that he was here to banter with. There was going to be no banter with Patrick. Just a one-way stream of me, me, me . . .

He emerged from the villa, clutching a bottle of Metaxa and two glasses. He poured two very generous measures and handed a glass to Frankie. She thought about reminding him that she didn't want any, then thought, what the was the point? Patrick wasn't interested in anything she had to say. He just wanted an audience. She suddenly realised that to him she could be anyone.

Chapter 28

Tor

Tor had pulled out all the stops tonight, desperate to remind Ed of what had attracted him to her in the first place, hence the uncomfortably tight red dress, hence flashing far more cleavage than usual, hence the high heels, hence trying to be fun Tor, suggesting they dance straight away, even though she would be far more comfortable sipping a non-alcoholic cocktail at a table, with her heels kicked off. Actually she would be far more comfortable in her PJs, with a cup of peppermint tea, watching something nice and unchallenging like *Downton Abbey*. But Ed's revelation about the return of Anise had been a wake-up call. She couldn't bear to lose him.

Last night in bed she had tried to initiate sex, ignoring her sore bazooka boobs, the weird metallic taste in her mouth, the fact that she felt like a beached whale . . . but he'd mumbled that he was too tired and had turned away from her. Ed had never in the short history of their relationship been too tired for sex before. He had cycled in the London to Brighton bike race and not been too tired for sex. He'd had barely four hours' sleep across the entire weekend in Glastonbury and not been too tired for sex on his return (once he'd showered off the layers of mud). He had worked a double shift, gone on to a party until five a.m. and not been too tired for sex.

All the rejection she had ever experienced with Harry felt like a rehearsal for that moment in bed when Tor was confronted with the sight of Ed's beautiful brown back, turning away from her. The pain had been searing; she'd felt as if someone had taken a blowtorch to her heart. She couldn't lose him. And at the moment she feared she most likely had, she admitted to herself what she had known for some time now. She loved him. This was not just a bit of fun, a fling, something to tick off her list of things to do. This was the real deal. This was it. She loved Ed. She couldn't lose him. She would not lose him.

'So do you like my new look?' she asked, as they took a break from dancing, channelling her most seductive voice, consciously batting her eyelashes and hoping that they wouldn't let her down at this crucial moment. No one could be seductive with wonky eyelashes. They said 'sad sorry lady', not 'confident sexy temptress'.

'I do,' he replied. 'Which is not to say that you don't look good all the time, but tonight you look extra sexy.' Thank God he sounded sincere, not sarcastic, not resentful. There was a chink of hope. Tor grabbed it and made a supreme effort not to bring up last night and ask him if he still desired her. That would be too needy, too desperate. She wound her arms round his neck, and murmured, 'So what are you going to do about it? How about a trip to the Gents', if you know what I mean?'

Early on in their relationship there had been a moment when a passionate snog in the corridor of a bar had led to something more in the men's loos. It had been an upmarket venue, with particularly stylish loos, lovely Fired Earth tiles, and hygienic enough for Tor who had high standards. But here and now she was prepared to slum it; she didn't give a fig what the state of the men's loos was. She wanted to show Ed how much she wanted him.

But she had reckoned without the kidney bean's influence. Clearly it had decided that sex in a loo was a no go. The kidney bean had decreed that there could only be one activity there for Tor, and that was throwing up. And so without even waiting for Ed's reply, she had to abandon her seduction routine and dash to the Ladies'. Typically there was a queue. There wasn't one for the men's. Also typical. A few minutes ago she had been contemplating having sex in a cubicle there, but she couldn't bear the thought of barging in to be sick.

She was in no fit state to work out what that said about her standards.

Oh, God! This was dire. She was going to have to throw up in the sink in front of all these women. But then she noticed Candy fixing her make-up in one of the mirrors. Candy paused midway through applying her lip gloss.

'Are you okay, Tor?'

No, I'm going to be sick,' she muttered, through the hand she had clamped over her mouth.

Candy immediately took control. 'Emergency! My friend is going to puke! She has to go next!'

And Tor got to throw up in the privacy of her very own cubicle.

She would explain it away as too much sun, she decided as she wiped her mouth with a tissue and prepared to face Candy. But as soon as she pushed open the door, Candy said, 'How are you feeling? Morning sickness is a bitch. My best friend Madison threw up every day, at least four times a day, for three months. She was absolutely fine after that though. So when are you due?'

Tor thought about trying to pretend that she didn't know what Candy was talking about, but she knew deep down that she couldn't pull off the lie – there was too much evidence stacked against her. And it would be such a relief finally to tell someone her big secret.

'I'm not entirely sure – I think it will be around February. I only found out I was pregnant the morning we flew out here. I haven't told anyone. I haven't even told Ed.'

'Shit!' Candy exclaimed. 'I didn't know! I'm sorry. I promise I won't say anything to anyone.' She paused. 'Though I'm surprised none of your friends have twigged. I knew the second day I was here.'

'You heard me throwing up?' Tor and the downstairs bathroom had become very well acquainted. Her knees had red marks on them from spending so long kneeling on the expensive marble tiles. Chic minimalism was all very well, but where was a nice fluffy pedestal mat when you needed it?

''Fraid so. And you're not drinking, and I overheard you ask Dimitri if the feta cheese was pasturised, and you haven't touched seafood. Bit of a giveaway. So why haven't you told Ed?'

That was the big question. And the Ladies' loo didn't exactly seem like the best place to be answering it, with women crowding round them to check out their make-up and others queuing to use the loo. Several of the women were English and were doing a very bad job of pretending not to eavesdrop. Tor was usually so private, but she found that she wanted to tell Candy and the words began tumbling out.

'I guess I need to work things out in my head first of all. It's so much to take in. There's the whole complication about him starting a new job in London, and me living in Brighton, and my business. And we don't live together. And he's younger than me.' She could go on. Every time she went through this it took on an even greater significance, and she felt that it was impossible for her and Ed to have any kind of future.

But Candy's reaction surprised her. It cut through all her worries, as if they were nothing. 'He'll be a brilliant dad. He's fantastic with kids. And all that other stuff doesn't really matter. Sure he's a bit younger than you, but it's not like he's young like Harry Styles! No one looks at you two together and thinks you're older and a cougar.' Candy smiled at Tor. 'And he adores you – anyone can see that. And you adore him.'

'I love him,' Tor declared, more loudly than she'd intended. The words seemed to echo around the tiled room.

The blonde woman standing next to them, who was applying bright fuchsia pink lipstick, stopped. Stabbing her lipstick enthusiastically in the air, she said, 'That is so romantic! I'm sorry, darling, but I couldn't help overhearing. You have got to tell him! This is better than *Jeremy Kyle*, and you're a lot posher than the people on that.'

She was slightly drunk, wearing too much make-up, and bit of a mutton number in a skin-tight hot pink bandage dress, but Tor beamed her thanks. And carried on.

'But I don't want him to feel that he *has* to be with me. We've only been seeing each other five months – that's nothing. This is the first holiday we've been on together. We've not talked about children, I don't even know if Ed wants them.'

'How will you know unless you tell him?' Candy persisted. 'He's a lovely guy. He's not going to flip out and refuse to have anything to do with you. Not like my best friend's boyfriend who fucked off when she told him she was pregnant and has never even seen his baby daughter.'

'Bastard!' declared the blonde with feeling.

Tor couldn't imagine Ed doing anything so brutal.

'I know you're right about him. He is lovely. I just need some time.' Time and someone to tell her how it was all going to work out. Preferably a Fairy Godmother with a wand who could grant her three wishes. She glanced at the blonde again who was now rearranging her boobs in her push-up bra. No, she didn't exactly have Fairy Godmother written all over her.

'So tell me about Madison, how old is her baby?'

She listened intently as Candy told her about being her friend's birthing partner, about how she'd had to live at her mum's but then managed to get a flat of her own and was now at college and had a new boyfriend, a nice one. Finally Candy showed her pictures of Madison's adorable little girl, that she kept on her phone.

'What would you like?' she asked.

And suddenly Tor felt a spark of excitement. She

had been suppressing it since she'd found out the news, but now she wanted to erupt. She was going to have a baby!

'I don't mind, but I think I'm having a boy. In fact, I'm sure I'm having a boy. I like the name Artie, what do you think?' She beamed. 'I never even thought I could get pregnant, that's why it was such a massive shock.'

'Well, congratulations!' Candy hugged her. 'I think it's fantastic. It's what life is all about, isn't it?'

It crossed Tor's mind that Candy, at twenty-two, was far more sussed than she was at thirty-four.

'It really is!' the blonde woman butted in. 'I've got three myself. Look.' she held up her long bleached-blonde hair and Tor and Candy saw three names tattooed in flowery letters at the base of her neck: *Connor, Bethany* and *Ryan*.

'Good luck! And remember, take as many drugs as you can while you're in labour. Screw all that natural birth shit, it hurts like hell! Worth it though,' she declared, as she tottered out of the door.

The two women grinned at each other. 'And on that bombshell, go and find that man!' Candy ordered.

Yes, that's exactly what Tor was going to do.

Even though the club was packed, it was easy for her to spot Ed standing by the bar as he was taller than most people there.

'Hey, where did you get to? I was about to send

out a search party in case you had gone off with another man. One minute you were promising me hot sex, the next you'd disappeared.'

Ah, yes, the hot sex might have to wait . . .

Tor linked her arm through his. 'I was gossiping with Candy in the Ladies'. Can we go somewhere quiet? I need to talk to you.'

'Oh?' Ed frowned. 'That sounds ominous.'

She shook her head. 'Just come with me.'

They made their way to the club entrance. The beefy bouncer insisted on stamping their hands with the image of a cocktail glass, and the letters BO so they could get back in, which slightly took the wind out of Tor's sails. This was going to be a momentous, life-changing moment. BO, standing for Blue Oasis, somewhat undermined that. As the club was in the middle of nowhere, there was nowhere to go except the car park. But she tracked down a spot under a tree which seemed a better option than hanging around by the door with the chain-smoking bouncers, who had a strong whiff of BO about them.

'What's on your mind?' Ed still looked worried.

'Well . . .' Tor folded her arms over her bazooka bosoms. She was so nervous that she was shaking. Her voice sounded thin and quavery. 'I have got something to tell you. Something huge. And before I do, I just want to say that, whatever you decide to do, it's okay. I'll understand.'

'Please, Tor, just get on with it,' Ed pleaded.

327

Oh God, oh God, oh God. This was it. She took a deep breath. 'I'm pregnant.' There, she had said it. She dared herself to look at Ed. He could not have looked more surprised if she had told him that she was an alien, who had arrived on earth with the sole intention of being impregnated by a human.

'What!' He leant against the tree as if he needed support. This didn't look good. He was going to do a runner like Madison's bastard boyfriend. Oh, well. Oh, shit . . .

'I'm having a baby. I found out the day we flew out here.'

'But we've always been so careful.'

He still looked dazed, and did that comment imply that he didn't think the baby was his? No, surely not.

'No, we haven't. Not always. Not on the night of Spencer's fancy dress party.' Tor paused, tilted her chin and said, 'And whatever you decide to do, I am having the baby.'

'Whatever I decide to do! Tor, this is incredible, awesome news! We're having a baby! It's brilliant. I thought you had brought me out here to dump me. I was getting ready to beg you not to. I know I've been giving you a hard time about moving in, but that's because I felt insecure.'

'Really?'

But Ed didn't reply. Instead he put his arms round Tor and kissed her. Kissed her like he meant it. Kissed her so that she was almost tempted to suggest the hot sex idea again – maybe this time al fresco.

'How could you doubt me, Tor?' he said when they finally stopped.

'I didn't want you to feel trapped – especially when I found out about your new job. It seemed completely the wrong time for you.'

'God, Tor, I hate to think of you keeping this to yourself. You don't have to any more. We're in this together.' He hesitated. 'Since this is a night of revelations, here goes with mine. I love you, Tor. And I have done for ages. I don't care if you think it's to soon, it's how I feel.'

'You do?' Now this she hadn't expected. But what a gift, what an absolutely gobsmackingly brilliant gift.

'I do. It's not something I would say for the sake of it.'

'Then we're even, because I love you too.'

Chapter 29

Candy

'I knew you'd be a good dancer,' Dimitri told her, his face pressed to Candy's, so he could make himself be heard over the music.

'What if I hadn't been?' she demanded, enjoying the feeling of being so close to him, so close she breathed in his citrus aftershave, felt the bristles on his jaw graze against her skin. They still hadn't kissed, just danced, danced for each other, revelling in being together.

'I would still have thought you were the most beautiful girl here and made it my mission in life to teach you how to dance.'

She laughed. Somehow Dimitri had the gift of making everything he said sound wonderful and romantic, not corny, or sleazy. She would never admit it out loud but maybe Patrick had done her a favour by nearly drowning her because now she was free of him and free to be with Dimitri. She had seen Frankie leading Patrick out of the club earlier, probably taking him back to the villa to sober him up. Whatever. Candy didn't care. The moment he had flung her into the water any feelings she might once have had for him had disappeared. She never wanted to see him again. Ever. The only thing she was sorry about was that Frankie couldn't be on the dance floor with her. She didn't deserve to be stuck with Patrick boring on, no one did.

She caught the eye of Leila, who was dancing with Tom, and waved at her. Leila beamed back. Until now Candy had had her down as being too in control, almost scarily so, which made her seem older, but tonight she seemed much younger, as if she had let go of something. And Tom, who so often this holiday had looked down, as if he had the weight of the world on his shoulders, seemed a different man, more confident, more relaxed. Candy had even noticed the married couple kissing in one of the booths, not a peck on the cheek either but a full-on snog, Leila sitting on Tom's lap. *Good for you*, Candy had thought, genuinely wanting them to be happy.

'I have to stop,' Dimitri told her, reaching for her hand, 'I can't dance any more.'

'Lightweight,' she teased, taking his hand and letting him lead her off the dance floor.

He rolled his eyes. 'I've been working all day, whereas you have been sunbathing by the pool. So d'you want a drink here? Or do you want to come back to my apartment?'

He caught sight of her raised eyebrows. 'To talk and have coffee. I wouldn't take advantage of you after what you've been through.'

Actually she would quite like him to do just that . . . but maybe he was right. 'A drink here would be good.'

She watched him make his way to the bar, and was just wondering if she could suggest that she cut his hair – or would that be way too shallow? – when a familiar figure stepped into view. Matt.

'Hiya,' she exclaimed.

'Candy, how are you doing?'

He was his usual polite, lovely self, but she sensed him looking around. No prizes for guessing who he wanted to see.

'Frankie's not here,' she told him. 'I think she's gone back to the villa with Patrick.'

The news seemed to take the spring out of Matt's step. 'Oh, I was really hoping to see her. Leila told me you were coming here. I've just driven back from the north of the island. I guess I'll get a drink, can I get you one?'

How like Matt to be polite when he was clearly gutted not to find Frankie. Candy thought of how well Frankie and Matt had been getting on before he went away, the start of something she was sure, and now he was giving up at the first hurdle.

'What I mean is, Patrick was steaming drunk as

usual and Frankie has taken him back to the villa. I'm sure she'd love to see you.'

Matt seemed less sure. God, these thirty-somethings were crap when it came to relationships! Age didn't bring wisdom, that was for sure. 'Um, well, I don't know.'

'You'll be saving Frankie from listening to Patrick moaning on! She only took him back as a favour to me. He's not my favourite person after nearly drowning me today. Fuckwit of the century.'

'Yes, she told me about that. Are you okay?'

Would he just leave now! 'I'm more than okay.'

Dimitri returned at that moment with their drinks, which further delayed Matt's departure as the two men chatted. She couldn't believe it when he started asking Dimitri if he knew the small fishing town he'd been staying at. She had to do something or at this rate Matt would never get his arse into gear. Dimitri was saying that, yes, he knew the town, and had Matt gone to such and such a taverna, which served the best fried halloumi? For fuck's sake, they were talking about cheese!

Candy cut across them. 'Matt, this is all very interesting, but will you please go and rescue Frankie! You can do the Good Cheese Guide tomorrow.'

He was about to say something else, but she held up her hand. 'Go!'

'Okay, okay, I will.' He smiled. 'Thanks, Candy, I'll see you both later.' He practically jogged out of the club.

Candy looked at Dimitri, 'I have a good feeling about Matt and Frankie.'

He put his arms round her waist. 'I know you are a people person who cares about your friends, but right now I only want you to think about me because I have a very good feeling about us.'

'Better than fried halloumi?'

He dipped his head down and kissed her by way of an answer.

Yep, definitely better than fried halloumi . . .

Chapter 30

Frankie

'So you and me, Frankie, alone at last.' Patrick sat down next to her, too close for comfort. She moved away fractionally, but couldn't get very far as she was already against the arm of the sofa.

'Love the hair by the way, very sexy.'

'Thanks,' she replied, feeling awkward with his proximity and the suggestion that they were there for something other than talking. 'So, in the morning we should sit down and draw up a list of editors you could contact about work, and we could spend some time over the rest of the holiday working on your novel synopsis.'

'Yeah, yeah, there's plenty of time for that.' He moved closer still. 'You know, I've always fancied you, Frankie. From the moment Leila introduced us, but Tom warned me not to get involved with you because you'd had that bad experience.'

Bad experience? That's what he called Ross dying? She felt the last of the attraction she had felt for Patrick shrivel up inside her.

He put his hand on her knee. 'But I've always thought you might feel something for me.' He moved his hand higher, reaching her thigh. Frankie clamped her legs together.

'Yeah, well, maybe . . . But we're friends now, Patrick. Just friends.'

'Don't be such a tease, Frankie.' He leaned closer. She was willing him to stop this and trying not to feel intimidated, but looking at him it was as if a switch had been thrown to change his mood from boring drunk to ugly drunk. 'I know you want me. I've seen the way you look at me. Well, now you can have me. It's your lucky night. The others won't be back for ages, it's just you and me.'

Then the scene seemed to be on fast forward. He was forcing her legs apart and pushing her against the arm of the sofa, attempting to kiss her and breathing vodka fumes and stale cigarette smoke in her face. She twisted her head away but he persisted, kissing her neck, tugging up the short dress, ramming his body against hers.

'Patrick, what are you doing?' She was trying to reason with him, but his hands were on her breasts, between her legs, and she had a rising feeling of panic that he wasn't going to stop and that she couldn't stop him.

'Get off me!' she shouted, feeling increasingly

desperate as she tried to push him away, but he grabbed her wrists and held them painfully tight.

'Come on, Frankie, we'll be good together.'

Fear was pulsing through her. 'I don't want this! Stop!' But along with the fear her survival instinct and anger kicked in. How dare he do this to her? And using all her strength, she shoved her knee as hard as she could into his groin.

Instantly Patrick recoiled from her in agony, groaning, 'My fucking balls! What the fuck did you do that for!'

She sprang up from the sofa, just as headlights illuminated the driveway and lit the terrace as if spotlighting a stage. The others were back, thank God.

But the car that pulled up alongside the villa was Matt's. She took a deep breath, aware that her hands were shaking and she could do with that brandy.

'Hi, Frankie, everything okay?' Matt asked, striding up the steps to the terrace and registering a still groaning Patrick.

She didn't get the chance to reply as he yelled out, 'She's a fucking nutter! Just attacked me for no reason.'

Matt looked at Frankie, who shook her head as if to say, don't ask.

'I find that hard to believe. I'm sure she had her reasons.'

'Bullshit! She's a frigid bitch! Leads me on,

asking me back to the villa, saying we need to "talk".'
Patrick actually had the audacity to make quotation
marks with his fingers when he said that. Bastard.

'And we all know what that means. I know she's
been after me for ages, but when it comes to it, she
changes her mind.'

Frankie could hardly bring herself to look at
Matt. Instead of feeling angry with Patrick she felt
as if her skin was crawling with humiliation and
shame. She was disgusted with herself for getting
into this situation with Patrick, disgusted that she
had ever had any feelings for him.

'But I see that she'd rather "talk" to you, so good
luck with that,' Patrick continued. Picking up the
brandy bottle, he staggered inside the villa.

'Are you okay?' Matt asked her again.

'I don't know what to say,' Frankie replied quietly.
'He was right about some of it.'

'You don't have to justify yourself to me.'

She folded her arms over her chest, feeling
vulnerable in the short dress. It seemed a very long
time since she had got glammed up, laughing with
Candy and Tor. It had all seemed so innocent, and
now she felt everything was ruined. 'He was drunk.
Very drunk and very upset. I should have realised
that at the club. I shouldn't have come back with
him.'

Matt walked towards her and gently took hold
of one of her hands. There was a red mark on her
wrist from where Patrick had restrained her.

'Stop beating yourself up, and stop defending him. You didn't do anything wrong.'

'I've done so many things wrong, Matt, that I've lost count.'

'Frankie, that's not true.'

And then she couldn't stand to talk about it. She tried to make a joke. 'Pity Jonas wasn't there tonight. He was probably at some all-night yoga convention and got stuck in an advanced position. It's going to be over before it even began. And, of course, Hector was out catching sardines. I really hate sardines. I know I shouldn't because they're a fantastic source of Omega 3, but I do.' She was rambling now.

'You don't have to make light of this, Frankie,' Matt sounded concerned. His sympathy made her want to cry.

'I'd rather I did. The alternative is too horrible. I'm going to bed.' She paused to say, 'I'm glad you came back.'

His blue eyes were warm. 'So am I, Frankie. Goodnight.'

Once she was inside her bedroom she wedged a chair under the handle. It was probably an illogical thing to do, but it made her feel better. She pulled off the gold dress and kicked it out of sight in the corner of the room – she would buy Candy another one. It wasn't a dress that should be worn again. She put on a long t-shirt and sat at the dressing table, wiping off all the make-up, peeling off the

339

lashes. Now she forced herself to confront the stark reality of what had happened. Patrick, the man she'd thought she loved, had tried to – God, she really didn't want to admit this, but there was no other word for this – rape her. There was no sugar coating it. That's what it had felt like.

She was too numb to cry. She sat on the bed and wished she was anywhere but here. Her phone beeped with a message and she reached for it. A message from Matt.

Hey again, Frankie, I meant to say that I only just got your message from earlier. You looked beautiful. xx

It was something, but it didn't feel like enough to banish the imprint on her mind of what had just happened. She didn't reply but curled up on the bed, hugging one of the pillows against her for comfort.

Frankie lay awake for much of the night, going over and over that scene with Patrick, despising herself for ever feeling anything for him. At six a.m. she finally gave up on sleep and tiptoed downstairs, intending to make herself a cup of tea. She paused by the living room. She had forgotten that Patrick had been banished from the bedroom. He lay sprawled out on the sofa, flat out on his back and snoring quietly, a sheen of sweat on his face. Not such a beautiful man now. He looked like what he had become – a drunk sleeping it off, oblivious to the pain he had caused.

The room reeked of alcohol. She forced herself to walk over to him and stared at his prostrate form. She wondered if he would even remember what had happened. If he did, he would no doubt laugh it off; deny it. '*Silly Frankie, I was drunk. It was just a bit of fun.*' She gave up on the tea and went back upstairs.

She stayed in her room until ten and then went down even though she was dreading seeing anyone, not knowing that she could pull off her 'I'm fine' routine. But somehow that seemed a better prospect than remaining with only her tortuous thoughts for company.

The villa seemed deserted as she crept downstairs; maybe everyone was still asleep or at the beach. She hoped so. There was no sign of Patrick in the living room, and his sheet and pillow had been thrown carelessly on the floor. But she heard voices coming from the kitchen, and froze. Shit, it was Patrick and Matt. The last two people she wanted to see. She should walk in and brazen it out, clear the air. But she couldn't, it was all too raw. Instead she leant against the cool stone wall in the hallway, and listened.

'Are you seriously going to keep up this tight-arse act for the rest of the day?' she heard Patrick say. 'Because, my God, it will be tedious for everyone. I've already told you, I was drunk.'

341

'We'd better not talk about it,' was Matt's curt reply. 'You shouldn't still be here as far as I'm concerned.'

'Yeah, yeah,' Patrick replied. 'Can't we just leave it?'

She really should go now. She had the strongest suspicion that nothing good was going to come of her eavesdropping on this conversation.

'I know, I messed up – again,' Patrick continued. 'But Frankie's okay, isn't she? We're good friends. I'll make it up to her.'

'Are you really this thick-skinned, Patrick?'

'Give it a rest, Matt, I've got a headache.'

'Frankie is in love with you. She's been in love with you for as long as I've known her.'

Patrick gave a disbelieving laugh. 'Frankie! No way. We're good mates, that's all. She's my one female friend.'

'Unluckily for her, it's true.'

'Well then, she must know me well enough by now to realise she's not my type. I mean, she's great and I love her company, but she's far too complicated for me. And I've had a text from Willow this morning. She wants us to give it another go.'

'What? Is she crazy or something?'

'Yeah, well, this time I'm not going to fuck it up. I'll break the news to Candy when she gets back from the beach. Funnily enough, I don't think she'll be too heartbroken, do you?'

'And Frankie?'

'She'll be cool with it. She's tough. And she'll understand that last night happened because I was drunk, feeling sorry for myself, and she was there. In a way it's good that she stopped things. It would have been awkward if it had gone any further.'

Frankie remained rooted to the spot in a daze. The hours, months, years she had wasted longing for this man, and he dismissed her feelings in a few trite sentences. He was not interested in her, he never had been. Nor would he face up to what he had done. *Awkward* if it had gone any further? She really had been deluding herself all this time. Patrick only cared about one person and that was himself. There was the sound of something being slammed down on the work surface and then a scuffle.

'Hey, what are you doing! Get your hands off me!' Patrick shouted.

'See, you can dish it out but you can't take it, can you? You fucking little shit! It should be beneath me to do this, but I can't help it,' came the response.

There was a loud thump and a yell from Patrick. Frankie raced into the kitchen where she saw him clutching his nose and Matt rubbing his knuckles.

'He just fucking hit me!' Patrick exclaimed. 'God! Has he broken it?'

'It would serve you right if he had,' she retorted. 'I heard everything. You deserved it.' And then she couldn't bear to be in the same place as him a second longer. She raced out of the door and into the garden.

The sense of waste, the shame, the humiliation, rushed through her like poison. She had to get away. The moped was parked on the driveway, the keys in the ignition. She wasn't wearing a helmet and she was in flip-flops and she'd only driven a moped once before, but she didn't care. She heard Matt calling her name, but nothing was going to induce her to stop as she got the bike started and careered down the drive.

She had no idea of where she was going; she only knew that she had to get as far away from the villa and Patrick as possible. Tears were streaming down her cheeks and she was sobbing, huge sobs that hurt her chest and made her feel as if she couldn't breathe. The wind was whipping her hair into her face, restricting her visibility, and she wobbled precariously every time a car overtook her.

She thought of how much she had been longing for this time away with Patrick, of how it had been all she had thought of every night, every single night for months and months. She thought of Patrick and Matt knowing all this. She didn't know how she was going to get through it, face anyone again. She thought of Ross, of sweet, funny, gentle Ross, who never would have hurt anyone, who had never hurt her. She thought of Ross who was lost to her. And realised with a burst of clarity that she had only fixed on Patrick because he was unavailable, because she knew she could never have him.

A sharp bend in the road caught her unaware, and she turned too late, hit a pothole and skidded across the road. She desperately tried to steer but she lost control and the bike slipped from under her. She was falling, falling, falling. This was it then. She experienced a searing, burning pain as she hit the tarmac, then nothing.

Chapter 31

Leila

Leila had a brilliant night. A brilliant, wonderful, liberating, totally fantastic night. She had spent much of it dancing with Tom – something that they hadn't done for years. Why hadn't they? She had forgotten what a good dancer her husband was. Not an embarrassing dad dancer, but a genuinely nifty mover, fluid, with rhythm. She had noticed the admiring glances sent his way by some of the other women close by and had felt a glow of pride that this man, this tall, sexy man with the moves, was her husband.

Tumbling off the dance floor, hot and sweaty, they had ordered cocktails – each daring the other to choose the one with the rudest name. Leila had a Screaming Orgasm, Tom a Blow Job – he bottled out of asking the waitress for a Cocksucking Cowboy. They'd enjoyed teasing each other that the night was young and anything was possible – flirting, yes, actually flirting together. Something else they hadn't done for far too long. They had talked and laughed and the conversation came easily. They were going to make changes to their lives, bold, important changes that were going to move them out of the suffocating dark place they had been surviving in for too long. She was going to cut down her hours, delegate more, employ a freelance director. Tom was going to work more. They were going to be a partnership again. They were going to try for another baby. Every time she thought of that Leila felt a smile a mile wide forming on her face.

She was still on a high after she had collected Gracie from Ellie and Nikos in the morning. She and her daughter sang along enthusiastically, though in fairness, more than slightly off key, to Eliza Doolittle's 'Pack Up' all the way back to the villa. Yes, her troubles were packed up now, she was certain of it.

Typically Patrick had left his sheet and pillow on the floor, and an empty bottle of wine and glass on the table. (And his last servant died of . . .?) But at least he wasn't still sprawled out on the sofa, stinking out the room with his booze breath, which was something.

Inside their bedroom the shutters were closed and Tom was still asleep, turned on his side, one arm flung across the bed as if reaching for her.

347

Leila couldn't resist tiptoeing over and kissing his shoulder. They were going to try for another baby . . . a flare of excitement kept igniting inside her at the thought.

Already they had racked up a session last night and this morning. Such passion had been unheard of for the last four years. She had also forgotten how much she loved sex with Tom. She was almost tempted to rip the cover off him and go for third time lucky. But Gracie ran in at that moment, clutching a squirming Buzz, to inform Leila that Matt was looking for her, reminding her precisely why sex had been less frequent and less spontaneous in recent years.

Leila tracked him down in the kitchen. He didn't even say hello but launched straight in with a question. 'Do you know where Frankie is?'

Leila smiled to herself. He must really have missed Frankie and their flirtation. She knew she hadn't been wrong about the spark she had seen between them. Good. 'She's probably still asleep or gone for a run. I'm sure you'll see her very soon.' She gave him a conspiratorial look that said that she knew all about the flirtation; knew and approved.

But Matt didn't bite. His blue eyes were serious.

'Neither of those. She tore off on the moped . . . she was terribly upset. I've no idea where she's gone and she hasn't taken her phone or her wallet.'

He didn't sound flirtatious. He sounded worried. 'Why would she do that?'

'Something Patrick said. If you don't mind, I'd rather Frankie told you herself.'

'She probably wants some headspace. You know what she's like. Just give her a bit of time. She'll be fine.' Leila reached for the kettle. 'Do you want a coffee? By the time you've had it, she'll be back.'

'I don't think so, Leila. I know she puts on this tough act, but it's all a front. I know how vulnerable she is underneath because of Ross.'

Leila's mood instantly shifted from euphoric to anxious. She couldn't help it; the mention of Ross triggered so many painful memories. She gave up on the coffee. 'What exactly did Patrick say to upset her?' she railed. 'Hasn't he caused enough problems with Candy? Jesus, that man!'

Matt shook his head, and scooped up the car keys. 'It's not for me to say. I'm going out to look for her. I can't stay here doing nothing. Call me if she comes back or if you hear anything from her.'

Two hours later there was still no sign of Frankie, and Matt was still out looking for her. Leila couldn't stop worrying, imagining the worst possible scenarios. She knew that her friend wasn't wearing a helmet – Frankie who always wore one when she cycled around Brighton. What had made her abandon her usual caution? Moped accidents were frighteningly common on the bumpy roads of the island. Every year the A&E department in Zakynthos Town hospital was full of injured tourists who had thrown caution to the wind and ridden a moped without wearing a helmet, as if being on holiday somehow made them invincible.

Everyone but Patrick was sitting on the terrace from where they had a clear view of the drive. He was the only one who seemed unconcerned and was lying by the pool, a bottle of beer in one hand, a cigarette in the other. Either he was a total bastard who couldn't care less or he was a total bastard who didn't want to let on how upset he was. Either way, every time Leila looked over by the pool she itched to march over and force a reaction from him. She wanted to pour the beer away, stub out his fag and make him sit up and take responsibility, for once.

It was way past lunchtime, Tom had made Gracie a cheese sandwich, but no one else was hungry. All they could do was take it in turns to make cups of tea or coffee and wait. Leila could barely look at Tor, whose strained expression mirrored her own anxiety.

'Do you really have no idea what Patrick said to upset Frankie so much?' Candy asked, loudly enough for him to hear. They had all asked variations on this question over the last two hours and were no closer to finding out the answer.

'I have no idea. Matt wouldn't tell me and Patrick claims not to know.' Leila replied.

They looked over at Patrick, who finally put down his beer. 'She'll be fine. She'll have stopped off at a café or a beach. Stop panicking.'

'But she doesn't have any money with her!' Leila snapped back.

'What's his problem?' Candy demanded. 'He doesn't care about anyone except himself, does he?'

'I heard that!' Patrick said peevishly.

'Good. You were meant to.'

Ed suggested a game of cards, but they were all distracted and it felt like too trivial an activity. The only sound was the cicadas and the squeak of Gracie's felt-tip pens against the paper as she drew a picture of a lizard, resembling an alien spaceship. Tom phoned Matt, but he had no news. The heat and the lack of breeze made the tension even more unbearable.

'I've had enough of this!' Candy got up and marched over to Patrick. Leila and Tor looked at each other and wordlessly did the same.

'How can you just lie there, acting as if nothing has happened, when your friend has gone missing! What did you say to her?' Candy stood in front of him, hands on hips, eyes blazing, an avenging angel in a gold bikini.

'Christ! I'm tired of being seen as the bad guy. First of all, I didn't say *anything* to her. She overheard Matt and me talking.'

'What about?'

A sigh from Patrick. 'Okay, you won't like this, but if it stops you going on at me, here it is – Matt claimed that Frankie was in love with me. How he knew I have no idea because I certainly didn't. I told him that I could only ever see her as a friend. I would have put it more tactfully had I known she was listening. And Matt's got anger-management issues – the bastard hit me!' Patrick raised his sunglasses and revealed an angry purple-and-black bruise circling his right eye.

Frankie in love with Patrick? How could she and Tor not have known this? Leila frantically replayed the last few times she had seen Frankie and Patrick together. Sure, she always let him off the hook and defended him whenever anyone criticised him, but there was nothing to suggest love, was there? And there was something glib about the way Patrick had just delivered his speech, as if he had glossed over something important.

'In love with *you?*' Candy sounded incredulous. 'Give us some credit. Frankie wouldn't fall for someone like you!'

'Yes, in love with *me*. Can you give it a rest now? My head is killing me, thanks to that thug Matt. I should bloody sue him – he's worth enough.' Patrick ground out his cigarette in the ashtray as if signalling an end to the matter.

Clearly Leila wasn't the only one enraged by his casual gesture as Candy exclaimed, 'You're such a shit, Patrick! I'm glad Matt decked you one.' She turned to Leila and Tor with a determined expression that said she meant to kick ass and quite possibly land Patrick another shiner.

'I was going to do this in private, but spending another second with this sorry bastard is doing my fucking head in! Apologies for swearing, but I can't fucking help it right now.'

'Swear all you want,' Leila told her. 'He's doing my fucking head in as well.'

'And my fucking head!' Tor added.

'What is this?' Patrick demanded. 'A swearing coven? An X-rated edition of *Loose Fucking Women*? You all need to chill the fuck out, you're supposed to be on holiday. Have you all got PMT?'

He seemed to be oblivious to the fact that he was digging himself into a deeper and deeper hole.

'Patrick, we're finished. Over. For good,' Candy declared. 'This has been one of the worst relationships of my life. Well, I call it a relationship but it was never that. It was a waste of space and time. You're a complete wanker. In fact, you give wankers a bad name.'

Go, girl! Leila only just resisted the urge to cheer and punch the air.

Patrick greeted the news with a shrug. 'Suits me. I was going to tell you the same thing – though in private – slightly more dignified, don't you think? My ex wants to get back with me.'

'God, she must need her head examined.' Candy shot back. 'You're a mistake I would never repeat. Never.'

He hauled himself up from the lounger. 'Well, this has been fun but I'm going inside to pack. My

353

flight leaves tonight. So you're free to go and shag Stavros – that's if you haven't already. Suck him off behind the bins last night, did you? I bet he thought it was his birthday. But then he's probably used to easy English girls who drop their knickers after one Piña Colada.'

He clearly intended to hurt Candy, but she shook her head as if she pitied him. 'We're not all like you, Patrick. But now I've dumped you, yes, I can do exactly what I like. I can guarantee that Dimitri will be way better in bed because he's not an alcoholic like you. He'll have more staying power. He won't be so pissed that he can't get it up. He won't be so blind drunk that he passes out after one grope. His breath won't stink like dead dog first thing in the morning. Oh, and he won't have the shakes until he gets the first drink of the day down his neck.'

Go, girl indeed! Leila looked at Tor who was struggling not to grin. But Patrick was livid, and hissed, 'Why don't you fuck off back to your council estate, you cheap little ho.'

'Patrick!' Leila was outraged by his comment.

'Oh, shut up, Leila, I know you feel the same. I saw the look on your face when Candy pitched up, all high heels and too much make-up. I know we're far too politically correct to admit it, but she's just a bit common, isn't she? A bit of a chav. I doubt she buys her linen from the White Company, or shops at Waitrose, or listens to Radio 4.'

Leila was about to launch into a hearty denial. On top of the insults aimed to Candy were the ones directed at her. Bastard. How dare he categorise her as a snob! And she didn't even shop at Waitrose. And she only ever bought anything from the White Company in the sale.

'You've got no right to say those things, Patrick. We've all accommodated your drinking for too long. You've got a serious problem and you need to address it or you're going to end up with no friends at all. And you'll finish up as a very lonely, sad fuck-up.' Now Tor was getting in there.

'Oh, it's Tor of the toyboy putting her oar in, is it? Well, you should be grateful that I won't be seeing Candy any more, I've seen the way little Eddie leers at her when he thinks no one is looking. His tongue's practically hanging out, you keep him on such a tight leash. But you can't blame him. Twenty-two-year-old pussy wins every time. And Tom no doubt feels exactly the same – but that's hardly surprising as you've completely emasculated the poor guy, Leila. You've lopped off his balls and turned him into a housewife. It's pitiful. You can't imagine that's what he wants.'

Leila couldn't believe that they had ever been friends with this vicious nasty misogynist. Invited him into their home, to their wedding, on their holiday. She felt violated by his presence.

'Ignore him. It's the drink,' Candy ordered. 'And he's really not worth it.' She looked set to return to the terrace, then she stopped. 'But there is one more thing.'

And before Patrick realised what was happening, Candy charged at him and gave him a hefty shove on the shoulder. Sober, Patrick would have kept his balance, but he was drunk and unsteady on his feet. He tipped into the pool with an almighty splash and a rather unmanly yelp.

'My work is done!' Candy declared, then high-fived Leila and Tor and all three of them fled to the terrace, giggling.

Tom was on the phone, serious-faced. Instantly the women stopped laughing. 'Frankie's had an accident. She's in hospital,' he called to them.

Chapter 32

Frankie

Frankie opened her eyes, winced in the light and then closed them again. Her head pounded, her shoulder throbbed, there seemed to be something wrong with her knee.

'Hey, Frankie, are you okay?'

It was Matt's voice. Even though the details of the accident were a blur she remembered exactly what had happened before it in crystal-clear high definition. She could not face seeing Matt. If she kept her eyes shut he would go away.

'I know you can hear me.'

Bugger. It was typical of him not to know when he wasn't wanted. She heard a curtain being pulled back and then she heard a man's voice. Nikos. God, who else was here? Surely not Patrick? No, she remembered how squeamish he was. Hospitals were not his thing.

'How is she? I've been speaking to the doctor and she says there is nothing broken. They will keep her in for a couple more hours for observation.'

'I still want them to do an MRI. She was unconscious for a few minutes. It's imperative that she has one.'

'Okay, the doctor's my cousin, I'll see what I can do. A lot of the staff are on strike here because they haven't been paid for months.'

'Then I'll go and pay them myself, in cash, but I need them to do the scan!'

Matt sounded so concerned that against her better judgment Frankie opened her eyes again. 'Not like you to throw money at a problem,' she mumbled, through a mouth that felt horribly dry and gritty as if she had been eating sand.

'Thank God! You're being sarcastic! Come on, say something else horrible. Anything you like.'

'I'm fine.' She didn't feel fine. She felt wobbly, undone. A mess. An epic mess. A gigantic fuck-up of a mess. She closed her eyes and a single treacherous tear sneaked out.

'I don't think you're fine,' Matt said gently, 'but you're going to be.' He reached out and held her hand. 'You had us all very worried – I'll save the lecture about wearing a crash helmet for when you're feeling up to it. I'm very glad to see you, Frankie.'

Was he really? How could he be after what had happened with Patrick? He must think she was an idiot for ever thinking herself in love with him. Briefly she opened her eyes, certain that Matt would be unable to hide what a fool he thought she was, but there was nothing like that in his expression. Concern, warmth, and the something bright there on the edges . . .

'So promise me that you're not going to waste any more time on Patrick? And that you're not still blaming yourself?'

She didn't have an answer but instead closed her eyes.

The images were still vivid in her head. A slide show of shame. A PowerPoint presentation of humiliation. She felt something cool and hard circle her wrist. Curiosity got the better of her and she opened her eyes. Matt had fastened a delicate bracelet of turquoises around her wrist.

'I saw this when I was away. I thought it would do until you got your other one re-threaded.'

She had a lump in her throat and feared more tears. 'Thank you.' She forced herself to meet his eyes. He didn't look as if he thought she was stupid. That made one less person in the room then.

'You're very welcome.'

Matt got his way and Frankie had her MRI scan – she had a feeling he usually got his way. The scan revealed that there was no damage. She supposed that the scan couldn't show damage to the spirit, to the heart; couldn't show when you felt as if you had been broken into pieces.

Instead of driving her back to the villa, Matt took her to Ellie and Nikos's house to give her time to recover and to ensure that Patrick would have packed up and left by the time she returned. She'd expected to feel something when Matt told her that Patrick was flying back to the UK and to Willow, but she felt only relief that she wouldn't come face to face with him. There had been no sense of loss, only a weary acknowledgement that she didn't know what she had ever seen in him. Whatever she had felt for him had not been love, it had been infatuation, obsession and a waste of three years. He had been her displacement activity when she should have been getting on with her life.

Ellie and Nikos were typically welcoming and insisted that Frankie and Matt should relax in their private garden, away from the busy taverna. It was a perfect sanctuary, the place where Ellie practised her yoga amidst the pots overflowing with brightly coloured flowers, and the sweet-smelling jasmine that cascaded over the wall. It was peaceful except for the soothing trickle of water through the conch-shaped stone water feature. It must have been the strong painkillers kicking in that made her see it as that, as usually water features irritated the hell out of Frankie and made her want to take an axe to them. She sat at one end of the wicker sofa, wrapped up in one of Ellie's shawls – a purple number – which she was sure must make her look like an ancient crone, about to tell someone's fortune. Matt sat at the other end. He was even more tanned after his trip away and Frankie wondered why she had never realised how compelling his blue eyes were. She had always thought blue eyes were cold, but Matt's were full of warmth.

Ellie had brought out a selection of food and a carafe of wine, ignoring Frankie's protests that she couldn't possibly eat anything. The bread had been freshly baked and smelt delicious and Frankie found herself reaching for a piece and discovered that she was starving.

'Good – you'll feel better if you have something to eat,' Matt told her, making her feel like a patient who needed to be monitored.

'Thank you, Dr Cartwright. I never usually eat bread, I'd forgotten how bloody lovely it is.' She paused. 'Ross used to make it. Way before baking was the "in thing". Said he found it relaxing after teaching all day.' She couldn't believe that she had mentioned Ross, usually she did all she could to avoid saying his name. It must be the accident.

'Do you miss him very much?'

She nodded and didn't say anything and hoped Matt would take the hint that she didn't want to go into details.

She looked around. 'Jonas would love it here, don't you think? He'd roll out a yoga mat and be in the downward dog position before you could say *Namaste.*'

361

Matt shook his head. 'You do know that Jonas isn't real, don't you?'

'Really? I'm not going to get my yogic master or my able seaman? Life is too cruel.'

'They weren't for you. And it's okay, you don't have to tell me about Ross, but I hope you will one day.' He didn't wait for her reply, which was fortunate as Frankie didn't even know what to make of that comment. But then nothing much was making sense to her. She felt as if her carefully structured world had been shaken up, turned inside out, and she was still trying to put it back together with pieces that didn't fit. Instead he asked her about her work, and they discussed their favourite films. His was *The Godfather*. That's so predictable, she told him; though when she revealed that hers was *The Piano*, he said that was true of her as well, which she supposed it was. Through their conversation it was as if he was helping her rebuild her image of herself as strong, in control Frankie. She appreciated his tact. At some time she would have to go back over what had happened with Patrick but not now. Now she wanted to let the warmth of the languid summer evening heal and restore her.

'So tell me about the people you stayed with?' Frankie asked, aware that she had been doing most of the talking.

'There was Pete and his wife Liz, and their two children. I work with Pete and Liz is a nurse who works in sexual health – the stories she can tell! Another couple I didn't know very well, and my friend Simon, who is a teacher, and Sara who is also a lawyer.'

There was something in the way he said 'Sara' that made Frankie wonder if she was anything more than a friend.

'Are Simon and Sara together?'

Matt grinned. 'Simon is gay, so no, they're not together.' He paused. 'Sara and I had a thing a couple of years ago, but we're just friends now.'

How long did the thing last? Frankie found herself wondering. Was it a thing that hadn't really mattered? Or was there still something there? And who was this Sara? She imagined a tall, slim blonde, bronzed and with a broad smile, always optimistic, embracing life. In other words, the complete opposite to her.

'Are you sure you're okay? You look exhausted.' Matt glanced at his watch, 'I could take you back to the villa, I'm sure he'll have gone by now.'

'It's okay, you can say his name. Patrick. He's not Voldemort, the one who can't be mentioned. And the accident wasn't his fault. That was all my doing. And before that, I left the club with him. I should have realised the state he was in.'

'You promised me that you weren't going to blame yourself!' Matt sounded wound up. He could hardly sit still, he was so agitated. She had never seen him like this before. 'It was entirely Patrick's fault. I blame him for being a drunk and for not caring about anyone except himself.'

'Actually I think he does care for someone else more – he cares about Willow. And as for the drinking, he definitely needs help, but maybe getting back with her will sort him out.'

Matt grimaced. 'You sound so forgiving and so calm. If it had been me, I would be raging against him.'

'I'm sure once he's home and sober he'll realise what he's done, and be sorry.' Frankie didn't know that for sure, but she hoped he would.

They were silent for a few minutes, sipped their wine, looked out over the garden. Frankie thought of Matt's unexpected arrival at the villa a week and a half ago. She couldn't possibly have imagined that they would end up like this.

She stretched out her left arm and winced slightly as her shoulder still throbbed from the impact with the road.

'I realised something just before I came off the bike. My Road to Damascus moment. I realised that I had spent all that time obsessing over Patrick, believing that I was in love with him, precisely because he was unavailable. It hurt not having him, but not as much as losing him would.'

'Because of Ross?'

'Very perceptive of you . . .Yes, because of Ross.' She managed a smile, in spite of her swollen, split lip. 'The truth is that I'm even more of a fuck-up than Patrick. I make him look normal and well adjusted.'

'That's not true! You're funny and loyal and clever and sexy. And you have the most beautiful eyes I have ever seen. And you're a terrible loser, and far too competitive, and a control freak over food and exercise . . . and it would be good if you wore something other than black. I love the fringe, though, it suits you.'

Matt said she was sexy? *Sexy?* She didn't feel sexy with a whacking great bruise on her forehead, a graze on the side of her face, and a split lip. She couldn't acknowledge the compliment but it glowed inside her.

Frankie suddenly felt overwhelmed with exhaustion, no doubt her body's survival strategy combined with the strong painkillers. She couldn't summon up the energy to say anything else. She wanted to sleep, to forget.

'Let me take you back to the villa,' Matt said, instantly switching off the banter.

'I'd rather stay here. Ellie mentioned that I could if I wanted. I'm not sure if I'm up to seeing the others.' She paused. 'Do they know everything that happened?'

'They only know that you overheard Patrick talking about you. I won't say anything else to them. You should get some rest. I'll see you in the morning.' And he leant over and kissed her lightly on the cheek, the one part of her face that didn't hurt.

'Thanks again for looking after me, and for the bracelet.' Frankie hesitated. 'And for being there last night.' She felt unusually shy, and hyper-aware of him being so close to her.

'Any time, Frankie.' He hesitated. 'You know I came back early from my trip because I wanted to see you? I missed our banter.' A beat. 'I missed you.'

'I can't imagine why, I feel as if you've seen the very worst of me.'

He shook his head. 'Ms Harper, I refer you to my previous comments. You're funny and loyal and clever and sexy. I love spending time with you. And you've no idea how many times I regretted walking out on you from that hotel room.'

Frankie suddenly didn't feel tired; all her senses were on high alert . . . She felt as if the next few minutes were going to be very significant indeed.

'In fact, I came back and knocked on the door, but you didn't answer. Probably very wise.' Matt gazed at her and she felt as if those blue eyes were seeing straight to the heart of her.

Frankie had no idea what might have happened next, but Ellie bustled out to ask if they wanted anything else. She seemed to register that she had gatecrashed something, but by then it was too late.

Matt stood up. 'I should go. Hurry up and get better so I can beat you at table tennis. I've got all these new moves to show you.'

'In your dreams,' Frankie called after him.

Ellie looked crestfallen as she exclaimed, 'So

sorry for barging in on you, my darling! I hope it wasn't at a crucial moment?'

'You should know, Ellie,' Frankie teased her. 'Aren't you supposed to be the oracle?'

'Well, it certainly looked as if you had revised your opinion of blond men. And now bed for you, young lady. It looks as if you might have an interesting finale to your holiday. First you need to sleep.'

Chapter 33

Tor

Tor was relieved to see that Frankie didn't look quite as bad as she had been anticipating, but it was still an emotional moment when she and Leila saw her the following day. She sat curled up on the seat in Ellie's garden. She looked as if she had been several rounds in a fight and lost – the bruise on her face was turning vivid shades of purple and lilac. Ellie had lent her an orange maxi dress in a floaty fabric patterned with the peace symbol, a most un-Frankie-like outfit. It was disconcerting.

'I'm really sorry I put you through all that worry,' she said, once they had hugged each other, carefully, mindful of Frankie's injuries. 'I wasn't thinking straight.'

'I can't believe you didn't wear a crash helmet!' Leila exclaimed. 'Promise me that you will never, ever do that again? You could have been killed! Or ended up with brain damage!' She had gone into anxious mum mode.

'I think Frankie's learnt her lesson,' Tor intervened gently.

'Has Patrick gone then?' Frankie asked, pleating the fabric of the dress with her fingers, the only sign that revealed she might have cared about the answer.

'Yep, he flew back last night, thank God,' Leila said briskly. 'Oh and before he left, Candy dumped him.'

'And pushed him in the pool,' Tor added.

'He totally deserved it!' Leila declared. 'He said some really terrible things.' She shook her head. 'Honestly, you think you know someone and then they behave in a way that shows you didn't at all.'

Frankie sighed. 'I think the drink has really messed him up. I guess he told you about me being in love with him?'

It was typical of her to get straight to the point.

'Yes, he said he hadn't realised,' Tor replied. She hesitated. 'Are you still?' She thought of Frankie carrying this secret for so long, never letting on to any of them. What a burden. And to be in love with Patrick of all people . . .

'I thought I was for so long, but I don't think I ever really was. It was like an obsession – I can hardly explain it. But I'm over it now, I really am. I know he's gone back to Willow. And I don't mind.'

Tor looked her anxiously. Was this just Frankie

putting on a brave face? It would be so typical of her. 'Are you sure?'

'I am. I hope he sorts himself out. He's not a bad person underneath it all. He lost his job just before he came on holiday, so that can't have helped his state of mind.'

Frankie stretched out her arms and Tor noticed a striking turquoise bracelet on her wrist that she hadn't seen her friend wear before. 'Is that new?'

She was certain that Frankie blushed as she replied, 'Yes, it was a present from Matt.'

Tor couldn't resist glancing at Leila, who smirked knowingly.

'I saw that look!' Frankie warned them. 'It was just a friendly gesture, nothing more. He was there when I broke the one Ross gave me.'

Tor held Frankie's wrist to examine the gift more closely. This was no cheap and cheerful number that Matt had bought from a market; this was a proper expensive piece of jewellery.

'A very friendly gesture, I'd say,' Tor told her.

'He really likes you, Frankie,' Leila put in. 'Really, really likes you. He was so relieved that you were feeling better, and he spent the whole night talking about you when he got back. That Sara woman called him three times and he didn't take any of her calls. You've got to him, Frankie – your unique brand of rudeness and charm has worked its magic. I knew that ultimately you'd get on.'

Frankie put up her hand. 'Stop it now! You've

only just found out that I've been suffering from unrequited love or whatever it was for the last three years. You can't be so quick to pair me off with Matt!'

But she was smiling and Tor didn't think that she minded in the slightest.

'You do like him though, don't you?' Leila persisted.

'I do, but that's all I'm going to say on the subject. And please tell me you brought me some clothes to change into? It's doing my head in wearing orange. I must look like a sarcastic Hare Krishna, except you probably don't get sarcastic ones – hard to chant and to sound those mini-cymbals in a sarcastic way.'

'If anyone could, you could – and I mean it as a compliment – but luckily for you I've brought your black dress,' Tor told her.

'Thank God for that! And how's Candy? She's not too upset, is she? God, poor girl, she's really been through it this holiday.'

'She's gone off with Dimitri to help out at the turtle project. She seems very happy and very relieved that Patrick's left,' Leila replied. 'I think she pretty much went off him from the moment they arrived in Greece. She's not the only one. I've been questioning why we were ever friends with him.'

'Because he wasn't always like this,' Frankie said quickly, and then seemed to want to change the subject as she asked Tor how she'd been getting on with Ed.

'We're really good. He's going to stay with me at the weekends. And . . .' Tor hesitated. There was absolutely no reason now not to tell Leila and Frankie her big news. She hadn't wanted to yesterday as they had all been so anxious about Frankie. 'And I've got something else to tell you.'

Leila and Frankie looked at her expectantly. Tor took a deep breath and announced: 'I'm pregnant.'

'Oh my God, Tor! That's brilliant!' Frankie exclaimed first as she flung her arms around her, then winced. 'Ouch, my shoulder!'

'Fantastic news, Tor!' Leila echoed.

Ellie chose this moment to bring out drinks and so there were more exclamations of delight, congratulations, hugs, questions about due dates and how she was feeling. Tor felt buoyed up by her friends' delight, optimistic and excited. She never should have tried to keep it a secret in the first place.

'It's all thanks to Candy. She realised that I was pregnant and when we talked she cut through all my wittering and told me that I should tell Ed. I had lost all sense of perspective until she said that.'

'That girl is a diamond,' Frankie commented. 'I adore her. Oh, Tor, I'm so happy for you! So anyone else got any other secrets that they'd like to share, as this seems to be confession time? Ellie?'

'Nothing on that scale, but I have just taken in

two more cats even though I promised Nikos that I wouldn't.'

'Ellie, that doesn't count, it's small fry. How about you, Leila? Any juicy secrets we should know about?'

Frankie had obviously intended this to be a light-hearted comment, but for some reason Leila looked taken aback and said defensively, 'No, why would I? I haven't got any secrets, you know me. My life is an open book. I wouldn't have time to have any secrets, for God's sake.'

There was a pause, then Frankie said quietly, 'Okay, Leila – I was only joking.'

Leila forced a smile. 'Well, there is something, but it's not really a secret – Tom and I have decided that we are going to try for another baby.'

More exclamations of delight, congratulations and hugs followed, but Tor had the feeling that Leila hadn't liked being put on the spot and she wondered why.

When Ed, Tom and Matt turned up around one and they all had lunch at the taverna, Tor was aware of Leila being unusually quiet. And yet everyone else was so happy, kicking back, glad to be without Patrick dragging them down with his nasty, bitter comments. Tom seemed more relaxed than she had seen him all holiday; Matt could hardly take his eyes off Frankie, and the two of them spent most of the meal teasing and bantering with each other.

There was definitely more than friendship between them, however hard Frankie tried to downplay it. Only Leila seemed subdued, but maybe she was imagining it – after all, it had been an emotionally charged twenty-four hours.

Ed put his arm around her. 'How are you feeling?' Since finding out about the pregnancy, he asked Tor this all the time.

She smiled at him. 'I'm feeling great. And at least we've got three more days of the holiday. I'm sorry I ruined the first part.'

'You didn't ruin it.'

'I very nearly did.' She kissed him lightly on the lips. 'I should have told you straight away. This whole thing has taught me that I have to be braver and come out and say what I feel, so here goes. Will you move in with me?'

Ed grinned. 'I'll let you know, I have to consider my options first.'

She swiped a punch at his shoulder.

The grin went. 'Of course I will, Tor, I want to look after you and the baby.'

Soon she would need to consider all the many practicalities: the store, the childcare, the working hours, the not having Ed around much in the week, and the really big things like becoming a mother and having a baby, but for now she wanted their time together to be happy and uncomplicated. And that was the wonderful thing about Ed; he wanted that too. Someone like Harry would have been calculating how the baby was going to impact on his life and his freedom, but Ed seemed to embrace everything about the news.

Tor was smiling as she made her way to the Ladies' – thankfully not to throw up for once – but she stopped when she saw Leila leaning over the sink and splashing water on her face. She turned round when she heard Tor. It looked as if she'd been crying.

Tor reached out and touched her arm. 'Hey, are you okay, Leila?'

'Fine.' She sniffed and brushed away the tears. 'It's just – oh, I don't know – those things that Patrick said were so awful . . . about me emasculating Tom and being such a nag. I can't seem to get them out of my head. Do you think Tom feels like that?'

Tor was stunned that Leila would be brooding about this; she had been so feisty when they had confronted Patrick. 'No, of course not! And forget about what he said anyway. He didn't mean any of it, he was lashing out at all of us. If anything he would be jealous of Tom, who has you and Gracie and a wonderful, happy life. What does Patrick have? Nothing except a very selfish, spoilt ex-girlfriend who may or may not be taking him back. He's lost his friends and he doesn't even have a job any more. He's really messed up.'

Leila bit her lip, she didn't seem convinced. 'Maybe. I just want everything to be good between Tom and me. I want it more than anything. It will be, won't it, Tor? I don't know what I would do without him.'

She had never seen Leila like this before. She was usually so confident, so in control, the person you went to when you were having a bad time. Tor put her arms round her friend and hugged her. 'Of course it will be, there's nothing to worry about. You've been through your bad patch. It's going to be great. It *is* great! That is such brilliant news about you and Tom trying for another baby. Imagine if we were pregnant together!'

'You're right, sorry. Just a funny five minutes.' Leila hugged her back. 'And I am so happy for you, Tor.' She finally managed a smile. 'This time next year you'll be a mother of one, and I might be a mother of two! We'll all have to come out here again.'

She was clearly doing her best to sound upbeat, but Tor felt she was putting on a front. When Frankie received a text message from Patrick, apologising for everything he had said and done, and saying that he was going to get help and sort himself out, only Leila seemed unmoved by it.

Chapter 34

Leila

It hadn't been Patrick's words that had upset her so much – vicious as they had been – she could deal with them, put them down to the alcohol and to the giant fuck-up his life had become. No, it had been Frankie's light-hearted quip that had really got under Leila's skin. She had been living in a bubble since the night out with Tom when they had decided to make another go of their marriage. Frankie's comment had effectively burst it and reminded her that she still had to deal with her toxic little secret. Now, back in her bedroom, where she was supposed to be gathering her things together for the beach, she found herself reaching once more for her phone. She had to confront the situation head on. It was naïve to pretend that the Jasper thing was going to go away. She would text him, telling him that she was very happy with her husband – she hadn't said this before because she hadn't been sure, but she was now – and she would repeat that she was sorry but she had made a mistake ever getting involved with him, and he had to leave her alone, once and for all.

This time there was just one message from him, but any sense of relief that he hadn't bombarded her with texts vanished as soon as she opened it. A picture filled the screen. For an instant her brain couldn't make sense of what she was seeing as she was so shocked, so unprepared for what confronted her. It was a picture of his dick. He had sent a picture of his erect dick. It made her want to be physically sick; she was repelled not just by the image but also by the thought that she'd ever been intimate with this man. Underneath the picture he had typed, *To remind you of me x.*

What warped universe was he living in? How did he think that this was in any way acceptable? Had she ever given the slightest indication that she would welcome something like this? No, never, she was certain. Ironically one of the dramas they had discussed working on together was about sexual harassment in the workplace – where a female boss pursues a younger male employee and sends him pictures of her naked body. They had both agreed how unsettling and threatening it would be to receive a picture like that.

'Mummy! Can we go now!' Gracie burst into the bedroom, already kitted out in her sunsuit and hat. The juxtaposition of her beautiful, innocent daughter with this sordid text was like a sucker punch to Leila, but she quickly deleted the message and once more stuffed the phone back in the drawer.

'I'm ready, darling,' she declared, taking Gracie's hand.

It was beautiful on the beach, and for the first time practically all holiday it was just the three of them there.

'This is all I want,' Tom told her as they watched Gracie building sandcastles, blissfully content. 'My family to be together again, and happy.'

He put his arm round Leila. She rested her head on his shoulder. 'That's all I want too.'

It should have been one of those moments she would look back on in the future, a moment when they were truly close. Instead the feeling of guilt had returned, tainting everything. Shouldn't she tell Tom? Confess what she had done? Would it make them stronger if she did? Then she thought of the pain it would cause him. He would never forgive her.

'I love you, Leila, don't ever forget that.'

'I love you too.' She couldn't tell him.

Frankie

Frankie was lying by the pool, along with Ed and Tor. Matt was getting them all a drink. Since his revelation about how he'd felt on the night of Tom and Leila's wedding she had been dying to talk to him alone, but there hadn't been the right moment – it seemed to be the story of her life. This morning she had woken up still woozy from the painkillers, but Matt's words had been the first thing she had remembered. Every time she thought of him saying that he thought she was sexy, and loved spending time with her, she felt a sense of anticipation that made everything that had happened with Patrick feel like a bad dream. She picked up her book and failed to get to the bottom of the page. Instead she flipped over on to her stomach and lay staring out at sea for a few minutes, then sat up. She had to talk to Matt.

There was no sign of him in the kitchen. 'Matt,' she called out. No answer. She found him upstairs in his bedroom. His suitcase was on the bed, and he had changed out of his swim shorts into jeans and a shirt.

'I was about to come and find you,' he told her as she stood in the doorway, feeling a crashing sense of disappointment to see what he was doing.

'I've just come off the phone with my office. I've got to fly back tonight, there's a major problem with one of our biggest clients. I have to deal with it personally.'

'Oh.' WTF!

He gave a rueful smile. 'Aren't you going to say that it's only what you would have expected? And what's so important that it can't wait? Because you'd be right.'

'Nope. I think that, of course, but I won't say it.'

'Go on, I could do with a bit of teasing from you. I'm gutted that I've got to go.' He threw the pile of t-shirts he was holding into the suitcase and walked over to her.

'I felt we were just starting to get to know each other better. And I want nothing more than to stay here and carry on doing that.'

He was giving her his most intense blue-eyed gaze. It was working.

'Yeah.'

'That's all I'm going to get from you? God, you're a tough audience, Frankie.'

She shrugged. 'You're the one who's leaving.' She was not going to give *anything* away.

'Regretfully. So regretfully. Do you want to know how much?' He had moved closer now.

Very slightly she moved her head and that was all the encouragement Matt needed to kiss her – a soft, tentative kiss at first that grew into a deep, probing, passionate kiss – where they both seemed to be signalling all the things that they wanted to do, longed to do. It was a staggeringly intense kiss that sent ripples of desire through Frankie. She abandoned her intention not to give anything away.

'God, I want you, Frankie. Want you so much,' he told her between kisses. 'Will you promise to see me when you get back?'

She couldn't resist those blue eyes. But neither

could she resist teasing him. 'I'll have to see where I can fit you in between Jonas and Hector. They're very demanding.'

Matt grinned. 'Yogi Boy and Fish Finger are no match for me.' He kissed her neck, then paused to say, 'Actually Hector's taken up with Alena, who shares his passion for sardines and has no sense of smell. She even has a sardine tattooed on her ankle. And he's given her his blue sweater. I think it's love.'

'That's not fair! I could never compete with Sardine Girl! And that sweater was *mine*.'

'I'll buy you one that doesn't stink of fish.'

She laughed, and then boldly put her arms round his neck and pulled him close to her. 'Do you really have to go now? Really, *really*? Like you'll lose your job if you don't?'

His body was telling her one thing, but he sighed and said reluctantly, 'I really, *really* have to go.' He gave a wicked grin. 'Just when I was going to show you all the many, *many* things I can do in a single bed.'

She felt another ripple of desire that made her want to push him back on the bed so he could demonstrate . . .

'What? With Our Lady looking at us?' She gestured at the kitsch Virgin Mary picture over the bed.

'I think she would approve. We've waited long enough.'

A car horn beeped from the drive. Matt kissed Frankie again. 'That's my taxi. I'll call you when I get back.'

'Won't you be going straight to the office to break someone's balls or whatever you say? Incidentally, what do you say when it's a woman? You can't say break someone's pussy, that sounds either too porno or a bit too Mrs Slocombe.'

Banter to hide how much she was going to miss him. How ironic when watching him leave would have been all she wanted at the beginning of the holiday.

'You say balls. And I *really* don't want to go. Will you say goodbye to everyone for me? And promise that you won't give Jonas and Hector a second chance? I want you all to myself, Frankie.' Another kiss and he was gone.

Chapter 35

Candy

Now Patrick was out of the picture, Candy felt as if her holiday was finally starting. No doubt he was back in his swanky Islington apartment, with his ex-girlfriend. He had left without saying goodbye to anybody, having behaved so incredibly badly, said such terrible things. She wondered if he fully realised, or whether he was even now drinking himself into oblivion. Whatever, he had to take responsibility for his behaviour. She had little sympathy for him as he had been the one systematically to ruin his life. Frankie had showed her his text and seemed ready to believe that he was going to sort himself out, Candy was less easily convinced. It would take more than a text to persuade her. Easy to send a text when it was actions that counted. But she didn't want to waste any more time thinking about Patrick.

She had spent the last two days with Dimitri. Ah, lovely, fit, sexy Dimitri, who made her heart beat faster, made her want to be reckless and pack in working in the beauty salon and move to Greece. Of course, she wouldn't – she had her sisters to think of. They had spent most of the time on the beach together, sunbathing, cooling off in the sea, stealing kisses. Yes, lots of kisses but nothing more. She had jumped straight into bed with Patrick and look where that had got her. Somehow she wanted it to be special with Dimitri, to mean something. But tonight was the last night of the holiday and, well, she was tempted. Very tempted.

Her phone beeped with a message and she instantly picked it up.

Will be with you in half an hour. Can't wait. Dxx.

Nor could she.

She wandered out of her bedroom and through to the kitchen where Tom and Ed were hard at work making dinner, accompanied by the sound of *The Beach Boys' Good Vibrations*. Yeah, that pretty much summed up how she was feeling now.

Ed was in the charge of the starters – aubergine and mint bruschetta, and baked mushrooms stuffed with ricotta; Tom the main course of asparagus and pea risotto. Everything smelt delicious. She reached out and sneaked a piece of bread.

'Oi, young lady, don't spoil your dinner!' Tom exclaimed. 'You can take these out to the others.' He handed her a bowl of shiny black olives and one of pistachio nuts.

God, she was going to miss everything about being here. She didn't want to think about her tiny flat and the undercooked baked potatoes for supper, the dead-end job, and above all no Dimitri . . . She felt a pang of sadness – this time tomorrow night she would be back home.

Tor and Frankie were outside. They had lit candles on the table, and in the silver hurricane lanterns arranged around the terrace, and on the steps leading to the pool. Candy paused in the doorway for a second, taking everything in, wanting to remember every single detail. Then she sat down next to Frankie who instantly poured her a glass of champagne. It seemed incredible to think that just two weeks ago Frankie would have been the last person she would have wanted to sit next to. It was no exaggeration to say that Candy now saw her as a real friend, and someone she could trust completely.

'Get this down you, girl,' Frankie told her, raising her glass and clinking it against Candy's. 'Cheers. To new friends. And when we get back to Brighton we're going to look into how you can get on to a midwifery degree. You'll need to go back to college and do A-levels or NVQs, but you should still be able to do that and work part-time. It should be manageable.'

Candy had a feeling that Frankie was going to be like a dog with a bone over the course. But maybe that's what she needed, and she was touched that Frankie would care enough to help her.

'Thanks, it's been great meeting you.' She grinned, 'Even if you were well fucking scary at first! Scared the knickers off me, in fact, with your icy stare and your sarcastic comments. The Woman in Black.'

Frankie screwed up her face. 'God, was I that bad? Sorry, I was such an old cow.'

'Yep,' Tor put in. 'And you missed out judgmental, Candy.'

'Ouch! I know, I know.'

'Ah, well, we're friends now,' Candy commented, and once more clinked her glass against Frankie's. 'D'you know, I think you might have a bit of a tan,' she continued. 'You're definitely not as ghostly white as you were. Have you been nicking my Fake Bake?'

'It's a Matt glow,' Tor teased. 'He just called her, and that's on top of who knows how many emails they've been exchanging. Was it his third call today? And him an important lawyer and all, with so many deals to oversee.'

Candy expected an eye roll from Frankie. Instead she replied, 'Fourth actually. And six emails.'

'Wow, that is keen! He must really like you, Frankie.'

'There's no need to sound so surprised. Believe

it or not, I'm not entirely unloveable.' But she was smiling.

'So when are you going to see him?'

'I don't know, I'll fix something up when I get back. I've got masses of work to do before the beginning of term. It's always a really full-on time for me.'

It was Candy's turn to be like a dog with a bone. 'It doesn't take long to go up on the train to London does it? Or he could come down. You don't want to play all hard to get. You want to see that man. And the rest! He's bloody gorgeous – I mean, not my type, but gorgeous.'

'Yeah, it would be too ironic if you and me fell for the same man again.' Frankie sighed. 'I hope Patrick is okay, wherever and whoever he's with.'

'I don't know if I can be as forgiving as you, Frankie.' The memory of Patrick's sneering face as he'd laid into her was still all too vivid for Candy.

'I wouldn't expect you to be. He treated you very badly.'

'Yeah, well, it's over. So when we get back to Brighton, I expect you to arrange that date with Matt. I'm going to be on your case.'

'Persistent, aren't you?'

'Very.'

Ed came out to tell them that the starter was nearly ready and Candy offered to go and let Leila know. She ran upstairs expecting to find her reading to Gracie, but the little girl was on her own, sitting cross-legged on her bed, setting out a tea party for her toys. Candy stopped to say goodnight and to have a sip of imaginary hot chocolate from one of the tiny plastic cups,

'Where's your mummy?' she asked.

'In her bedroom.'

She found Leila sitting on the edge of her bed, staring into space.

'Are you feeling okay? It's time for dinner.'

'I'm fine, thanks.'

She didn't seem fine; she seemed distracted.

'I've just got a bit of a headache.' She stood up and tucked her hair behind her ears. 'Do you by any chance know how to block phone numbers? I keep getting all these spam texts.'

'It depends on what sort of phone you've got. I did it for my friend when her shit of an ex kept bombarding her with obscene messages and pictures.'

Leila seemed to change her mind. 'Oh, don't worry. I'll just delete them and sort it out when I get back home.'

'It's no trouble, honestly.'

'No really, forget I said anything. Come on, we're missing out on the champagne, I don't trust the others not to guzzle it all.'

'That was delicious,' Dimitri declared as he finished the last of the risotto on his plate – his second helping.

'Tom is the best at making risotto,' Leila said. 'I

don't order it in restaurants as it's never as good as the ones he makes.'

'But you've left half of yours,' he commented.

'I know, sorry, I've still got this wretched headache. But it was lovely, darling.' She smiled at him. 'I think we should have a toast, to friendship and love.'

'That's very profound of you,' Frankie teased. 'Not just to the holiday?'

'That too, but it feels like so much has happened in such a short space of time.' Leila held up her glass. 'To friendship and love.'

'To friendship and love,' everyone repeated, clinking glasses with each other.

And soon this will all be over, Candy thought to herself, and catching Dimitri's eye managed a smile. He had already given her his Skype details, his email address and they were Facebook friends. He had insisted they would stay in touch, that he would come and see her in the autumn and that she must come over to Athens. But would she really see him again? It seemed a lot to ask of a holiday romance . . . too much perhaps. She should probably just put it down to experience.

'And now I must excuse myself and Candy as I promised I would take her to Turtle Beach,' Dimitri said unexpectedly as he stood up.

That was news to her, but she welcomed any chance to be alone with him.

*

Fifteen minutes later they had reached the turning for the beach, but Dimitri kept going.

'Hey, shouldn't we have gone that way?' Candy shouted to make herself heard over the over the putt-putt of the moped's engine. Dimitri pulled over to the side of the road and turned to face her.

'You didn't seriously think that I wanted to spend my last night with you looking at turtles, along with all the other volunteers and moody Naida?'

It was hard to look sexy in a white crash helmet but Dimitri pulled it off. His eyes were alight with desire and longing.

'Maybe I did!' she teased. But right now she couldn't care less about the cute endangered reptiles taking their first tentative steps towards the sea and swimming away to wherever turtles went.

'You will see plenty of them next year when you spend the summer with me.'

'Will I?'

He didn't answer but attempted a kiss that caused their crash helmets to bump together.

'Okay, let's go back to your place,' she murmured. 'Bugger the turtles.'

'That's probably not the slogan we'll be putting on our t-shirts. But for now, I agree.'

Chapter 36

Leila

As soon as Leila walked through the front door she was hit by the smell – a horrible musty odour of decay and rot.

'God, what's that?' Tom exclaimed. 'I hope we haven't had a leak somewhere.'

'I don't know,' she replied, dumping her bag in the hallway. 'You check the living room and I'll do the kitchen.' The feeling of foreboding that she'd had since Jasper had sent her that picture intensified. Something bad was going to happen, she just knew it, knew it in her gut. The holiday was over.

She walked briskly along the hall to the sound of Gracie swinging on the banisters and shouting, 'Yuck! Mummy, what's that bad smell?'

Switching on the kitchen lights, she froze. There on the oak table arranged in all the vases she owned were four bouquets of lilies, roses and freesias in various stages of wilting and decay. The water in the vases had turned a slimy, murky green. This was the something bad, here in her house. There was only one person she knew who was capable of making such a theatrical and threatening gesture. She imagined Jasper plotting it out like a scene from one of his plays, manipulating all his characters into doing exactly what he wanted.

She caught sight of a neatly handwritten note in the middle of the table. It was from her neighbour, who had watered the garden while they were away.

There were three more of these but I had to chuck them. I've left the envelopes on the side. Hope you had a fab hols! Can't wait to hear all about it! Hxx

A chirpy note from Hazel who had no idea what she had unleashed by accepting the bouquets.

'Who the hell are these from?' Tom asked, wandering into the kitchen and making a beeline for the pile of post, thoughtfully stacked up by Hazel.

'I've no idea. Maybe they've been sent by mistake. Maybe they're from an actor who wants a part. But I'm not open to bribery – not with dead flowers anyway. It would have to be a crate of champagne, Vintage Bollinger at the very least.' Leila hoped Tom was too tired to pick up on how false and strained her voice sounded.

He finished flipping through the post.

'Well, I'm guessing they're for you. Aren't you going to find out who they're from? Bit odd that they would send them when you were away, and so many of them.' He ripped off one of the tiny envelopes pinned to one of the bouquets and gave it to her, waiting for her to open it. It felt as if he had handed her a live grenade. Leila dropped it back on the table.

'Ugh! I've got to get some air in here, that vile smell is making me feel sick.'

She unlocked the back door and stepped outside. The night air already had a hint of autumn chill to it. It was usually her favourite season, but now this too felt like a threat. The summer was over; it was time to face reality, and Jasper.

When she went back inside Tom was sorting out Gracie and getting her ready for bed and Leila took the opportunity to get a bin bag and shove every single bouquet and envelope into it, including the one that was still lying on the table like an accusation. Then she carried the bag and dumped it in the wheelie bin outside. *That's what I think of your gesture and of you, Jasper.*

'So who were they from?' Tom asked later as she got into bed. Of course he would want to know. She would too in his position.

She lowered her head, unable to meet his gaze. 'This writer called Jasper. He's very ambitious. Bit of a wanker, to be honest. He knows that we've got a season on the Brontës coming up and he's desperate to be part of it.'

'I'm surprised he hadn't done his homework properly and found out when you were away. He must have wasted so much money.'

'Like I said, he's a bit of a wanker. I don't want to work with him again anyway. He wasn't the easiest person to have around. Very arrogant. An egomaniac.'

'Oh? He wrote those last two plays you produced, didn't he? I thought you said he'd been brilliant to work with. Inspiring, I seem to remember. Hugely talented.'

Fuck. All the lies were coming back to haunt her. 'He started out well, but became difficult. I probably didn't want to go on about it.' She snuggled up next to Tom. 'We had a brilliant holiday, didn't we?'

He kissed her. 'We did. Love you.' He switched off the light.

'You too.'

Tom fell asleep immediately while Leila lay awake, trying to work out what she should do. She would have to confront Jasper face to face. She should have done it as soon as he began sending the texts, but she had been too cowardly. She was paying the price for that now.

She finally fell asleep around half-past four, and as a result slept until ten. When she padded downstairs she discovered that Tom and Gracie had gone out, possibly to buy food, but they hadn't left a note. Tom had gathered the vases in the sink and filled them with soapy water to try and get rid of the green scum marks. Hating the sight of them, she quickly emptied them and stacked them in the dishwasher, not caring if they were dishwasher safe or not. She felt out of sorts, on edge. She made herself a cup of tea – black because there was no milk – had a shower, unpacked, loaded the dirty clothes into the washing machine. And all the time there was that feeling of foreboding gnawing away inside of her. Two hours later on there was still no sign of Tom and Gracie. Where the hell were they?

She was just about to call Tom when she heard the sound of his keys in the door. Relieved, she walked into the hall. But he was alone and he wasn't carrying any shopping bags.

'Hey, I wondered where you were. And where's Gracie?'

'I dropped her off at my mum's.'

'D'you want a coffee? We don't have any milk but you're okay with black, aren't you?' There was something about Tom's serious expression and flat tone that was making her feel anxious, as if she needed to fill all the silences, as if she needed to stop him from saying anything.

In the kitchen Leila only got as far as filling the kettle when Tom said quietly, 'I don't want a coffee.

I want you to tell me the real reason Jasper sent you those flowers.'

There it was, the question that she had been dreading. She forced herself to look at Tom, make eye contact, appear as if she had nothing to hide. But she already knew that she wouldn't succeed.

'I told you, he wants to write one of the new dramas.' Her voice sounded brittle. Liar, liar, liar.

Tom put his head in his hands. 'One of the things I always loved you for was your honesty and the fact that you're a terrible liar.' He looked up at her. 'But, God, right now I wish you were a better liar. I went through the bin this morning and found this.' He pulled out a white envelope from his pocket, opened it and began reading, struggling to keep it together as he read out Jasper's words: '"I can't wait to see you, Leila. I want you. I long for you, I must—"'

'Please don't read any more,' she cut across him. *'Please.'*

Tom slammed his hand down on the table. 'Then fucking tell me the truth! Stop treating me like an idiot.'

She was shaking as she sat down at the kitchen table, the table where they'd had so many meals together, shared good times, bad times, indifferent times and now this. The past had caught up with her. She clasped her hands together. 'Whatever happened it doesn't change the way I feel about you. I love you, Tom.'

'You had an affair with him, didn't you?'

'No, it wasn't like that. I slept with him once, and as soon as I did I regretted it. I told him it was over then, but he kept on sending me texts. I don't want anything to do with him. Please, Tom, I made a mistake, a huge mistake but it was at the time when we weren't getting on. I felt lost and—'

'Don't fucking blame this on me!' Tom shouted, standing up. 'You were the one who fucked someone else! And all the time I felt desperate because we were getting on so badly and I thought it was all down to me.'

His anger and hurt was like a wave roaring towards her. She didn't know how to stop it, how to make it right. All her words sounded so feeble and self-serving.

'I'm sorry. I'm really, truly sorry.'

'Why? Because you've been found out? Christ, Leila, I believed we had a second chance on holiday, but you've ruined everything.'

'It doesn't *have* to ruin everything. I don't want to be with Jasper, I want to be with you. What happened on holiday wasn't a lie, it was the truth, we do have that second chance. I love you, Tom.'

'Yeah, well, you're got a funny way of showing it, Leila. I'll be staying with a friend until I decide what I want to do.'

'Don't go, Tom. We can work this out, I promise.' She could hardly get the words out, she was crying so hard.

'I've had enough of your promises for a while. I'm going to pack some things. Gracie can stay at my mum's tonight, I don't want her being upset by any of this. I'll drop her off tomorrow morning.'

She remained where she was, listening to the sound of Tom gathering his things together upstairs, then unable to bear it any longer, she went and sat at the bottom of the stairs, clutching on to the banister. She got up when she heard him on the landing and watched him walk down, carrying his laptop and a rucksack. She tried to take some comfort from the fact he hadn't taken a suitcase. There wasn't much to be had.

'Please, Tom, I'm begging you not to go.'

But he walked past her without a word and Leila could only watch him shut the door behind him.

Chapter 37

Frankie

Frankie opened her front door to sign for a delivery still in her PJs, at nine o'clock. She was going to have to start getting up earlier. In four days' time she would be back at school, and by nine o'clock would be ten minutes into her first lesson. PJs were not such a good look for that.

'Interesting parcel you've got,' the courier said cheerily, handing her a triangular-shaped package.

'I've no idea what it is, I'm not expecting anything.'

'Surprises . . . always the best things.'

And Frankie was about to say that she hated surprises when she stopped herself. Her post-holiday resolution was to be more open to things and people.

She ripped open the paper to find a layer of bubble wrap and then a table tennis bat – a snazzy red number with a black-and-red handle. It could only be from Matt. She smiled as she opened the accompanying note.

Looking forward to playing with you tonight. Missing Greece, missing the sun, missing you. Matt x

Instantly she felt a rush of lust. Was it wrong to feel a sexual frisson from holding a table tennis bat?

'That is so sweet!' Candy exclaimed when Frankie met her for coffee a couple of hours later and told her about the gift.

They were sitting in one of Frankie's favourite cafés, a large airy space, with quirky photographs of Brighton on the walls. She and Candy had managed to nab one of the much-coveted squashy leather sofas. They were supposed to be checking out midwifery degrees on Frankie's laptop, but gossip had to take precedence.

'He'll probably have you playing strip table tennis.'

An eye roll from Frankie. 'Please – can't you imagine everything wobbling around?'

A smirk from Candy. 'I bet his everything won't be wobbling around, it'll be rock hard.'

Frankie didn't reply, she suddenly had an image of Matt stark naked. Even playing table tennis and brandishing a bat and a ping-pong ball, he would still look sexy. She imagined lying back on the table, Matt bearing down on her with his rock hard— Phew! Since her last encounter with him and that kiss, she hadn't been able to stop thinking about him. Specifically of what she would like to do with him. It was a long list . . .

'Sorry, that sounds like I'm perving after him, and I promise I'm not. So what time are you going up?'

Frankie shrugged, as if it was hardly significant, as if she wasn't counting the hours. 'Sixish, I guess.'

'Why are you sounding so low-key?'

Because mixed with her desire to see him and the rest . . . she was horribly nervous. 'I don't know, maybe it was just a holiday thing – not that anything happened.'

'Bollocks! You two had such strong chemistry between you. Every time you were together it was like the air had turned electric.'

'I think you're mixing your sciences there,' Frankie joked.

'Shut up, you know I'm right!'

Candy twirled a strand of hair around her finger. She had replaced the red with a rich brunette that suited her. She had also ditched the fake lashes and the heavy make-up, all in preparation for applying for her midwifery course. The fake nails were still there, though, in all their white-tipped glory.

'I told you those would have to go,' Frankie commented.

Candy sighed, 'Yeah, I know. I'm going to leave

it until the last possible moment, though, before I get them taken off.'

'And have you heard from Dimitri?'

'We Skyped each other last night. He's back in Athens. He's really pleased that I'm applying for the course. I guess it sounds better to Mummy and Daddy that he's dating a student and not a beautician.'

'All right, Ms Chip on Her Shoulder, you shouldn't be so down on yourself.'

'You're one to talk, Ms Play Hard to Get. Straight out of the school of treat them mean. And don't think that I don't realise what you've just done, changing the subject. Back to Matt, please, and what are you going to wear for your date?'

'I was thinking of my black skater dress with my black ankle boots.'

'Black!' Candy sounded disgusted. 'Always black with you. Nope, I do not approve. Drink your latte and get that pain au chocolat down you, because as soon as we've filled in my form, lady, we are going shopping!'

Yes, Frankie had decided to ease up on the no carbs rule. Sometimes a pain au chocolat was exactly what you needed, and a friend like Candy to make you do something different. Which wasn't to say that their subsequent shopping trip went smoothly. They argued over every single garment Candy picked up – too mutton, too glitzy, too short – and every single one that Frankie picked up – too boring, too safe, too black. It was only when she was about to give up that finally they found a dress they both agreed on in French Connection, a stunning fitted red crepe number, with a zip at the back and a slit at the neck to give a hint of cleavage.

'Perfect,' Candy told her when she emerged uncertainly from the changing room. 'Absolutely bloody perfect. And now I have to go to work and wax a few fannies. Are you in need of my services?'

Frankie rolled her eyes. 'All good to go, but thanks for the offer.'

She was still smiling as she strolled back to her flat. She had almost arrived home when her mobile rang. It was Leila. She was crying so hard Frankie hardly recognised her voice.

'Tom's left me. Please come round. I don't know what to do.'

A distraught-looking Leila opened the door to Frankie some twenty minutes later. Her eyes were puffy from crying, mascara streaked her cheeks, her hair was unbrushed and she was still wearing her pyjamas. Frankie had never seen her friend in such a state. On seeing Frankie she burst into more tears.

'Sorry,' was all she kept saying.

Frankie hugged her and took her into the living room where the blinds were still drawn. Leila sat hunched on the sofa and between sobs blurted out what had gone on. Frankie was stunned. She'd had absolutely no idea, had never suspected, not for a second.

'I'm a dreadful person. You're shocked, aren't you?'

'I admit that I am shocked, but not because I'm judging you. It happened and it must have happened for a reason.'

Leila covered her face with her hands. 'It happened because I was stupid and selfish, and I've ruined my marriage and I've destroyed my family . . . and it was all over a man who I hate.' She looked up at Frankie. 'I hate him.' And promptly burst into tears again.

Frankie made her a cup of tea, ran her a bath, tidied up the kitchen, emptied the washing machine, wondered if Tom could forgive Leila . . . After her bath she seemed a little more together; she had put on clean clothes and washed her hair. She instantly checked her phone when she walked into the kitchen and Frankie could see her disappointment when there was nothing from Tom.

'He's supposed to be dropping Gracie round later. She starts school next week. This is a great beginning for her, isn't it?' Tears again.

'What can I do, Frankie, to make him see that it was a mistake, that it didn't mean anything?'

'Oh, God, Leila, I don't know. He probably needs time to work things out. He's bound to be hurt and angry.'

405

'Do you think he will ever forgive me?'

Frankie thought of Tom who was so straight-down-the-line honest about everything, who had always impressed her with his loyalty to Leila and to his friends. It would be a big ask.

'I don't know. In time, it's not something you can expect instantly. I'm sorry, Leila, I'm not saying anything helpful.'

'Just having you here is helpful. Will you stay? I don't think I could bear to be on my own.'

'You know I will.' There were so many times that Leila had been there for her.

Tom dropped Gracie off but didn't stay. Leila did her very best to keep it together while she made Gracie tea, bathed her and read her bedtime story, but Frankie could see what an immense effort it was.

As soon as Gracie was settled Leila came downstairs into the kitchen where Frankie had prepared a snack of pitta, hummus and salad. Leila ignored the food and instead poured herself a large glass of red wine. Getting drunk wasn't going to make anything better, but right now it was possibly what she needed. Frankie poured herself a smaller glass. It was likely to be a long night.

It was after one by the time she finally managed to persuade Leila to go to bed and she suddenly remembered where she should have been tonight, in her red dress. Fuck! She pulled her phone out of her bag and saw all the missed calls from Matt and the text he had finally sent at nine o'clock.

Where are you? I'm trying not to take this personally, but it's hard not to when the woman you've been longing to see stands you up. Call me, it doesn't matter how late xx

She selected his number.

'Hey, Frankie,' he said sleepily. 'What happened to you?'

She quickly detailed what had gone on. 'I'm sorry, I should have called but it's been full on here, and I thought Tom might have told you.'

'He hasn't been in touch. I'll call him in the morning. Shit, not Tom and Leila, my favourite couple. I don't suppose there's any chance you could come up and see me tomorrow?'

She really, *really* wanted to but she couldn't leave Leila, not like this. 'I can't, and next week's going to be difficult as I'm back at school.'

The earliest they could meet was next Friday. It seemed a very long way away.

Chapter 38

Tor

'Shall we go for a zombie theme this Hallowe'en or vampires again? Zombies are hot right now, though it has to be said not nearly as glam as your cheeky bloodsucker.'

Tor looked up from the computer screen to see Spencer, her assistant, in full zombie get-up. He was working a putrefying green face, a fake eye falling out of its socket, dried blood dribbling out of the side of his mouth, a filthy blood-stained bandage around his head. Spencer absolutely adored Hallowe'en and took it very seriously indeed. The beginning of September was about the time he began planning for it even though Tor refused to allow him to display anything in the window until October, she didn't care what every other store was doing.

'Well, it's all in the mad stare, isn't it? You could

wear an evening dress and still be a zombie, with the right amount of fake blood . . . maybe an axe stuck in your chest.'

'I guess – so what's it going to be?'

She shrugged. 'I don't mind, it's up to you.' Ordinarily Tor would mind very much but she had too many other things to think about. Top of her list was the baby – she had her scan this afternoon – and then there was the bombshell news about Leila and Tom, and Ed was moving into her flat tonight. Zombies versus vampires didn't exert the same hold on her as it did on Spencer. She expected him to be overjoyed at being given the opportunity to choose. Instead he seemed oddly deflated.

'Are you sure? Normally we argue over this for days until you get your own way.'

'Well, I'm cool with zombies. Just remember not to mention it to Frankie, she hates them. They're the only things that give her the heebie-jeebies.' She was keen to get back to ordering stock, but Spencer remained where he was. 'Is there anything else?'

'You tell me, Tor. You've been acting differently since you got back from Greece. You barely checked the sales figures, you didn't notice my window display and you don't care if we go for vampires or zombies! Please don't tell me you're selling the store? I love working with you . . . for you . . . I'll never get another job. Only you understand my foibles. And what about Maud? Who's going to employ her? I don't want you to feel guilty – all right, I *do* want you to feel guilty. We need you. Please don't sell! I'll take a pay cut. I'll work longer hours. I'll do the cleaning as well. I'll get you a latte every single morning from that café you like, I'll—'

It was quite something watching a zombie make such a passionate entreaty.

'Spencer! Will you shut up for once and listen to me!'

He looked stunned by her sounding so assertive.

'I don't know where you've got the idea that I'm selling the boutique. I have been distracted but that's because of something different.' She stopped; she hadn't planned to tell anyone else until after the scan.

'Something good or something bad?' Spencer persisted.

Oh, for God's sake! She wouldn't get any peace until she came out with it.

'I'm pregnant.'

Her disclosure achieved something that she had never thought possible – Spencer was actually lost for words.

Then he shouted out, 'I'm going to be an uncle! Fucking ace news!' He hugged her and raced straight into the back room. 'Maud, get knitting, Tor is going to have a baby!'

Tor lay back and winced as the sonographer, a young woman called Ruth, gently rubbed cold gel on to her tummy and then moved the hand-held device to and fro. She and Ed were riveted to the screen and its black-and-white images – was that the kidney bean's leg? An arm? A head? They had no idea and Ruth was disconcertingly silent as she paused to take measurements and then moved the device around again.

'Is everything okay?' Ed asked anxiously after a few minutes.

Ruth stopped what she was doing and looked at Tor. Oh, God, she was going to say that the baby had died. She should have known that the pregnancy was too good to be true. Ed reached out for Tor's hand as tears filled her eyes.

'I just wanted to check all the details. Congratulations, you're having twins! From what I can tell at this stage – and I estimate that you are between twelve and thirteen weeks – both babies look absolutely fine.

Twins! Tor couldn't even begin to imagine that. Ruth had delivered the news as if it was the most normal announcement, when it was the most astounding, astonishing thing Tor had ever heard in her life. Ever! Twins! Two babies!

For a second Ed was quiet then he burst out with, 'Wow, that's brilliant! Tor, we're having twins, how incredible is that?' And as if to answer all the worries that were bubbling up in her mind, he kissed her.

'It's going to be okay, Tor. It's going to be amazing.'

411

Chapter 39

Leila

Tom had been gone over a week now. He wouldn't talk to her or reply to her texts and emails where she poured out her feelings, told him how much she loved him and how much she wanted to be with him. She had no idea where he was staying. Leila supposed she deserved that. She spent the first three nights after he'd gone downing bottles of wine – until the shame of Gracie catching her throwing up in the morning stopped her.

Drawing on reserves of strength that she didn't know she possessed, she put on the bravest of faces for her daughter; she went to her office and went through the motions of working; she organised play dates for Gracie, cooked tea for her and her friends; researched and found out where there were some kittens for sale, took Gracie to chose two – a black one and a tortoiseshell, exactly as she had wanted. She had a frenzy of house tidying and got rid of all the piles of magazines that drove Tom mad and whole bagfuls of clothes that she never wore. She functioned.

She was dying inside. People said they were 'devastated' too easily; they said it when they really weren't. She was devastated. She felt as if her very being had been ripped out. Nothing made sense without Tom. Jasper the bastard continued to send her texts, telling her that he had to see her. There would be one every morning, taunting her when she switched on her phone, even though she had told him to leave her alone.

Wednesday was Gracie's first morning at school. Leila made sure she got up extra early so she could take pictures of her, make her favourite breakfast of pancakes, yoghurt and fruit, and generally make a fuss of her. At eight-twenty the doorbell rang. It was Tom. As soon as she saw him standing there Leila wanted so badly to put her arms around him. She ached for him.

But he barely looked at her.

'Hi, I hope it's okay but I wanted to take Gracie to school?' He paused. 'I thought we should both be there for our daughter.'

Leila ignored the judgmental tone. 'That would be great, she'll love that.'

He remained standing where he was. It was all wrong to be asking her own husband to come inside his own house but she was going to have to do it.

413

'Come in, she's playing with the kittens.'

That had his attention. 'You got them then?'

'Yes, she's been dying to tell you, but she wanted to surprise you.'

Gracie raced down the stairs at that moment and grabbed Tom's hand, desperate to show off Buzz and Jessie Mk 2.

They bumped into Polly and her daughter India on the walk to school, and while the two little girls chatted to each other Tom talked to Polly the entire way, making Leila feel like an outcast as she walked behind them, trying not show how much she minded. After all, she had caused this; she couldn't blame him.

'Who's going to pick me up?' Gracie asked when it was time to say goodbye.

Leila was about to say that she would, but Tom got there first. 'It'll be me, Gracie, and we'll go to the park with India, if you like.'

'Can't Mummy come too?'

'Mummy's probably got to work,' Tom answered for her.

Leila cried all the way back to the house: tears because her daughter starting school seemed like such a milestone, tears because of Tom. The text message from Tor with her incredible news about having twins made her cry even more. All her own excitement about the prospect of having another baby . . . all gone.

Unable to settle to any work, she went into the living room and pulled out one of the photo albums. There were the pictures of her pregnant, looking radiantly happy out for a walk by the sea with Tor and Leila, two weeks before Gracie was born; the Demi Moore-style shot that Tom had taken of her in black-and-white, where he had wanted her to look sexy and moody but she had been giggling because she could feel Gracie squirming away and it felt completely ridiculous to be standing there naked, except for her strategically placed arms; maybe only Hollywood stars could pull off sexy and moody when they were up the duff; then the pictures of a newborn Gracie, her scrunched-up face still covered in vernix; of Leila holding her daughter in her arms, with Tom next to her, both of them smiling away and looking insanely knackered after the twelve-hour labour; Gracie's first outing in a sling strapped to her proud dad, eyes wide open; looking stunned by her first bath . . . All her firsts shared by both parents; Leila wondered how much longer that would last.

Chapter 40

Frankie

Friday evening on the six-nineteen train to London, Frankie felt as jittery and jumpy as a teenager. She couldn't settle down to anything. She had abandoned her magazine and paper, and couldn't even listen to music. All she could think about was that in less than two hours' time she would be seeing Matt again. At his house. The what ifs were whizzing round in her head. What if she didn't feel the same way about him? What if he didn't feel the same way about her? What if she stayed? What if she didn't?

She had her back-up plan in place. If it didn't work out then she would have one drink, make an excuse and head off – either to Brighton or to her friend Em in Archway. Will they? Won't they? murmured the train. Christ, she was going mad if she was imagining an inanimate object having thoughts. It was one of her pet hates to see buses displaying the sign, 'Sorry, I'm not in service'. She always had to fight the urge to shout, 'It's a fucking bus, not a human!'

She checked her phone and saw there was a message from Candy.

Hope you're on the train. Hope you're wearing the red dress. Hope you have a gr8 night. Want to hear all about it xx

Matt opened the door to her wearing a black t-shirt and jeans, and all the what ifs went out of Frankie's head as a rush of lust took over and she was left with the single thought, *I want you.* He shut the door behind her and slipped off her jacket. She shivered at his touch.

'Stand still, I want to look at you.' He was giving her the blue intense stare.

'Red – I can't believe I've never seen you wear it before. You look stunning, Frankie. Beautiful.'

Somehow she silenced the inner voice that wanted to deflect the compliment.

He ducked down to kiss her, a hi there kiss, that became a want you, must have you kiss, and Frankie who had spent so long resisting, found herself murmuring, 'Where's your bedroom?'

He took her hand and led her upstairs. She kicked off her heels on the way. He had already lit candles on the mantelpiece and she could have commented that that seemed contrived but she didn't, she appreciated the gesture. And then he was unzipping the red dress, it was falling to the ground, she was pulling off his t-shirt, unbuckling his belt. He was naked, gorgeous, they were on the bed, and Frankie, who had always been the one in control with men before, abandoned herself to his touch, and abandoned herself to him.

Afterwards they lay in each other's arms, a first for Frankie who usually couldn't wait to extricate herself after having sex with someone because it had never felt right. But this felt perfect. She wanted to wrap herself round Matt, never let him go.

'What are you thinking?' he asked, lightly kissing her.

She wasn't ready to reveal that, so she kissed him back and murmured, 'Nothing, just being.'

'Oh? Because I was thinking that was bloody amazing and I want to spend all weekend making love with you, kissing you, tasting you, pleasing you, fucking you.'

'Yeah, that sounds good to me.' It sounded off-the-scale incredible to her . . . but she couldn't resist teasing him, 'So when are we going to fit in that game of table tennis?'

Matt laughed, 'Fuck that! Did you really think I'd asked you here to play? I've got many other games in mind.' And he kissed her again. He paused. 'Mind you, I suppose we could play strip table tennis. I quite like the thought of that.'

'Wouldn't everything be wobbling around?'

He gave a wicked grin that she was certain he didn't use on his corporate clients. 'Nope. Check it out.'

She trailed her hand down the length of his body. Candy had been right, rock hard just about covered it – not that Frankie was going to tell her that.

Chapter 41

Leila

Leila had come to dread the evenings, when Gracie was tucked up in bed and it was just her, on her own with her thoughts, rattling round the house, unable to settle. She was grateful to Frankie and Tor who made sure they regularly came over. Tonight, Frankie had come, which was a relief as earlier that day Tom had been round when she was out and had taken more of his clothes. He was staying with a friend, and three weeks on he still wouldn't talk to her. Leila kept hoping that he would change his mind, kept hoping that he could forgive her, but it was hard to hold on to that hope when he wouldn't even reply to her messages.

She felt cold all the time, as if even her body was missing being close to Tom, who was always warm. It was a chilly night and she had lit the fire in the living room, trying not to think about how this was usually his job, and trying not to think about how in two months' time it would be Gracie's birthday, and then it would be Christmas. The summer holiday seemed a very long time ago . . .

Her phone beeped with a message. Immediately she picked it up, always hoping against hope that it would be Tom. But it was Jasper, asking her if they could meet.

'Why does he keep texting me!' she exclaimed. 'I've told him so many times now to leave me alone.'

'D'you know where he lives?' Frankie unexpectedly asked.

'In London. I've got his address somewhere in the office. Why?'

'I've been thinking about this and I reckon you need a more direct approach. I think he's getting a kick out of sending you those messages. It will freak him if you turn up out of the blue.'

Leila shook her head. 'There is no way I want to see him again.'

'I'll come with you. We can go after school tomorrow. You've got to sort this out, Leila.'

Leila felt sick with anxiety on the train the following day. She hadn't been able to eat anything, such was her dread of seeing Jasper again. Thank God for Frankie who was so calm and together, and made her drink a cup of tea. She nearly bottled out at Clapham Junction when they arrived, thought of staying on the train to Victoria and then jumping on the first one back to Brighton. But Frankie took her arm. 'Come on, it's just a ten-minute walk away.'

Jasper was obviously doing well for himself because he lived in a smart double-fronted Victorian terrace house, which had been beautifully and stylishly renovated. Leila was surprised; she had imagined a flat where he lived the ideal bachelor life. This looked more like a family house. A home. She hesitated at the wrought-iron gate, but Frankie was already pushing it open and walking towards the dark grey door, and before Leila could say *I don't know if I can do this*, she had pressed her finger on the bell.

They could hear shouting inside the house and the sound of footsteps. 'It's okay,' Frankie murmured reassuringly as the door swung open, and they were confronted by a blond-haired three-year-old boy wearing a Spider-Man outfit and brandishing a light sabre.

'Who are you?' he demanded, then spun round and shouted, 'Daddy, Daddy some people are here.'

Jasper had a son? She'd had no idea. He had never mentioned having a family. He had always led her to believe that he was single.

A harassed-looking Jasper ran down the stairs, calling out, 'Cosmo . . . I've told you not to answer the door without me!' He froze when he saw Leila.

Guilt flared in his eyes as he put a protective hand on Cosmo's head.

'Leila, I wasn't expecting to see you.'

Seriously? That was the best line he could come up with? And him a writer? She suddenly felt entirely in control.

'We were in the area and we thought we'd pop by. I really wanted to thank you for the flowers. That was quite something, finding them all when I got back from my holiday.'

'Well, it's not really convenient. I'm expecting my wife back any minute. So another time.' He was all set to close the door in their faces and scuttle back into his house, thinking he'd got away with it.

His *wife?*

'It won't take long. We really can't leave until we've talked.'

Jasper seemed to wilt under the strength of her gaze. How could she ever have been attracted to him? He was still good-looking, but now she could see that his face entirely lacked the character of Tom's.

Cosmo took that opportunity to dart away upstairs.

'So can we come in?' Frankie asked briskly. 'Or do you want to have the conversation outside?'

Looking defeated, Jasper led them into the large living room, which was at least twice the size of Leila's and furnished with expensive-looking

423

pieces of furniture. Frankie sat on one of the grey velvet sofas, while Leila remained standing and Jasper took position by the black marble fireplace and attempted to assert himself.

'Look, Leila, I don't know why you're here but it's really not a good time.'

She ignored this. 'You've got a lovely home, Jasper, I had no idea you were doing so well as a writer. Or is it your wife who's the main breadwinner? The wife you never mentioned to me.'

'Leave my wife out of this.'

'What? Like you left my husband out of things?'

She was wrong to think that he was defeated as he gave a nasty smile and said, 'You were perfectly happy to leave him out of it that night in the hotel room. And then what? You think you can just dump me? Airbrush me out of your life? Women like you make me sick.'

He sounded so bitter; Leila was taken aback by his tone. For a moment she almost said that she was sorry, when she realised what she was doing. There was no excuse for what he'd done. He had wrecked her marriage. Bastard.

'You are never to contact me again. Not a text, not a phone call, no flowers.'

When he remained silent, an almost sneering expression on his face, she continued, 'And if you do, I will come here and tell your wife everything. You've already fucked up my marriage so I really

424

won't have any problem in returning the favour. Understand?'

He still didn't say anything. This wasn't meant to happen. Leila looked at Frankie, what did she do now? Her friend spoke, 'You've done this before, Jasper, haven't you? Got your kicks out of harassing women?'

'You don't know anything about me,' he shot back.

'Yeah, well you've left Leila with nothing to lose. She really will tell your wife everything. Also, the world of radio drama is a very small one, and Leila is well respected. It would be easy for her to put the word out that you were unreliable and difficult to work with.'

Jasper's 'Fuck you' was lost as the door swung open and in marched a thirty-something woman, in a chic navy suit, her long blonde hair pulled back in a ponytail.

'Hello, I didn't know you were having a meeting J. It wasn't on the calendar.' She smiled warmly at everyone.

For a second Leila was tempted to tell her the real reason they were there, but she just couldn't do it. Not out of any regard for Jasper, but for the woman standing before her, who clearly had no idea what her husband was really like.

'Actually we're just finished,' Leila replied, standing up along with Frankie. 'I'm Leila by the way and this is Frankie.'

'Are you sure? Don't leave because of me. I'm Helen.' Her open friendly manner only made Leila despise Jasper even more.

'I hope it was a productive meeting. I'm sure J won't mind me saying that it's been a little quiet for him lately and you know what that does for writers.'

'Oh yes, it was very productive, wasn't it, Jasper? I think we've covered everything and it's clear to everyone what will happen?'

Leila looked at Jasper for what she hoped would be the last time. He had moved next to his wife.

'Yes. Thank you, Leila, it's perfectly clear.' The sneer had gone.

Frankie chatted to Helen as they walked to the front door, asking what she did for a living (university lecturer in Economics). Perhaps in their other lives she and Frankie could come back as actors . . .

They didn't say a word until they had reached the end of Jasper's road, and then Frankie stopped and hugged her.

'You're shaking,' she exclaimed.

'Yes, but it's over. Now I just need to work out how to save my marriage.'

It was a month before Tom would actually agree to meet up and talk about something other than arrangements for looking after Gracie. They met at Tom's favourite café, the one he was convinced served the best coffee in Brighton. Leila arrived early. She was far too wound up to order her usual espresso and had a peppermint tea instead. She sat at a table for two, facing towards the door. Tom arrived ten minutes later. He was wearing a new dark brown leather jacket; it looked good on him. He looked good. She yearned to run over to him and hug him, feel his body next to hers, show him how much she loved him. Instead she raised her hand and smiled. He nodded when he saw her and mouthed that he was going to grab a coffee.

She sipped her tea and tried to calm herself, though she was a mass of anxiety. What if Tom had agreed to this meeting so that he could tell her to her face that he wanted a divorce? He would do it face-to-face; he was decent like that.

He took a seat opposite her, making no attempt to kiss her. He had shaved, which she tried to see as a positive sign as he knew that she preferred him clean-shaven. But set against that was his serious expression. Oh, God, maybe he was going to say that their marriage was over. She felt sick. Immediately she had to fill the silence, stop him coming out with the announcement.

'So, everything's on track for Gracie's party. My mum's made the cake – it's a *Toy Story* theme with Buzz and Jessie – please God, let Gracie not go off it before next week. I've bought all the presents for the party bags and for pass-the-parcel. I was trying to persuade Gracie that there should only be one present for the winner, like in our day, but she wasn't having any of it and so—'

'Do you love that man?' Tom interrupted.

For a moment she had no idea what he could be talking about as Jasper was so far from her thoughts, especially as he had stopped texting. 'I never want to see him again,' she said passionately. 'Not ever. He means nothing to me.'

For the first time since that terrible night when Tom had found out, he looked at her, and seemed to see her. 'This has been the worst time of my life. I was so angry with you, so full of blame. I wanted to lash out and hurt you. Christ, I even thought about sleeping with someone else – just to get even, for all the good that would have done.'

'Oh.' Polly, she supposed. But knew that she couldn't say anything; she'd forfeited that right.

'But I realised that I didn't want to, because you were right, we weren't getting on, I know I had left you feeling isolated and although I didn't sleep with anyone else, in some ways I might as well have.'

Leila felt as if she hardly dared breathe; everything, her whole future and Gracie's, depended on what Tom went on to say.

'What I'm trying to say, incredibly badly, is that I don't want our marriage to end because of one mistake.'

'Nor do I, Tom.'

'It's not going to be easy, I'm still angry and hurt

and jealous and if I think about you with him then I want to punch someone, him preferably.'

'I'll do everything I can to make it work,' she said quietly.

He reached out for her hand, 'We both will.'

Chapter 42

August, one year later

Tor looked at the two rucksacks bulging with baby-related paraphernalia, the two buggies, the two car seats, at Ed struggling to close one of the two enormous suitcases, at her two babies sitting in their inflatable play ring . . . and felt a great longing to go back to bed. Their first family holiday at this moment seemed more like an endurance test. Were they mad to be going to Greece? They'd never be able to get out of the front door with all this lot, never mind board a plane . . .

The last year had been a rollercoaster. So much had happened, with Ed moving in and starting his new job, with having the twins in March – a boy and a girl as it turned out – Artie and Zoe – with juggling the shop – with being a mum. But Ed had been brilliant throughout it – she had never doubted him for a second. All her doubts and anxieties about him being younger than her, about him feeling trapped by the babies, had been blown away by seeing what a fantastic dad he was.

Ed finally managed to close the case just as the doorbell rang. 'That'll be Candy,' he said. 'Right on time.'

Candy, their marvellous part-time nanny. She had started working with them when the babies were only three weeks old. A natural with children, she had been reassuring, practical, kind, constantly good-humoured, had saved Ed and Tor from going under from lack of sleep. A total Godsend.

She walked into the living room. Her long brown hair was in plaits, she wore a minimal amount of make-up, a pair of denim cutoffs, red Converse and a blue-and-white polka-dot t-shirt. She had given up the waxing and fake tanning and gone back to college to study for her A-levels part-time. She was still seeing Dimitri and frequently claimed that it wouldn't last, but no one was buying that. He had been over to visit her regularly and there was talk of him moving over here to study. Candy was going to be dividing her time between the villa and Dimitri's apartment while they were in Greece.

'Ready, guys?' she asked. She looked at Tor and registered her anxious expression. 'Stop worrying, it's going to be fine. You'll have five adults to look after Zoe and Artie on the flight.'

'Yeah, and one of them is Frankie – she'll be able to scare them into submission,' Ed joked. Actually

Frankie had been a revelation with the twins. She was amazing with them and often when Ed was working late, and Tor was feeling frazzled, would come over to help give them their baths and put them to bed.

Ed put his arms around Tor. 'We're going to have a great holiday, I promise.'

While Candy knelt down to talk to the twins, he whispered, 'And who knows? We might even get to have sex.'

She punched him on the shoulder. 'We nearly did the other week, but you fell asleep, remember? I tried not to take it personally.' Sleep had become a highly prized commodity in their household.

He looked pained at the thought of what he'd missed out on. 'That doesn't sound like me. You know I'm always up for it.'

'True. But I went to check on Artie, and when I came back to bed, you were out for the count. I think you might even have been snoring.'

'I am making up for that when we're away,' he murmured, and kissed her neck, and suddenly Tor wanted to go back to bed again, but this time not to sleep . . .

'When will everyone get here?' Gracie demanded, spinning round and round with her arms outstretched, as you do when you're five and very, very excited.

Leila smiled at her daughter. It was only about

432

the tenth time in the last half-hour that she'd asked that question.

'Soon, sweetie, I promise.'

She was sitting in the shade of the terrace, attempting to stay cool. At five months pregnant she was finding the heat much harder to tolerate than she had anticipated, but it felt wonderful to be here on the island again. Tom came out of the villa with a carrot, orange and ginger juice for her. She had developed a craving for the drink and at one time during her pregnancy was on about five a day – now she had cut down to three. Still, at least it wasn't packets of Cadbury's mini chocolate fingers as it had been when she was pregnant with Gracie.

'Thanks,' she said gratefully. He sat down next to her and rubbed her lower back.

'How are you feeling? Not too tired? It is going to be full on when everyone gets here. Are you sure you're up to it?'

'I'll be fine, I'm so looking forward to seeing everyone.'

The last year had been one of the most challenging of their marriage. The pain she had caused Tom over Jasper was not something that could easily go away. He might have forgiven her, it was the forgetting that was hardest. There had been days when he was moody and withdrawn, when she was tempted to retreat into herself in retaliation. But they were getting through it, and her becoming pregnant had felt like an affirmation.

'They're here!' Gracie shouted, 'Can I open the gate?'

'Let the fun begin,' Tom said dryly, but he was smiling.

'What kind of idiot wears a white t-shirt to travel with babies?' Frankie asked, looking at the front of Matt's top which was covered in banana stains, smeared there by Artie.

'Thanks so much for your sympathy,' Matt replied, peeling off the offending item of clothing and dropping it on the floor.

A sexy idiot, she was tempted to say, not able to resist putting her arms round him and leaning against him. This past year with Matt had been a revelation. She had fallen completely in love with him. It was scary opening herself up to that emotion again, knowing what it was to lose someone, but brilliant, exciting, intoxicating as well. And to know that this was the real thing, not the infatuation she had once felt for Patrick. As for him, he was living in the South of France with Willow, and claimed he hadn't had a drink for six months. He had been in touch with each of them to apologise, part of the Twelve Steps programme he was following. And maybe one day they could all go back to being friends again . . .

Matt glanced at Frankie's shoulder. 'What kind of idiot wears black? You've got regurgitated biscuit all over you.'

'It's not biscuit, it's one of those repellant organic sugar-free rusks. I ate one by mistake, thinking it was going to be a biscuit. No wonder Zoe spat it out.' She adored the chubby-cheeked, curly-haired twins, but God they were messy. Angels of destruction, she privately called them.

She pulled off her shirt, dropped it on the floor and fell back on the bed. 'I don't know how Tor and Ed do it. I'm knackered, and I've only been with them for less than a day.'

Matt grinned and lay down next to her. 'I think we might need to go to bed. But, just to let you know, I've no intention of sleeping. You know, last year I spent my whole time in that single bed next door fantasising about you, and about what it would be like to be with you. And now here you are. My brown-eyed girl.'

'Yes, here I am.' Frankie curled her arms round his neck. She hadn't told him that Ross used to call her that. Somehow she thought that Matt was someone Ross would have approved of . . .

He kissed her and gazed at her. 'I guess we don't need to go down for a while . . . This is a holiday, after all.'

A Funny Thing About Love

Rebecca Farnworth

The funny thing about love is that just when you think you've got it sorted, it turns round and bites you. Which is exactly what's happened to Carmen Miller.

Her ex-husband's girlfriend is pregnant, her career as a comedy agent is going down the pan, she's made a fool of herself with fellow agent Will Hunter, a man she's fancied for ages, and to cap it all she has to move out of her flat. Surely things can't get any worse.

Moving down to Brighton to write the TV comedy series that she's always dreamed about, Carmen meets the divine Daniel. A man so gorgeous, she doesn't even mind that he's got long hair. It seems that Carmen's life is on the up again. Until, that is . . . love bites again. Looks like Carmen's back where she started.

But could it be that love isn't the problem? Maybe she's just been choosing the wrong men.

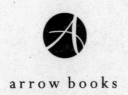

arrow books

A Funny Thing About Love

Rebecca Farnworth

The funny thing about love is that just when you think you've got it sorted, it takes a turn and takes you 'wheee' to exactly what's happened to Carrie's tables.

Valentine

Rebecca Farnworth

Will a shocking secret cause a rising star to fall?

Valentine Fleming dreams of making it as an actress but after years of failed auditions and bit parts her hopes are fading fast – so too is her self-esteem. She is staring into the abyss and a large jar of peanut butter. Her love life is faring no better, with too much time wasted with an ex who has bad news written all over him.

So when she gets a call from her agent telling her she has a part in a play with a sexy leading man, she's over the moon. She's not packing her bags for the Hollywood hills just yet but could this be her lucky break?

But just as it seems that her luck might be set to change she learns a shocking secret and Valentine's world is turned upside down...

arrow books

A Quite Interesting Book

THE SECOND BOOK OF OF GENERAL IGNORANCE

John Lloyd and John Mitchinson

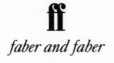
faber and faber

First published in 2010
by Faber and Faber Ltd
Bloomsbury House
74–77 Great Russell Street
London WCIB 3DA

Typeset by Palindrome
Printed in England by CPI Mackays, Chatham

All rights reserved
© QI Ltd, 2010
Illustrations © Mr Bingo, 2010

The right of QI Ltd to be identified as author of this work
has been asserted in accordance with Section 77 of
the Copyright, Designs and Patents Act 1988

A CIP record for this book
is available from the British Library

ISBN 978-0-571-26966-2

2 4 6 8 10 9 7 5 3 1

CONTENTS

FORETHOUGHT | Stephen Fry

Now, what I want is facts. Teach these boys and girls nothing but Facts. Facts alone are wanted in life. Plant nothing else, and root out everything else. You can only form the minds of reasoning animals upon Facts: nothing else will ever be of any service to them. This is the principle on which I bring up my own children, and this is the principle on which I bring up these children. Stick to Facts, sir!

Nothing but a shudder runs up the spine of the sensible man, woman or child as they read these well-known words of Thomas Gradgrind in Dickens's novel *Hard Times*.

'But surely, Stephen,' you say, in that *way* of yours, 'QI and General Ignorance and all that they are or hope to be represent nothing more than the triumphant distillation of Gradgrindery, fact-dweebiness, trivia-hoarding and information-hugging. The world of noble ideas falls before your world of grinding facts. Facts are the abrasive touchstones on which we test the validity of concepts! Surely, Stephen. Surely, surely, surely! I'm right, aren't I? Aren't I? Oh *do* say I am!'

Well now, bless you and shush and oh you dear things. Calm yourselves and sit down in a semicircle on the play mat while we think about this.

I know it must seem sometimes that QI is a nerd's charter

that encourages boring dorks to vomit undigested boluses of fibrous factoid. QI and its volumes of General Ignorance might appear to some to be nothing more than provisioners of ammunition for tiresome gainsaying did-you-knowers and tedious trotters out of turgid trivia. But look beneath the surface and I hope you will agree that the volume that you hold in your delicate hands is in truth a *celebration*, a celebration of the greatest human quality there is. Curiosity. Curiosity has wrongly, by those with a vested interest in ignorance and their own revealed truths, been traduced and eternally characterised as a dangerous felicide, but you, dearest of dear, dear readers, know that Curiosity lights the way to glory.

Let us put it another way: the *lack* of curiosity is the Dementor that sucks all hope, joy, possibility and beauty out of the world. The dull torpid acedia that does not care to find out, that has no hunger and thirst for input, understanding and connection will desertify the human landscape and land our descendants squarely in the soup.

Do we want our species to makes its way, foreheads thrust out, knuckles grazing the ground, into a barren of tedium and brutish unquestioning blindness, or do we want to skip through the world filled with wonder, curiosity and an appetite for discovery?

This screamingly overwrought preface that is even now embarrassing you to the encrimsoning roots of your scalp, is called *Forethought* in honour of Prometheus, the greatest of the Titans of Greek mythology. Prometheus, whose brother Atlas was busy holding up the world, looked at us poor newly made humans and loved us and felt sorry that we were animals so close to gods yet still lacking . . . *something* . . .

Prometheus climbed up Olympus and stole that something from the gods, bringing it down carefully preserved in a fennel stalk. It was fire. Fire that gave us technology, but more than that, it was *iskra,* the spark, the divine fire, the quality that drove us to *know.* The fire that allowed us to rise up on a level with the gods.

The Greeks rightly understood that if there *were* such creatures as gods, they were (it is self-evident) capricious, inconsistent, unjust, jealous and mean. And indeed Zeus, their king, was outraged that Prometheus, one of their own, had given humans great creating fire. He punished the Titan by chaining him to the Caucasus mountains. Every day an eagle (or vultures depending on your source) came to peck out his liver, which (Prometheus being an immortal) grew back each night. This eternal torture he underwent for humans, that we might, each one of us, have the divine spark, the immortal fire that drives us to ask Why? Who? When? What? Where? and How?

The name Prometheus means Forethought. We can repay him his daily agony by being, every day, curious, wondering and entirely on fire.

I adore you widely.

SECOND THOUGHTS |
John Lloyd and John Mitchinson

When we compiled the original Book of General Ignorance in 2006 – aided by the doughty and indefatigable QI Elves – we laboured under the misconception that we might have mined the Mountain of Ignorance to exhaustion, depleting its resources forever.

Nothing could be further from the truth.

Four years on, four series later, there is so much more ignorance available that we've had to deliberately cull it in order to make this *Second Book of General Ignorance* tolerably portable.

We hope you'll have as much fun reading it as we've had putting it together.

It is a wonderful thing that we, 'The Two Johnnies' (aged 58 and 47 respectively) can honestly say that we genuinely do 'learn something new every day'.

Thank you for allowing us to do that.

THE SECOND BOOK
OF
GENERAL IGNORANCE

Everybody is ignorant, only on different subjects.
Will Rogers (1879–1935)

Who made the first flight in an aeroplane?

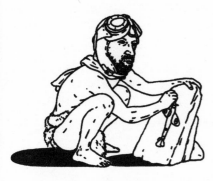

We don't know his name but he beat the Wright Brothers to it by fifty years.

He worked for Sir George Cayley (1773–1857), an aristocratic Yorkshireman and pioneer of aeronautics, who carried out the first truly scientific study of how birds fly. Cayley correctly described the principles of 'lift, drag and thrust' that govern flight and this led him to build a series of prototype flying machines. His early attempts with flapping wings (powered by steam and gunpowder engines) failed, so he turned his attention to gliders instead.

In 1804 he demonstrated the world's first model glider and, five years later, tested a full-sized version – but without a pilot. More than three decades passed before he finally felt ready to trust his 'governable parachute' with a human passenger. In 1853, at Brompton Dale near Scarborough, the intrepid baronet persuaded his reluctant coachman to steer the contraption across the valley. It was this anonymous employee who became the first human ever to fly in a heavier-than-air machine.

The coachman, so the story goes, was not impressed. He handed in his notice as soon as he landed, saying, 'I was hired to drive, not to fly.' A modern replica of Cayley's glider, now on show at the Yorkshire Air Museum, successfully repeated the flight across Brompton Dale in 1974.

But wings weren't Sir George's only legacy. With his work on the glider's landing gear, he literally reinvented the wheel. Needing something light but strong to absorb the aircraft's impact on landing, he came up with the idea of using wheels whose spokes were held at tension, rather than being carved from solid wood. These went on to transform the development of the bicycle and the car and are still widely used today.

And that wasn't all. Cayley was a remarkably prolific inventor, developing self-righting lifeboats, caterpillar tracks for bulldozers, automatic signals for railway crossings and seat belts. Even more remarkably, he offered all these inventions for the public good, without expecting any financial reward.

The Wright Brothers made their famous flights half a century later, in 1903. They were inspired by Cayley and by another unsung hero of aviation, Otto Lilienthal (1848–96), a Prussian known as the 'Glider King'. He was the first person to fly consistently: in the decade before the Wright Brothers, he made over 2,000 glider flights before falling to his death in 1896. His last words were humble and poignant: 'Small sacrifices must be made.'

STEPHEN *Who invented the aeroplane?*
RICH HALL *It's Orville and Wilbur Wright.*
KLAXON *'The Wright Brothers'*
PETER SERAFINOWICZ *Is it the Wrong Brothers?*

How many legs does an octopus have?

Two.

Octopuses have eight limbs protruding from their bodies, but recent research into how they use them has redefined what they should be called. Octopuses (from the Greek for 'eight

2

feet') are *cephalopods* (Greek for 'head foot'). They use their back two tentacles to propel themselves along the seabed, leaving the remaining six to be used for feeding. As result, marine biologists now tend to refer to them as animals with two legs and six arms.

An octopus's tentacles are miraculous organs. They can stiffen to create a temporary elbow joint, or fold up to disguise their owner as a coconut rolling along the sea floor. They also contain two-thirds of the octopus's brain – about 50 million neurons – the remaining third of which is shaped like a doughnut and located inside its head, or mantle.

Because so much of an octopus's nervous system is in its extremities, each limb has a high degree of independence. A severed tentacle can continue to crawl around and, in some species, will live for several months. An octopus's arm (or leg) quite genuinely has a mind of its own.

Each arm on an octopus has two rows of suckers, equipped with taste-buds for identifying food. An octopus tastes everything that it touches. Male octopuses also have a specialised arm in which they keep their sperm. It's called the hectocotylus and is used for mating. To transfer the sperm, the male puts his arm into a hole in the female's head. During copulation the hectocotylus usually breaks off, but the male grows a new one the following year.

The way octopuses mate was first described by Aristotle (384–322 BC) but for over 2,000 years no one believed him. The French zoologist Georges Cuvier (1769–1832) redis-covered the process in the nineteenth century and gave the hectocotylus its name. It means 'a hundred tiny cups' in Greek.

Genetic variations sometimes cause octopuses to grow more than eight limbs. In 1998 the Shima Marineland Aquarium in Japan had a common octopus on display that had 96 tentacles. It was captured in nearby Matoya Bay in December 1998 but died five months later. The multi-armed cephalopod managed to lay a batch of eggs before its death. All the offspring hatched with the normal number of arms and legs, but none survived longer than a month.

Octopuses occasionally eat their own arms. This used to be blamed on stress, but is now thought to be caused by a virus that attacks their nervous system.

MEERA SYAL *Do you know how octopuses mate?*
STEPHEN *Tell, tell.*
ALAN *With difficulty.*
MEERA *They mate with their third right arm.*
ALAN *Do they?*
MEERA *Yes!*
CLIVE ANDERSON *We all do that.*

What colour are oranges?

That depends.

In many countries, oranges are green – even when ripe – and are sold that way in the shops. The same goes for lemons, mangoes, tangerines and grapefruit.

Oranges are unknown in the wild. They are a cross between tangerines and the pomelo or 'Chinese grapefruit' (which is pale green or yellow), and were first grown in South-East Asia. They were green there then, and today they still are. Vietnamese oranges and Thai tangerines are bright green on the outside, and only orange on the inside.

Oranges are subtropical fruit, not tropical ones. The colour of an orange depends on where it grows. In more temperate climes, its green skin turns orange when the weather cools; but in countries where it's always hot the chlorophyll is not destroyed and the fruits stay green. Oranges in Honduras, for example, are eaten green at home but artificially 'oranged' for export.

To achieve this, they are blasted with ethylene gas, a by-product of the oil industry, whose main use is in the manufacture of plastic. Ethylene is the most widely produced organic compound in the world: 100 million tons of it are made every year. It removes the natural outer green layer of an orange allowing the more familiar colour to show through.

Far and away the world's largest producer of oranges is Brazil (18 million tons a year), followed by the USA, which grows fewer than half as many. American oranges come from California, Texas and Florida. They were often synthetically dyed until the Food and Drug Administration banned the practice in 1955.

You can't tell the ripeness of an orange by its colour, no matter where it's from. If an orange goes unpicked, it can stay on the tree till the next season, during which time fluctuations in temperature can make it turn from green to orange and back to green again without the quality or flavour being affected.

The oranges you see on display in your supermarket certainly *appear* to be completely orange, but you may now start to worry they've been gassed. Don't.

Ethylene is odourless, tasteless and harmless, and many fruits and vegetables give it off naturally after they're picked. Ethylene producers include apples, melons, tomatoes, avocados and bananas. The gas isn't bad for you, but it can affect other kinds of fruit and veg – which is why you should keep apples and bananas separate from, say, lemons or carrots (and, of course, oranges).

Ethylene has other uses apart from making plastics (and

detergents and antifreeze) and altering the colour of an orange. If you want to speed up the ripening process of an unripe mango, keep it in a bag with a banana.

What's the name of the most southerly point of Africa?

It's not the Cape of Good Hope.

The residents of nearby Cape Town often have to explain this to visitors. The southernmost point of the continent is the altogether less famous Cape Agulhas, 150 kilometres (93 miles) south-east of the Cape of Good Hope.

The usual reason given for the Cape of Good Hope's fame (and its name) is that it was the psychologically important point where sailors, on the long haul down the west coast of Africa on their way to the Far East, at last began to sail in an easterly, rather than a southerly, direction.

On the other hand, it might have been an early example of marketing spin.

Bartolomeu Dias (1451–1500), the Portuguese navigator who discovered the Cape of Good Hope and became the first European to make the hair-raising trip around the foot of Africa, named it Cabo das Tormentas ('Cape of Storms'). His employer, King John II of Portugal (1455–95), keen to encourage others to adopt the new trade route, overruled him and tactfully rechristened it Cabo da Boa Esperança ('Cape of Good Hope').

The King died childless, aged only forty. Five years later Bartolomeu Dias also died. He was wrecked in a terrible storm – along with four ships and the loss of all hands – off the very cape he had so presciently named.

Cape Agulhas is equally treacherous. It is Portuguese for 'Cape of Needles', after the sharp rocks and reefs that infest its roaring waters. The local town is home to a shipwreck museum that commemorates 'a graveyard of ships'.

Because of its isolation and rocky, inaccessible beach, the area is rich in wildlife. On land, it is home to the critically endangered micro-frog (*Microbatrachella capensis*) and the Agulhas clapper (*Mirafra (apiata) majoriae*), a lark whose mating display involves much noisy wing-flapping.

In the waters offshore, between May and August, the sea boils with billions of migrating South African pilchards (*Sardinops sagax*). These shoals form one of the largest congregations of wildlife on the planet, equivalent to the great wildebeest migrations on land, and can stretch to be 6 kilometres (3.7 miles) long and 2 kilometres (1.2 miles) wide. Hundreds of thousands of sharks, dolphins, seals and seabirds travel in the fishes' wake, snacking on them at will but making little impact on the overall numbers.

Cape Agulhas is at 34° 49' 58" south and 20° 00' 12" east and it is the official dividing point between the Atlantic and Indian oceans. If you sailed past it, along the relatively unimpressive, gradually curving coastline, you probably wouldn't even notice it but for the cairn that marks the tip's exact location.

What's the hardest known substance?

It's not diamonds any more.

In 2005 scientists at Bayreuth University in Germany created a new material by compressing pure carbon under extreme heat. It's called hyperdiamond or aggregated diamond nanorods (ADNR) and, although it's incredibly hard, it looks rather like asphalt or a glittery black pudding.

It's long been known that one form of pure carbon (graphite) can be turned into another (diamond) by heat and pressure. But the Bayreuth team used neither. They used a third form of pure carbon, fullerite, also known as buckminsterfullerene or 'buckyballs'. Its sixty carbon atoms form a molecule shaped like a soccer ball, or like one of the geodesic domes invented by the American architect Richard Buckminster Fuller (1895–1983).

The carbon atoms in diamond are arranged in cubes stacked in pyramids; the new substance is made of tiny, interlocking rods. These are called 'nanorods' because they are so small – *nanos* is Greek for 'dwarf'. Each is 1 micron (one millionth of a metre) long and 20 nanometres (20 billionths of a metre) wide – about 1/50,000th of the width of a human hair.

Subjecting fullerite to extremes of heat (2,220 °C) and compression (200,000 times normal atmospheric pressure) created not only the *hardest*, but also the *stiffest* and *densest* substance known to science.

Density is how tightly packed a material's molecules are and is measured using X-rays. ADNR is 0.3 per cent denser than diamond.

Stiffness is a measure of compressibility: the amount of force that must be applied equally on all sides to make the material shrink in volume. Its basic unit is the pascal, after Blaise Pascal (1623–62), the French mathematician who helped develop the barometer, which measures air pressure. ADNR's stiffness rating is 491 gigapascals (GPa): diamond's is 442 GPa and iron's is 180 GPa. This means that ADNR is almost three times harder to compress than iron.

Hardness is simpler to determine: if one material can make a scratch mark on another, it's harder. The German mineralogist Friedrich Mohs (1773–1839) devised the Mohs Hardness scale in 1812. It starts at the softest end with talc (MH1). Lead is fairly soft at MH1½; fingernails are graded MH2½ (as hard as gold); in the middle are glass and knife blades at MH5½. Ordinary sandpaper (which is made of corundum) is MH9, and right at the top end is diamond at MH10. Since ADNR can scratch diamond, it is literally off the scale.

And there's more disappointing news for diamond fans: they aren't 'forever'. Graphite (which, oddly enough, is one of the *softest* known substances, as soft as talc) is much more chemically stable than diamond. In fact all diamonds are very slowly turning *into* graphite. But the process is imperceptible. There's no danger of anybody suddenly finding their earrings have become pencils.

What's the strangest substance known to science?

H_2O.

Water, or hydrogen oxide, is the strangest substance known to science. With the possible exception of air, it's also the most familiar. It covers 70 per cent of the earth and accounts for 70 per cent of our own brains.

Water is oxygen linked to hydrogen (the simplest and most common element in the universe) in the simplest way possible. Any other gas combined with hydrogen just produces another gas: only oxygen and hydrogen make a liquid.

And it's a liquid that behaves so differently from any other that theoretically it shouldn't exist. There are sixty-six known ways in which water is abnormal, the most peculiar being that nothing else in nature is found simultaneously as liquid, solid and gas. A sea full of icebergs under a cloudy sky may appear natural, but in chemical terms it is anything but. Most substances shrink as they cool, but when water falls below 4 °C it starts to expand and become lighter. That's why ice floats, and why wine bottles burst if left in the freezer.

Each water molecule can attach itself to four other water molecules. Because water is so strongly bonded, a lot of energy is needed to change it from one state to another. It takes ten times more energy to heat water than iron.

Because water can absorb a lot of heat without getting hot, it helps keep the planet's climate steady. Temperatures in the oceans are three times more stable than on land and water's transparency allows light to penetrate its depths, enabling life in the sea. Without water there would be no life at all. And, though you can put your hand right through it, it's three times harder to compress than diamonds and water hit at speed is as hard as concrete.

Although the bonds between water molecules are strong, they aren't stable. They are constantly being broken and remade: each molecule of water collides with other water molecules 10,000,000,000,000,000 times a second.

So many things can be dissolved in water that it's known as the 'universal solvent'. If you dissolve metal in acid, it's gone forever. If you dissolve plaster in water, when all the water has evaporated, the plaster is still there. This ability to dissolve stuff without eradicating it also paradoxically makes water the most destructive substance on the planet. Sooner or later, it eats away everything – from an iron drainpipe to the Grand Canyon.

And it gets everywhere. There are substantial deposits of ice on the moon and on Mars: traces of water vapour have even been detected on the cooler patches of the sun's surface. On Earth only a tiny fraction of all the water is in the atmosphere. If it fell evenly throughout the world, it would produce no more than 25 millimetres or an inch of rain. Most of Earth's water is inaccessible, locked deep inside the planet, carried down when tectonic plates overlap, or held inside the mineral structure of the rocks themselves.

If this hidden water were released it would refill the oceans thirty times over.

At what temperature does water freeze?

Pure water doesn't freeze at 0 °C, nor does seawater.

For water to freeze, it needs something for its molecules to latch on to. Ice crystals form around 'nuclei', such as small particles of dust. If there are none of these, you can get the temperature of water down to −42 °C before it freezes.

Cooling water without freezing it is known as 'super-cooling'. It has to be done slowly. You can put a bottle of very pure water in your freezer and supercool it. When you take the bottle out and tap it, the water will instantly turn to ice.

Cooling water extremely fast has a completely different effect. It bypasses the ice stage (which has a regular crystalline lattice structure) and transforms into a chaotic amorphous solid known as 'glassy water' (so called because the random arrangement of molecules is similar to that found in glass). To form 'glassy water' you need to get the water temperature down to −137 °C in a few milliseconds. You won't find glassy water outside the lab on Earth, but it's the most common form of water in the universe − it's what comets are made of.

Because of its high salt content, seawater regularly falls below 0 °C without freezing. The blood of fishes normally freezes at about −0.5 °C, so marine biologists used to be puzzled by how fish survived in polar oceans. It turns out that species like Antarctic icefish and herring produce proteins in the pancreas that are absorbed into their blood. These prevent the formation of ice nuclei (much like antifreeze in a car radiator).

Given the peculiarities of water at low temperatures, it won't surprise you to learn that the boiling point of water, even at normal pressure, isn't necessarily 100 °C either. It can be much more. Again, the liquid needs to be warmed slowly and in a container that has no scratches. It is these that contain the small pockets of air around which the first bubbles form.

Boiling happens when bubbles of water vapour expand and break the surface. For this to happen, the temperature must be high enough for the pressure created by the vapour bubble to exceed the atmospheric pressure. Under normal conditions this is 100 °C, but if the water is free of places where bubbles could form, more heat is needed to overcome the surface tension of the bubbles as they struggle into life. (It's the same reason that blowing up a balloon is always harder at the beginning.)

This explains why a boiling hot cup of coffee in the microwave can explode all over you once removed or stirred. The movement sets off a chain reaction, so that all the water in the coffee vaporises at high speed.

One last watery oddity: hot water freezes faster than cold water. Aristotle first noted this in the fourth century BC, but it was only accepted by modern science in 1963. This resulted from the persistence of a Tanzanian schoolboy called Erasto Mpemba, who proved it by repeatedly demonstrating that a hot ice cream mixture set more quickly than cold. We still don't know why it does.

Where is the largest known lake?

It's 842 million miles away, halfway across the solar system.

In 2007 the Cassini–Huygens space probe sent back pictures of Titan, the largest of Saturn's moons. Near the moon's northern pole, radar imaging revealed a giant lake estimated to cover 388,500 square kilometres (150,000 square miles), significantly bigger than the Caspian Sea, the largest lake on Earth at 370,400 square kilometres (143,244 square miles).

The lake is called Kraken Mare – *mare* is Latin for 'sea' and the kraken is a sea monster from Norse mythology.

Titan has many lakes and they are the only bodies of stable liquid known to exist anywhere other than on Earth. But the liquid isn't water: Titan's average temperature is −181°C, so any water would be frozen solid. They are lakes of liquid gas – methane and ethane, the main ingredients of natural gas on earth – and they are so cold that they may even contain frozen methane-bergs.

Titan's chemical composition is thought to be very similar to that of Earth during the period when life first appeared here, and it is the only moon in the solar system with an atmosphere.

In 2004 Ladbrokes the bookmaker, in a joint publicity stunt with *New Scientist* magazine, offered odds of 10,000 to 1 against life being discovered on Titan. Would this be worth risking a titan on? (A 'titan' is the £100 million note used by the Bank of England for inter-bank accounting purposes.)

On balance, probably not. The development of DNA on Titan is unlikely because of the extreme cold and the lack of liquid water. However, some astrobiologists have suggested that Titan's hydrocarbon lakes might sustain forms of life that would inhale hydrogen in place of oxygen. Another theory is that life could have reached Titan from Earth, through microbes clinging to rocks smashed out of Earth's orbit by asteroid impacts. This theory is called panspermia (from *pan* 'all' and *sperma* 'seed' in Greek) and was used to explain the presence of life on Earth as long ago as the fifth century BC, when the Greek cosmologist Anaxagoras first proposed it.

What is certain is that, as the sun gets hotter, the temperature on Titan will also rise, making the conditions for life more likely. Whether, in six billion years or so, Ladbrokes will still exist to pay out any winnings is much less probable.

The Cassini–Huygens probe is named after the Italian astronomer Giovanni Domenico Cassini (1625–1712), who discovered four of Saturn's smaller moons between 1671 and 1684, and the Dutch polymath Christiaan Huygens (1629–95), who discovered Titan in 1654. Among Huygens's other achievements were working out the theory of centrifugal force, publishing a book on the use of probability in dice games, building the first pendulum clock and writing the first ever physics equation.

Where is the world's saltiest water?

Not in the Dead Sea.

The saltiest water in the world is found in Don Juan Pond in the Dry Valleys of north-eastern Antarctica. Also known as Lake Don Juan, it's really more of a puddle, with an average depth of less than 15 centimetres (6 inches). Its water is so salty that it doesn't freeze, despite the surrounding air temperature of −50°C. The water is 40 per cent salt – eighteen times saltier than seawater and more than twice as salty as the Dead Sea (which is only eight times saltier than the oceans).

Don Juan Pond was discovered by accident in 1961 and

named after two US Navy helicopter pilots, Lieutenants Donald Roe and John Hickey (hence Don John or 'Don Juan' in Spanish), who carried in the first field party to study it.

It's probably the most interesting puddle on Earth. Given that Antarctica's Dry Valleys are the driest, coldest places on the planet, it's astonishing that there's water there at all. It didn't come from the sky — it's too cold and windy there for rain or snow — it seeped up from the ground, slowly becoming saltier as the top layer of water evaporated. In spite of these unpromising conditions, the first researchers were amazed to discover it contained life: slender mats of blue-green algae that harboured a flourishing community of bacteria, yeast and fungi.

Since that first expedition, for reasons that are unclear, the water level in the pond has more than halved and no life remains. But even this is significant, because its waters still contain nitrous oxide (better known as laughing gas), a chemical previously believed to require organic life to produce it. This has now been shown to be a by-product of the reaction between the salts in the pond and the volcanic basalt rock that surrounds it.

If liquid water is found on Mars, it is likely to be in the form of cold, briny pools, just like Don Juan Pond. And we now know that at least some of the nitrogen-rich chemicals needed to produce life can occur in even the harshest environment.

Unlike Don Juan Pond, there is still plenty of life in the Dead Sea. There are no fish, but it is teeming with algae. This supports microbes that feed on it called *Halobacteria*. They belong to the Archaea domain, the oldest life forms on the planet. Archaea are so ancient that, on the evolutionary timescale, human beings are closer to bacteria than bacteria are to Archaea. Like the former inhabitants of Don Juan Pond, *Halobacteria* are 'extremophiles', surviving in conditions once believed impossible for life.

The *Halobacterium* is also known as the 'Renaissance Bug' because it can mend its own DNA (which is damaged by high salt concentrations). If this can be harnessed, it could be of great benefit to cancer sufferers. It might even enable manned space flight to Mars, by helping astronauts protect their DNA from exposure to the fierce radiation of interplanetary space.

Where did most minerals in the world come from?

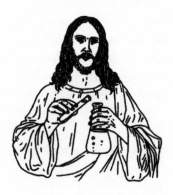

Life on Earth.

There are about 4,300 minerals in the world today, but in the primordial dust that was to become the solar system there were fewer than a dozen. All the chemical elements were already there, but minerals were very rare before the sun and the planets formed.

Unlike all the other planets, Earth's crust is a patchwork of constantly moving tectonic plates ('tectonic' is from the Greek for 'construction'). No one knows why, but one theory is that all the water on the earth's surface caused cracks in it, like damp from a flooded bathroom seeping through a plaster ceiling. As the plates of the young Earth jostled together, they created immense heat and pressure, pushing the number of minerals up to perhaps a thousand.

Then, 4 billion years ago, life appeared. Microscopic algae began using sunlight to convert the carbon dioxide that made up most of the atmosphere into carbohydrates for food. This released oxygen as a by-product. Oxygen is both the most abundant and the most reactive element in the planet's crust. It forms compounds with almost anything. As it bonded with silicon, copper and iron, hundreds of new minerals were created. Although we think of oxygen as a gas, almost half the rocks on Earth are made from it.

While oxygen was being released into the atmosphere, carbon was also being sucked into the sea. Carbon, the basis of life, is as stable as oxygen is reactive. Its stability has made it the core of millions of organic compounds, including all the proteins, fats, acids and carbohydrates that go to make up living things. As the complexity of life on Earth increased, new minerals were created. Marine creatures died and drifted to the seabed, the thick layers of their shells and skeletons destined to become limestone, chalk and marble. Meanwhile, over millions of years, the sludge of rotting plants provided the ingredients for coal and oil. More life, and more diversity of life, meant more minerals. Two-thirds of all the minerals on earth were once alive.

This 'parallel evolution' of life and rocks gives clues to what we should look for on other planets. If certain minerals are detected, it's a good bet that they came into being alongside particular types of organism.

Are we depleting the world's mineral reserves? Oil aside, none of the evidence suggests so. Although vegetables grown in the UK and the USA over the past fifty years have shown significant drops in the levels of the trace minerals they contain, this is the result of artificial fertilisers, which promote faster growth at the expense of the plants' ability to absorb nutrientsfrom the air and soil.

This may explain why people say that food 'tasted better during the War'. They're probably right.

Which came first, the chicken or the egg?

The egg. Final answer.

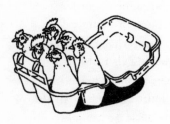

As the geneticist J. B. S. Haldane (1892–1964) remarked, 'The most frequently asked question is: "Which came first, the chicken or the egg?" The fact that it is still asked proves either that many people have never been taught the theory of evolution or that they don't believe it.'

With that in mind, the answer becomes obvious. Birds evolved from reptiles, so the first bird must have come out of an egg – laid by a reptile.

Like everything else, an egg is not as simple as it looks. For a start, the word 'egg' is used in two different ways. To a biologist, an egg is an ovum (Latin for egg), the tiny female reproductive cell which, when fertilised by a male sperm (Greek for seed), develops into an embryo. Both the ovum and the sperm are called gametes (from the Greek *gamete*, 'wife', and *gametes*, 'husband').

In a hen's egg these two tiny cells merge in the 'germinal spot' or blastodisc (from *blastos*, Greek for 'sprout'). Around this is the yolk, which provides most of the nutrition for the growing chick. The word 'yolk' comes from Old English, *geolca*, 'yellow' (until the late nineteenth century it was often spelt 'yelk'). Around the yolk is the egg white or albumen (from the Latin *albus*, 'white') which is also nutritious but whose main purpose is to protect the yolk, which is held in place in the centre of the egg by two twisted threads called chalazae. (*Chalaza* is Greek for 'hailstone': the knotted white cord looks like a string of minute pearls or balls of ice.) Around the albumen is the shell, which is made from calcium carbonate – the same stuff that skeletons and indigestion pills are made from. It's porous so that the chick can breathe, and the air is kept in a pocket between the albumen and the shell. Membranes separate each part and together it's known as a cleidoic egg – from the Greek *kleidoun*, meaning 'to lock up'. A chicken makes the whole thing from scratch in a single day.

Because its shell is porous, if you keep an egg for a long time, the yolk and albumen dry out, sucking air inside. That's why rotten eggs float. To find out what colour egg a hen will lay, examine her earlobes. Hens with white earlobes lay white eggs; hens with red earlobes lay brown ones. The colour of a hen's egg depends on the breed of the chicken: it has nothing to do with diet.

In 1826 the Estonian biologist Karl Ernst von Baer (1792–1876) proved that women produce eggs like other animals. Since the time of Aristotle, everyone had thought that a male seed was 'planted' in the woman and nurtured in the womb. (The first observation of semen under a microscope by Anton van Leeuwenhoek (1632–1723) in 1677 seemed to confirm this: he thought he had seen a miniature *homunculus*, or 'little man', in each sperm.) It wasn't until the 1870s that the embryo was proven to develop from the union of egg and sperm and it took another twenty years before German biologist August Weismann (1834–1914) discovered that sperm and ovum carried only half the parent's genes. The sperm is the smallest cell in the human body – it's only a twentieth the size of an ovum – whereas the ovum is the largest. It's a thousand times bigger than the average cell, but still only the size of a full stop on this page.

Can you name a fish?

Don't even try: there's no such thing.

After a lifetime's study of the creatures formerly known as 'fish', the great palaeontologist Stephen Jay Gould (1941–2002) concluded they didn't exist.

The point he was making is that the word 'fish' is applied indiscriminately to entirely separate classes of animal – cartilaginous ones (like sharks and rays); bony ones (including most 'fish', from piranhas and eels to seahorses and cod); and ones with skulls but no backbones or jaws (such as hagfish and lampreys). These three classes split off from one another far longer ago than the different orders, families and genuses did from each other, so that a salmon, for example, has more in common with (and is more closely related to) a human than a hagfish. To an evolutionary biologist, 'fish' is not a useful word unless it's on a menu.

And this isn't just a quirk particular to Gould. The *Oxford Encyclopedia of Underwater Life* comments: 'Incredible as it may sound, there is no such thing as a "fish". The concept is merely a convenient umbrella term to describe an aquatic vertebrate that is not a mammal, a turtle, or anything else.' It's equivalent to calling bats and flying lizards 'birds' just because they happen to fly. 'The relationship between a lamprey and a shark', the *Encyclopedia* insists, 'is no closer than that between a salamander and a camel.'

Still, it's better than it was. In the sixteenth century seals, whales, crocodiles and even hippos were called 'fish'. And, today, cuttlefish, starfish, crayfish, jellyfish and shellfish (which, by any scientific definition, aren't fish at all) still are.

Stephen Jay Gould made the same point about trees. The 'tree' form has evolved many times in the course of history: its ancestors were unrelated plants such as grasses, roses, mosses and clovers – so, for Gould, there's no such thing as a tree either.

One fish that absolutely doesn't exist is the 'sardine'. It's a generic term used for around twenty different small, soft-boned, oily fish. And only once they're in a can. In the UK, they're usually pilchards, often called – optimistically – 'true sardines', although the Latin name (*Sardina pilchardus*) points up the confusion. Sometimes what you get in a sardine can is a herring, sometimes it's a sprat (which glories in the scientific name *Sprattus sprattus sprattus*).

What it isn't, is a 'sardine'. Nor even, as we now know, a fish.

ALAN *At night all the ugly fish come out. And it's really interesting.*

STEPHEN *You don't need to be pretty out there.*

ALAN *That's right. You go to the Red Sea and, in the day, the fish are beautiful, colourful fish. And then at night, they're all bug-eyed. They limp around and you're not allowed to touch them. And they all kind of look at you. And you shine a light at them and they go 'No! No! Don't look at me, don't look at me!'*

How does a shark know you're there?

You don't have to be bleeding for one to track you down.

Sharks have an astonishingly powerful sense of smell. They can detect blood at a concentration of one part in 25 million, the equivalent of a single drop of blood in a 9,000-litre (2,000-gallon) tank of water.

It's the currents that determine the speed and direction of a smell's dispersal in water, so sharks swim into the current. If you are bleeding, even slightly, a shark will know. If the current is running at a moderate 3½ kilometres per hour (about 2¼ miles per hour), a shark 400 metres (a quarter of a mile) downstream will smell your blood in seven minutes. Sharks swim at nearly 40 kilometres per hour (25 miles per hour), so one could reach you in sixty seconds. Faster currents make things worse – even allowing for the fact that the shark has more to swim against. In a riptide of 26 kilometres per hour (16 miles per hour), a shark less than half a kilometre (a quarter of a mile) downstream would detect you in a minute and take less than two to reach you – giving you three minutes in total to escape.

Sharks also see very well, but even a short-sighted shark with a bad head cold (not that it happens) would still be able to find you. Sharks have excellent hearing in the lower frequencies and can hear something thrashing about at a distance of half a kilometre (a third of a mile). So you could try being very quiet indeed.

A blind, stone-deaf shark with no nose would still find you without breaking stride. Sharks' heads are riddled with jelly-filled canals by the name of the 'ampullae of Lorenzini' after Stefano Lorenzini, the Italian doctor who first described them in 1678. We've only recently discovered what their purpose is: to register the faint electrical fields generated by all living bodies.

So, as long as you're not bleeding, not moving and your brain and heart aren't working, you should be fine.

And there's some more good news – sort of. Californian oceanography professor Dr Jamie MacMahan has found that the standard view of a riptide is wrong – it doesn't run out to sea but is circular, like a whirlpool. If you swim parallel to the shore, he says, there's a 50 per cent chance you'll be swept out into the ocean deeps. But, if you just tread water, there's a 90 per cent chance of being returned to shore within three minutes – perhaps just in time to escape the shark.

If a shark does find you, try turning it upside down and tickling its tummy. It will enter a reflex state known as 'tonic immobility' and float motionless as if hypnotised. Killer whales exploit this by flipping sharks over on to their backs and holding them immobile in the water until they suffocate. You have about fifteen minutes before the shark gets wise to your ruse. Careful, though: not all species of shark react the same way. Tiger sharks, for example, respond best to a gentle massage around the eyes. According to shark expert Michael Rutzen, it's just like tickling trout: 'All you have to do is defend your own personal space and stay calm.'

Having said all this, relax. Sharks almost never attack people. Figures from all twenty-two US coastal states, averaged over the last fifty years, show that you are seventy-six times more likely to be killed by a bolt of lightning than by a shark.

Does the Mediterranean have tides?

Yes it does, despite what every tour guide tells you.

Most of them are very small: just a few centimetres back and forth on average. This is because the Mediterranean is cut off from the Atlantic (and the huge effect of the pull of the moon on it) by the narrow Straits of Gibraltar.

Right next door to the entrance to the Med, sea levels can change by around 80 centimetres (3 feet) but in the Gulf of Gabes off the coast of eastern Tunisia, the tidal elevation can be as much as 2.5 metres (8 feet) twice a day.

This is because tides are caused not only by the gravitational effect of the moon but also by atmospheric pressure, depth, salinity, temperature and the shape of the coastline.

The relatively big tides in the Gulf of Gabes result from its shape. It is a wide, shallow basin, about 100 kilometres (60 miles) wide by 100 kilometres long. The gulf acts as a funnel, the tidal energy forcing water into a progressively smaller space, thereby increasing the rise in sea level – and, correspondingly, lowering it on the way out. The same thing happens on a much greater scale in the Bristol Channel, which has a tidal range of over 9 metres (30 feet).

Tidal effects are at their strongest when the sun and moon are on the same side of the earth (new moon), or on the opposite side (full moon), and their gravitational pulls combine to create the strong 'spring' tides ('spring' in the sense of 'powerful forward movement', not the season).

The Phoenicians founded Gabes in about 800 BC. Pliny the Elder first noted its unusually large tides in AD 77 in his *Natural History*. He also recorded that Gabes was second only to Tyre in the production of the expensive purple dye made from murex shells, which the Phoenicians discovered (hence the Greek for purple, *phoinikeos*), and which was highly prized by the Romans: the *toga purpurea* was worn only by kings, generals in triumph and emperors.

The Mediterranean is bigger than you might think. At 2,500 square kilometres (965 square miles) it covers the same area as Sudan, the largest country in Africa, and would comfortably swallow Western Europe (France, Spain, Germany, Italy, Greece, Britain, the Netherlands, Belgium, Switzerland and Austria combined). Its coastline stretches for 46,000 kilometres (28,000 miles) or about twice the length of the coastline of Africa. Nor is it particularly shallow: its average depth is over 1½ kilometres (about a mile) while the North Sea's is a mere 94 metres (310 feet) and, at its deepest point, in the Ionian Sea, it reaches down nearly 5 kilometres (over 3 miles), substantially deeper than the average depth of the Atlantic.

Six million years ago, the Mediterranean dried out completely in the so-called Messinian Salinity Crisis. This created the largest salt basin that ever existed and raised the sea level of the rest of the world by 10 metres (33 feet). Three hundred thousand years later, the rock barrier at the Straits of Gibraltar gave way – in a cataclysm called the Zanclean Flood – producing the world's largest-ever waterfall and refilling the whole of the Mediterranean in as little as two years. The tide would have risen 10 metres every day. But it wouldn't have gone out again.

STEPHEN *The Mediterranean was once the biggest dry lake in the world. In the late Miocene era.*

ALAN *The water came rushing in over the Strait of Gibraltar.*

STEPHEN *You're quite right. Six million years ago.*

ALAN *I know this because I saw it in the Plymouth Aquarium.*

JIMMY CARR *That must have been fabulous for all the towns around Spain and Portugal that rely on tourism. When that came in, they went: 'This is fantastic. Finally these jet-skis are going to get an outing.'*

Which birds inspired Darwin's theory of evolution?

Many smart people would answer 'finches', but actually it was mockingbirds.

The great passion of the young Charles Darwin (1809–82) was killing wildlife. As a student at Cambridge, when the shooting season started, his hands shook so much with excitement he could hardly load his gun. Though studying medicine and divinity to please his father, he dismissed lectures as 'cold, breakfastless hours, listening to discourses on the properties of rhubarb'.

But he was also an enthusiastic amateur biologist and fossil-hunter and was keen to see the tropics, so he signed on as a 'gentleman naturalist' for HMS *Beagle*'s second survey expedition (1831–6). He almost didn't get the job: the captain was keen on physiognomy and thought that Darwin's nose indicated laziness. Charles later noted that 'I think he was afterwards well satisfied that my nose had spoken falsely'.

The story goes that, during the voyage, Darwin noticed that finches on different islands in the Galapagos had distinctive beaks, which led him to guess that each type had adapted for a specific habitat and evolved from a common ancestor. It's true that Darwin's theory of evolution by natural selection originated aboard the *Beagle*, but it had nothing to do with finches. Though Darwin did collect finch specimens from the Galapagos, he showed very little interest in them until years later. He was no ornithologist in those days and wasn't even aware that the finches were of different species. It wouldn't have helped much if he had been, because he didn't label them to show where they'd been caught. He mentioned them only in passing in his journals and they are not mentioned once in *On the Origin of Species* (1859).

The mockingbirds were a different matter. Intrigued by the variations between the populations on two nearby islands, Darwin took careful note of every mockingbird he encountered. Gradually, as his journals show, he began to realise that species were not immutable: they could change over time. Out of that insight all his subsequent theories on evolution grew.

Because the finches are a perfect example of Darwin's theories in action, later scientists assumed that they must have been the birds that inspired him. One of these was the evolutionary biologist David Lack (1910–73) whose 1947 book, *Darwin's Finches,* fixed the idea (and the term) in the popular consciousness.

Darwin's book on the voyage of the *Beagle* was an immediate best-seller, and the trip made the captain's name too. Robert Fitzroy (1805–65) went on to become a vice-admiral, Governor General of New Zealand and the inventor of weather forecasting – one of the sea areas in the Shipping Forecast is named after him.

The finches got famous, too, as we know. The fifteen species of *Geospizinae* are still popularly known today as Darwin's Finches – although it turns out they're not finches at all, but a different kind of bird called a tanager.

Where's the most convenient place to discover a new species?

In your own back garden.

You can cancel that expensive (and possibly dangerous) trip up the Amazon.

In 1972 an ecologist called Jennifer Owen started to note down all the wildlife in her garden in Humberstone, a suburb of Leicester. After fifteen years she wrote a book about it. She had counted 422 species of plant and 1,757 species of animal, including 533 species of parasitic Ichneumon wasp. Fifteen of these had never been recorded in Britain, and four were completely new to science.

Suburban gardens cover 433,000 hectares (well over a million acres) of England and Wales. If so many new species can be found in just one of them, this must be true of others. Between 2000 and 2007, the Biodiversity in Urban Gardens in Sheffield project (BUGS) repeated Dr Owen's work on a bigger scale. Domestic gardens account for some 23 per cent of urban Sheffield, including 25,000 ponds, 45,000 nest boxes, 50,000 compost heaps and 360,000 trees. These present, as Professor Kevin Gaston, BUGS' chief investigator, put it '175,000 separate conservation opportunities'. One of BUGS' discoveries was what may be a new, minuscule species of lichen, found in the moss on an ordinary tarmac path.

To more or less guarantee discovering a new species, all you need is a garden, a lot of time and patience, and a lot of expertise. In the words of the eighteenth-century naturalist Gilbert White (1720–93), 'In zoology as it is in botany: all nature is so full, that that district produces the greatest variety which is the most examined.' In 2010 London's Natural History Museum found a new species of insect in its own garden. They are baffled by what it is, as it doesn't match any of the more than 28 million specimens inside the museum itself.

Part of the fun of discovering a new species is that you get the chance to choose what it's called. A recently discovered beetle with legs resembling overdeveloped human biceps was named *Agra schwarzeneggeri*; a fossilized trilobite with an hourglass-shaped shell was called *Norasaphus monroeae* after Marilyn Monroe; and *Orectochilus orbisonorum* is a whirligig beetle dedicated to singer Ray Orbison because it looks like it's wearing a tuxedo. In 1982 Ferdinando Boero, now a professor at Lecce University in Italy, but then a researcher at Genoa, had a more underhand motive in naming the jellyfish he discovered *Phialella zappai* – it was a cunning plan to persuade his hero Frank Zappa to meet him. It worked: they remained friends for the rest of the musician's life.

British-born astrobiologist Paul Davies of Arizona State University urges us all to search for new unknown forms of life. 'It could be right in front of our noses – or even in our noses,' he says.

The one thing you don't want to find in your nose is an Ichneumon wasp. These unpleasant insects caused Darwin to lose his religious faith. 'I cannot persuade myself', he wrote, 'that a beneficent and omnipotent God would have designedly created the Ichneumonidae with the express intention of their feeding within the living bodies of caterpillars.'

What kind of bird is *Puffinus puffinus*?

Before you answer, bear in mind that *Rattus rattus* is a rat, *Gerbillus gerbillus* is a gerbil, *Oriolus oriolus* is an oriole, *Iguana iguana* is an iguana, *Conger conger* is a conger eel and *Gorilla gorilla gorilla* is emphatically a gorilla.

And *Puffinus puffinus*?

Bad luck, that's the Manx shearwater. It's unrelated to the puffin.

Scientific names for animals are usually composed of two words: the genus comes first, followed by the species. The species of a living thing is defined as that group with which it can reproduce. Its genus is analogous to its tribe: a group of species that are clearly related to each other. When the names of an animal's genus and its species are the same that's called a tautonym (from the Greek *tautos* 'same' and *onoma* 'name'). For example, the bogue fish is *Boops boops* and *Mops mops* is the Malayan Free-tailed bat.

Where there is a third part to the name of a species, it is used to indicate a subspecies. So the triple tautonym *Gorilla gorilla gorilla* (the Western Lowland gorilla) is a subspecies of *Gorilla gorilla* (the Western gorilla). The Tiger beetle subspecies *Megacephala (Megacephala) megacephala* has a name that translates as 'bighead (bighead) bighead'. Sometimes a subgenus is also given in brackets such as *Bison (Bison) bison bison*, which (for the avoidance of doubt) is a kind of bison.

Tautonyms for animals are not uncommon, but are strictly forbidden for plants under the International Code of Botanical Nomenclature.

There are three species of puffin and they belong to the genus *Fratercula*, Latin for 'little brother', because their plumage resembles monastic robes.

There are about thirty species of shearwater, all of which share the genus name *Puffinus*, which comes from an Anglo-Norman word meaning 'fatling'. This refers to the chubbiness of the young birds, and hints at their culinary uses. They were eaten both fresh and pickled and, because they swim so well under water, were for a long time thought to be half fish, which allowed Catholics to eat them on Fridays and during Lent. Shearwater chicks are easily mistaken for puffins: which probably explains the confusion over the name. Puffins (and particularly their hearts) are a national delicacy in Iceland.

The oldest living bird ever recorded in Britain was a Manx Shearwater. It was found by chance in 2002 by the staff of the bird observatory on Bardsey Island in North Wales. They were delighted to discover that ornithologists had ringed it in 1957, when it must already have been at least five years old. It's reckoned to have covered around 8 million kilometres (5 million miles) over more than half a century, flying to South America in the winter and back again to Britain for the *Puffinus puffinus* breeding season.

JEREMY CLARKSON *You don't want to listen to this, but I once had some whale. And they said to me: 'Would you like me to grate some puffin on that?'*

Can you name three species of British mouse?

Two points each for Harvest mouse, House mouse, Field mouse and Wood mouse – and four points for Yellow-necked mouse – but minus ten for dormouse.

The dormouse is more of a squirrel than a mouse.

Admittedly, it does look rather mouse-like – except for its tail, which is furry. (Mice have scaly tales.) It also has fur inside its ears – which mice don't. In fact, the dormouse is generally furrier all round. This to keep it warm in winter: it's the only British rodent that hibernates.

The 'dorm-' part of its name means 'sleepy' and sleeping is what it's best at. The golden-coloured Common (or Hazel) dormouse can spend three-quarters of its life asleep. It's also known as the 'seven-sleeper' because it regularly spends seven months of the year dormant, though warmer winters now mean its hibernation lasts five and a half weeks less than it did twenty years ago.

If you want to get involved with dormice, you'll need to go on a Dormouse Handling Course and apply for a government dormouse licence. The British dormouse population has fallen by 70 per cent in the last quarter century and it is now strictly illegal to disturb, let alone kill, this rarely seen nocturnal creature.

The much larger Edible (or Fat) dormouse (*Glis glis*) is even less common in Britain than the Common dormouse (*Muscardinus avellanarius*). It's grey and white and could easily be mistaken for a small squirrel with big ears. It was introduced to Britain in 1902 by Lord Rothschild, as part of his wildlife collection in Tring Park, Hertfordshire – since when escapees have spread across the Chilterns. They can be a serious pest in lofts and outbuildings and can cause fatal damage to young trees. It's legal to shoot them.

The Romans were very keen on eating Edible dormice,

though there's no evidence that they brought them to Britain. They kept them in earthenware pots called *dolia*, fattening them up on a diet of walnuts and currants, and storing the pots in special dormouse gardens or *glisaria*. Recipes included roast stuffed dormouse and honey-glazed dormouse with poppy seeds.

It's a taste that survives in many parts of Europe, where dormouse hunting is illegal but often done. In Calabria in southern Italy, where tens of thousands are eaten annually, the Mafia allegedly controls the lucrative dormouse trade.

In 2007 fifteen Calabrian restaurateurs were charged with serving *Glis* stewed in wine and red pepper. They all denied the allegations. Their defence was that the meat in the casseroles wasn't dormouse – it was only rat.

How far are you from a rat?

It's much further than you think.

The idea that you are 'never more than 6 feet away from a rat' is wrong by a factor of ten. Of course, it depends where you live: some of us live close to hundred of rats, others live near none. But rats, although they happily 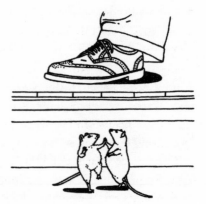 live off our rubbish, don't like to get too close. Rentokil, the pest control company, estimates that the average city dweller is at least 21 metres (70 feet) from the nearest one.

The bad news is that rats in the UK now outnumber people. According to the National Rodent Survey, there are around 70 million rats in the country: 10 per cent more than the current human population.

Rats carry seventy or so infectious diseases including salmonella, tuberculosis and Weil's disease. They are also responsible for consuming a fifth of the world's food supply each year. Their sharp teeth (which never stop growing) enable them to gnaw through almost anything, causing a quarter of all electric cable breaks and disconnected phone lines in the process.

Plus, they brought the fleas that gave us bubonic plague. And they have those nasty, scaly tails.

It was the Black or Ship rat (*Rattus rattus*) that brought the plague. It sought out human company because our living conditions were so squalid. Slovenly disposal of food waste causes 35 per cent of rat infestations: broken sewers only 2 per cent.

Today, *Rattus rattus* is one of the UK's rarest mammals. Only small clusters remain, around big ports like London and Liverpool and on remote islands like Lundy, where they still are regularly (and legally) culled. The Black rat doesn't appear on any endangered lists – presumably because it's a rat.

Any rat you see today is almost certain to be the larger, stronger Brown or Norway rat (*Rattus norvegicus*), which arrived in the UK less than 300 years ago. They have nothing to do with Norway (they originated in northern China) and they don't carry plague. In fact, their use in laboratory experiments saves many human lives.

The dreaded rat's tail is actually a device for regulating body temperature. It acts as a long, thin radiator (rather like an elephant's ears), which is why it isn't covered in hair.

ALAN *You know, all the rats in England all face the same direction at any given time . . .*

What kind of animal is 'Ratty' from *The Wind in the Willows?*

You won't be surprised to hear that he's not a rat.

The Wind in the Willows by Kenneth Grahame (1859–1932) began as a series of letters to his young son, Alistair (nicknamed 'Mouse'). After being rejected by several publishers, it came out in book form in 1908 – the same year that Grahame retired after thirty years working at the Bank of England.

Ratty, one of the main characters, is a water vole (*Arvicola amphibius*), colloquially known as a 'water rat'. As a child, Kenneth Grahame would have seen plenty of water voles, nesting in the riverbanks near his grandmother's home at Cookham Dean on the Thames – but today they are one of Britain's most endangered species. Water voles underwent a catastrophe after the fur trade started farming imported American mink in the 1920s. Unlike native predators, mink can follow voles right into their tunnels. Escaped mink (and their descendants) have been eating vast numbers of voles ever since, wiping them out entirely in many places.

This is bad news for future archaeologists. Voles are the world's fastest-evolving mammals, dividing into new species up to a hundred times faster than the average vertebrate. This allows archaeologists to use the so-called 'vole clock'. Carbon dating only works up to about 50,000 years ago. For older digs, the investigators use fossilised vole teeth – tiny things about the size of a fingernail clipping. The ways they have altered at different stages in voles' evolution are so specific that items found alongside them can be dated with great accuracy.

Water voles are vegetarian but, in 2010, researchers in Berkshire were amazed to discover they had been eating the legs of toads. It's thought that pregnant voles needing extra protein were responsible, but it seems like poetic justice given all the trouble that Toad caused Ratty in the book.

Early reviews of *The Wind in the Willows* were damning. Arthur Ransome (1884–1967), author of *Swallows and Amazons*, wrote that it was 'like a speech to Hottentots made in Chinese'. It only started to sell after Grahame sent a copy to US President Theodore Roosevelt (1858–1919), who adored it.

Grahame's own life was much less delightful than the riverside idyll he wrote about. His mother died when he was five, causing his father to drink himself to death. As Secretary to the Bank of England, he spent his time collecting fluffy toys and writing hundreds of letters in baby language to his equally strange fiancée, Elspeth. In 1903 he survived an assassination attempt when a 'Socialist Lunatic' shot him at work (the Governor wasn't available). Luckily, the fire brigade managed to subdue the terrorist by turning a hose on him.

The life of his troubled son, Alistair ('Mouse'), was even worse. Blind in one eye from birth, his childhood hobbies included lying down in front of passing cars to make them stop. He had a nervous breakdown at school and then took to calling himself 'Robinson' – the name of his father's would-be assassin. In 1920, while an undergraduate at Oxford, Alistair lay face down across a railway track in Port Meadow and was decapitated by a train.

What kind of animal did Beatrix Potter first write about?

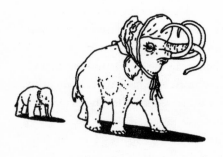

It wasn't a rabbit – or a hedgehog, or a frog – or anything remotely cute. The first living things that Beatrix Potter wrote about were fungi.

Fungus is Latin for mushroom. You might think it's pushing it a bit to call a mushroom an animal, but fungi are biologically closer to animals than they are to plants. Since 1969 they've had their own kingdom (along with yeasts and moulds) and they're neither plant nor animal.

The English author and illustrator Beatrix Potter (1866–1943) was educated by governesses and grew up isolated from other children. From the age of fifteen she recorded her life in journals, using a secret code that wasn't unravelled until twenty years after her death. She had lots of pets: a bat, newts, ferrets, frogs and two rabbits (Benjamin and Peter), whom she took out for walks on leads. She spent her summers in Scotland and the Lake District where her close observation of nature led her to become an expert on fungi or 'mycologist'.

Although an amateur, Potter kept up with all the latest advances in mycology.

Her first published work, presented at the Linnaean Society in 1897, was *On the Germination of Spores of Agaricineae*. It had to be read out for her by her uncle, because women were not allowed to address meetings. She applied to study at the Royal Botanic Gardens at Kew, but was turned down for the same reason – and the Royal Society refused to publish at least one of her papers. A hundred years later, the Linnaean Society, at least, had the grace to issue a belated posthumous apology.

Potter was an early pioneer of the theory that lichens were a partnership between fungi and algae – two separate organisms rather than one – and she produced a series of detailed drawings to support her hypothesis. This idea, later confirmed as correct, was considered heretical by the British scientific establishment at the time, but her scientific illustrations were greatly admired. This proved useful when she came to write her children's books.

The first of Beatrix Potter's twenty stories for children began life in 1893, as a letter to a young boy named Noel Moore, whose mother had been one of her governesses. The ex-governess loved the story and persuaded her to publish it. Frederick Warne brought it out in 1902, and by Christmas *The Tale of Peter Rabbit* had sold 28,000 copies. Within a year, Peter Rabbit was so popular he had become a soft toy, making him the world's first licensed character.

Peter Rabbit was inspired by a pet rabbit named Peter Piper, bought for the young Beatrix in Shepherd's Bush for 4s 6d. He was trained to 'jump through a hoop, and ring a bell, and play the tambourine'. Although he brought her fame and financial security, Potter was baffled by the success of her creation: 'The public must be fond of rabbits! What an appalling quantity of Peter.'

Beatrix Potter borrowed the names for many of her characters from tombstones in Brompton Cemetery in London, which was near the family home in South Kensington. Peter Rabbett, Jeremiah Fisher, Mr Nutkins, Mr Brock and Mr McGregor are all buried there.

Which animal dreams most?

You might think it's the ones that sleep most, like the dormouse or the sloth, or perhaps humans, who have the most complex brains. But it's none of these. The greatest dreamer of all is the duck-billed platypus.

All mammals (but only some birds) dream. What happens to them when they do, or why they do it at all, is much less well understood.

The dream state is known as Rapid Eye Movement (REM) sleep and it was discovered in 1952. Eugene Aserinsky, a graduate physiology student at the University of Chicago, used a device called an electroculogram to record the eye-movements of his eight-year-old son. He noticed a distinct pattern as he slept during the night and pointed it out to his supervisor, Dr Nathaniel Kleitman. An electro-encephalograph (EEG) was then used to measure the brain activity of twenty sleeping people. To the researchers' amazement, this showed that, when the subjects' eyes were moving rapidly, their brain activity was so vigorous that they should really have been awake. Waking them from REM sleep led to vivid recall of their dreams – which didn't happen when their eyes were still.

Zoologists soon found that many animals also undergo the same process. Cats, bats, opossums and armadillos all have extended periods of REM sleep but, surprisingly, giraffes and elephants get very little and dolphins have none at all. The animal with by far the longest REM sleep is the duck-billed platypus (*Ornithorhynchus anatinus*), one of the oldest of all mammals. They spend eight hours a day in the dream state, four times as much as an adult human.

REM sleep is different from either normal sleep or waking: it is a third state of existence in which the brain is racing, but the body is virtually paralysed. It seems that the animals most at risk from predators dream least. Ruminants like elephants and sheep have few dreams; a platypus, with few enemies, can afford plenty. Dolphins, who need to rest while afloat but still keep breathing, don't sleep at all in the traditional sense. One half of their brain and body goes to sleep at a time, while the other half is fully awake – including one of their eyes. This may explain why they don't have REM: the conscious eye would be jiggling about all over the place.

Platypuses sleep so deeply that you can dig open their burrows without waking them. Though much of this is REM sleep, unlike almost all other animals, the brains of sleeping platypuses aren't as active as when they were awake. So we can't say for certain that they are dreaming.

But then, we can't be absolutely sure that any animal dreams – because we can't ask them – we can only say it of ourselves. No one knows why we dream. Assuming an average life of sixty-five years, with two hours' REM a night, we would spend 8 per cent of our lives dreaming (about five years).

Eugene Aserinsky got his doctorate but, angry at having to share the credit for REM with Dr Kleitman, gave up sleep research for ten years. He died aged seventy-seven when his car ran into a tree. Kleitman kept at it, earning himself the title the 'Father of Sleep Research', and outlived Aserinsky by a year. He died aged 104.

Which animal drinks most?

The biggest boozer after man is the Pen-tailed tree shrew of Malaysia.

Ptilocercus lowii, a rat-sized animal with a tail shaped like a quill pen, gets through nine units of alcohol a night (the equivalent of nine single whiskies, five pints of beer or five 175-millilitre glasses of wine).

Its staple diet is nectar from the flowers of the Bertram palm, which ferments as a result of natural yeasts in the plant's spiky buds. This brew weighs in at 3.8 per cent ABV (alcohol by volume) – about the strength of a decent pale ale – and the Pen-tailed tree shrew spends an average of two hours a night sipping it.

The nectar of the Bertram palm is among the most alcoholic of any naturally occurring food. German researchers from the University of Bayreuth were first alerted to the presence of alcohol in the plant by its wafting, yeasty aroma, and what looked very much like a foamy 'head' on the nectar.

Analysis of the tree shrew's hair revealed blood-alcohol levels that would be dangerous in most mammals, but it never gets drunk. If it did, it wouldn't have lasted long as a species. Being small and edible makes for a tough enough life, but being small, edible and permanently confused would be fatal.

The Pen-tailed tree shrew has somehow evolved to break down the alcohol without becoming intoxicated, and it may also have benefited from the so-called 'aperitif effect'. First noted in humans, this is the fact that alcohol stimulates the appetite, so we eat more. The higher an animal's calorie intake, the more energy it has and the more likely it is to survive. As the Pen-tailed tree shrew appears to have discovered, the smell of fermentation in a fruit indicates that it has reached its peak calorific level.

The first record of humans drinking alcohol dates from 9,000 years ago, when brewing was invented in Mesopotamia. But the Bayreuth research suggests we may have inherited the taste for it from our pre-human past. The common ancestor of shrews and man was a small mammal that lived between 55 and 80 million years ago. The closest living match to this nameless creature is thought to be the Pen-tailed tree shrew. If we can work out why it likes alcohol so much (and why it never gets drunk), we may reach a better understanding of why humans like to drink, how we can do it without becoming legless, and maybe discover a hangover cure along the way.

In the oldest surviving work of literature on earth – the 4,000-year-old *Epic of Gilgamesh* – Shamhat, a temple prostitute, tames Enkidu, a hairy wild man raised by animals, by taking him to bed for a week and plying him with seven jars of beer. The result that is he starts to wash, puts on clothes for the first time and abandons his former animal friends, 'having acquired wisdom'.

STEPHEN *Name a green mammal*
BILL BAILEY *A really, really jealous shrew.*

How do elephants get drunk?

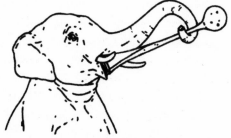

African tourist bro-chures often tell of elephants blundering around drunk after eat-ing the fermented fruit of the marula tree, but it's a complete myth.

The marula tree (*Scelerocarya birrea caffera*) is a member of the mango family and elephants do indeed love its plum-sized yellow fruit. And it's not just the elephants' favourite – warthogs, monkeys, antelopes, giraffes and zebras all enjoy eating both the fruit and the bark of the tree.

In fact they like the fruit so much that none of them leave it lying on the ground long enough to allow it to rot and start to ferment. Elephants like their fruit fresh and visit the trees often to check whether their lunch is ripe. They are so eager that they will sometimes push the tree over to get what they want. Even if elephants liked rotten fruit, there's none on the ground because it's all been eaten by other species.

A study by Steve Morris of the University of Bristol calculated that, even if there *were* rotten fruit on the ground and the elephants *did* eat it, they would have to consume about 1,500 marula fruit, all at the same time, to get tipsy.

The myth can be traced back to a wildlife movie called *Animals Are Beautiful People* (1974) by the South African film director Jamie Uys (1921–96). His scenes of elephants, warthogs and baboons getting drunk on marula fruit were almost certainly staged. All Uys's other films were comedies, and one, *Funny People* (1978), was a spoof show similar to *Candid Camera* or *Beadle's About*.

The Bristol University study suggested that any odd behaviour by elephants around marula trees might be due to another form of 'intoxication' altogether. The bark is host to the grubs of the Lebistina beetle, traditionally used by the San Bushmen to poison their arrows.

Elephants can get drunk – but only by drinking alcohol. They can detect the pleasant smell of ethanol (pure alcohol) up to 10 miles away. In 1999 a herd of elephants broke into thatched huts in a village in India and polished off several vats of fermenting rice wine. They then went on a drunken rampage through the other huts, killing four unlucky villagers.

People have been eating marula fruit, which is rich in vitamin C, for 10,000 years. The tree has many other uses. The wood is used for carvings, the inner bark is made into rope and the skin of the fruit into substitute coffee. The bark also contains antihistamines (used to cure dysentery, diarrhoea and malaria), and caterpillars (which are collected and eaten roasted).

Marula beer is the favourite drink of the people of Swaziland. Drinkers claim it doesn't give you a hangover but, in 2002, the Swazi authorities banned it, citing a huge increase in drink driving, street brawls and absenteeism at work.

Amarula Cream, a sweet liqueur distilled from the fruit, is a speciality of South Africa, where it is served as an after-dinner *digestif*. It has a picture of an elephant on the label.

What's the world's most aggressive mammal?

It's not tigers or hippos.

According to *Scientific American* in 2009, the world's most fearsome land mammal is the Honey badger (*Mellivora capensis*). The *Guinness Book of Records* also lists it as 'the most *fearless* animal in the world'.

Honey badgers live in Africa and Asia in vacant burrows abandoned by other creatures such as aardvarks, and they aren't badgers. They're called that because they bear a superficial resemblance to regular badgers (*Meles meles*) and because they love honey. Badgers and Honey badgers are unrelated members of the weasel family, *Mustelidae*, the largest group of carnivores. It includes ferrets, polecats, minks and wolverines, but the Honey badger is a one-off: the only species in the genus *Mellivora*, which means 'honey-eaters'.

Honey badgers use their large and powerful claws to ravage termite mounds, rip through the wire round chicken coops and, especially, tear beehives apart. They are led to the hives by honeyguide birds, which call out when they find one, and take their share when the Honey badger has eaten its fill.

One of the things that makes the Honey badger such an indomitable adversary is its very loose-fitting skin: if it's caught from behind it is able to twist around inside its own skin and fight back. As a result, they have few predators and will attack most animals when provoked, even humans. They have fought or killed hyenas, lions, tigers, tortoises, porcupines, crocodiles and bears. They eat venomous snakes, which they grab in their jaws and devour in fifteen minutes. They also eat young Honey badgers: only half the cubs survive to adulthood.

Legend has it that a Honey badger's attack methods are below the belt. The first published record of this was in 1947 when a Honey badger was allegedly observed to castrate an adult buffalo. They are also said to have emasculated wildebeest, waterbuck, kudu, zebra and man. In *Top Gear's* 2009 Botswana special, Jeremy Clarkson reported: 'The honey badger does not kill you to eat you. It tears off your testicles.'

In Pakistan, they are called 'Bijj' and are said to take away dead bodies from graves. Such is the animal's terrifying reputation that, during the Iraq war, British troops in Basra were accused of having unleashed a plague of man-eating bear-like beasts to terrify the locals. They turned out to be Honey badgers, which had been driven into the city by the flooding of marshland.

ROSS NOBLE *You know what annoys me, right, is the term to 'badger' somebody. Because badgers don't actually badger. If you were going to badger somebody you'd move into their garden and you'd just sleep a lot...*

Which animal has saved the most human lives?

It's not the faithful dog, the loyal horse or the brave carrier pigeon, but the oldest surviving species on the planet: the horseshoe crab.

If you've ever had an injection you quite possibly owe your life to the North American horseshoe crab (*Limulus polyphemus*). An extract of its blood, Limulus amebocyte lysate, or LAL, is used by the pharmaceutical industry to test drugs, vaccines and medical devices like artificial kidneys to ensure they are free of dangerous microbes. No other test works as easily or reliably.

Horseshoe crabs live in shallow coastal seas, which are often polluted. A litre of such seawater can contain over a thousand billion toxic bacteria. Horseshoe crabs have no immune system and can't develop antibodies to fight infection. Instead, their blood contains a miraculous ingredient that disables invasive bacteria and viruses by clotting around them, and it is this that is used to make LAL. To find out if anything intended for medical use is contaminated or not, all you have to do is expose it to some LAL: if it doesn't clot, it's fine.

Unlike humans, the blood of horseshoe crabs has no haemoglobin – which uses iron to carry oxygen – instead it has haemocyanin, which uses copper. As a result, their blood is blue. It sells for about $15,000 a litre.

To obtain the blood, horseshoe crabs are 'harvested' rather than killed. Up to a thousand of them a week are collected by hand from small boats with a clam rake, and brought to the lab alive. Although 30 per cent of their blood is taken, they recover quickly when put back in the water. The crabs are bled once a year and their blood is freeze-dried and shipped around the world.

Horseshoe crabs aren't, in fact, crabs. They're not even crustaceans. More closely related to ticks, scorpions and spiders, they are the last surviving members of the once thriving *Xiphosura* ('sword-tail') order, and they've been scuttling around the Atlantic coast of America and the seas of South-East Asia unchanged since the Ordovician era, 445 million years ago. That's 75 per cent of the entire time that animal life has existed on the planet and 200 million years before the dinosaurs arrived. Not bad for something that looks like a fancy computer mouse or a small tin hat.

It's their smooth, curved shells that helped them survive for so long. They're hard for predators to overturn and expose the soft underside, though Native Americans once used them as bailers to scoop water out of their canoes.

As well as their extraordinary blood – now known to be able to detect meningitis and cancer as well – horseshoe crabs can endure extremes of heat and cold and go for a year without eating.

They also have ten eyes. Which is odd, because Polyphemus, the giant of Greek mythology they're named after, only had one.

STEPHEN *It's the blood of the horseshoe crab.*

JACK DEE *When you get given it, do you walk out sideways?*

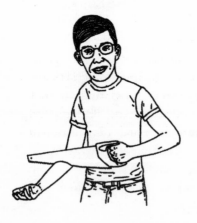

What's the best way to treat a jellyfish sting?

Don't urinate on it!

There's a well-established urban myth that urinating on a jellyfish sting relieves the pain.

In fact, it doesn't – and could make it worse.

The sting of a jellyfish comes from specialised cells in the skin of its tentacles called cnidocytes (literally 'nettle-jars', from Greek *cnide,* 'stinging nettle', and *cytos,* a 'vase' or 'vessel').

Each small, bulb-shaped capsule holds a coiled, barbed, thread-like tube, filled with poison and sealed in under high pressure. On the outside of each cell is a tiny hair called a cnidocil (Latin *cilia* for eyelashes). Touching this 'hair-trigger' explodes the cell's minuscule toxic harpoon into your skin in 700 billionths of a second.

It is the fastest known mechanism in nature.

Feeling or scratching a jellyfish sting is not a good idea. It sets off any other unfired sting cells clinging to the skin, and you get stung on your hand as well.

Brush off any loose tentacles with a towel and splash the sting with salt water to wash away any unfired cells. Fresh water is no good: the change in the salt content of the water also activates the cells and injects more venom.

There's a lot of fresh water in urine – you can survive by drinking it if you have to – and, depending on who's doing the urinating, a lot of other stuff as well. It may contain harmful bacteria that can infect the wound. (Don't be fooled by the 'fact' that human urine is sterile. It is when it leaves the bladder, but it has to pass through the urethra which contains plenty of germs, all of them waiting to multiply in a warm, hitherto unoccupied medium like urine.)

Many Australian beaches have supplies of vinegar (5 per cent acetic acid) available in case of jellyfish stings. This can work – if you know the species you've been stung by. But some jellyfish have acid stings and some have alkaline ones. Vinegar is a good temporary remedy for the deadly Australian box jellyfish, but only exacerbates the sting of the Portuguese man of war.

Pain is not necessarily the worst thing about jellyfish

stings. They can cause anaphylactic shock. Watch out for swelling, itching, rashes or shortness of breath. If you spot any of these symptoms, don't waste valuable time urinating on the patient – call a doctor.

What causes pins and needles?

Ordinary pins and needles have nothing to do with poor circulation.

They happen when pressure on a part of the body compresses the nerve cells and impedes the blood flow. When the pressure is released and the blood flow returns to normal, numbness gives way to tingling as oxygen and glucose are restored to the nerves. This can affect anywhere on the body – though it's usually found in arms, legs, hands or feet – and passes within a few minutes. The technical term for it is 'transient paraesthesia', Greek for 'altered feeling'.

If you suffer from *chronic* pins and needles, however, you might want to get a professional opinion. It can be symptomatic of a stroke, brain tumour, brain abscess, multiple sclerosis, rheumatoid arthritis, HIV, Lyme disease, cancer, alcoholism, malnutrition, exposure to radiation or whiplash injury.

Disturbing though that list is, it won't lead to the onset of belonephobia, the 'fear of pins and needles'. That only applies to fear of sharp points (*belone* is Greek for 'needle'). There is no such word as paraesthesiaphobia – at least, there wasn't until just now.

The indescribably peculiar feeling you get when you bang your 'funny bone' is a close relative of transient paraesthesia. The 'funny bone' isn't a bone – it's the ulnar nerve, which is unusually near the surface. The twinge comes from it getting jammed up against an actual bone, the humerus, which starts at the shoulder and ends at the elbow. Banging it produces dysaesthesia, meaning an unpleasant sensation, as opposed to paraesthesia, which is merely an unusual one.

A good way to get pins and needles is to sit on one of your feet, a pose that was very popular in nineteenth-century Turkey. In the travel book *Constantinople in 1828* by Charles Macfarlane, the author noted that the polite sitting position for ladies in Smyrna was 'with one leg on the sofa bent under them, and the other hanging over the edge'. This led a visiting Frenchman to ask whether 'this unipedal exhibition' meant that 'all the women in the city had but the one leg'.

In the USA 27 November is official Pins and Needles Day, though few people know why. It commemorates the opening night, in 1937, of a unique Broadway musical. *Pins and Needles* was produced by the International Ladies' Garment Workers' Union, and the cast was made up of union members. Despite being ignored by mainstream theatre critics, the show ran for 1,108 performances, a record only overtaken by *Oklahoma!* in 1945.

Finally, in case you're wondering, acupuncturists *do* claim to be able to treat pins and needles. They may not ask you how you got them: paraesthesia is one of the side effects associated with acupuncture.

What causes a hernia?

It's not the strain of lifting something heavy.

Hernia is Latin for 'rupture' and is the condition in which a bodily organ (or part of one) breaks through into a part of the body it shouldn't be in. This could be the brain pro-truding through a defect in the skull, or a loop of intestine escaping from the abdominal cavity and ending up in the chest.

The most common use of the word hernia refers to tissue that has protruded through the abdomen. Heavy lifting never *causes* this – although straining the abdominal muscles by lifting something heavy might make an existing, unnoticed hernia more prominent.

A hernia is caused by a lack of collagen (the protein in skin and muscle tissue that makes it flexible) in the affected area. This can be the result of genetic abnormalities, of smoking (which breaks down the collagen in your body) or just the general wear-and-tear of advancing age. Only one in ten people who are diagnosed with a hernia will have discovered it by straining themselves.

The most common type of hernia in the UK is the inguinal hernia (from Latin *inguen*, 'groin'), in which a segment of bowel slips down into the scrotum, using the same route as the descending testes during puberty. If it gets caught, and cannot return easily, it can 'strangulate' – causing vio-lent vomiting and abdominal pain and requiring immediate surgery.

But this misfortune is a weakness that you are born with: it's not caused by strenuous exercise.

Why should you avoid the free peanuts in bars?

You'll have heard about the scientists who tested a bowl of peanuts in a bar and found traces of urine belonging to twenty-seven different people. Johnny Depp certainly has; he mentioned it during an appearance on *The Tonight Show* with Jay Leno in July 2005.

This alarming tale is trotted out again and again, and it's in the back of many people's minds every time they reach for the bar snacks.

As far as we know, there has never been any such scientific study but, in 2003, the London *Evening Standard* conducted an informal tour of six London bars and took away samples of the free snacks. Tests showed that four of the six contained enterobacteria, which are also found in faeces.

There is certainly cause for concern about many people's attitudes to toilet hygiene. In 2000 the American Society for Microbiology asked a thousand people whether or not they washed their hands when visiting a public lavatory and 95 per cent said they always did. The Society's researchers weren't convinced and so they set up hidden cameras to see how people actually behaved. The percentage of those who really *did* wash their hands turned out to be 58 per cent.

Another US survey produced the even odder statistic that 8 per cent of Americans are so frightened of catching germs from lavatories that they flush with their feet.

The French, at least, are more honest – or perhaps less paranoid: 56 per cent of men and 66 per cent of women admitted to researchers that they *never* wash their hands after visiting *les toilettes*. This prompted a French engineer to develop a device that locked users inside restaurant lavatories until they'd done so.

The peanut factoid is sometimes told about bowls of complimentary mints in restaurants, with exactly the same wording. When the news of this reached Canada and was reported in the *Ottawa Sentinel* in 1994, the regional health authorities sent out their inspectors to ensure that all such mints were either ready-wrapped, or were offered in such a way that they could 'only be handled by one person at a time'.

Which is riskier: nuts or mints? The answer turns out to be ice cubes.

Recent official studies of both hotels and pubs in Cardiff and fast-food joints and bars in Chicago found that at least 20 per cent of all ice cubes were contaminated with 'faecal matter' caused by staff failing to wash their hands.

In January 2010 a study at Hollins University in Roanoke, Virginia reported that almost half the drinks from ninety local soda fountains tested positive for coliform bacteria, indicating possible faecal contamination.

On a more optimistic note, they also noted that there were no reported outbreaks of food-related illness in Roanoke at the time of the study.

But please, now wash your hands. And don't shake anyone else's.

What is household dust made from?

The composition of house dust has been extensively studied because of its role in allergies. Not much of it is dead skin.

It's quite difficult to get meaningful data because dust varies so widely from country to country, house to house, and even room to room. It also depends on the season and on the lifestyle of the householder – whether you have a pet, how often you clean, whether you open the windows etc.

What is clear is that the allegation that house dust is 70 per cent human skin is wildly exaggerated. More common sources of dust include flakes of animal skin, sand, insect waste, flour (in the kitchen) and lots and lots of ordinary dirt.

The dead skin we shed each year would be enough to fill a

small flour bag, but most of it is drained away in bathwater or eaten by dust mites.

Dust mites are tiny, fat, eight-legged members of the spider family. They live in beehives and in birds' nests as well as in human homes. Half a teaspoon of dust may contain as many as 1,000 mites and 250,000 droppings.

They also live in beds, but the idea that dead dust mites and their waste products make up half the weight of your mattress or pillow is nonsense.

Bedding manufacturers (particularly in the USA) are in no hurry to discourage these rumours.

Most people who react badly to dust are actually allergic to dust mite faeces. Enzymes excreted from the mite's gut attack the respiratory passages, causing hay-fever-like symptoms or asthma.

Such allergies aside, there's no reason to worry about mites: you're already supporting a thriving community of them on your face.

Follicle mites (*Demodex follicularum*) live exclusively on human beings. They are long (about a hundredth of an inch) and slim (to fit snugly into the follicles). They have microscopic claws and needle-shaped mouthparts, which they use to pierce skin cells. They can't walk backwards, so once they've burrowed head first into somewhere comfortable like the base of your eyelashes, they're stuck for life. They eventually dissolve away harmlessly *in situ*, rear end last.

This rear end is an interesting sight: unlike dust mites, follicle mites create so little waste that they don't even need an anus.

STEPHEN *Now, what is house dust mostly composed of?*
VIC REEVES *Rust.*
STEPHEN *'Rust'! I don't think mostly of rust, no.*
VIC *If you live in an iron house like me . . .*

What might land on your head if you live under a flight path?

A huge block of frozen urine? It has never happened and it never will.

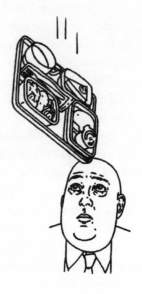

Aeroplanes do not dump the contents of their lavatories overboard. The waste is contained in a holding tank, which is emptied when the aircraft lands. Great care is taken to ensure that this tank is secure. Even if a mad pilot wanted to jettison it, access to the tank is located on the outside of the plane.

On very rare occasions, ice can fall from aeroplanes. Some 3 million flights pass through British airspace every year; in the same period, the Civil Aviation Authority gets just twenty to thirty reports of possible icefalls. The CAA investigates all such complaints by checking the relevant flight paths. Over the past twenty years, they estimate that five people have been hit by small amounts of falling ice.

In July 2009 a lump of ice the size of a football crushed the roof of a car in Loughborough, Leicestershire, but no flights were in the area at the time and the incident has been put down to a freak conglomeration of hailstones.

If ice does fall from a plane, it is either water that has frozen on the wings owing to the high altitude (which melts off as the plane comes into land) or water from the air-conditioning system that has leaked through a faulty seal on to the fuselage. Aircraft toilets often add a blue chemical to the water to deodorise the waste and break down any solids, but any blue ice that falls to the ground is a result of a fault in the input pipe. It cannot come out of the toilet itself or from the holding tank, which is a fully integrated, sealed unit.

In the USA the Federal Aviation Authority is equally adamant. No American has ever been hit by anything falling from an aircraft lavatory. Phone calls to the FAA complaining about brown droplets coming from the sky always increase during the bird migration season. The FAA also blames so-called 'blue ice' on incontinent birds that have been eating blueberries.

Like planes, modern trains in the UK carry chemical retention tanks, but some older rolling stock still offloads its toilet waste straight on to the tracks.

Around Britain's coastline, there are 20,000 pipes pumping untreated sewage into the sea. These 'combined sewer overflows', or CSOs, are intended as a last resort when there is a danger of an urban sewage system flooding. But heavy rainfall in recent summers means that some have been in almost constant use. As a result, in 2009, almost half of Britain's beaches were 'not recommended' for swimming by the Marine Conservation Society's *Good Beach Guide*.

Resorts that failed to come up to scratch included fashionable destinations such as Rock in Cornwall, Sandgate in Kent and West Sands in St Andrews. It was the worst result for Britain's beaches for eight years and bad enough for the European Commission to decide to take the UK to court to try to get CSO discharges banned.

ALAN *Urine. Frozen urine. It kills you and you just look like you've pissed yourself. To death.*

What are your chances of surviving a plane crash?

They're very good indeed: especially if you're in the cheap seats.

In the USA, between 1983 and 2000, there were 568 plane crashes. In 90 per cent of them there were survivors and, out of a total of 53,487 people onboard, 51,207 survived. According to *Popular Mechanics* magazine the safest place to be in the event of a crash is at the back, well behind the wings, where there is a 69 per cent survival rate. Sitting over (or just in front of) the wing reduces your chances of getting out alive to 56 per cent. The worst place to be is right up at the front in first class, where the survival rate falls to 49 per cent. Which is an outrage, considering how much you have to pay to sit there.

According to the world's leading 'fire safety engineer', Professor Ed Galea of the University of Greenwich, the biggest danger is seatbelts. In an emergency, passengers panic and revert to what they are familiar with: they struggle to open them like a seatbelt in a car, resulting in (sometimes fatal) delay. Fire is, of course, a major problem, largely because of smoke inhalation. Your safest bet is to sit on the aisle close to an exit. Before take-off, make a note of how many rows there are between you and the nearest door. That way, even if the cabin is filled with smoke, you'll still be able to crawl your way out by feel.

Until recently, it was thought impossible for a passenger airliner to make a successful emergency landing on water. The margin for error is so small. To prevent the plane breaking up on impact, the pilot must slow down as much as possible – but without losing lift – and raise the nose of the plane to 12 degrees so that the tail hits the water first. The wings must be perfectly level: if one wing-tip hits the water before the other the plane will cartwheel and break up. The fuel must be used up or dumped: its weight would cause the plane to sink even if it did land successfully. Then there's the weather, and sea conditions, either of which could wreck the plane, no matter how calmly the pilot behaves.

Despite such unnerving obstacles, there have been at least half a dozen successful emergency landings by airliners on water, including one off the coast of Sicily in 2005. The most recent and spectacular example occurred in January 2009 when an Airbus A380, US Airways Flight 1549, ditched in the Hudson River in New York. Shortly after take off, the plane hit a flock of geese and Captain Chesley 'Sully' Sullenberger III had to make a forced landing on the water. He did this perfectly, saving the lives of all 155 people on board.

Airline statisticians like to say that you are ten times more likely to be hit by a comet than to die in a plane crash. This is because, once every million years or so, an extraterrestrial body collides with Earth. The next time this happens it will probably wipe out half the world's population but, as far as we know, the last time anyone was hit by a comet was 12,900 years ago.

It is the case, however, that you are many times more likely to die in the taxi on the way to and from the airport than you are on the flight itself.

DAVID MITCHELL *I imagine your survival swings on the whistle that you get on the life jacket.*

JIMMY CARR *It does rather rely on someone having quite selective hearing, and going, 'I didn't hear that plane go down,' but . . .*

What's the word for the fear of heights?

It's not vertigo.

The fear of heights is called acrophobia (from the Greek *akros*, 'highest').

Reactions include clinging, crouching, or crawling on all fours as well as the usual symptoms associated with other phobias such as sweating, shaking and palpitations. Acrophobia is unusual among phobias in that it can actually cause what the person is frightened of. A panic attack at height may lead them to lose control and fall.

Vertigo (Latin for 'whirling') is a recognised medical condition. It's a type of dizziness where sufferers feel they are moving when they are in fact stationary. Women are two to three times more likely to suffer from it than men and it gets more common with age. Up to 10 per cent of people experience some form of vertigo in their lives. Vertigo doesn't necessarily take place high above the ground and it's not the same thing as acrophobia.

The confusion wasn't helped by Alfred Hitchcock's film *Vertigo* (1958). In the movie, an ex-police detective (Jimmy Stewart) suffers from acrophobia as a result of witnessing a fellow officer fall to his death in a rooftop chase. His condition haunts him and the film comes to a climax when he apparently fails to prevent the woman he loves falling from a bell tower. He is unable to climb the stairs due to his crippling fear of heights and an attack of vertigo.

In real life, people with acrophobia may never suffer from vertigo – and vice versa.

A sensible caution towards high places seems to be built into all of us. In 1960, psychologists E. J. Gibson and R. D. Walk created the 'visual cliff experiment' in which infants from different species (including human babies) had to cross a transparent glass panel with an apparently sharp drop-off point beneath it. They found that all the species in the experiment saw and avoided the cliff as soon as they were old enough to manage independent movement – six months for a human or one day in chicks.

While not everyone is frightened of heights, acrophobia appears to be the second most common human phobia of all.

The first is fear of public speaking.

What's the world's second-highest peak?

Actually, it's also Everest.

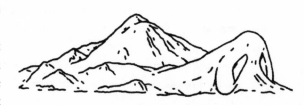

Mount Everest's main summit is the highest point on the Earth's surface measured from sea level. It rises 8,850 metres (29,035.4 feet) into the sky. The second-highest separate mountain is K2, but the unremarkable bump of Everest's south summit is in fact higher, at 8,750 metres (28,707 feet). This beats K2 – 8,611 metres (28,250 feet)– by almost 140 metres (460 feet).

K2 is not in the Himalayas. It's in a range called the Karakorum – the initial K of which gives K2 its rather functional name.

K2 was a temporary label given to it by Lieutenant Thomas Montgomerie (1830–78) a young officer in the Great Trigonometric Survey of India, which lasted through most of the nineteenth century. He named the biggest peaks he saw in the Karakorum range K1, K2, K3, etc., in the order that he came across them.

K1, which he first saw in 1856, is only the twenty-second highest mountain in the world, but it already had (and has) a local name: Masherbrum. And so, as it eventually turned out, did all the others in Montgomerie's list – except K2.

K2 hadn't been given a local name (and still hasn't) by either the Pakistanis in the south or the Chinese in the north. The reason for this is the mountain's remoteness. Despite its majestic height, it cannot be seen from any of the villages in the area – and it's possible that no one even knew of its existence until the Great Trigonometric Survey. An early attempt to name it Mount Godwin-Austen – after another surveyor, Henry Godwin-Austen (1834–1926) – was rejected by the Royal Geographical Society. But K2 is informally known as 'The Savage Mountain' – one in four people who attempt to get to the summit die, and it has never been conquered in winter.

The south summit of Everest may be a long way up, but it is only a cone of snow and ice about the size of an ordinary dinner table. For most climbers it is just another stop on the way to the highest point on Earth, a time to change oxygen bottles and admire the view of the final slopes of the main summit.

The south summit is inside what mountaineers call the 'Dead Zone' (above 8,000 metres or 26,246 feet). Although Everest kills fewer people proportionately than K2, many more people climb it. As a result, the Dead Zone is full of rubbish and frozen corpses. In 2010 a team of twenty Sherpas began a concerted effort to tidy it all up. As well as removing several bodies, they expect to clear 3,000 kilograms (about 3 tons) of old tents, ropes, oxygen cylinders, food packaging and camping stoves from the mountain.

Pedants should be aware that the English name for the world's highest mountain should be spoken aloud as *EEV-uh-rest*, not *EV-uh-rest*.

This is how Sir George Everest (1799–1866), the Welsh-born Surveyor General of India, after whom it is named, pronounced his surname.

How can you tell how high up a mountain you are?

Make some tea.

The traditional method of estimating the height of a mountain while you're on one is by taking the temperature of a pot of boiling water.

Water boils when the pressure of the steam trying to escape from it exceeds the pressure of the air above it.

Air pressure decreases with altitude in a rather neat (if non-metric) way. For every 300 metres (1,000 feet) gained in height, the boiling point of water reduces by 1 °C.

So, at 4,500 metres (15,000 feet, the summit of Mont Blanc) water boils at 84.4 °C. At the top of Everest it boils at 70 °C and at nearly 23,000 metres (75,000 feet) it would boil at room temperature (not that any room would be at room temperature at that altitude).

This form of measurement is called hypsometry (from the Greek *hypsos*, 'height' and *metria*, 'measure').

In his travelogue *A Tramp Abroad* (1880), Mark Twain (1835–1910) tells how, on an expedition to the Swiss Alps, he tried to calculate the altitude by boiling his barometer in bean soup. This gave 'a strong barometer taste to the soup' which was so unexpectedly popular he had the expedition cook make it every day. The cook used two barometers, one in working order, the other not – the soup from the former went to the Officers' Mess, the latter to the Other Ranks.

The Challenger Deep in the Marianas Trench in the Pacific is the deepest known part of the world's oceans.

The pressure there is 1,100 times that at sea level, so if you wanted to make a cup of tea you'd have to wait awhile.

The kettle would start to boil at 530 °C.

How can you tell which way is north in a forest?

It's old woodsman's lore that moss always grows on the north side of the trees, but it doesn't.

Mosses prefer shady places but they can grow on the south, west and east of trees (as well as the north), if there's enough moisture to sustain them. The presence of moisture depends as much on the direction of the prevailing wind as on being out of the sun. And, although a tree in isolation tends to have more shade on its northern side, trees in wooded areas throw shade on one another, making it perfectly possible for the south side to be the mossy one.

Can you tell which way is north from the sun? If you face the sunrise in the east, north is 90° to your left, isn't it?

This isn't foolproof either. The sun only rises *exactly* in the east on two days a year, at the spring and autumn equinoxes, when night and day are of equal length. (*Equinox* is Latin for 'equal night'.) In Britain, as a general rule, the sun rises in the south-east and sets in the south-west in winter; and rises in the north-east and sets in the north-west in the summer.

A more reliable method is to wait for nightfall and use the stars. Find the constellation of Ursa Major (Latin for 'Great Bear'), better known as the Plough or Big Dipper. It looks a like a pan with a handle. Make a line between the two stars on the side of the pan opposite the handle and follow it upwards.

Polaris – the North Star – is the next bright star you find along that line. It's not *exactly* north; but it's good enough for someone hopelessly lost in a forest.

Unfortunately, this doesn't work so well in the southern hemisphere. The nearest star to the celestial South Pole, sometimes called *Polaris Australis*, or the 'Southern Pole star', is Sigma Octantis in the constellation Octans, but it's barely visible without a telescope.

The North Star isn't always due north, either. This is because Earth wobbles as it spins. Think of the Earth as a ball, spinning round an imaginary stick that passes through each pole. Because of the gravitational pull of the Sun and Moon, the stick moves slightly over time, slowly tracing a circle in the sky. This means that the end of the stick isn't always pointing directly at Polaris: it's either moving slowly towards or away from it.

You don't need to worry about that for a while yet, though. The movement is *very* slow: each rotation of that circle takes 25,765 years to complete. For our Bronze Age ancestors in 3000 BC, the star Thuban in the constellation of Draco was closer to north. In 12,000 years time it will be Vega in the constellation Lyra. Polaris will be back in pole position again by AD 27800.

Meanwhile, a neat trick is to use your watch. Point the hour hand at the sun. Taking the middle of the angle formed between that and the number twelve gives a fairly good approximation to south.

STEPHEN *You can float a razor blade on water and, if it's magnet-ised, it would act as a compass.*

ROB BRYDON *But if you were lost in the forest and you were getting pretty despondent, and you thought, 'I'll float a razor blade on the water', you would be tempted, wouldn't you, as you looked at that razor blade, to end it all?*

Do people really go round and round in circles when they're lost?

Yes, they do. In situations where there are no navigational clues – such as in a snowstorm or thick fog – human beings who are convinced they're walking in a straight line always end up going round in circles.

Until very recently this peculiar effect was explained away by the not very convincing theory that one of our legs is stronger than the other, so that over a period of time we tend to veer in the direction of the weaker leg. But research carried out in 2009 by the Max Planck Institute for Biological Cybernetics in Tübingen has shown that it's not our legs, but our brains, that are at fault.

Volunteers were set down in a particularly empty bit of the Sahara in southern Tunisia or the dense, flat Bienwald Forest in south-west Germany and tracked as they walked, using GPS (the Global Positioning Satellite). When the sun or moon was out, they were perfectly capable of walking in a straight line. As soon as these were absent, the volunteers started to walk in circles, crossing their own path several times without noticing it. When another group of volunteers was blindfolded, the effect was even more obvious and immediate: the average diameter of the circle they walked was only 20 metres (66 feet).

This is far too rapid a change of course for the 'stronger leg' theory to explain. What the research proved is that, deprived of any visual points of reference, people have no instinctive sense of direction.

Vision is by far the most important of all human senses. Processing visual information uses 30 per cent of the brain's activity, whereas smell, the directional aid used by most mammals, accounts for just 1 per cent. Only birds are as visually dependent as we are, but they navigate using 'magnetoception', the ability to plug into the Earth's magnetic field. Embedded in their brains are crystals of an iron-based mineral called magnetite.

The bones of human noses also contain traces of magnetite, which suggests we may once also have had 'magnetoception' but have forgotten how to use it.

In 2004 Peter König, a cognitive scientist at the University of Osnabrück in Germany, made a belt that he wore round his waist constantly, even in bed. It had thirteen pads linked to a sensor that detected Earth's magnetic field: whichever pad was pointing north vibrated gently like a cellphone. Over time, König's spatial awareness radically improved. Wherever he was in the city, he found he knew intuitively the direction of his home or office. Once, on a trip to Hamburg, over 160 kilometres (100 miles) away, he correctly pointed towards Osnabrück.

When he finally removed the belt, he had a powerful sensation that the world had shrunk and that he had become 'smaller and more chaotic'. The belt had reactivated – or perhaps re-educated – a sense he didn't realise he had. It may be that our bodies have been faithfully sending out magnetoception signals all the time, but that our brains have lost the ability to interpret them.

STEPHEN *Why do we walk in circles if we're lost?*
ALAN *Homing pigeons: we're descended from homing pigeons.*

What's the best way to weigh your own head?

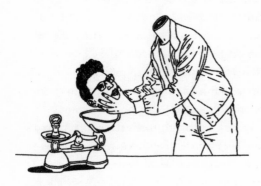

Self-decapitation? Are you sure?

A severed head has left than five seconds of consciousness left, so you wouldn't have much time to enjoy the results of your experiment.

Resting your head on the bathroom scales is another idea but it's very inaccurate: your neck would still be supporting some of the weight.

The simplest way is to stick your head in a bucket.

The density of most people's heads is very close to that of water. Put a bucket in a large tray, fill it to the brim with water and then dunk your head in it. Weighing the water that spills over into the tray will give you a fairly good approximation of the weight of your head.

For an encore, you can repeat the experiment with your whole body, using larger containers. You can then compare the amount of water displaced by your head to the amount displaced by your whole body, and work out what fraction of your total body weight your head is.

To ensure 100 per cent accuracy, though, what you really need is a CT scan.

Computed Tomography (CT) scanners use X-rays to produce an extensive series of images of objects in cross-section. (Tomography is Greek for 'writing in slices'.) The information can be used to analyse any part of the human body and determine the exact density at each point within it. From this, a SAM – or Specific Anthropomorphic Mannequin

– can be generated: a 3-D computer model that, among other things, will tell you the exact weight of your head.

If you're not particularly bothered about accuracy and only want to know *roughly* what your head weighs, according to the anatomy department at Sydney University the weight of an adult human head (with hair removed), cut off at the third vertebra down, is between 4.5 and 5 kilograms (9.9 and 11 pounds).

If you like to be accurate to the point of extreme pedantry, you might be able to use this. It was the Greek mathematician Archimedes (about 287–212 BC) who discovered you could measure the volume of irregular objects by seeing how much water they displaced. He supposedly found this out while he was sitting in his bath and was so excited that he jumped out and ran naked through the streets of Syracuse yelling 'Eureka!' (Greek for 'I've found it!')

How do snakes swallow things bigger than their heads?

They don't, as you may have heard, 'dislocate their jaws': they stretch them.

Most of the bones in a snake's head – including the two halves of the jaw – are not locked in position, as in mammals, but are attached by a flexible ligament.

One of these bones links the snake's lower jaw to its upper jaw in a double-jointed hinge. It's called the quadrate bone because it is connected at four points.

We have this quadrate bone too, but it's no longer attached to our jaw. Instead, it has migrated up into the ear and shrunk down in size to become the incus, or 'anvil', bone. This combines with two other bones called the malleus (or 'hammer') and the stapes ('stirrup'), to produce the miracle of efficiency that is the human middle ear.

The three-bone arrangement amplifies sound and is capable of much more acute hearing than the reptile system, where the eardrum is connected directly to the inner ear by just the single 'stirrup' bone. So, while we can't swallow a goat whole, we can at least hear much better than snakes can.

Despite their big mouths, snakes sometimes bite off more than they can chew.

In 2005 the remains of a 1.8-metre (6-foot) alligator were found in the Florida Everglades National Park, protruding from the stomach of a 4-metre (13-foot) Burmese python. The python had tried to swallow the alligator whole and had then exploded. The alligator is thought to have clawed at the python's stomach from the inside, leading it to burst.

Burmese pythons come from South-East Asia and are one of the six largest snakes in the world. In their natural habitat, they can grow to more than 6 metres (20 feet) long. They now infest the Everglades: all of them are pets that have been abandoned by, or escaped from, their owners.

In 1999 a study at Cornell University estimated that the control of invasive species cost the US a staggering $137 billion a year. In the following five years 144,000 more Burmese pythons were blithely imported into the United States.

In 2010 Florida finally passed a law banning the importation of Burmese pythons, but too late. They thrive in the hot, wet climate of the local swamps (along with dozens of other non-native species like monitor lizards and vervet monkeys). Fights between alligators and Burmese pythons are a not uncommon sight and are a popular tourist attraction. The result is quite often a draw.

Where does a snake's tail begin?

You might think a snake is just one long tail with a head at one end, but in fact only about 20 per cent of a snake is tail.

The word *vertebra* is Latin for 'joint'. Human beings have thirty-three vertebrae, which form the spinal column and the bones in the neck. Depending on the species, snakes can have over ten times as many. The great majority of these sprout a pair of ribs. Just as with people, snakes don't have ribs in their head. And, at the other end (also as with people), where the ribs stop, the tail begins. The human 'tail' is called the coccyx; in a snake, its tail starts after its cloaca.

All reptiles, birds and amphibians have a cloaca. It's named after the Cloaca Maxima, an early sewage system that ran through the Forum in ancient Rome. In snakes the cloaca is a small, flexible vent on its underside: the reptilian equivalent of a bottom. So a snake's tail starts, just like a lizard's or a pheasant's, behind its behind.

Although controlled by a sphincter muscle, as in mammals, it differs from a mammal's anus by providing a common passage for the removal of both urine and faeces. It's also used for mating and egg laying. Stored inside a male snake's tail are his two penises (known as hemipenes or 'half-penises'). To mate, he turns each one inside out, so that they poke out of his cloaca. They look rather like exotic varieties of mollusc, adorned with various knobs, spines and protuberances. Each is inserted, in turn, into the female's cloaca, which is of a matching design to deter interlopers from other snake species.

Recent studies have shown that, while a snake can't be referred to as 'right-handed', they are definitely 'right-penised': the hemipenis on the right side tends to be larger and is the one inserted first. Another use for the cloaca in some snake species is 'popping'. This is where air is expelled from it in a series of sharp bursts, indistinguishable in timbre and volume from high-pitched human farts. The foul smell (and surprise value) helps keep predators at bay.

If a snake is kept in too small a space, it may attack and eat its own tail, thinking it's a rival. Some snakes have been known to choke on their own tails.

The Ouroboros (Greek for 'tail-eater') is an ancient symbol of a snake swallowing its own tail. It appears in Egyptian, Greek, Norse, Hindu and Aztec mythology and represents the cyclical nature of things. In the *Timaeus* (360 BC), Plato credited the origin of life in the universe to such a circular, self-consuming creature and the Swiss psychologist Carl Jung (1875–1961) believed it was an archetype, a concept hard-wired into our unconscious.

The Ouroboros unlocked one of the great scientific puzzles of the nineteenth century: the chemical structure of benzene. Found in crude oil, benzene is a powerful solvent used in the manufacture of dyes and plastics. First isolated in 1825, it was used as paint stripper, aftershave and to decaffeinate coffee before it was discovered to be dangerously toxic. Though its chemical formula, C_6H_6, was known, its atomic structure baffled everyone until the German chemist August

Kekulé (1829–96), after years of work, had the sudden insight that it was a ring of six carbon atoms. These were attached to each hydrogen atom with a single bond, but to each other with alternating single and double bonds.

Kekulé's solution transformed organic chemistry. The breakthrough came to him in a daydream, when the image of a snake with its tail in its mouth suddenly came to mind.

ALAN *When I was a kid, there was a rattlesnake on TV, every week. It was, like, a big thing in the '70s. Every week, in something, there was always a rattlesnake. And nowadays, there's never a rattlesnake on TV.*

What are the chances of a coin landing on heads?

It isn't fifty–fifty.

If the coin is heads up to begin with, it's more likely to land on heads. Students at Stanford University recorded thousands of coin tosses with high-speed cameras and discovered the chances are approximately fifty-one–forty-nine.

The researchers showed that coin tossing is not a strictly random procedure, but a measurable event that obeys the laws of physics. If each coin is subject to exactly the same initial conditions and exactly the same initial force, then its spin will produce an even chance of landing on heads or tails.

However, the slightest difference in the conditions – speed and angle of spin, height of the coin from the ground, which side is facing up to start with – will affect the result. The Stanford research showed that, averaged over many tosses, these changes were significant enough to prevent a fifty—fifty probability.

The toss of a coin can be a serious matter. In the third European Football Championships in 1968, Italy and Russia drew 0–0 in the semi-final. There were no penalty shoot-outs in those days (and there was no time in the schedule to fit in a replay), so the result was decided by the toss of a coin. Russia lost and Italy went through to the final and won the Championship.

In cricket, although winning the toss doesn't seem to affect the results of daytime cricket matches, statistical analysis from University College London suggests that, in day—night games, winning the toss and batting first (during daylight) increases the chances of victory by almost 10 per cent.

Under British electoral law, if a vote finishes in a dead heat, the result is determined by lot.

In the 2010 UK council elections, there were tied votes in Great Yarmouth and Bristol. In one, the victory went to the candidate who drew the highest card from a pack; in the other, the returning officer drew the name from a hat.

Perhaps they'd seen the Stanford research and decided to give the coin-toss a miss . . .

SEAN LOCK *I still can't get my head round the notion that it's just as likely to be 1, 2, 3, 4, 5, 6 on the lottery – and I still go 'it just wouldn't happen'. You know why? You know why? Because it's a lottery. I mean, the clue's in the title.*

What does biting a coin prove?

If you can leave teeth marks in a gold coin, it's almost certainly a fake.

People who've watched too many old pirate movies think that, because gold is a soft metal, the way to prove a gold coin is genuine is by biting into it. While this theoretically works with a pure gold coin, it ignores the fact that all 'gold' coins minted for circulation in the UK and America since Tudor times have contained copper. This made them more durable (and hard to the bite).

In 1538 Henry VIII set the levels of purity and weight for the gold sovereign. By law, the coin had to contain 91.6 per cent gold – the rest being copper – and weigh half a troy ounce. ('Troy weight' was a French system of measurement named after the famous Troyes fair, the medieval version of an international trade convention.) Each coin was minted to a standard diameter and thickness.

Gold is very difficult to counterfeit, but its high value made it worth trying. The simplest method was to mix lead with gold, or to gild lead coins.

But, though gold is relatively soft, it's also denser than almost all other metals – almost twice as dense as lead. To test a coin, all a merchant or banker had to do was weigh and measure it and compare it to the royal standard. Because gold is so heavy, a fake coin would either be too light or too big. A lead coin of the same *thickness* and diameter as a sovereign would be only a third as heavy. A lead coin of the right *weight* and diameter would be twice as thick.

A much more successful ploy for forgers was adulteration. The trick was to remove small amounts of metal from legal coinage, melt down the scraps and recast new coins. There were three ways of doing this: 'clipping' (filing tiny fragments from the coin's edges); 'drilling' (taking the coin and punching small holes in it, which were then hammered shut); and 'sweating' (shaking a bag of coins for long enough to create a dust of gold and copper).

Sir Isaac Newton (1643–1727) became obsessed with the underworld of counterfeiting gangs after he was made Warden of the Royal Mint in 1696. His secret career as an alchemist had made him something on an expert at assessing the purity of metals. By his reckoning, one in five coins in circulation in England were false. He took on the criminal networks, collecting evidence by frequenting taverns and brothels in disguise. In 1699 he ensnared the master forger William Chaloner, who once boasted he had 'coined' 30,000 guineas of false gold (the equivalent of £50 million today). Chaloner was convicted of treason and publicly hanged, drawn and quartered.

About 40,000 gold sovereigns are still minted in the UK every year, to the same purity standard laid down under Henry VIII. Sovereigns are no longer legal tender but are kept as gold bullion, which is a tradable commodity. The average world market price of gold in 2009 was about £20,500 per kilogram.

Who invented the catflap?

It wasn't Sir Isaac Newton.

It's an appealing idea that the father of gravitation, the leading theoretical scientist of his day and arguably the most famous celebrity in Europe at the start of the eighteenth century, invented something as mundane as the cat flap. Sadly, the evidence doesn't stack up.

To this day, students at Cambridge are told that, while an undergraduate at Trinity College, Isaac Newton cut two holes in the door of his lodgings – a large one for his pet cat and a smaller one for its kittens. The story plays on a classic stereotype, the genius with no common sense – because there's no need for the smaller door. But we know it never happened. Newton's secretary and distant relative, Humphrey Newton, was explicit: his master 'kept neither dog nor cat in his chamber'. Also, the doorways of most Cambridge lodgings of the period had a system of double doors. The outer doors were thick and heavy, and usually carved from a large piece of oak. The inner door acted as a draught excluder. Sawing holes through both would have been a major DIY project. And a self-defeating one – turning Newton's rooms into a wind tunnel.

Nobody knows where the catflap myth started, but we do have a source for the legend of the apple tree: Newton himself. Never one for self-deprecation, he likened his discovery of gravity to Adam being expelled from the Garden of Eden, as both featured the sudden acquisition of knowledge through an apple.

Newton often told the story during his lifetime, but, over a century later, the German mathematician Karl Friedrich Gauss (1777–1855) offered his own version of events. 'Undoubtedly,' he said, 'the occurrence was something of this sort: There comes to Newton a stupid importunate man, who asks him how he made his great discovery. Newton wanted to get rid of the man, told him that an apple fell on his nose; and this made the matter quite clear to the man, and he went away satisfied.'

Newton certainly had a reputation for grumpiness. He didn't suffer fools (or anyone else) gladly, and preferred solitary study to human company. At times his eccentricities seem to have shaded into genuine mental illness, particularly in 1692, when he complained of 'great disturbance of mind'. Historians have variously ascribed the other symptoms he exhibited – insomnia, obsessive behaviour, lack of appetite and the delusion that his friends were turning on him – to depression, Asperger's syndrome and even mercury poisoning. Recent tests on a lock of his hair showed abnormally high levels of mercury, perhaps caused by decades of secret alchemical experimentation.

Whatever afflicted him, it didn't prevent Newton from producing *Principia Mathematica* (1687), the most influential scientific book of all time, or from building a successful second career as a civil servant and administrator. He lived until he was eighty-four and died a very wealthy man, leaving assets worth £31,821 (equivalent to £49 million in today's money).

STEPHEN *There are people in history who were said to be agelastic, including Isaac Newton, who was supposed to have laughed only once in his life.*

CLIVE ANDERSON *When an apple fell on his head.*

STEPHEN *No, when someone asked him what was the point of studying Euclid, and he burst out laughing.*

JIMMY CARR *Yeah, that is a good one, though.*

What did Molotov invest?

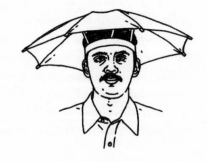

Molotov didn't invent his 'cocktails'. They were named after him as an insult.

Vyacheslav Mikhailovich Skriabin (1890–1986) took the pen name 'Molotov' (*molot* means 'hammer' in Russian) as a young Bolshevik party organiser and underground journalist in pre-Revolutionary Russia. He became Stalin's most loyal deputy, and was one of only four members of the 1917 revolutionary government to survive Stalin's purges of the 1930s.

The story of the Molotov cocktail begins in 1939 when, as Soviet foreign minister, Molotov secretly authorised the illegal invasion of Finland, weeks after the Second World War had started. In the early phases of the invasion, he claimed in radio broadcasts that the cluster bombs Soviet planes were dropping were actually food parcels for starving Finns.

The Finnish resistance was stronger than the Soviets had anticipated and the invasion lasted through the bitter winter of 1940. The Finns' secret weapon was a handmade incendiary device made from a bottle filled with flammable liquid and stoppered with a wick. They had borrowed the idea from General Franco's Fascist troops, who had recently emerged as victors in the Spanish Civil War. The Fascists had produced these hand-held bombs to disable the Soviet-built tanks used by the left-wing Republican government forces. The Finns christened them 'Molotov's cocktails', the joke being that they were 'a drink to go with his food parcels'. They used a government vodka distillery to produce more than 450,000 of them. Their fame spread and, by the end of the War, combatants on all sides knew them as 'Molotov cocktails'.

The disinformation about food parcels was typical of Molotov. He wasn't a soldier; he was a bureaucrat, skilled in the use of propaganda. The Finnish war resulted from the Molotov–Ribbentrop pact that he had signed with the Nazis in August 1939. (Von Ribbentrop was Molotov's opposite number, the German foreign minister.) This was a secret agreement for the USSR and Germany to carve up Poland and the Baltic states between them. It wasn't made public until after war had ended – Molotov went to his grave denying it had ever existed – but it made possible the German invasion of Poland (which began the Second World War) as well as the Soviet invasion of Finland. It also allowed Molotov to destroy Polish resistance by authorising the murder of all 22,000 members of the Polish officer corps at Katyn forest in March 1940.

The short-lived pact with Germany wasn't Molotov's only legacy. During the Soviet purges of the 1930s, it had been his idea to use lists to sentence people to death, greatly speeding up the process. In 1937–8, he personally signed 372 orders for mass executions – more than Stalin himself – leading to the murder of more than 43,000 people.

Vegetarian, teetotal and a studious collector of first editions (many were dedicated to him by authors he later sent to the Gulag), Molotov was the last surviving Bolshevik. He died, an unrepentant Stalinist, in 1986, just after Mikhail Gorbachev announced the *perestroika* (restructuring) reforms that would lead, five years later, to the dissolution of the USSR.

Why was the speed camera invented?

It was designed to speed cars up, not slow them down.

A Dutch engineer called Maurice Gatsonides (1911–98) devised the first speed camera. Far from being a road-safety campaigner, Gatsonides was Europe's first professional rally driver. The pinnacle of his career came in 1953 when he won the Monte Carlo Rally in a Ford Zephyr by just three seconds.

His world-famous invention was driven by a desire to improve his speed round corners. The first 'Gatsometer' consisted of two pressure-sensitive rubber strips stretched across the road. Driving over the first strip started a stop-watch; crossing the second stopped it. This was the world's first reliable speed-measuring device. Gatsonides then added a flash camera which made it even more accurate. It enabled him to see just how much extra speed he could squeeze out of a corner by approaching it along a different line.

Gatso soon realised that his camera could also be used to catch speeding motorists. He founded Gatsometer BV in 1958 and over the next twenty years gradually refined his invention, introducing a radar beam to replace the rubber pressure strips in 1971. The 'Gatso 24' is now installed in more than forty countries. In many languages, speed cameras of any kind are simply known as 'Gatsos'.

The first Gatsos in the UK were installed in Nottingham in 1988, after a triple fatality at a traffic-light-controlled junction. Having been slow to adopt the new technology, the UK now leads Europe in the use of speed cameras. In 2007 the UK had 4,309 of them (compared with 1,571 in 2001), more than France and Italy combined.

Do they work? The evidence suggests that they do. A four-year survey by the UK Department for Transport, published in 2006, reported that the overall speed past camera sites was reduced by an average of 6 per cent, and the number of people killed or seriously injured by 42 per cent. While the motoring lobby points out that driving too fast is the main cause in only 14 per cent of fatal accidents – compared with 'driver distraction' which accounts for 68 per cent – the enforcement of speed limits has had a massive impact on the number of collisions. In the ten years since 32 kilometres per hour (20 miles per hour) limits were introduced in London, the number of accidents has halved.

Dislike of speed cameras is nothing new. The Automobile Association was established in 1905 to help motorists avoid police speed traps which (then as now) many felt were more to do with extorting money than road safety. All drivers speed at some point: 75 per cent admit to doing it regularly. But for all the grumbling, according to the Department for Transport, 82 per cent of us think speed cameras are a good thing.

Gatsonides certainly thought so. 'I am often caught by my own speed cameras and find hefty fines on my doormat,' he once confessed. 'I love speeding.'

JEREMY CLARKSON *There's a marvellous new club in Holland called the Tuf Tuf Club that goes around destroying speed cameras.*

STEPHEN *Oh, really?*

JEREMY *You get prizes if you can think of the most imaginative way. My favourite one was to put some of that builders' foam in. It just bursts and then sets in a rather ugly, Dr Who-y special effect. Which is quite good.*

What's the word for a staircase that goes round and round?

It's not 'spiral', it's helical.

A spiral is a two-dimensional curve which radiates out from a fixed, central point. The longer it gets, the less curved it becomes, like a snail shell. A helix is a three-dimensional curve, like a spring or a Slinky, which doesn't change its angle of curve no matter how long it gets.

In the Scottish Borders there's a legend that the Kerr family built their castle towers with helical staircases that went round in the opposite direction to everybody else's. Because most of the male Kerrs were left-handed, this gave them an advantage in defending the stairs against a right-handed swordsman.

Sadly, it isn't true: Kerrs are no more left-handed than any other family. A 1972 study in the *British Medical Journal* reported a 30 per cent incidence of left-handedness among Kerrs against a 10 per cent incidence in the British population generally, but the research turned out to be flawed. It had been based on a self-selecting sample, i.e. left-handed people with the surname Kerr were encouraged to come forward, and so the results were badly skewed. A later and more careful study in 1993 found no such tendency.

What's more, the staircase trick wouldn't work: if a defender was left-handed then an anticlockwise staircase would indeed allow him to use his sword more effectively, but it would also give a right-handed attacker the same advantage. So, a staircase that twisted the other way would only be useful when defending against another Kerr (not impossible given their bloodthirsty reputation).

The Chateau de Chambord in the Loire Valley has a double-helix staircase: two staircases which wind around each other so that people going up don't bump into people coming down – and the cliff-top fortifications at Dover have a *triple*-helix staircase (known as the 'Grand Shaft') designed to get three columns of troops down to harbour level simultaneously.

The most famous of all double helixes is the molecule called deoxyribonucleic acid, better known as DNA. Francis Crick and James Watson first described its structure in 1953, although they were inspired by an X-ray photograph of DNA taken by Rosalind Franklin (1920–58), who almost beat them to it.

If you unravelled all the DNA strands in your body they'd stretch for 1,000 billion kilometres (620 billion miles), which is nearly 7,000 times further than the distance to the sun, and further away in the other direction than the edge of the Solar System.

To put that in perspective, to count to 620 billion you would have to have started 20,000 years ago, in the middle of the last ice age.

What's so great about the golden ratio?

Every Dan Brown fan has heard of this mysterious figure that crops up everywhere – in the human body, in ancient architecture, in the natural world – and whose appeal nobody can explain. The truth is that it doesn't appear in most of the places it's supposed to, and many of the claims about it are false.

The golden ratio (also known as 'the golden mean' or the 'divine proportion') is a way of relating any two quantities – such as the height (a) of a building to the length (b) – in the following simple way.

$$\frac{a+b}{a} = \frac{a}{b}$$

If a=1, then b=1.6180339887 . . .

In the nineteenth century, this ratio was given the name phi – φ – after the great Greek sculptor Phidias (490–430 BC), who supposedly used it in the proportions of his human figures. The reason that such a simple formula produces such a complicated, unharmonious looking number is that phi (φ), like pi (π), cannot be written as a neat fraction, or *'ratio'*, so it is called an *irra*tional number. Irrational numbers can only be expressed as an infinite string of decimal places that never repeat themselves. A prettier way of expressing phi in maths is: ($\sqrt{5}+1$) divided by 2.

A 'golden spiral' is one that gets further from its central point by a factor of φ for every quarter turn it makes. A frequently quoted example of this is the beautiful shell of *Nautilus pompilius*, a member of the octopus family. But in fact this is a 'logarithmic spiral', not a golden one. In 1999 the American mathematician Clement Falbo measured several hundred shells and showed quite clearly that the average ratio was 1 to 1.33: a long way from 1.618. (If you did want to use a shell to demonstrate the golden mean, the abalone would do well, but they're not nearly as photogenic as the nautilus.)

The Greeks knew about the golden ratio, and the Parthenon is the usual example given of its use in architecture. But any diagrams showing how its side or front elevations demonstrate a 'golden rectangle' always either include some empty air at the top or leave out some steps at the bottom.

The golden ratio was forgotten for hundreds of years after the fall of Rome, until Luca Pacioli (1446–1517), a Franciscan monk and Leonardo da Vinci's tutor, wrote about it in *De Divina Proportione* (1509). Leonardo did the illustrations for the book but, despite what it says in *The Da Vinci Code*, he did not use the golden ratio to compose either the Mona Lisa or his famous 1487 drawing of a man in a circle with his limbs extended.

The latter is called Vitruvian Man after the Roman architect Vitruvius, who lived in the first century BC and is sometimes called 'the world's first engineer'. He based his buildings on the proportions of the ideal human body, where the height is equal to the span of the arms and eight times the size of the head. He didn't use φ at all, whether or not Phidias once used it for a similar purpose.

What kind of stripes make you look slimmer?

Vertical ones, surely?

Nope.

According to research carried out in 2008 at the University of York, it is stripes running *across* 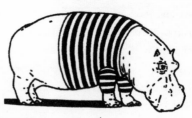 the body that make the wearer appear more trim.

The experiment asked people to compare over 200 pairs of pictures of women wearing dresses with either horizontal or vertical stripes and say which of them looked fatter.

The results showed conclusively that, with two women of the same size, the one wearing the horizontal stripes appeared to be the thinner of the two. In fact, to make the women *appear* to be the same size, the one in the horizontal stripes had to be 6 per cent wider.

Led by psychologist Dr Peter Thompson, the York team had been puzzled that the conventional view that vertical stripes are 'slimming' went against a famous optical illusion, the Helmholtz square, in which a square filled with horizontal lines appears taller than one filled with vertical ones.

Hermann von Helmholtz (1821–94) was a German polymath. Not only was he a qualified physician and a theoretical physicist, he also helped found the discipline of experimental psychology and transformed the science of optics, writing the standard textbook on the subject and, in 1851, inventing the ophthalmoscope, an instrument which enabled people to see the inside of the eye for the first time.

On the matter of striped dresses, von Helmholtz was absolutely categorical: 'Frocks with cross stripes on them make the figure look taller.'

For some reason, everyone has steadily ignored him for well over a century. When Sheriff Joe Arpaio of Maricopa County,

Arizona, reintroduced striped prison uniforms in 1997, female inmates begged him to make the bars vertical so they wouldn't look fat. He said: 'I told them I am an equal-opportunity incarcerator – the men have horizontal stripes, and so will the women.'

Striped prison uniforms, first introduced in the early nineteenth century, made it easier to spot escapees in a crowd. But they were also intended as a psychological punishment. In the Middle Ages, striped clothes were the pattern of choice for prostitutes, clowns and other social outcasts – whether or not they were overweight.

One piece of received fashion wisdom the York team did confirm was that black really does make you look slimmer. This research was provoked by another famous optical illusion, in which a black circle on a white background appears smaller than a white circle on a black background.

ROB BRYDON *I have a friend who's quite short and he likes to wear vertical stripes because they make him look taller.*
DAVID MITCHELL *Only when he's not standing next to anyone. It's not going to make him look taller than a taller man. It's all relative. You won't just say: 'Oh, there's a normal size man next to an enormous man' and then go: 'Oh thank God, he's taken his striped shirt off, it's actually a tiny man next to a normal man.'*

How many eyes do you need to estimate depth and distance?

One.

You'd think that we need both eyes, but we don't.

It is true that most depth perception is created by the different angles of vision produced by each eye. It's the way that 3-D film works, combining the output of two different cameras. When we look at something we create a single 'field of view', with the visual information split between the right and the left eye. The right-hand field from both eyes is sent to the right side of the brain; the left half of the field is sent to the left side. The brain merges them into a single solid-looking image.

However, our brains can still judge distance with a single eye. If you lose sight in one eye, the brain processes information from the remaining eye and plots it against the motion of your body. It then combines these visual and non-visual clues to create a sense of depth.

In fact, it turns out that you don't need eyes to 'see' at all.

Over thirty years, US neuroscientist Paul Bach-y-Rita (1934–2006) experimented with 'sensory substitution'. He had noticed that, although different parts of the body collect different types of sensory information, the way they're transmitted – electrical nerve impulses – is always the same. In theory, this meant the nervous system could be rewired, swapping one sense for another.

In 2003 he began to test a device called the BrainPort. This uses a camera attached to the head to record visual images, which are translated into electrical signals that are sent to electrodes attached to the tongue. (The tongue has more nerve endings than anywhere on the human body except the lips.) What the tongue feels is a sequence of pulses of different length, frequency and intensity, which corresponds to the visual data. Gradually the brain learns to 'see' the image being sent to the tongue. The results are remarkable: after a while, people wearing the device can recognise shapes, letters – even faces – and catch balls that are thrown to them. Brain scans show that even blind people using it are having their visual cortex stimulated.

Darting movements of the eyes are called saccades (from the French *saquer* 'to twitch', and pronounced 'suck-hards'). They are the fastest movements produced by the human body.

Our eyes are also continually vibrating. These tiny, imperceptible movements, each covering 20 arcseconds (or 1/5,000th of a degree) are called microsaccades. They are an essential component of vision: without them we'd be blind. In order to send nerve impulses to the brain, the rod and cone cells need to be continually stimulated by light. Microsaccades ensure that light keeps striking the retina, but the brain edits them out as unnecessary.

One spooky way of demonstrating how much the brain edits our sight is to stand facing a mirror and look at one eye and then the other. You won't be able to see your eyes moving (although it's quite obvious to anyone else).

What's the natural reaction to a bright light?

Squinting or shading the eyes is instinctive for most people, but at least a quarter of us respond to bright lights by sneezing.

This is called the photic sneeze reflex (from *photos*, Greek for 'light') or, with rather heavy-handed humour, the ACHOO syndrome (Autosomal-dominant Compelling Helio-Ophthalmic Outburst).

It was first medically described in 1978, but people have been known to sneeze after looking at the sun since Aristotle; he blamed the effect of heat on the nose. Francis Bacon (1561–1626) disproved Aristotle's theory in the seventeenth century by going out into the sun with his eyes closed; he suffered from photic sneeze reflex, but with his eyes shut nothing happened. Since the heat was still there, he decided that the sneezing must be caused by light; he guessed that the sun made the eyes water and this water irritated the nose.

In fact, the disorder is caused by confused signalling from the trigeminal nerve, the one responsible for sensation in the face. (Trigeminal means 'triple-origin' because the nerve has three main branches.) Somewhere along its passage to the brain the nerve impulses from around the eye and inside the nose become scrambled, and the brain is tricked into thinking that a visual stimulus is a nasal one. The result is that the body tries to 'expel' the light by sneezing.

Photic sneeze reflex affects between 18 per cent and 35 per cent of people. It most often occurs when someone leaves a dark place such as a tunnel or a forest and emerges into bright sunlight. The usual number of sneezes is two or three, but it can be as many as forty. This surprisingly common trait is inherited. Both men and women can get it, and they have a fifty–fifty chance of passing it on to their children. Because it's genetic, it isn't equally distributed but occurs in geographical clusters.

'Honeymoon rhinitis' is another genetic condition where people are attacked by uncontrollable sneezing during sex. One theory is that the nose is the only part of the body other than the reproductive system (and, strangely, the ears) to contain erectile tissue. It may be that the 'arousal' impulse, in some people, triggers both the nose and the genitals simultaneously.

An interesting side effect of this is that, like Pinocchio, our noses really do get bigger when we lie. Guilt causes blood to flow to the erectile tissue in the nose. This is an automatic reflex, and explains why people who are not very good liars often give themselves away by touching or scratching their noses or ears.

How do you know when the sun has set?

'When it has disappeared below the horizon' is the wrong answer.

The sun has already set when its lower edge touches the horizon.

As the setting sun falls in the sky, its light passes through the atmosphere at an increasingly shallow angle and is bent more and more as the amount of air it has to pass through increases. At the end of the process, the light is bent so much that we can still apparently see the sun even though it's physically below the horizon. By coincidence, the degree of bending is almost equal to the width of the sun – so when we see the lower rim of the sun kiss the horizon, the whole of it has in fact completely disappeared.

What we're looking at is a mirage. The bending of the light also has the effect of reducing the apparent distance between the top and bottom of the sun. This can cause the sun to appear oval.

When sunlight travels through the atmosphere, green light is bent very slightly more than red light – as when passing through a prism. This means that the top of the setting sun has a very thin green rim – too thin to be seen by the naked eye. Very occasionally, when atmospheric conditions are right, this green rim can be artificially magnified and it shines for a second or so just as the sun disappears from view. This phenomenon is known as the 'green flash' and is considered a good omen by sailors.

Another common mirage is the one you see on a road in summer. Hot tarmac heats the air above it, producing a sharp shift in its density, which causes light to bend. You think you see water; what you're actually seeing is a reflection of the sky. The brain tells you it's water, because water also reflects the sky.

Desert mirages are the same: the thirsty adventurer only ever 'sees' water.

Any other images of the type associated with mirages in cartoons and films (palm trees, ice-cream vans, dancing girls, etc.) are just figments of a heat-addled imagination.

STEPHEN *Light from the setting sun passes through our atmosphere at a shallow angle; it is gradually bent as the air density, i.e. the pressure, increases. Not dissimilar to the image of your legs when you sit in a swimming pool. Our brains cannot accept that light is bent. The effect is to artificially raise the sun in the last few minutes of its decline, through the thickness of the atmosphere at that shallow angle there. And by coincidence, the amount of bending is pretty much equal to the diameter of the sun, so it's exactly, exactly as it is there, that it's actually disappeared.*

PHILL JUPITUS *I hate this show.*

What are the highest clouds called?

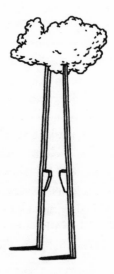

'Everyone knows' that the wispy cirrus clouds are the highest – but they aren't.

Clear midsummer evenings can occasionally reveal one of the loveliest and least understood phenomena of the night sky. Noctilucent ('night-shining') clouds are silvery blue streaks that form so high up in the atmosphere they catch the sun's light, even at night. At over 80 kilometres (50 miles) in altitude, they are seven times higher than the highest cirrus clouds.

The word atmosphere is Greek for 'globe of vapour'. Earth's atmosphere is a succession of layers of gas, stretching about 100 kilometres (62 miles) into space. We live in the troposphere (*tropos* is Greek for 'change'), which is warm and moist and is where all the clouds (except the noctilucent ones) form. At 11 kilometres (7 miles) up, the stratosphere starts (*stratum* is Latin for 'covering'): it contains the protective ozone layer. The outermost layer is the mesosphere, somewhat confusingly called the 'middle sphere' because it's between the other, inner layers and space. It starts nearly 5 kilometres (about 3 miles) up and is 32 kilometres (20 miles) thick. It's too high for most aircraft and too low for space flight, and it's nicknamed the 'ignorosphere' because we know so little about it.

Noctilucent clouds form right on the boundary of the mesosphere and space. Clouds need water vapour and dust particles to form and the mesosphere is so dry and cold (about −123 °C) it was first thought that noctilucent clouds must be made of something other than water vapour. Now we know they are made of tiny ice crystals – a fiftieth of the width of a human hair – but we still don't understand how they form.

Another thing we don't know about them is whether they have always existed or not. No one had ever reported seeing them until 1885 when they were first named by Otto Jesse, a German cloud enthusiast. This was just two years after the eruption of Krakatoa and at a time when the industrial age was at its peak. It seems that this was the first time dust had ever got high enough for clouds to form in the mesosphere.

Today, the mesosphere is getting cooler still, as a result of increased carbon dioxide (CO_2) emissions. At the same time, ironically, carbon dioxide is busy heating up the troposphere.

CO_2 naturally absorbs heat. In the thin air of the mesosphere, it simply sucks it up. But, in the troposphere, nearer the Earth's surface, where the gases are more densely packed, CO_2 collides continually with other substances (such as water vapour). This releases heat and causes global temperatures to rise and is known as the 'greenhouse effect'.

Over the past three decades, the number of noctilucent clouds has more than doubled, which has led some scientists to liken them to miner's canaries: their eerie beauty warning of the dangers of climate change to come.

How much does a cloud weigh?

A *lot*.

A popular unit of measurement for cloud-weight seems to be the elephant. According to the National Center for Atmospheric Research in Boulder, Colorado, an average cumulus cloud weighs about 100 elephants, while a big storm cloud tips the scales at 200,000 elephants.

This is nothing compared to a hurricane. If you extracted the water from a cubic metre of hurricane, weighed it and then multiplied it by the number of cubic metres in the whole hurricane cloud, you would find that a single hurricane weighs *40 million* elephants. That's twenty-six times more elephants than exist on the planet.

Which raises an obvious question: how can something that weighs as much as even *one* elephant float in the sky? The answer is that the weight is distributed across a vast number of tiny water droplets and ice crystals spread over a very large area. The biggest droplets are only 0.2 millimetre (less than

0.008 inch) across: you'd need 2 billion of them to make a teaspoon of water. Clouds form on top of updraughts of warm air. The rising air is stronger than the downward pressure of the water droplets, and so clouds float. When the air cools, and sinks, it begins to rain.

In order to rain, the water in the clouds has to freeze before it falls. If the air temperature is low enough, it will fall as snow or hail; if not, the frozen drops melt on their way down. One puzzle is why there is so much rain in temperate climates like Britain, where clouds rarely get cold enough to freeze pure water. Catalysts like soot and dust help, providing nuclei around which ice can form, but there isn't enough pollution of that kind to create all the rain.

The answer seems to be airborne microbes. Certain kinds of bacteria are first-class 'ice nucleators', to the extent that they have the magical ability to *make* water freeze. Adding *Pseudomonas syringae*, for example, to water, makes it freeze almost instantly, even at relatively warm temperatures of 5–6 °C.

The rain they 'seed' carries the bacteria to earth where they use their ice-making powers to mush up plant cells, including many crops, so they can feed on them. Air currents then sweep them back up into the atmosphere again, causing more rain.

If this theory is right, the implications are enormous: merely growing the kind of crops that these ice-making bacteria like could wipe out droughts forever.

How much of the Moon can you see from the Earth?

It's not half.

Because the Moon takes exactly the same amount of time to revolve around its own axis as it does to orbit the Earth, we only ever see one face of it.

But the Moon's motion is not quite regular. As it goes round, it shifts backwards and forwards and side to side, revealing rather more of itself than half. This is known as 'libration', from the Latin *librare*, 'to swing', after the balancing movements of a pair of scales, or *libra*.

Galileo Galilei (1564–1642) discovered it in 1637, and it comes in three forms.

Latitudinal libration is caused by the fact that the Moon is slightly tilted on its axis. This means that from a fixed point on the Earth's surface the Moon appears to rock first towards and then away from us as it passes by, allowing us to glimpse a little more of its top and bottom in turn.

Longitudinal libration, or side-to-side motion, results from the fact that Moon travels round the Earth at a slightly uneven speed. It always *rotates* at the same rate but, because it's travelling round the Earth in an ellipse rather than a circle, it's going faster when it's closer to the Earth and slower when it's further away. We can see more of its trailing edge when it's going away from us, and more of its leading edge when it's coming towards us.

Finally, there's *diurnal* ('daily') *libration*. Because the Earth is also rotating on its axis, at different times of day we're looking at the moon from a different angle. This allows us to see a bit round the back of the Moon's western edge as it rises, and a bit more round the back of its eastern edge as it sets.

The net result is that in any one month (each twenty-eight-day orbit of the Moon) we see 59 per cent of the Moon's surface. The Soviet spacecraft Luna 3 took the first pictures of the 'dark' side of the Moon in 1959.

The fact that the Moon always shows the same face to the Earth is known as 'tidal locking'. Many of the 169 known moons in the solar system are synchronised in this way: including both the moons of Mars, the five inner moons of Saturn and the four largest of Jupiter's moons, known as the 'Galilean satellites' after Galileo who also discovered them in 1610.

Earth has a similar relationship with Venus. Despite spinning in the opposite direction to Earth, when Venus is closest to us (every 583 days) it always presents the same face. No one knows why. Astronomical bodies become tidally locked when they are relatively close to each other: Venus never gets nearer to us than 38 million kilometres (24 million miles). So it might just be chance.

STEPHEN *There is this strange thing called libration, which is like vibration beginning with an 'l'. It was a thing that was noted by quite a few of the early astronomers . . .*

ROB BRYDON *Can I say, sorry Stephen, but that's not an acceptable way of defining a word: 'Libration, it's like vibration but beginning with an l.'*

What can you hear in space?

In space, no one can hear you scream, but that's not to say that there's no noise there.

There are gases in space, which allow sound waves to travel, but interstellar gas is much less dense than Earth's atmosphere. Whereas air has 30 billion, billion atoms per cubic centimetre, deep space averages fewer than two.

If you were standing at the edge of an interstellar gas cloud and a sound came through it towards you, only a few atoms a second would hit your eardrums – too little for you to hear anything. An extremely sensitive microphone might do better, but humans are effectively deaf in space. Our ears aren't up to it.

Even if you were standing next to an exploding supernova, the gases from the explosion would expand so rapidly that their density would decrease very fast and you'd hear very little.

Sound doesn't travel well on Mars, either: its atmosphere is only 1 per cent as dense as ours. On Earth, a scream can travel a kilometre (⅔ of a mile) before being absorbed by the air; on Mars, it would be inaudible at a distance of 15 metres (50 feet).

Black holes generate sound. There's one in the Perseus cluster of galaxies, 250 million light years away. The signal was detected in 2003 in the form of X-rays (which will happily travel anywhere) by NASA's Chandra X-ray Observatory satellite.

No one will ever hear it, though. It's 57 octaves lower than middle C: over a million billion times deeper than the limits of human hearing.

It's the deepest note ever detected from any object anywhere in the universe and it makes a noise in the pitch of B flat – the same as a vuvuzela.

How do you open a parachute?

Not with a ripcord any more.

The traditional way of opening a parachute was to pull a handle attached to a stainless steel cable known as a ripcord.

Since the 1980s, pilot chutes, packed into a pocket in the parachute harness, have replaced ripcords. The pilot chute is much smaller than the main parachute – about a metre or 3 feet in diameter – and is usually released by the jumper pulling it out of its pocket and throwing it into the air. The sudden jerk as the pilot chute inflates removes the release pin for the main chute, which then opens. This is much safer than ripcords, as there is less chance of jamming.

Modern parachute canopies aren't shaped like jellyfish any more, either. They are rectangular and made of a double layer of parallel tubular cells, a bit like an airbed. The back and sides of each cell are closed, but open at the front. As the tubes fill with air, the canopy forms a wedge, similar to the shape of a hang-glider. And, just as with hang-gliders, parachutes can be steered. The control cords also allow the jumper to slow down or speed up the rate of descent.

If the main parachute fails, there is a second or 'reserve' parachute to open and, even if the jump causes a loss of consciousness, there is an AAD, or Automatic Activation Device, which automatically releases the reserve parachute at about 230 metres (750 feet). The fatality rate for parachute jumps is one in 100,000, but almost none of these are caused by faulty equipment. Most result from reckless manoeuvres or from landing too fast; changes in wind conditions; or 'canopy collisions', where two parachutes get entangled.

Modern parachutists descend at about 40 kilometres per hour (25 miles per hour). In freefall, a body's terminal velocity – where air resistance prevents it from falling any faster – is about 200 kilometres per hour (125 miles per hour). In normal atmospheric pressure, and with an un-controlled posture, it takes about 573 metres (1,880 feet) or 14 seconds to reach this speed.

At higher altitudes, where the air is much less dense, a faster fall is possible. In 1960 US air force pilot Joseph

Kittenger leapt from a balloon at 31,333 metres (102,800 feet) and reached a speed of 988 kilometres per hour (613 miles per hour), close to the speed of sound. Despite continuing to dive head first, he began to spin rapidly and blacked out, coming round when his chute opened automatically around 1.6 kilometres (a mile) above the ground. He is now helping skydiver Felix Baumgartner prepare to break his fifty-year-old record. Baumgartner plans to dive from a balloon at 36,500 metres (120,000 feet or 23 miles). He aims to reach a speed of 1,110 kilometres per hour (690 miles per hour). This will make him the first person to break the sound barrier outside an aircraft. No one knows what the physical effects of supersonic speed will be on a human body.

Leonardo da Vinci is often credited with inventing the idea of a parachute, but the concept predates his famous 1485 drawing. An anonymous manuscript from a decade earlier shows a man wearing rather comical Italian dress and a nonchalant expression, holding on to a cone-shaped canopy. One can only hope it was never tested: it was much too small to slow his descent at all.

STEPHEN *I believe, Pam, that you felt some erotic feelings towards your instructor. Is that correct?*

PAM AYRES *I did. I took a shine to the instructor. I think that's why I jumped out the aircraft, really, 'cause I wanted to impress him.*

JOHNNY VEGAS *I often do that. If I like a woman, I jump out the window. Just to show 'em I really care.*

Why shouldn't you touch a meteorite?

It's not because you might burn your fingers.

A *meteorite* is an object that has fallen to Earth from space. *Meteors*, or 'shooting stars', are objects passing through the Earth's atmosphere. Hundreds of tons of meteors bombard the Earth every day, but most of them are smaller than a grain of sand and burn up on entry.

Both words come from the Greek for celestial phenomena, *ta meteora*, which translates literally as 'things suspended high up'. In films and comics, meteorites are hot – they hiss and sizzle as they land in the snow. In reality, they're usually cold: some are even covered in frost.

This is because space is extremely cold. Although the friction of entering the atmosphere heats meteorites up, it also slows them down. They can take several minutes to fall to the ground: quite long enough for them to lose all the heat their outer surface has temporarily gained.

Meteorites are either stony or metallic – metallic ones ring like a bell when struck with another piece of metal. Most of them are as old as the Earth itself. A few are found immediately after their fall, many have lain in the ground for tens of thousands of years before being discovered. You are most unlikely to come across one. In the whole of the USA between 1807 and 2009, only 1,530 verified examples were found – that's fewer than eight a year. Actually seeing a meteorite falling, and then finding it, is even rarer. In the same period, it only happened 202 times – by coincidence, exactly once a year. The latest edition of the Natural History Museum's *Catalogue of Meteorites*, published since 1847 and listing every known meteorite, records just twenty-four as ever being found anywhere in the British Isles. Meteorite experts get hundreds of calls from the public every year: they rarely turn out to be the real thing.

The reason for not touching one is that you may contaminate any organic matter it might carry. If you do find a fresh one, you should put it in a sealed plastic bag (without touching it) and send it to your nearest research group.

The 'Bolton Meteorite' was found in the backyard of a house in the high street of the Lancashire town in 1928. It caused great excitement, which was rather dampened by the verdict of the British Museum in London – that it wasn't a meteorite at all, just a piece of burnt coal. Even so, it's still on display at the Bolton Museum.

When the first Europeans came to northern Greenland, they were amazed to find the local Inughuit, or polar Inuit, people using metal knives, despite having no idea how to either mine or smelt metal. They had chipped iron flakes off a meteorite using volcanic stones, and set them into handles made of walrus tusks.

The meteorite was one of three that were the centrepieces of their religion. They were 4.5 billion years old and the largest weighed 36 tons. In 1897, the American explorer Admiral Robert E. Peary stole them, selling all three to the American Museum of Natural History in New York for $40,000.

STEPHEN *Around 50,000 meteorites larger than 20 grams fall from space to Earth every year. But more have been found on which continent than any other?*

RICH HALL *Antarctica.*

STEPHEN *Antarctica, yes.*

ALAN *Bit tough on the penguins really, isn't it.*

PHILL JUPITUS *That's why they always stand up, because there's less of a surface area.*

What is a 'brass monkey'?

It's got nothing to do with cannonballs.

The phrase 'cold enough to freeze the balls off a brass monkey' is often said to refer to a metallic grid with circular holes in it, set under a pyramid of cannonballs on a ship's deck to keep it stable. When this 'brass monkey' got cold enough, the metal contracted and the cannonballs all popped out.

In fact, the phrase means exactly what it says; the fake nautical euphemism is an attempt to make its rude humour more acceptable.

First of all, it doesn't make any sense to stack piles of cannonballs on the deck of a pitching warship. And they weren't: they were kept in long thin racks running between the gunports, with a single hole for each cannonball.

Second, these frames were called 'shot-racks' or 'shot garlands' and they were made of wood, not brass.

Third, for one of these imaginary 'brass monkeys' to contract even 1 millimetre (0.3 inch) more than the iron cannonballs it was supposed to hold, the temperature would have to drop to −66 °C, 8 degrees colder than ever recorded in Europe.

Fourth, naval slang from the days of sail abounds in expressions that involve the word monkey, but the phrase 'brass monkey' is nowhere among them. *The Sailors Word Book of 1867*, the comprehensive dictionary of nautical terms compiled by the naval surveyor and astronomer Admiral W. H. Smyth (1788–1865), records monkey-block, monkey-boat, monkey-tail, monkey-jacket, monkey-spars, powder-monkey and monkey-pump (an illegal device for illegally sucking rum through a hole drilled in the cask). The only entry under brass reads: 'BRASS. Impudent assurance.'

Fifth, according to Dr Stewart Murray, a professional metallurgist and Chief Executive of the London Bullion

Market Association, the difference in thermal contraction between brass and iron in such a situation is 'absolutely tiny', even at extreme temperatures, and 'far too insignificant to have that kind of effect'.

'Cold enough to freeze the balls off a brass monkey' began life demurely as 'cold enough to freeze the tail off a brass monkey'. It was first recorded in mid-nineteenth-century America and variants of it were used as often about extremes of heat as they were of cold. In Herman Melville's novel *Omoo* (1850) one of the characters remarks that 'It was 'ot enough to melt the nose h'off a brass monkey'.

Michael Quinion of www.worldwidewords.org suggests that the 'monkey' element originated in the popular nineteenth-century brass ornaments featuring the three monkeys that 'hear no evil, see no evil, speak no evil'.

Clustering round a roaring Dickensian fire on a winter's night, far inland from the sea, what better reminder could there be of how cold it is outside than the line of cheeky brass monkeys sitting on the mantelpiece?

What would you find on the ground at the northernmost tip of Greenland?

You will struggle to find any snow or ice at all. You are most likely to bump into a large, malodorous beast known as the musk ox.

Peary Land is a mountainous peninsula extending from northern Greenland into the Arctic Ocean. It is the most northerly ice-free land on Earth. Lying 725 kilometres (450 miles) south of the North Pole and covering 57,000 square kilometres (22,000 square miles), it is bigger than Denmark.

It was first mapped in 1892 by the American explorer Robert E. Peary (1856–1920), who modestly named it after himself.

Dry enough to be counted as a desert, it is frost-free for three months in the summer, when temperatures often exceed 10°C and can reach 18°C. Winter is very cold, though: usually around −30°C. Rain is rare and the very occasional snow that falls is so dry it simply drifts away and never forms into ice.

Vegetation covers only 5 per cent of the total area but thirty-three species of flowering plant have been recorded and this is enough to support the population of 1,500 musk oxen.

Despite their names, musk oxen are actually large, shaggy members of the goat family. They get their name from the intense smell the males secrete from glands under their eyes when aroused. Musk-ox hair can grow almost 60 centimetres (2 feet) long, covering them in a thick-fringed pelt that reaches to the ground. This keeps them warm but it also means they aren't particularly fast on their feet.

Their defensive strategy is to form a circle around the younger and more vulnerable members of the herd and try to stare down any predators.

Historically, this worked well with Arctic wolves and bears, but wasn't much use against men with rifles. At the turn of the twentieth century, they had been hunted to the brink of extinction. They are now a protected species and the Arctic population has recovered to 150,000 individuals.

Musk oxen are ancient. They evolved over 600,000 years ago and were contemporaries with the woolly mammoth, the giant ground sloth and the sabre-tooth tiger. They are one of very few large mammal species to have survived the last Ice Age, which reached its peak 20,000 years ago.

How cold is 'too cold to snow'?

It's never too cold: at least, not in this world.

Anyone who lives in a country where it snows in winter will have heard people say, 'It's been trying to snow all day, but it's just too cold!'

This is never the case. Snow has been recorded in Alaska at below −41°C and there are reports of snow falling at the South Pole at an incredible −50°C. Flakes have even been made in the lab at −80°C, which is as cold as the coldest parts of Antarctica ever get. It is true that, at temperatures below −33°C very little ordinary 'snow' is produced. Instead, individual ice crystals fall to Earth in a phenomenon known as 'diamond dust'. These are so cold they can't clump together to form the familiar snowflakes, but they are still snow.

The reason why it doesn't always snow when it's cold is that, in northern Europe, very cold weather is usually associated with high pressure. In an area of high pressure, there is little air movement, so the cold air gradually sinks, warming as it falls. This means that any water in the air evaporates completely rather than forming into clouds. In summer, this produces hot, clear weather. In winter, it allows heat from the ground to rise upwards, because there is no insulating cloud layer. This lowers the ground temperature, particularly at night, when there is no sun to warm it. Although it's bitterly cold, there are no clouds to produce snow.

Not that this means it is necessarily warmer when it's snowing.

The coldest temperature ever recorded in England was −26.1°C at Newport, Shropshire on 10 January 1982 – a day also notable for its heavy snowfall.

Where do you lose most of your body heat?

Not necessarily, as Mummy warned you, from the top of your head.

The amount of heat released by any part of the body depends largely on how much of it is exposed. On a cold day, you could easily lose more body heat from a bare arm or leg.

That myth about the head is not only persistent, it's official. The current field manuals for the US Army recommend a hat in cold weather, stating: '40 per cent to 45 per cent of body heat' is lost through the head. The idea is thought to stem from the 1950s, when military scientists put subjects in Arctic survival suits (that didn't cover the head) to measure heat loss in extremely low temperatures.

According to Professor Gordon Giesbrecht, at the University of Manitoba, the world's leading expert on cold-weather survival, the head and neck are only 10 per cent of our body surface area and are no more efficient at losing heat than the rest of our skin.

If our heads *seem* to get colder it's because the concentration of nerve cells in our head and neck makes them five times as sensitive to changes in temperature as other areas. But information from our nervous system (feeling cold) isn't a direct indication of heat loss. This depends on the circulation of the blood – and there isn't a corresponding increase in blood vessels in the head and neck.

Our bodies respond to cold by closing the blood vessels in exposed skin and reducing blood flow to the extremities. This makes the fingers, toes, nose and ears susceptible to frostbite, while the brain and vital organs are unaffected. The other response to cold is shivering: our muscles shake involuntarily to generate heat by using up energy. Both responses are automatic, controlled by a cone-shaped part of the brain called the hypothalamus, which also governs other instinctive processes such as hunger, thirst and tiredness.

Professor Giesbrecht is no armchair theorist. Since 1991, he has put himself into states of hypothermia at least thirty-nine times to study the effects of cold on the human body. Hypothermia (from Greek *hypo* 'under'. and *therme*, 'heat') is the point at which our internal temperature drops below 35 °C, and the body's key processes start to slow down. This has led the redoubtable Dr Giesbrecht to plunge repeatedly into frozen lakes and hurtle a snowmobile at night into freezing seas. This, and the survival guides he has published, has earned him the nickname 'Professor Popsicle', after North America's favourite iced lolly.

Dr Giesbrecht advises that the key to survival if you suddenly find yourself in an icy lake is to master your breathing in the first minute. Once your breathing is steady, you have ten minutes before the cold starts affecting your muscles and an hour before hypothermia sets in. Other tips: hot drinks do not help beat the cold (though sugary drinks do, as they provide fuel for the body to generate heat). And don't blow on your hands to keep warm. The moisture in your breath makes them colder and increases the risk of frostbite.

DAVID MITCHELL *Is it not just a fact that your head is a bit of you that is more naked than the rest of you?*

STEPHEN *Well, that's right, if your arm was exposed, more would escape from your arm than from your head.*

DAVID *If people went around with bare buttocks a lot, they would say: 'Well, in the cold you really should put on a buttock hat.'*

What colour should you wear to keep cool?

We're all told at school that white reflects sunlight and black absorbs it, so that the paler your clothes are, the cooler you'll be.

But it's not quite that simple.

In many hot countries, locals often wear dark colours. Peasants in China and old ladies in southern Europe, for instance, traditionally wear black, and the Tuareg, the nomadic people of the Sahara, favour indigo blue.

Dark clothes are effective because there are two thermal processes happening at once. Heat is coming downwards from the sun but it is also going outwards from the body. Though light clothes are better at *reflecting* the *sun*'s heat, dark clothes are better at *radiating* the *body*'s heat. Given that no one born in a hot climate willingly stands in direct sunlight, the dark clothing has the edge because it keeps you cooler when you're in the shade.

Then there's the wind factor. People who live in really hot places don't wear tight jumpers or tailored suits. They wear loose robes that enable maximum air circulation. In 1978 a study examining the significance of colouring in birds' plumage found that, in hot and still conditions, white feathers were best at letting heat escape; but as soon as the wind got above 11 kilometres per hour (7 miles per hour), black feathers – provided they were fluffy – were the most efficient coolers. Experiments on black and white cattle have reached similar conclusions.

Applying this to humans, given even a modest breeze, loose black clothes will carry heat away from your body faster than they absorb it.

In less extreme climates, one of the best ways to keep cool is to learn how to use windows properly. Physicists at Imperial College, London have shown that optimum air flow in a room comes from opening both the top and bottom sections of a sash window.

If the two openings are of equal size, colder, heavier air coming in through the lower gap pushes the warmer, less dense air out of the top, much as a cooling gust ventilates a Tuareg's flowing garment, known as a *k'sa*.

The equivalent robe in French-speaking West Africa is called a *Grand Boubou*.

Is there any land on Earth that doesn't belong to any country?

Yes, there are two such places.

The first is Marie Byrd Land in western Antarctica, which is so remote that no government seems to want it.

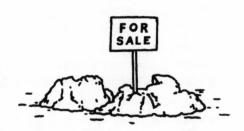

It's a vast swathe of the Earth's surface, spreading out from the South Pole to the Antarctic coast and covering 1,610,000 square kilometres (622,000 square miles). This is larger than Iran or Mongolia, but it's so inhospitable that it supports only one permanent base, which belongs to the USA. Marie Byrd Land is named after the wife of US Rear-Admiral Richard E. Byrd (1888–1957), who first explored it in 1929. The remote research station was the inspiration for John Carpenter's classic horror film, *The Thing* (1982).

The rest of Antarctica is administered by twelve nations under the Antarctic Treaty system established in 1961, which made the continent a scientific preserve and banned all military activity there. The biggest territories belong to the nations that first explored the continent (Britain, Norway and France) and those that are closest (New Zealand, Australia, Chile and Argentina). The ocean beyond Marie Byrd Land stretches up into the empty reaches of the South Pacific, where no one nation is close enough to claim it as their own.

The legal term for a territory outside the sovereign control of any state is *Terra nullius*, literally 'no-man's-land'. Although Marie Byrd Land is the biggest remaining example, there is one small tract of Africa that can claim the same status.

The Bir Tawil Triangle lies between Egypt and Sudan and is owned by neither. In 1899, when the British controlled the area, they defined the border between the two countries by drawing a straight line through a map of the desert. This put Bir Tawil in Sudan and the piece of land next door, called the Halai'b Triangle, in Egypt. The boundary was redrawn (using wigglier lines) in 1902. Bir Tawil ('water well' in Arabic) went to Egypt, and Halai'b to the Sudan.

Bir Tawil is the size of Buckinghamshire – 2,000 square kilometres (770 square miles) – and you'd think both countries would be fighting over it, but they're not. What they both want is Halai'b. Whereas Bir Tawil is mostly sand and rock, Halai'b is fertile, populated, on the Red Sea coast and ten times larger. Egypt currently occupies it, citing the 1899 boundary. Sudan disputes the claim, citing the 1902 amendment. Both disown Bir Tawil for the same reason.

The world's most disputed territory is the Spratly Islands, an archipelago of 750 uninhabited islets in the South Pacific: 4 square kilometres (1½ square miles) of land spread over 425,000 square kilometres (164,000 square miles) of sea. Rich fishing grounds and potential oil and gas fields mean that six nations claim them: the Philippines, China, Taiwan, Vietnam, Malaysia and Brunei. Apart from Brunei, all maintain a military presence in the area. To strengthen their claim, the Philippines pay a rotating team of public sector employees to live on one of the Spratlys. It isn't a popular posting: the charm of a tiny tropical rock that can be walked round in thirty minutes soon fades.

Which country is the river Nile in?

Despite its timeless association with Egypt, most of the Nile is in Sudan.

The Nile rises in Rwanda, in the Great Lakes area of Central Africa, and flows through Ethiopia, Uganda, the Democratic Republic of Congo and Egypt, but the largest section traverses Sudan. The river's two great tributaries – the Blue and White Niles – meet in Khartoum, the country's capital.

Sudan is the largest country in Africa, covering 2,505,813 square kilometres (967,500 square miles), making it bigger than Western Europe and a quarter of the size of the USA. It is also the largest country in the Arab world. Because of its political and military precariousness, no one is quite sure what its current population is, but most estimates suggest 40 million, with four times as many living in the Arabic-speaking Muslim north as in the largely Christian south.

The northern Muslim population is descended from Arab invaders and the indigenous Nubian people, one of black Africa's earliest civilisations. The name 'Nubia' comes from the Egyptian *nbu*, 'gold', as the region was famous for its gold mines. From the seventh century AD, waves of Arab invaders spread out from Damascus and Baghdad, establishing Islam throughout north-west Africa. The first Nubian Muslim ruler ascended to the throne in AD 1093 and northern Sudan has been a part of the Islamic world ever since.

'Sudan' means 'black' in Arabic. It comes from the Arabic *bilad as-sudan* meaning 'land of the black people' and southern and western Sudan contains a complex mix of almost 600 black African tribal groups, speaking over 400 different languages and dialects. Many of them are Christian, or practise traditional African religions. The Dinka – whose name means 'the people' and who are, at over a million strong, Sudan's largest tribal group – practise both.

For over thirty years, the northern government and the southern tribes like the Dinka were locked in civil war. Ending in 1989, the war cost the lives of more than 2 million people and displaced another 4 million. It is estimated that 200,000 southern Sudanese have been forced into slavery in the north. Most of them are Dinka. In 2005 Southern Sudan was finally granted autonomy and this is being implemented by the United Nations.

In the meantime, the Northern Islamic government has been accused of genocide by using terrorist militias to destroy three tribal groups in the western region of Darfur. In 2008 the International Criminal Court (ICC) issued an arrest warrant for President Omar al-Bashir, charging him with war crimes and crimes against humanity. This is the first time the court has brought charges against a serving head of state.

Sudan is 150th out of 182 nations on the UN's human development index. One in five Sudanese lives on less than £1 a day. In the 2009 Happy Planet Index, which measures well-being and environmental impact, Sudan is ranked 121 out of 143, though this beats both Luxembourg and Estonia.

What was Cleopatra's nationality?

She was Greek.

Cleopatra (literally meaning 'renowned in her ancestry') was a direct descendant of Ptolemy I (303–285 BC), the right-hand man to Alexander the Great. On Alexander's death in 325 BC, Ptolemy's loyalty was rewarded with the governorship of Egypt. Like Alexander, Ptolemy came from Macedon, north of Greece. The Macedonians had hereditary, all-powerful kings and despised the newfangled ideas of the south, crushing democracy in Athens in 322 BC. In keeping with his heritage, Ptolemy appointed himself Pharaoh of Egypt in 305 BC, founding a dynasty that would last 275 years.

The Ptolemaic court spoke Greek and behaved as an occupying foreign power, rather like the British in India. The Ptolemies, like all Pharoahs in Egypt, were also gods and they were a close-knit bunch. All the male heirs were called Ptolemy and the women were usually either Cleopatra or Berenice. Brothers and sisters often married each other, to keep things in the family and reinforce their aloofness from their subjects. This makes the Ptolemaic family tree almost impossible to follow.

For example, the Cleopatra we know is Cleopatra VII (69–30 BC), but her mother might have been either Cleopatra V or VI. Our Cleopatra's father, Ptolemy XII (117–51 BC), married his sister, who was also his cousin. It was a tiny gene pool: Cleopatra had only four great-grandparents and six (out of a possible sixteen) great-great-grandparents. The sculptures and coins that survive make clear that she wasn't as beautiful as Shakespeare painted her, but nor did she have the classic Ptolemy look — fat with bulging eyes — that resulted from centuries of inbreeding. And, though no one knows exactly which of her relatives gave birth to her, ethnically she was pure Macedonian Greek.

Despite this, she identified strongly with Egypt. She became queen at eighteen and ruled the country for most of four decades. She was the first Ptolemy to learn the Egyptian language and had herself portrayed in traditional Egyptian dress. She was ruthless in removing any threats to her power, arranging for the murder of two siblings and plunging the country into civil war to take on the third, her brother (and husband), Ptolemy XIII.

When senior courtiers backed Ptolemy, she responded by seducing Julius Caesar, recently elected as *dictator* (senior magistrate in the Roman Senate), and commander of the most powerful army in the world. Together they crushed all opposition. When Caesar was assassinated, leading to civil war in Rome, Cleopatra seduced his second-in-command, Mark Antony. In the midst of all this, she still found time to write a book on cosmetics.

The war ended when the Roman fleet under Octavian (later the Emperor Augustus) defeated Mark Antony at the battle of Actium (31 BC). Antony committed suicide in the belief that Cleopatra had already done so and she poisoned herself (though the latest research suggests no asps were involved). She was the last pharoah. The Romans made off with so much Egyptian gold that the Senate was immediately able to reduce interest rates from 12 per cent to 4 per cent.

STEPHEN *Donkeys' milk is very nutritious indeed; it contains oligosaccharides, which are very, very good for you and have all kinds of immuno-helpful things, don't they, Dr Garden?*

GRAEME GARDEN *I'm sure they do, yes. Very good for bathing in, too. Wasn't Cleopatra in ass's milk?*

STEPHEN *She was in ass's milk, absolutely, and Poppaea, the wife of Nero: 300 donkeys were milked to fill her bath.*

GRAEME *Big girl, was she?*

Why did Julius Caesar wear a laurel wreath?

Not victory, but vanity.

According to the Roman historian Suetonius in *On the Life of the Caesars* (AD 121), Julius Caesar 'used to comb forward his scanty locks from the crown of his head' and was thrilled when the Senate granted him the special privilege of being able to wear a victor's laurel wreath whenever he felt like it.

Caesar's baldness bothered him a lot. During his affair with Cleopatra, she recommended her own patent baldness cure, a salve made from burnt mice, bear grease, horse's teeth and deer marrow, rubbed on the head until it 'sprouts'. Clearly, it wasn't very effective.

Caesar wasn't the only general with hair-loss problems. According to the Greek historian Polybius, the Carthaginian commander Hannibal (247–183 BC) found a way to get round this: 'He had a number of wigs made, dyed to suit the appearance of persons differing widely in age, and kept constantly changing them.' Even those closest to Hannibal had trouble recognising him.

Before the establishment of the Empire, Roman hair was worn simply. Only afterwards did hair styles become more elaborate and wigs more popular. The Empress Messalina (AD 17–48) had an extensive collection of yellow wigs, which she wore when moonlighting in brothels. (By law, Roman prostitutes had to wear a yellow wig as a badge of their profession.) Wigs continued to be worn after Rome became Christian in AD 313) but the Church soon condemned them as a mortal sin.

The tradition of a laurel wreath being given to the victor began at the Pythian Games in Delphi in the sixth century BC. These were held in honour of the god Apollo, usually portrayed wearing a wreath of laurels in memory of the nymph Daphne, who turned herself into a laurel tree to escape his amorous advances.

As well as indicating victory, the laurel had a reputation as a healing plant, so doctors who graduated also received a laurel wreath. This is the origin of the academic expressions baccalaureate, Bachelor of Arts (BA) and Bachelor of Science (BSc). They all come from the Latin *bacca lauri*, 'laurel berries'.

No one knows where the Latin surname Caesar comes from.

Pliny the Elder thought it was because the first Caesar (like Macbeth) was 'cut from his mother's womb' – *caesus* means 'cut' in Latin. Pliny's idea is the origin of the term 'Caesarian section'. But this can't be true: such operations were only ever performed to rescue a baby whose mother had died, and Caesar's mother, Aurelia, is known to have lived for many years after his birth.

The most likely meaning of 'Caesar' is that it's from the Latin *caesaries*, which means 'a beautiful head of hair'.

What was Caesar talking about when he said '*Veni, vidi, vici*'?

Most of us think '*Veni, vidi, vici*' ('I came, I saw, I conquered') – Julius Caesar's second most famous line after '*Et tu, Brute*' – refers to his invasion of Britain.

In fact, as every schoolboy knows, he was summing up his victory over King Pharnaces II of Pontus at the battle of Zela in 47 BC.

At the time the Roman civil war was at its height, with Caesar leading the Senate's modernisers and Gnaeus Pompeius Magnus (better known as Pompey) commanding the traditionalist forces.

The kingdom of Pontus, on the southern coast of the Black Sea, had proved a troublesome enemy to Rome over the years. Knowing Caesar was preoccupied fighting Pompey in Egypt, King Pharnaces spotted his chance to regain some lost territory and invaded Cappadocia, in what is now northern Turkey. He inflicted a heavy defeat on the depleted Roman defence, and rumours spread that he had tortured Roman prisoners.

When Caesar returned victorious from Egypt, he decided to teach Pharnaces a lesson. At Zela he defeated the large, well-organised Pontic army in just five days and couldn't resist crowing about it in a letter to his friend Amantius in Rome: hence the quote. Suetonius even claims Caesar paraded the famous phrase around after the battle itself. It was to prove a decisive moment in the civil war against Pompey and his supporters, and in Caesar's career.

Caesar's attempted invasion of Britain was a much less satisfactory affair. He invaded twice, in 55 and 54 BC. The first time, he landed near Deal in Kent. The lack of a natural harbour meant his troops had to leap into deep water and wade towards the large British force that had gathered on the shore. Only the on-board Roman catapults kept the blue-painted natives at bay. After a few skirmishes, Caesar decided to cut his losses and withdrew to Gaul.

The following year he returned with 10,000 men and sailed up the Thames, where he tried to establish a Roman ally as king. He left shortly afterwards, complaining there was nothing worth having in Britain and that the locals were an ungovernable horde of wife-swapping, chicken-tormenting barbarians. No Romans stayed behind.

The whole invasion was staged for the Senate's benefit: conquering the 'land beyond the ocean' made Caesar look good at home. This set the pattern for Rome's involvement with Britain: trade and Roman influence continued to grow without the need for full occupation. When that finally happened, ninety-six years later under the Emperor Claudius, it took four legions – 15 per cent of the whole Roman army – to do the job.

The phrase *'veni, vidi, vici'* lives on today in the scientific name of the Conquered lorikeet, an extinct species of South Pacific parrot discovered in 1987. A member of the *Vini* genus, its full name is *Vini vidivici*.

How many men did a centurion command in the Roman Empire?

Eighty.

The actual number of soldiers in each Roman legion changed over time and in different places, and the army was always short of men. Legions were at first divided into ten cohorts, each consisting of six centuries of a hundred men, or 6,000 men in all. But well before Julius Caesar came along, and right through the Roman Empire that followed him, the full strength of a legion had settled at 4,800 men. Each cohort was made up of 480 men and each of its six centuries comprised eighty soldiers, led by a centurion.

The smallest division of the Roman army was the *contubernium*, originally a unit of ten men who lived, ate and fought together. The word is from Latin *con*, 'together' and *taberna*, 'a hut' – military tents were made from boards, or *tabulae*. Such intimacy had the effect of transforming the soldiers into comrades, or *contubernales*, and it was the basis of the Roman army's legendary *esprit de corps*. We know there were ten of them in each tent, because the man in charge was called the *decanus*, meaning 'a chief of ten, one set over ten persons'.

Each century was made up of ten *contubernii*.

By Caesar's time, though, the number of men in each *contubernium* had shrunk to eight, although their leader was still called a *decanus*. It seems that, although a fighting unit of ten men worked well enough when near to home, as the Romans expanded far beyond Italy military experience in distant, dangerous and unfamiliar places found that an eight-man unit was the ideal size for close bonds between soldiers. So, because army rules had always decreed ten *contubernii* in a century, a century became eighty men.

Another Roman official, who might have been in charge of 100 men but wasn't, was the *praetor hastarius*, or 'president of the spear'. Praetors were judges, and the spear was the symbol of property. The *praetor hastarius* presided over a court that dealt with property disputes and resolving wills. Court members were drawn from a pool of *centumviri*, or Hundred Men. But there were never exactly 100 of them. Originally there were 105 – three from each of the 35 Roman tribes – and this later grew to 180.

A hundred of anything is rarer than you might think. The English language has, buried within it, a numbering system that used twelve rather than ten as a base. That's why we say eleven (*endleofan*, which meant 'one left') and twelve ('two left') instead of *tenty-one* and *tenty-two*. The Old English word for 'a hundred' was *hund*, but there were three different kinds – *hund teantig* (a hundred 'tenty' is 100); *hund endleofantig* (a hundred 'eleventy' is 110) and *hund twelftig* (a hundred 'twelfty' is 120). These lasted for many centuries. The expression 'a great hundred' meant 120 well into the sixteenth century and a 'hundredweight', today meaning 112 pounds, was once 120 pounds.

By coincidence, each legion of Roman infantry had a detachment of (much less important) cavalry. There were 120 of them in each legion.

What language was mostly spoken in ancient Rome?

It was Greek, not Latin.

A *lingua franca* is a language used between two people when neither is using their mother tongue. Rome was the capital city of a fast and expanding empire, a commercial hub of over a million people. Although the native language of Rome (capital of Latium) was Latin, the *lingua franca* – the language you would use if you were buying or selling or generally trying to make yourself understood – was *koine* or 'common' Greek.

Greek was also the language of choice for Rome's educated urban elite. Sophisticated Romans saw themselves as the inheritors of Greek culture. Virgil's *Aeneid* – the epic poem that tells the story of Rome's foundation – makes it explicit that contemporary Rome grew directly out of the mythical Greece that Homer had written about. Speaking Greek at home was essential. Most of the literature that upper-class Romans read was in Greek; the art, architecture, horticulture, cookery and fashion they admired was Greek; and most of their teachers and domestic staff were Greeks.

Even when they did speak Latin it wasn't the classical Latin that we recognise. For speaking native Romans used a form of the language called 'Vulgar Latin'. The word vulgar simply meant 'common' or 'of the people'. Classical Latin was the written language – used for law, oratory and administration but not for conversation. It was the everyday version that the Roman army carried across Europe and it was Vulgar, not classical Latin that spawned the Romance languages: Italian, French and Spanish.

But Vulgar Latin was only the daily language of Latium, not the Empire. Greek was the first language of the eastern Empire, based around Constantinople and of the cities in southern Italy. The name Naples (*Neapolis* in Latin) is actually

Greek (*nea*, new, and *polis*, city). Today, the local dialect in Naples, Neopolitana, still shows traces of Greek and the Griko language is still spoken by 30,000 in southern Italy. Modern Greek and Griko are close enough for speakers to be able to understand one another. Greek, not Latin, was the popular choice for the Mediterranean marketplace.

Lingua Franca was originally an Italian – not a Latin – term for the specific language that was used by people trading in the Mediterranean from the eleventh to the nineteenth century. Based on Italian, it combined elements of Provencal, Spanish, Portuguese, Greek, French and Arabic into a flexible lingo everyone could speak and understand.

Lingua Franca doesn't mean 'French language', but 'Language of the Franks'. It derives from the Arabic habit of referring to all Christians as 'Franks' (rather as we once referred to all Muslims as 'Moors'). *Franji* remains a common Arabic word used to describe Westerners today.

Where is English the official language?

There are many countries in which English is the Official Language, but England, Australia and the United States aren't among them.

An official language is defined as a language that has been given legal status for use in a nation's courts, parliament and administration. In England, Australia and over half the USA, English is the *unofficial* language. It is used for all state business, but no specific law has ever ratified its use.

Bilingual countries such as Canada (French and English) and Wales (Welsh and English) do have legally defined official languages. National laws often recognise significant minority languages, as with Maori in New Zealand. Sometimes, as in Ireland, an official language is more symbolic than practical: fewer than 20 per cent of the population use Irish every day.

English is frequently chosen as an alternative 'official' language if a country has many native languages. A good example is Papua New Guinea where 6 million people speak 830 different languages. In the USA the campaign to make English the official language is opposed by many other ethnic groups, most notably the Hispanic community who account for more than 15 per cent of the population.

Perhaps the most interesting case of an English-speaking country that doesn't have English as its official language is Australia. As well as large numbers of Greek, Italian and South-East Asian immigrants, Australia is home to 65,000 native Maltese speakers. There are also 150 aboriginal languages which are still spoken (compared to the 600 or so spoken in the eighteenth century). Of these, all but twenty are likely to disappear in the next fifty years. Attempting to declare English the official language risks looking insensitive.

The Vatican is the only country in the world that has Latin as an official language.

When did Parliament make slavery illegal in England?

6 April 2010.

With a few minor exceptions, slavery was abolished throughout the British Empire in 1833, but it wasn't thought necessary to outlaw it at home.

In 1067, according to the Domesday Book, more than 10 per cent of the population of England were slaves. The

Normans, perhaps surprisingly, were opposed to slavery on religious grounds and within fifty years it had virtually disappeared. Even serfdom (a kind of modified slavery) became increasingly rare and Queen Elizabeth I freed the last remaining serfs in 1574.

At the same time, Britain was becoming a colonial power and it was the height of fashion for returning Englishmen to have a 'black manservant' (who was in fact, of course, a slave). This unseemly habit was made illegal by the courts in 1772 when the judge, Lord Mansfield, reportedly declared: 'The air of England is too pure for any slave to breathe', with the result that thousands of slaves in England gained their freedom.

From that moment, slavery was arguably illegal in England (though not in the British Empire) under Common Law, but this was not confirmed by Parliament until the Coroners and Justice Act.

Previous acts of Parliament dealt with kidnap, false imprisonment, trafficking for sexual exploitation and forced labour, but never specifically covered slavery. Now, Section 71 of the Coroners and Justice Act (which came into force on 6 April 2010) makes it an offence in the UK, punishable by up to fourteen years' imprisonment, to hold a person in 'slavery or servitude'.

'Servitude' is another word for serfdom. A serf is permanently attached to a piece of land and forced to live and work there, whereas a slave can be bought and sold directly like a piece of property. It's a fine difference: in fact, the English word 'serf' comes from the Latin word *servus*, 'a slave'.

Until now, the lack of a specific English law has made it hard to prosecute modern slave-masters. There's a difference between 'abolishing' something and making it a criminal offence. Although slavery was *abolished* all over the world many years ago, in many countries the *reality* only changed when laws were introduced to punish slave owners.

You might think slavery is a thing of the past and isn't relevant to modern Britain, but there are more slaves in the world now – 27 million of them – than were ever seized from Africa in the 400 years of the transatlantic slave trade. And forced labour, using migrant workers effectively as slaves (and also outlawed by the Act), is widespread in Britain today.

Under the Criminal Law Act 1967, a number of obsolete crimes were abolished in England including scolding, eavesdropping, being a common nightwalker and challenging someone to a fight.

It is odd to think that, in the year England won the World Cup, eavesdropping was still illegal but slavery wasn't.

ALAN *I bet it was one of these odd little New Labour laws in about 1996, 7, 8 . . .*

STEPHEN *What an odd law, to outlaw slavery. It's political correctness gone mad!*

Why doesn't Britain have a written constitution?

It does have one.

The idea that Britain has an 'unwritten constitution' has been described by Professor Vernon Bogdanor, the country's leading constitutional expert, as 'misleading'.

The rules setting out the balance of power between the governors and the governed *are* written down. They're just not all written down in *one place*.

The British constitution is composed of several documents, including Magna Carta (1215), the Petition of Right Act (1628), the Bill of Rights (1689), the Act of Settlement (1701), the Parliament Acts (1911 and 1949) and the Representation of the People Act (1969). Between them, they cover most of the key principles that, in other countries, appear in a single formal statement: that justice may not be denied or delayed; that no tax can be raised without parliament's approval; that no one can be imprisoned without lawful cause; that judges are independent of the government; and that the unelected Lords cannot indefinitely block Acts passed by the elected Commons. They also say who can vote, and how the royal succession works.

There's also 'case law', in which decisions made by courts become part of the constitution. An important example is the Case of Proclamations (1611), which found that the king (and thus his modern equivalent, the government) cannot create a new offence by merely *announcing* it. In other words, nothing is against the law until proper legislation says it is.

The reason why Britain doesn't have a single written document (and almost every other parliamentary democracy does) is to do with its age. The British state has evolved over a millennium and a half. It had no founding fathers, or moment of creation, so its constitution has continued to develop bit by bit.

This has left some surprising gaps. The Cabinet has no legal existence; it is purely a matter of convention. The law established neither of the Houses of Parliament and, although the office of Prime Minister was formally recognised in 1937, British law has never defined what the PM's role actually is.

But that's not as unusual as it might sound. There is no constitution anywhere whose authors have thought of everything. The US Constitution does not contain one word on the subject of how elections should be conducted.

Whether that would surprise many US citizens is hard to say. In 2002 a survey by Columbia Law School found that almost two-thirds of Americans identified the phrase 'From each according to his ability, to each according to his needs' as a quotation from the US constitution rather than coming from the pen of the founder of communism, Karl Marx (1818–83).

What does a British judge bang to keep order in court?

British judges do not, and never have, used gavels – only British auctioneers.

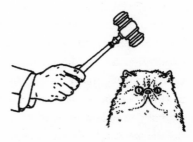

Actors playing judges on TV and in films in Britain use them because their real-life American counterparts do. After decades of exposure to US movies and TV series, they have become part of the visual grammar of the courtroom. Another self-perpetuating legal cliché is referring to the judge as 'M'Lud'. Real British barristers never do this: the correct form of address is 'My Lord'.

The origin of the word *gavel* is obscure. The original English word *gafol* dates from the eighth century and meant a 'payment' or 'tribute', usually a quantity of corn or a division of land. The earliest known use of the word *gavel* to mean 'a chairman's hammer' dates from 1860, so it's hard to see a connection. Some sources claim it might have been used earlier than this among Freemasons (as a term for a mason's hammer), but the evidence is faint.

Modern gavels are small ceremonial mallets commonly made of hardwood, sometimes with a handle. They are used to call for attention, to indicate the opening (call to order) and closing (adjournment) of proceedings, and to announce the striking of a binding bargain in an auction.

The US procedural guidebook – *Robert's Rules of Order Newly Revised* (1876) – provides advice on the proper use of the gavel in the USA. It states that the person in the chair is never to use the gavel in an attempt to drown out a disorderly member, nor should they lean on the gavel, juggle or toy with it, or use it to challenge or threaten, or to emphasise remarks.

The handleless ivory gavel of the United States Senate was presented by the Republic of India to replace one that had been in continuous use since 1789. The new one was first used on 17 November 1954. The original had been broken earlier in 1954, when Vice-President Richard Nixon brandished it during a heated debate on nuclear energy. Unable to obtain a piece of ivory large enough to replace the historic heirloom, the Senate appealed for help to the Indian embassy, who duly obliged.

The gavel of the United States House of Representatives is plain and wooden and has been broken and replaced many times.

STEPHEN *British judges have never had gavels. Never.*

JACK DEE *Sometimes, if they're conducting an auction at the same time, they do.*

What does European law force British fishermen to do?

If you read the British popular press, your answer is bound to be: 'wear hairnets'. This isn't true.

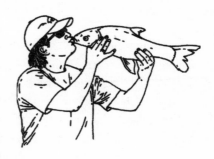

Under EU rules only people who work in fish-processing factories must have their heads covered, to prevent their hair ending up in our fish fingers.

This particular Euro-myth is unusual in having an identifiable beginning. Former Euro MP Wayne David told the House of Commons in July 2002 that he had overheard a group of British journalists joking about it in a Brussels bar: 'They had invented the story about fishermen's hairnets and sent it back to the UK, and to their amazement, it hit the front pages.'

One of the 'myths' most quoted by pro-Europeans is the belief that the EU has banned bent bananas. Their Eurosceptic counterparts point out that rules governing banana shape certainly do exist. Commission Regulation (EC) 2257/94 decrees that bananas must be 'free from malformation or abnormal curvature', even though no bananas have ever been 'banned' as such.

Unhelpfully this rule does not define or quantify 'abnormal curvature', whereas Commission Regulation (EEC) 1677/88 does specify that the permissible bend of Class I cucumbers may be up to 10 mm per 10 cm (0.4 of an inch per 4 inches).

Nevertheless, many of the myths are entirely unfounded. In 1997 British newspapers announced that it was to be made compulsory for motorway bridges to carry works of art glorifying leading EU figures. The *Daily Mail* voiced the concerns of Tory MEP Graham Mather that, if the scheme were to get off the ground, Britain could be inundated by more statues and busts of former EU Commission President Jacques Delors than there were of Winston Churchill. 'It's a terrifying prospect,' said Mr Mather, 'and might frighten people.' The actual proposal was entirely reasonable. It was to set aside 1 per cent of the EU public works subsidy to spend on art that would 'bring people together and promote human dignity and a spirit of tolerance'.

There was also a notorious *Daily Telegraph* report that official notices would have to be displayed on mountains warning climbers that they were 'in a high place'. The Commission explained that this was a misinterpretation of safety rules. It applied only to people *working* at heights, such as scaffolders — not to those engaged in leisure activities.

Perhaps the strangest example of a genuine EU regulation is the ambiguous message printed on tins of nasal snuff: 'EEC Council Directive (992/41/EEC) CAUSES CANCER', which suggests that it's the directive itself that is deadly, rather than the snuff.

DAVID MITCHELL *Well, it makes practical sense as well, of course, because the hairnet could also catch any smaller fish, like, you know, whitebait or scampi that might get in the hair of the fisherman, and then at the end of the day . . . 'Oh, that's dinner!'*

Why have firemen's poles been banned?

They haven't. 'Health-and-safety-mad' bureaucrats still allow fire stations to be built with the traditional poles in them.

Firefighters on the night shift spend their time in dormitories or rest rooms. When the call to action comes, they leap out of bed and dash to their engines. To get there from the upper floor of the station, sliding down a pole is quicker (and safer) than hurtling down stairs. But, either way, a bunch of half-asleep people trying to get down in a tearing hurry can still lead to a twisted ankle – which isn't much use in an emergency.

The obvious solution is not to use poles *or* stairs, but to build the fire station entirely on the ground floor, and this is now standard practice. However, in built-up areas where land is scarce, new stations are still multilevel. In those, poles are generally installed and old stations have mostly retained their poles.

The 'poles banned' myth can be traced to a flurry of misleading newspaper reports published in the summer of 2006, about a refurbished, pole-free station that had opened in Plymouth. The *Daily Mail* began its shock exposé with the words: 'Barmy fire chiefs came under a blaze of criticism today after they banned the traditional fireman's pole – because it posed a "health and safety hazard".' Meanwhile, the *Mirror* found a 'local pensioner' eager to provide the voice of common sense: 'It's barmy. Can't they just put a pile of cotton wool at the bottom of the pole?' The truth was less sensational: the shape of the renovated building had simply made a pole impractical. The Devon Fire Brigade had not adopted a 'no-pole' policy.

Some basic safety measures arrived surprisingly late in firefighting history. The London Fire Brigade continued using brass helmets until 1936, when it occurred to someone that a non-conductive material might be less of a risk when electric cables were flailing around the firemen's heads. (New York firemen, by contrast, had worn leather helmets for over a century.) Yellow helmets and trousers (for visibility) weren't issued in the UK until the 1970s, and fireproof jackets only replaced woollen ones in 1989.

You may have heard that the fire brigade – and fire insurance – was invented by the US founding father, Benjamin Franklin (1706–90). It's not true: when he started Philadelphia's first fire brigade in 1736 (and the first fire insurance scheme in 1751) such things had long existed in Britain and other countries, and were already established in several US cities. Nor did Franklin invent the fireman's coat; when called to fires, his men wore whatever was to hand. They were well equipped, though: with leather buckets, hoses, fire hooks, ladders and water-pumping engines – all of them imported from Britain.

STEPHEN *What happened to the fireman's pole?*
ROB BRYDON *He tiled the fireman's bathroom.*

Why was absinthe made illegal?

It was never illegal in Britain and it doesn't send you mad.

Few drinks have attracted the hysteria that surrounded absinthe at the end of the nineteenth century. Known as the 'Green Fairy', it was supposed to have enslaved and then destroyed the minds of a whole generation of artists and writers. Vincent van Gogh, Arthur Rimbaud, Charles Baudelaire, Paul Gauguin, Henri de Toulouse-Lautrec, Oscar Wilde and Aleister Crowley were all dedicated *absintheurs* and every kind of depravity was ascribed to its hallucinogenic effects. Alexander Dumas (1802–70) even claimed that absinthe had killed more French soldiers in North Africa than Arab bullets.

The high point of 'absinthe madness' came in 1905, when a Swiss alcoholic called Jean Lanfray shot his wife and two young daughters while drunk (he said he did it because his wife had refused to clean his shoes). He had drunk copious amounts of wine, cognac, brandy and crème de menthe that day, but it was the two glasses of absinthe he'd also had that got the blame. A storm of temperance-led moral outrage followed, which led to absinthe being banned in the United States and across most of Europe (though never in the UK). The prohibition has only recently been lifted.

The crack-cocaine of its day was (and is) made from daisies. Wormwood, or *Artemisia absinthium*, is a member of the daisy family and was prized as a medicinal herb from ancient times. Among many other things, it was used as a cure for intestinal worms, though this wasn't the origin of the name 'worm' wood. It comes from the Old English *wermod* – literally 'man-courage' (it was once also used as an aphrodisiac). Before absinthe came along, wormwood was already a popular flavouring for alcoholic drinks. Vermouth, invented in Italy in the late eighteenth century, took its name from the German for wormwood (*wermut*) and many contemporary brands (Punt e Mes, Green Chartreuse, Bénédictine) still include wormwood in their recipes.

The active ingredient in wormwood is thujone (pronounced 'thoo-shone'), so called because it was first found in the aromatic Thuja tree, a sort of cedar also known as Arborvitae ('tree of life'). Similar in chemical structure to menthol, thujone can be dangerous in high doses and does have a mild psychoactive effect, but not at the 10 milligrams per litre concentration that most absinthe contains. Sage, tarragon and Vicks VapoRub all contain similar levels of thujone, but no one has yet linked them to depraved behaviour.

The legendary effects of absinthe are almost certainly due to its high alcohol content, which, at 50–75 per cent by volume, comfortably exceeds most other spirits (usually 40 per cent). Preparing a glass of absinthe involved an elaborate ritual in which water was poured into the spirit through a special perforated spoon holding a sugar cube. This diluted it, and took the edge off any bitterness.

The clouding effect the water produces was known as the louche, It isn't certain that it is connected to the Old French word *lousche* which originally meant 'to squint' and gave us the modern louche, meaning shady or disreputable. But whether used to mean squinting, cloudy or dubious, louche is the perfect adjective for a dedicated *absintheur*.

ALAN *I had some absinthe in a bar in Manchester, and they made it over a hot spoon. And it was trannie night. And I enjoyed it much more after the absinthe than before.*
STEPHEN *What was it Ernest Dowson said? 'Absinthe makes the tart grow fonder.'*

How many countries are represented in the G20 group of leading economies?

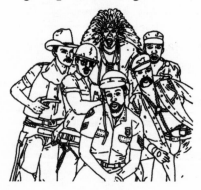

It's not twenty, but it is The Answer.

The G20 group was created after the financial crises of the late 1990s, in an attempt to bring stability to the global economy. Previously known as the G33 and, before that, the G22, its formal title is 'The Group of Twenty Finance Ministers and Central Bank Governors'. The representatives are drawn from nineteen countries: Argentina, Australia, Brazil, Canada, China, France, Germany, India, Indonesia, Italy, Japan, Mexico, Russia, Saudi Arabia, South Africa, South Korea, Turkey, the UK and the USA.

The twentieth seat is held by the European Union.

There are currently twenty-seven members of the EU, but France, Germany, Italy and the United Kingdom are already in the original list of nineteen. So, adding the remaining twenty-three countries of the EU to the original nineteen members, gives us the total number of countries represented by the G20.

Rather pleasingly, it is forty-two.

According to Douglas Adams in *The Hitchhiker's Guide to the Galaxy*, forty-two is The Answer to Life, the Universe and Everything. Whether or not that is true, it's definitely the answer to The Number of Countries in the G20.

And forty-two is also the number of dots on a single dice, the number of years winter lasts on Uranus and the length in inches of the penis of the Argentinian Lake duck.

Fully extended and relative to its size, this is the longest of any vertebrate.

Which European country has the lowest age of consent?

Vatican City. You can legally have sex there with a twelve-year-old.

This bizarre situation goes back to the time when the Vatican was established as a sovereign state (separate from the papal diocese of the Holy See) under the Lateran Treaty of 1929.

Until 1930 the age of consent in the whole of Italy was twelve. The fact that it still is in the Vatican has more to do with death than sex. The death penalty had been abolished in Italy in 1889, but Mussolini reintroduced it in 1926. When the Vatican City State was born three years later – and had to choose a legal system – it decided against capital punishment and adopted the laws in force in Italy on 31 December 1924. From then on, as an independent country, the Vatican had no further connection with Italian law. When Italy raised its age of consent from twelve to fourteen in 1930, the Vatican saw no need to follow suit. Over half its population consisted of celibate Catholic priests and no children lived there at all, so it can't have seemed particularly relevant.

Today, outside Europe, the age of consent in Angola is also twelve, as it is in parts of Mexico. In most Arab states sex is illegal outside marriage, but children can be married at younger than twelve. An exception to this is Tunisia, which has the world's oldest age of consent (twenty). North Korea has no age of consent at all.

The Vatican has its own banking system, coinage, telephone network, post office and radio station. Banking operations are shrouded in secrecy. There is no income tax and no restriction on the export or import of money. Its small size results in several statistical anomalies. For example, it has the highest crime rate in the world: with a population of barely 800, more than 1,000 offences are recorded each year. (Fortunately, this is mostly pick-pocketing and purse-snatching rather than sex crimes.) The Vatican also has the highest number of helipads and TV stations per capita in the world, and also the most restricted voting system (you have to be a cardinal under eighty years of age). It is also the only country in the world that has no hotels.

English law first imposed a legal age of consent in 1275. It, too, was set at twelve, but the law was muddied by the anti-witchcraft frenzy of the sixteenth century. Men accused of underage sex could plead 'bewitchment'. The mere mention of the word was often enough for them to escape conviction. In 1875 the age of consent was raised to thirteen and it reached its present level of sixteen ten years later.

An age of consent for homosexual sex was first proposed in 1957, after a three-year inquiry headed by Sir John Wolfenden (1906–85). He suggested twenty-one as a suitable age but it took another decade before this was finally made law in 1967. In 1994 the age of same-sex consent was lowered to eighteen and it was reduced again in 2001 to sixteen, bringing it into line with the consensual age for everyone else.

The 1994 bill was also the first British legislation ever to mention lesbian sex, setting the age of consent between two women at sixteen.

Who lives in Europe's smallest houses?

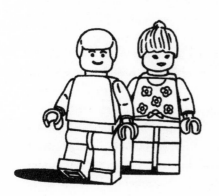

We do.

According to a survey by the *Commission for Architecture and the Built Environment* (CABE), the British build the pokiest homes in Europe. The UK has both the smallest new houses and smallest average room size.

The average size of a room in a new house in France is 26.9 square metres. The equivalent in the UK is 15.8 square metres – only a smidgeon larger than a standard parking space (14 square metres).

In terms of overall floor space, the UK average for new homes is a miserly 76 square metres, less than a third of the size of the average tennis court. This compares to: Ireland (88 square metres); Spain (97 square metres); France (113 square metres) and Denmark (137 square metres).

Outside Europe, the comparisons are even less flattering. Australian homes cover an average area of 206 square metres and American homes are nearly three times as big as ours at 214 square metres.

There have been attempts to alter things for the better. In 1961 Sir Parker Morris (1891–1972), an urban planner and founder of the Housing Association's Charitable Trust, chaired a government report called *Homes for Today and Tomorrow*. Out of this came a set of specifications, called the 'Parker Morris' standards. These went though each room in a standard house, laying down what the minimum floor space per inhabitant should be, the number of flushing toilets required, the acceptable standard of heating to be installed and a sensible amount of space for each essential piece of furniture. By 1967 the specifications had been adopted by all new towns, all local authority housing departments and most private developers.

The Parker Morris standards were abolished in 1980. Under Mrs Thatcher's iron rule, local authorities were urged to give priority to market forces instead. There are still no national minimum space standards for the UK, though in 2008 Boris Johnson, the Mayor of London, pledged to reintroduce them for the capital in an updated, 10 per cent more generous form.

Today almost three-quarters of UK residents say there's not enough space in their kitchen for three small recycling bins, while half complain they don't have enough space to use their furniture comfortably. More than a third claim their kitchens are too small even for a toaster or microwave and almost half say they don't have enough space to entertain visitors.

The expression 'not enough room to swing a cat' does not, as some people think, refer to the space needed to brandish a 'cat o'nine tails' whip. The first recorded use of the phrase (1665) is three decades earlier than the first use of the term 'cat o'nine tails' (1695).

In Britain, when we say 'not enough room to swing a cat', we mean it literally.

Which country is the most successful military power in European history?

France.

If you enter 'French military victories' on Google, a cheeky bit of software pops up with the message: 'Did you mean French military defeats?' This, plus the 'cheese-eating surrender monkeys' tag immortalised by *The Simpsons*, plays on the enduring reputation of the French army as cowardly losers. *Mais, ce n'est pas vrai!* France has the best military record in Europe.

The French have fought more military campaigns than any other European nation and won twice as many battles as they have lost.

According to historian Niall Ferguson, of the 125 major European wars fought since 1495, the French have participated in fifty – more than both Austria (forty-seven) and England (forty-three). And they've achieved an impressive batting average: out of 168 battles fought since 387 BC, they have won 109, lost forty-nine and drawn ten.

The British tend to be rather selective about the battles they remember. Our triumphs at Waterloo and Trafalgar and in two World Wars easily make up for losing at Hastings. But the school curriculum never mentions the battle of Tours in 732, when Charles the Hammer, king of the Franks, defeated the Moors and saved the whole of Christendom from the grip of Islam. While every English schoolboy was once able to recite the roll-call of our glorious wins at Crécy (1346), Poiters (1356) and Agincourt (1415), no one's ever heard of the French victories at Patay (1429) and (especially) at Castillon in 1453, where French cannons tore the English apart, winning the Hundred Years War and confirming France as the most powerful military nation in Europe.

And what about Duke of Enghien thrashing the Spanish at Rocroi late on in the Thirty Years War in 1603, ending a century of Spanish dominance? Or the siege of Yorktown, Virginia, in 1781 in which General Comte de Rochambeau defeated the British and paved the way for American independence? Under Napoleon, France crushed the might of Austria and Russia *simultaneously* at Austerlitz in 1805, and, at Verdun in 1916, the French pushed the Germans back decisively in one of the bloodiest battles of all time.

The British always prided themselves on superiority at sea, but this was only because they realised they could never win a land war on the Continent. The French army has, for most of history, been the largest, best equipped and most strategically innovative in Europe. At its best, led by Napoleon in 1812, it achieved a feat that even the Nazis couldn't repeat: it entered Moscow.

These remarkable achievements help explain another French military victory. Whether it is ranks (general, captain, corporal, lieutenant); equipment (lance, mine, bayonet, epaulette, trench); organisation (volunteer, regiment, soldier, barracks) or strategy (army, camouflage, combat, esprit de corps, reconnaissance), the language of warfare is written in one language: French.

In which country was Alexander the Great born?

It depends who you're asking. The simple answer is Greece. After that it gets complicated.

Before the fourth century BC, Macedonia (or Macedon, meaning 'land of the tall') was a small kingdom in the northeast corner of the Greek peninsula. When Alexander the Great (356–323 BC) succeeded his father Philip II in 336 BC, Macedonia had already conquered all the other city-states and kingdoms of ancient Greece. The town of Alexander's birth, Pella, then in the kingdom of Macedonia, is now in the area of Greece still known as Macedonia. But, by the time of his death, aged thirty-three, Alexander ruled more of the world than anyone before him, and the Macedonian empire had spread beyond Europe, into the Middle East and Asia. This is where the problems start.

After Alexander's empire disintegrated, Greece and the southern Balkans were ruled by the Romans, invaded by Slavs and conquered by the Ottoman Turks. Ethnic identities became entangled and rarely coincided with national boundaries. Nowhere was this more complicated than in Macedonia. Pella, Alexander's home town, became Turkish, then Bulgarian, and then, in 1926, it was returned to Greece. Today, an estimated 4.5 million people claim to be Macedonian. They are spread across Greece, the Former

Yugoslav Republic of Macedonia (FYROM), Bulgaria, Serbia and Kosovo.

Nineteenth-century diplomats called this 'The Macedonian Question' and you might think the answer to it would be the establishment of a Macedonian state. In fact, you might think that that's what FYROM was. If only it were that simple. 'Ethnic' Macedonians are split into three main groups: Greek Macedonians (about 2.5 million, most of whom live in Macedonia in Greece); Macedonian Slavs (1.3 million, who live in FYROM); and Macedonian Bulgarians (about 370,000, who are also Slavs, but speak a different language from 'Macedonian Slavs', and live in the Bulgarian province of Pirin Macedonia). All three groups are Orthodox Christians, but there is no love lost between them.

The Greeks refuse to accept the name FYROM, suggested as a compromise by the United Nations. They claim the only 'true' Macedonia is in Greece and that Macedonian culture, the legacy of Alexander the Great, is Greek and the Slavs can't 'steal' it. The Macedonian Slavs say they can call their own country what they damn well please. The Bulgarians are more pragmatic. They recognise FYROM but claim that most of 'their' Macedonians are proud Bulgarians first. In the meantime, they busily grant citizenship to thousands of immigrants from FYROM who want to live in Bulgaria since it joined the European Union in 2007.

It's an ironic legacy for Alexander, revered in his time as a great unifier. But his legend nonetheless endures. If you happen to be sailing in the Aegean when a mermaid stirs up the sea, don't worry. Do as Greek fishermen still do. When she calls out, *'Where is Alexander?'* just shout back, *'He lives and reigns and keeps the world at peace,'* and you'll get home safely.

Who killed Joan of Arc?

It was the French, not the English, who executed the 'Maid of
Orléans'. They burnt her for being a cross-dresser.

Jeanne d'Arc (1412–31) was a peasant girl from Domrémy
in north-east France who inspired a remarkable series of
victories during the Hundred Years War – England's long and
doomed attempt to conquer France.

By 1420 the King of France, Charles VI (known as 'Charles
the Mad' because he suffered from the delusion that he was
made of glass) was too ill to rule. His queen, Isabeau of
Bavaria, took charge. She agreed to the marriage of her
daughter Catherine to the English king, Henry V, transferring
the French succession to their offspring and declaring her own
son Charles illegitimate.

The French king Charles VI and the English king Henry V
died within weeks of each other in 1422, and the infant son of
Henry V and Catherine, Henry VI, was declared king of both
England and France. The disinherited Charles of France still
had the support of a group of French nobles, but his coffers

were empty and he had fallen out with the powerful Duke of Burgundy, who threw in his lot with the English. By 1428, the Anglo-Burgundian alliance controlled all of northern France, including Paris, and had ventured as far south as the Loire, where they began laying siege to the city of Orléans.

Then fate intervened. An eighteen-year-old illiterate farm girl presented herself to the future Charles VII. She said God had spoken to her and that she would drive out the English and install Charles as king. Whether it was divine will that was on her side (an old French prophecy said that a young maid would save France) or her tactical nous (she favoured pre-emptive attacks) her impact was immediate. Dressed as a man, with cropped hair and wearing white armour, she broke the five-month English siege at Orléans in a week. More triumphs followed. Charles VII was crowned at Reims seven weeks later.

In early 1430 Jeanne fell into the hands of Burgundian troops. They sold her to the English for a ransom (worth £4.5 million today) and the English persuaded a French ecclesiastical court to bring charges of heresy against her.

When she came to trial eight months later, she had suffered torture and probably rape at the hands of her captors. She confessed, but then recanted, claiming she'd only done so 'out of fear of the fire' and reappeared dressed in men's clothes. Given that the most serious charge against her was dressing as a man – an 'abomination unto the Lord' (Deuteronomy 22:5) – this was all the French judge, Pierre Cauchon, the Bishop of Beauvais, needed.

On 30 May 1431 Joan was burnt at the stake at Rouen. She was nineteen. To prevent people from building a shrine in her honour, her remains were dumped in the Seine. In 1453 Charles VII avenged her memory by expelling the English from France and ending the Hundred Years War. Soon afterwards Pope Callixtus III ordered a retrial in which Joan of

Arc was found 'not guilty'. Sadly, it was too late to find her 'not dead' as well.

How tall was Napoleon?

He wasn't short.

The universal belief that Napoleon Bonaparte (1769–1821) was tiny came about from a combination of mistranslation and propaganda.

Napoleon's autopsy, carried out in 1821 by his personal physician Francesco Antommarchi, recorded his height as '5/2'. It is now thought this represents the French measurement '5 pieds 2 pouces', which converts to English measurement as 5 feet 6½ inches (1.69 metres).

The average height of Frenchmen between 1800 and 1820 was 5 feet 4½ inches (1.64 metres), so Napoleon would have been taller than most of the people he knew and taller, in fact, than the average Englishman, who was then 5 feet 6 inches (1.68 metres). Napoleon was only 2½ inches shorter than the Duke of Wellington – tall for his day at 5 feet 9 inches (1.75 metres) – and 2½ inches taller than his other great rival Horatio Nelson, who was only 5 feet 4 inches (1.62 metres).

Shortly after seizing power in 1799, Napoleon imposed height requirements on all French troops. In the elite Imperial Guard, Grenadiers had to be at least 5 feet 10 inches tall (1.78 metres) and his personal guard, the elite Mounted Chasseurs, had to be a minimum of 5 feet 7 inches (1.7 m). So, for much of the time, the soldiers around him would have been noticeably taller, creating the impression that he was small.

The great British caricaturist James Gillray (1757–1815)

produced the first and most damaging image of a diminutive Napoleon in 'The King of Brobdingnag and Gulliver', inspired by *Gulliver's Travels*. In the cartoon George III holds Napoleon in the palm of his hand, inspects him with an eye-glass and comments, 'I cannot but conclude you to be one of the most pernicious little odious reptiles that nature ever suffered to crawl upon the surface of the Earth.'

The survival of the 'short Napoleon' myth is perpetuated by the widespread use of the term 'Napoleon complex' to describe short people who supposedly make up for their lack of stature by being aggressive.

There isn't much scientific evidence for this commonly held theory, however. It's not an officially recognised psychiatric syndrome and it doesn't seem to occur in the animal kingdom. Although one study found that, in contests between males in some species of swordtail fish, the smaller fish started 78 per cent of the fights, this is very much the exception.

Napoleon may have been aggressive, but he wasn't small.

STEPHEN *Nelson was three inches shorter than Napoleon.*

ALAN *Nelson was five foot four?*

STEPHEN *Yeah.*

ALAN *Like Danny de Vito?*

STEPHEN *Yes. He was a very short chap.*

ALAN *No wonder they put him on such a big column.*

What did Mussolini do?

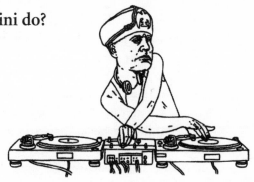

He certainly didn't make the trains run on time. If anything, he made them less reliable than before.

As early as 1925 European and American fascist sympathisers said of Mussolini, 'At least he makes the trains run on time.' It defused criticism of his despotic policies. Even if all the stories about him were true, only a strong leader could bring order to the chaos in Italy after the First World War.

Today, the cliché is used to belittle a useless person or as a sarcastic complaint about the shortcomings of one's own country: 'Even Mussolini managed to get the trains running on time!'

When Mussolini arrived on the political scene in the early 1920s, the Italian railways were already working as well as any in Europe. The credit for this largely belongs to Cavaliere Carlo Crova, general manager of Italian State Railways in the 1920s, who built an effective, nationalised rail system from the ruins of several private companies. His life's work merely happened to coincide with Mussolini's ascent to power.

Contemporary reports by foreign journalists and diplomats say that, under the Fascist government of the 1930s, the trains didn't operate particularly well, especially on local lines. Fuel and staff were diverted from the railways to mount the invasion of Ethiopia in 1935. Once the Second World War started, coal had to be imported by land instead of sea, and the railways weren't up to the job.

Italian government propaganda – and its banning of any

reporting of rail delays – meant that none of the problems were addressed. Italy's railways were officially excellent and no one dared suggest otherwise.

Interestingly, even in his most detailed and boastful biographical writings, Il Duce himself never claimed to have made the trains run on time. But he may have been the origin of the myth. According to his authorised biography, when the king summoned him to form a government in 1922, Mussolini told his local station master: 'We must leave exactly on time – from now on everything must function to perfection!'

A number of railway stations were built or renovated under Mussolini, notably Ostiense in Rome, specially designed so that Hitler could arrive at somewhere suitably 'ancient Roman' when he visited the city.

Among Mussolini's many unfulfilled ambitions was straightening the Leaning Tower of Pisa, which he felt gave the wrong image of the new Italy. On his orders in 1934 tons of liquid concrete were poured into the wonky landmark's foundations. The result was that the concrete sank into the wet clay, and the tower began leaning even more.

Who thought Waterloo was won on the playing fields of Eton?

Apparently, it was Adolf Hitler.

The Duke of Wellington would have been horrified by the suggestion that he thought cricket had anything to do with his famous victory. Wellington hated sport. Furthermore, he was unhappy at Eton and during his time there the school didn't have any playing fields.

According to the historian Sir Edward Creasy, the misunderstanding came about in the following way. Decades after the battle of Waterloo, the Duke passed an Eton cricket match and remarked: 'There grows the stuff that won Waterloo.' But this was purely a general comment about the qualities of the British officer class, not an appreciation of his old school's cricket coaching.

Adolf Hitler, it seems, took a very different view. In 1934, Anthony Eden went to meet him in Berlin. Eden was then the British cabinet minister responsible for the League of Nations and hoped to find common ground with Hitler by reminiscing about the old days (they had fought in opposite trenches at Ypres in the First World War). Eden described him as 'reasonable, charming and affable', but the Führer only wanted to talk obsessively about one thing: Eton.

Hitler was convinced Britain owed its victory in the First World War to strategic skills acquired at Eton. Eden, an Old Etonian himself, disagreed. He pointed out that the Eton College Officer Training Corps was a shambles.

His protests were in vain: one of the first things Hitler did after the outbreak of the Second World War was to arrange for Eton to be bombed.

Two bombs fell on the school. One shattered all the glass in the college chapel; the other narrowly missed a library full of boys studying. There were no reported casualties. When parents asked for the pupils to be moved to a safer location, the Headmaster, Charles Elliott, refused. If London's poor couldn't leave London, he said, Etonians wouldn't leave Eton.

Eton College was founded in 1440 by Henry VI. Called the 'King's College of Our Lady of Eton beside Wyndsor' it was originally intended as a charity school, providing free education for seventy poor students using scholars from the town as teaching staff. Henry VI lavished upon it a substantial income from land, and a huge collection of priceless holy relics – including alleged fragments of the True Cross and the Crown of Thorns.

Today Eton has 1,300 pupils and 160 masters and the annual school fee is £29,682. The Officer Training Corps still exists and the current British Prime Minister is a former member of it. By his own account, David Cameron's favourite song is 'The Eton Rifles' (1978), a scathingly anti-public school composition by The Jam.

STEPHEN *When the railway was being built through that particular part of Buckinghamshire, who was it that said, 'We won't have a station here?' What school is nearby?*

ROB BRYDON *Oo-oh, erm . . . It's Eton.*

STEPHEN *Eton College, of course, is there, and yes, they thought the boys would be tempted to go into London and visit prostitutes and so on.*

BILL BAILEY *'I'd like a Prostitute Super-Saver, please!'*

JIMMY CARR *[baffled expression] 'But this prostitute seems to be a woman.'*

Which revolution ended the First World War?

The German Revolution of November 1918. It's much less well known than the Russian Revolution of 1917, but the repercussions were just as significant.

By the middle of 1918, most Germans knew they had lost the First World War. So when Admiral Franz von Hipper (1863–1932), commander of the German battlecruisers at the Battle of Jutland, proposed a last do-or-die engagement with the British Navy, the reaction was less than enthusiastic and several ships mutinied. Although the revolt was short-lived, it persuaded the German High Command to rescind the battle order and return the fleet to Kiel.

There, convinced they were back in control, the authorities arrested forty-seven of the mutineers. Local union leaders, outraged by the treatment of the sailors, called for a public demonstration. On 3 November, several thousand people marched through Kiel under banners demanding 'Peace and Bread'. The military police opened fire on the march and seven protestors were killed.

Within twenty-four hours there was a mass uprising of soldiers, sailors and workers all over Germany, demanding an end to the war, the abdication of the Kaiser and the establishment of a republic. At this point, most states in the German Federation still had individual royal families but, in less than a week, they had all abdicated in favour of democratically elected Workers' and Soldiers' Councils.

In Berlin Friedrich Ebert (1871–1925), leader of the Social Democrats, the main left-wing political party, was worried that this might spark a communist revolution along Russian lines, plunging the country into civil war. To appease the rebels, he asked the Kaiser to abdicate. By this time even the troops on the Western Front were refusing to fight, but the Kaiser refused. Exasperated, the liberal Chancellor of the Reichstag, Prince Max von Baden, took matters into his own hands and sent a telegram announcing the Kaiser's abdication.

The Kaiser promptly fled to the Netherlands where he remained until his death in 1941. Baden resigned and, on 9 November, Ebert declared a republic with himself as Chancellor. The Armistice was signed two days later.

Ebert then tackled the revolutionaries, who wanted the entire mechanism of the old state abolished. In early 1919 the newly formed German Communist Party provoked armed insurrections in many German cities. Ebert had them brutally suppressed by the army. To the Left Ebert was now a traitor, and the militaristic Right hated him just as much for signing the infamous 'war guilt' clause in the Treaty of Versailles.

On 19 January 1919 Ebert established a new constitutional government, not in Berlin but at Weimar, the base of the great writers Goethe and Schiller and the spiritual home of German humanism. For the next fourteen years the Weimar Republic battled political instability and hyper-inflation caused by punishing war debts. In one year, between 1921 and 1922, the value of the German Mark fell from 60 to 8,000 against the dollar. The German Revolution that had ended the First World War created the chaos out of which Nazism was born.

Which country suffered the second highest losses in the Second World War?

The worst were in the USSR. The second worst were in China.

The Soviet–German war of 1941–45 was the largest conflict in human history. When Hitler sent three million troops into the Soviet Union, he expected a quick victory. Four years later, an estimated 10 million Soviet troops and 14 million Soviet citizens had died. The Germans lost over 5 million men too: it was in Russia that the outcome of the Second World War was really decided.

It was a vast theatre, fought over thousands of square miles. The Red Army were untrained and hopelessly underequipped in the early stages of the war, with infantry often pitted against tanks. The initial German advance was swift, destroying countless towns and villages, and wrecking the infrastructure of agriculture and industry. This left millions of Russians homeless and hungry. As the German advance became bogged down, the troops were ordered to show no mercy, systematically butchering prisoners and civilians alike.

It was a very similar set of factors that produced the war's second largest death toll. Very little is known in the West about the Sino-Japanese War of 1937–45, yet even the lowest estimates suggest 2 million Chinese troops and 7 million civilians died. The official Chinese death toll is a total of 20 million.

The Japanese invaded China in 1937 to provide a buffer between themselves and their real enemy, the USSR. China had no central government: much of it was still controlled by warlords and Chiang Kai-Shek's Nationalists and Mao Zedong's Communists hated each other almost as much as they did the Japanese. Chinese troops were pitifully short of weapons and modern military equipment (some still fought with swords) and they were no match for the disciplined and ruthless Imperial Japanese army.

The invasion turned into the greatest, bloodiest guerrilla war ever fought. Both sides pursued horrific scorched earth policies, destroying crops, farms, villages and bridges as they retreated, so as to deny their use to the enemy. Widespread famine and starvation were the result. As in Russia, a lack of military hardware was made up for by the sheer numbers of Chinese willing to fight and die. And, by the end of the war, 95 million Chinese were refugees.

Early on in the conflict, after capturing Chiang Kai-Shek's capital, Nanking, Japanese troops were sent on an officially authorised, six-week spree of mass murder, torture and rape that left 300,000 dead. Over the course of the war, 200,000 Chinese women were kidnapped to work in Japanese military brothels. Another 400,000 Chinese died after being infected with cholera, anthrax and bubonic plague dropped from

Japanese aircraft. But, no matter how appalling the casualties, the Chinese refused to give in.

All Japan's military forces surrendered after the dropping of the atomic bombs on Hiroshima and Nagasaki. In China Mao Zedong's Communist Party swept to power. In 1972 Mao expressed his gratitude to the Japanese prime minister, Kakuei Tanaka. 'If Imperial Japan had not started the war,' he said, 'how could we communists have become mighty and powerful?'

Which nationality invented the 'stiff upper lip'?

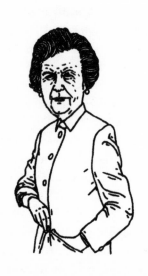

It wasn't the British. Unlikely as it may sound, it was the Americans.

To keep a stiff upper lip is to remain steadfast and unemotional in the face of the worst that life can throw at you. Though long associated with Britain – and especially the British Empire – the oldest-known uses of the term are all from the USA, beginning in 1815. Americans were going around with 'stiff upper lips' in Harriet Beecher Stowe's *Uncle Tom's Cabin* (1852) and in the letters of Mark Twain (1835–1910) and it was only towards the end of the nineteenth century that the expression first appeared in print in Britain. By 1963, when P. G. Wodehouse published his ninth Jeeves and Wooster novel, *Stiff Upper Lip, Jeeves!*, the phrase, if not the concept, had become almost entirely humorous.

The idea behind the expression is that a trembling lip is the first sign you're about to start crying. Why it should be the *upper* lip, in particular, that needs to be stiff is not clear. It may be because the saying originated in an age when most men wore moustaches, which would make shakiness more obvious in the upper lip than in the lower one; or perhaps 'stiff bottom lip' just sounded odd, like some obscure naval flogging offence.

Is a stiff upper lip good for you? That depends on whose research you choose to believe. Cancer Research UK recently published a survey conducted by the University of Leeds that showed that British men were 69 per cent more likely to die of cancer than women. This is due in part, they claimed, to men adopting 'a stiff upper lip attitude to illness': in other words, they ignore persistent symptoms and refuse to have regular check-ups.

On the other hand, psychologists in the USA, studying the aftermath of the terrorist attacks of 11 September 2001, found that — contrary to their expectations, and to popular belief — people who 'bottled up' their feelings suffered fewer negative mental and physical symptoms than those who were keen to talk openly about their experiences.

In Victorian times, the 'stiff upper lip' had a practical application: it was attached to a German contraption called the *Lebensprüfer* ('Life-prover'). This was a device intended to prevent premature burial. Wires were clipped to the upper lip and eyelid of someone who had apparently died. A mild electrical current was sent through their body and, if the patient's muscles twitched, you knew not to bury them quite yet.

What did George Washington have to say about his father's cherry tree?

We don't know. We don't even know if his father *had* a cherry tree.

The story of Washington and the cherry tree was entirely the invention of a man known to Americans as 'Parson' Weems, who wrote and published the first biography of the first US President just months after he died in 1799.

In Weems's tale, the six-year-old George Washington was given a small axe as a present and amused himself with it for hours in the garden of the family's plantation, Ferry Farm in Stafford, Virginia. One day George went too far and hacked the bark off his father's favourite cherry tree, condemning it to death. Though his father, Augustine Washington, was furious, George confessed at once: 'I can't tell a lie, Pa; you know I can't tell a lie. I did cut it with my hatchet.' George's honesty so impressed his father that he gave him a hug and congratulated him on 'an act of heroism that is worth a thousand trees'.

It's a good story, but it appears in no other accounts of Washington's life and was never mentioned by Washington himself. Even Weems was evasive about his sources: 'I had it related to me twenty years ago by an aged lady, who was a distant relative' was as far as he was prepared to go.

Mason Locke Weems (1756–1825) was born in Maryland but studied medicine and theology in London. Ordained by the Archbishop of Canterbury in 1784, he returned to America to take services at Pohick church in Virginia. Both George Washington and his father had once been members of the governing body there and Weems later falsely inflated his role into 'Former Rector of Mount Vernon', Washington's country estate nearly 10 kilometres (6 miles) from Pohick.

In 1790 a shortage of cash forced Weems to leave the ministry and become an itinerant bookseller. He cut an eccentric figure riding through the southern states, peddling his wares at fairs and markets. He was part preacher and part entertainer, talking up the quality of his merchandise as if delivering a sermon, then pulling out his fiddle for a rousing finale.

When Washington died, Weems had been working on his biography for six months. He wrote to a friend that 'millions are gaping to read something about him. I am very nearly prim'd & cock'd for 'em.' The outpouring of grief at the President's death (some people wore mourning clothes for months afterwards) confirmed Weems's view that what the American people needed was a heroic yarn, not a balanced political biography. Washington's modesty, his refusal to join a political party, his adoption of the homely 'Mr President' as his title, his rejection of a third term in office – all needed a mythic context that Weems's fantasy supplied.

A History of the Life and Death, Virtues and Exploits of General George Washington (1800) was one of the first American best-sellers, appearing in twenty-nine editions by 1825, and finding a place next to the Bible in almost every farm in the land. Although it's the source of most half-truths told about Washington, it's also the book that confirmed him as the 'Father of his Country'.

How many men have held the office of President of the United States?

Forty-three. (Not forty-four, as Barack Obama claimed at his inauguration.)

Barack Obama is the forty-fourth president of the USA, but only the forty-third *person* to become president. This is because Grover Cleveland held the position twice – with a four-year break in between – making him both the twenty-second and the twenty-fourth president of the United States.

Stephen Grover Cleveland (1837–1908) was the only Democrat in an otherwise unbroken fifty-year run of Republican presidents from 1860 to 1912. Almost no one has a bad word to say about him. 'He possessed honesty, courage, firmness, independence, and common sense,' wrote one contemporary biographer. 'But he possessed them to a degree other men do not.'

In the 1888 presidential contest Cleveland should have been elected for a second consecutive term. He actually polled more votes than John Harrison, but Republican electoral fraud in Indiana cost him the election. As she left the White House, Cleveland's young wife Frances – at twenty-one the youngest ever First Lady, and the only one to have been married in the White House – told her staff: 'I want you to take good care of all the furniture and ornaments in the house, for I want to find everything just as it is now, when we come back again.' When asked when that would be, she said: 'We are coming back four years from today.'

Which is just what happened. In the 1892 campaign, universally considered the cleanest and quietest since the Civil War, Grover Cleveland beat President Harrison by a landslide. He decided not to fight for a third term, which he was then still allowed to do. (President Roosevelt served for four consecutive terms from 1932–44.) It wasn't until the 22nd Amendment to the US Constitution was passed in 1951 that presidents were limited to a maximum of two terms.

Cleveland died in 1908. His last words were: 'I have tried so hard to do right.'

He is the only president to appear on two different $1 bills.

Despite putting a cross next to the name of the candidates on the ballot paper, the American people do not directly elect their president and vice-president. This is done a month after the popular vote by a 'college' of 538 state electors, allocated according to the size of the state's population: California (55) and Texas (34) have most; Vermont (3) and Alaska (3) the fewest. This system dates back to the beginning of the Union and was adopted because George Washington hoped it would reduce the amount of divisive party politics.

It's not perfect. The 'electors' have no power: they are a constitutional formality, pledged to vote for whichever candidate wins the popular vote in their state. Just as in British general elections, where votes don't always translate into seats, so in America. As long as a candidate wins the eleven biggest states they can be elected president with fewer votes overall. This is how Cleveland lost in 1888 and how George W. Bush defeated Al Gore in 2000.

STEPHEN *Barack Obama is currently known as the forty-fourth, just as Bush was known as the forty-third, but ... but they aren't. Bush was the forty-second and Obama is the forty-third. Do you know why this is?*

SEAN LOCK *One of them was invisible?*

Which country ritually burns the most American flags?

The USA.

Every year, the Boy Scouts of America and military veteran organisations like the American Legion burn thousands of US flags between them.

This is because Section 176(k) of the US Flag Code (a set of rules on the correct treatment of the Stars and Stripes) provides that: 'The flag, when it is in such condition that it is no longer a fitting emblem for display, should be destroyed in a dignified way, preferably by burning.' Flag burnings (or 'retirements', to use the official term) are usually held on Flag Day, 14 June.

Although the Code allows for burning the flag 'in a dignified way', it also warns sternly against (and lays down the legal penalties for) anyone who 'knowingly mutilates, defaces, physically defiles, burns, maintains on the floor or ground, or tramples upon' the flag for other, possibly nefarious reasons. However, in 1990 the Supreme Court ruled that this was a restriction of 'freedom of speech' and thus violated the First Amendment to the US Constitution. So, even though the US Flag Code says you mustn't, you can legally burn the US flag in America for any reason you like.

The US Flag Code is a comprehensive document. Among other things, it sets out in precise detail how to fold the flag, showing where all of the twelve folds must be made and the symbolic reasons for each fold. It also makes it clear that the flag is not to be embroidered on to cushions or handkerchiefs; not to be 'used as a covering for a ceiling' or as 'a receptacle for receiving, holding, carrying, or delivering anything'; or to be used in advertising; or to form part of a 'costume or athletic uniform'.

Contrary to myth, the flag does not have to be burned if it ever touches the ground, and it's perfectly OK to clean it if it gets a bit grubby, rather than rushing straight to the burning option.

The anxious concern of Americans for the well-being of their flag strikes many foreigners as faintly comical or even fetishistic. But in the USA, where the President serves as both head of state *and* head of the government, there is no symbolic figurehead (such as a ceremonial monarch) to unite the nation. For many Americans, the flag plays that role, providing a non-partisan rallying point for all patriotic citizens, irrespective of their political differences.

That explains why the US Flag Code insists that the Stars and Stripes 'is itself considered a living thing'.

In which country is the Dutch city of Groningen?

The Netherlands.

Groningen is definitely not in Holland and, even if it were, Holland isn't a country.

The city of Groningen is capital of the northern Dutch province of Groningen. It is one of twelve provinces into which the Netherlands is divided. 'Holland' refers only to the two western provinces, North Holland and South Holland, which together represent an eighth of the country's total land mass. To call the Netherlands 'Holland' is like calling the UK 'England' or 'the Home Counties'.

The reason Holland is commonly used in this way is that it punches above its weight in the Netherlands – both in terms of population (40 per cent), and economic and political power (the three largest cities in the Netherlands – Amsterdam, Rotterdam and The Hague – are all in Holland). In the sixteenth century, when the Dutch navy ruled the waves, most Dutch ships came from these three ports, so any Dutchmen found abroad usually came 'from Holland'.

'Holland' is from Middle Dutch *holtland* ('wooded land'). The origin of 'Dutch' is more complicated. Its original meaning was 'of the people': the word 'Dutch' is a corruption of the ancient Indo-European root *teuta* 'people', from which we also get 'Teutonic'. In Old High German this became *duit-isc* ('people-ish' or 'the language of the people') and was used about Germanic languages generally.

The Old English variant of *duit-isc* ('people-ish') was *þeodisc* (pronounced 'thay-odd-ish'). It originally meant 'English' and then, in about the ninth century, came to mean 'German'. As *þeodisc* evolved into 'Dutch' it continued to mean 'German' right up until the early sixteenth century. At that point English rivalry (and frequent war) with the Hollanders or 'Low Dutch' meant the word 'Dutch' was exclusively applied to them, usually as part of a term of abuse. Examples from the time include 'Dutch courage' (bravery brought on by alcohol) and 'Dutch widow' (a prostitute).

For this reason, even as late as 1934, Dutch government officials were advised to avoid using the expression 'the Dutch' in international communications, in favour of the officially sanctioned 'of the Netherlands'.

Confusingly, but entirely logically, the Dutch word for Germans is *duitsch*.

Groningen, the Netherlands's eighth largest city, is the Dutch equivalent of Manchester: a lively university town full of bars. Students make up more than a quarter of its 185,000 population. As Groningen is the only city of any size in the northern Netherlands, locals simply refer to it as 'Stad', which means 'city'. Until Groningen's sugar beet factory closed recently, it gave the city a distinct sweet smell during the summer.

ROB BRYDON *The photo of Groningen that you showed looked like Guildford, didn't it.*

ALAN *Are you suggesting we have more in common with our European neighbours than otherwise?*

ROB *I'm suggesting the world is becoming homogenised and*

indistinct and I for one think that's a bad thing.
STEPHEN *Hear hear hear, quite right, quite right. Very good.*
JIMMY CARR *I think we all think like that, we're all the same.*

What language is the Spanish national anthem sung in?

It isn't.

Despite having one of the oldest tunes of any national anthem, *La Marcha Real* is the only one with no words. They were dropped in 1975 on the death of Generalissimo Francisco Franco, dictator of Spain for forty years. In 2007 the Spanish Olympic Committee, inspired by a performance of 'You'll Never Walk Alone' by visiting Liverpool football fans, held a competition to find new words for the national tune. The winner, called – believe it or not – *¡Viva España!* was dropped after just five days. Several Spanish regions (many of which have their own anthems) denounced the words as 'too nationalistic'.

> *Long live Spain!* (it went)
> *We sing together, with different voices,*
> *and only one heart.*

This seems pretty bland compared to France's bloodthirsty 'La Marseillaise':

> *Do you hear in the countryside*
> *The roar of those ferocious soldiers?*
> *They come right here into your midst*
> *To slit the throats of your sons and wives!*

Or the long-since hushed-up sixth verse of 'God Save the Queen'

> *Lord grant that Marshal Wade*
> *May by thy mighty aid*
> *Victory bring*
> *May he sedition hush*
> *And like a torrent rush*
> *Rebellious Scots to crush*
> *God save the King*

The oldest (and perhaps the oddest) national anthem of all belongs to the Dutch and dates from 1574. Here it is in its entirety:

> *William of Nassau, scion*
> *Of a Dutch and ancient line,*
> *Dedicate undying*
> *Faith to this land of mine.*
> *A prince I am, undaunted,*
> *Of Orange, ever free,*
> *To the King of Spain I've granted*
> *A lifelong loyalty.*

The Dutch seem to have no problem singing about being loyal subjects of Spain, despite not having been so for more than 350 years. Maybe the Spanish should sing the Dutch anthem instead?

Which city has the most Michelin stars in the world?

Not Paris, but Tokyo.

In the 2010 Michelin Guide, Tokyo has eleven 3-star restaurants to Paris's ten. The Japanese capital also has more Michelin stars altogether than any other city in the world – 261 across 197 restaurants – three times more than Paris.

At least some of this is do with scale: Tokyo is a much larger city with 160,000 restaurants. Paris has only 40,000. And France still tops the country listings, with twenty-five 3-star restaurants to Japan's eighteen. (The UK currently has four.)

Though two of Tokyo's eleven 3-starred restaurants are French, most of the 197 starred restaurants in the city specialise in classical Japanese cuisine, including three *fugu* houses, where the deadly poisonous puffer fish is rendered edible by specially trained chefs. The raw ingredients for this (and for all the *sushi* and *sashimi*) come from Tsukiji, the world's largest fish market, which handles 2,000 tons of fish a day. The Japanese are obsessed with good food – about half the output of Japanese television is food-related.

In 1889, two brothers from Clermont-Ferrand, André and Édouard Michelin, founded the Michelin Tyre Company. In 1891 they patented the world's first removable pneumatic tyre. The company is still based in the Auvergne and is the world's second largest tyre manufacturer, with over 109,000 employees and revenues of £12.3 billion.

André published the first Michelin guide in 1900, when there were just 300 cars in France. The guide was intended to stimulate road travel (more cars meant more tyres) and was given away free to motorists to encourage them to explore France by road. As well as listing hotels and restaurants, the first guides had practical tips on how to change tyres and where to find mechanics.

Michelin stars started in 1926. One star is 'a very good restaurant in its category'; two means 'excellent cooking, worth a detour'; three means 'exceptional cuisine, worth a special trip'. Just seventy-five Michelin inspectors cover all of Europe and many fewer the rest of the world. They eat out on 240 days in a year, file over 1,000 reports, and must order the maximum number of courses and always clear their plates. To remain anonymous they never return to the same place for several years, and never reveal what they do – even to their parents.

The Michelin man is over a century old. His name is 'Bibendum'. His inspiration was a stack of tyres that reminded Édouard Michelin of a human torso. In the first poster featuring him, in 1898, he drained a champagne glass full of nails and glass, making the point that 'Michelin tyres drink up obstacles'. His name comes from the strapline on the poster: *'Nunc est bibendum'* ('Time to drink!').

He isn't tyre-coloured because tyres weren't dark grey until 1912, when carbon black was added to preserve them. They were originally grey-white or beige. The Michelin man is not as racy as he was – he gave up cigars in 1929 after a TB epidemic – but he remains much loved. In 2000 he was voted the best-ever corporate logo, just ahead of the symbol for the London Underground.

STEPHEN *Which city has the most Michelin stars?*

REGINALD D. HUNTER *I know for a fact it ain't London. And I'm not just trying to offend London . . . I'm trying to offend the UK in general.*

STEPHEN *Ha ha.*

REG *But I feel like any country that can produce Marmite, they started later than everybody else in trying to make food taste good.*

STEPHEN *This from a country that has spray-on cheese.*

Where was football invented?

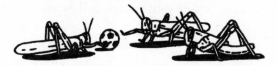

Not in England, but in China.

The Chinese played football for over 2,000 years before the English claimed it. *Cuju* or *tsu' chu* – literally 'kick-ball' – began as a military training exercise but was soon popular all over China. It used a leather ball (stuffed with fur or feathers) and two teams trying to score goals at opposite ends without using their hands. According to some accounts, each goal was a hole cut into a sheet of silk hung between bamboo posts. *Cuju* was first recorded in the fifth century BC and was at its peak during the Song Dynasty (AD 960–1279), when *cuju* players became the world's first professional footballers. The sport eventually fell into oblivion during the Ming period (AD 1368–1644).

In twelfth-century Japan *cuju* was adapted into a new game called *kemari*. Essentially a formal version of 'keepy-uppy', it was played in a square with trees at the corners. The eight players, in pairs, had to keep the ball in the air as long as possible, bouncing it off the trees. There was an umpire who gave extra points for particularly stylish play.

There are also claims of a game even older than *cuju*, called *marngrook* ('game ball'), played by the Aboriginal peoples of Western Australia. Involving over fifty players, the aim was to prevent the ball (made of possum-skin) from touching the ground. The long punts and high catches of Australian Rules football may owe something to *marngrook*.

In medieval England football involved so many players, so few rules and so much violence that it was regularly banned: no fewer than thirty royal and local laws were enacted against it between 1314 and 1667. This didn't reduce its popularity among all classes – even the young Henry VIII shelled out 4 shillings for a pair of leather football boots (worth about £100 today).

Modern football started in England in 1863, when rugby football and association football (or 'soccer' for short) diverged and England's Football Association was founded. The world's oldest football club is Sheffield FC, founded six years earlier (in 1857) as an amateur club.

Although the 1863 rules of the English game provided the template for today's international sport, it took a long time to shake off its violent origins. In the nineteenth century you could shoulder-barge players even if they didn't have the ball, and if a goalkeeper caught the ball, he could be shoved over the line to score.

One of the rules proposed in 1863 allowed players to approach the man with the ball and 'to charge, hold, trip or hack him, or to wrest the ball from him'. This was eventually dropped, despite the objections of Blackheath FC who argued that, without it, 'you will do away with the courage and pluck of the game, and it will be bound to bring over a lot of Frenchmen who would beat you with a week's practice'.

How prescient that has proved to be.

Who was the first Olympian to score a 'perfect 10'?

It wasn't Nadia Comăneci at the Montreal Games in 1976 – in fact, at the time of the first 'perfect 10', she wasn't even born.

In 1924 in Paris, a French gymnast named Albert Sequin (1891–1979) won the individual Gold in a vaulting event called the Men's Sidehorse, which has only been contested at one other Olympiad (St Louis in 1904). His score was listed as 10.000, which makes him the first to score a perfect 10.

The 1924 Olympics was Albert Sequin's only Games, but he made the most of it: also picking up silver medals for the Men's Team All-Around – and for the Men's Rope-Climbing, which hasn't appeared at the Olympics since 1932.

Rope-climbing Olympians began by sitting on the floor, with the lower end of an 8-metre (26-foot) rope dangling between their outstretched legs. Only their hands and arms could be used in climbing: the use of feet and legs was banned, even in the initial push-off. The key to success was the momentum gained by an explosive, upper-body surge from the floor. In some forms of the competition, the climbers were required to keep their bodies L-shaped – that is, with their legs sticking out horizontally – throughout the climb.

At the top of the rope was a 'tambourine', a flat plate covered with soot. Back on the ground, the competitor would show his stained fingers to prove that he had touched the tambourine. In 1904 the rope-climbing Gold went to the legendary American George Eyser who won six Olympic medals that year, despite his wooden leg.

Nadia Comăneci, the first female Olympian to score a perfect 10, did so at the age of fourteen in 1976. The youngest female gold medallist was Marjorie Gestring of the USA, who took a diving Gold in 1936, aged thirteen.

Sports that are no longer part of the Games include live Pigeon-shooting: nearly 300 birds were killed during the event at the 1900 Paris Olympiad. However, Pistol Duelling at the 1906 Athens Games produced no fatalities: competitors shot at mannequins dressed in frock coats with bull's-eyes on their throats. The Diving Plunge (St Louis, 1904) – which tested how far athletes could travel in the water without actually swimming – and the Long Jump for Horses (Paris, 1900) are other modern non-runners. In 2008 the official Beijing Olympic website announced the introduction of Olympic Poodle-Clipping – but this turned out to be an April Fool's joke, included in the agenda by accident after first being printed by the *Daily Telegraph*.

Perhaps the most unusual Olympic record-breaker of all time was Japanese runner Shizo Kanakuri. In 1912 he began the marathon at the Stockholm Games but, being exhausted after his eighteen-day journey to Sweden, stopped for a rest after 30 kilometres (nearly 19 miles) and asked at a local house for a glass of water. Having drunk it, he fell asleep on the sofa and woke up the next morning. In 1967, aged seventy-six, he was invited to return to the city and complete his run. His finishing time was therefore 54 years, 8 months, 6 days, 32 minutes and 20.3 seconds.

Why did sportsmen start going into huddles?

It had nothing to do with team-building.

The huddle was invented at Gallaudet University, a college for the deaf in Washington DC, as a way of hiding hand signals from other deaf teams.

In American football, the 'line of scrimmage' is an imaginary line across the pitch where the two sides face each other before commencing the next part of the game, or 'play'. Until the 1890s, the signal caller on each team shouted out his team's strategy for the next play. Nothing was hidden from the opposite team's defence.

When the forerunner of Gallaudet College (founded in 1864) started playing American football with an all-deaf team, their quarterback, Paul Hubbard, used American Sign Language

(ASL) to call a play at the line of scrimmage. His team therefore had a distinct advantage when they played non-deaf colleges, but other deaf schools could easily read his intentions. So in 1894 Hubbard began concealing his signals by gathering his attacking players into a cluster before each play.

This worked brilliantly and became a regular habit. In 1896 the huddle started showing up on other college campuses and it is now considered an essential part of the game.

Gallaudet was the first University for deaf people, set up by Edward Milner Gallaudet, the son of Thomas Hopkins Gallaudet (1787–1851), the man who brought sign language to America. Because Thomas Gallaudet (who wasn't deaf himself) based American Sign Language (ASL) on the French sign language that he had learned in Paris, American and French sign languages share 60 per cent of the same gestures.

This has the strange result that it is much easier for a deaf American to make himself understood in Paris than in London.

STEPHEN *Do you know where the sports huddle originated?*
JACK DEE *Glenn Huddle?*

What's a bat's eyesight like?

No, they aren't blind at all.

Of the 1,100-odd species of bat in the world, not one is sightless – and many can see very well indeed. The notion that bats don't need eyes because they get about exclusively using echolocation or 'sonar' is complete nonsense.

Fruit bats (also called Megabats) don't use echolocation at all. They have large eyes, which they use both to navigate and to find their food – which is, as you might expect, fruit. Echolocation isn't much help in finding food that doesn't move around. Instead, for fruit-location, they also have a keen sense of smell.

The Common Vampire bat (*Desmodus rotundus*) is the only bat that feeds on the blood of mammals. It is such a very long way from blind that it can see a cow 120 metres (400 feet) away: in pitch darkness, in the middle of the night.

Even microbats – which eat insects and include all British bats, and which *do* use sonar to hunt – use their (much smaller) eyes for avoiding obstacles, for spotting landmarks, and for working out their flying height. Microbats have good night vision. They see in black and white because they're nocturnal, whereas fruit bats see in colour because they're active in the daytime.

In the Americas there are several species of 'fishing bats', such as the Greater Bulldog bat (*Noctilio leporinus*), which lives by using its keen eyesight and immense feet to drag fish out of the water. It is easily identified, not only by its 66-centimtre (26-inch) wingspan, but also by the repugnant odour of its roosts.

Very few humans find bats palatable but, for special occasions like weddings, the Chamorro people of Guam like to boil giant fruit bats or 'flying foxes' in coconut milk and eat them whole – wings, fur and all. This may explain why so many Chamorro suffer from a rare and terrible neurological condition – ALS-Parkinson dementia complex.

The bats feed on poisonous cycad plants, whose dangerous neurotoxins are passed on (now lightly flavoured with coconut) to the unfortunate diners.

Can you name an animal that only eats bamboo?

Meet the bamboo mite.

Bamboo mites (*Schizotetranychus celarius*) eat bamboo and bamboo alone. They are tiny creatures related to spiders and are only 0.4 mm (1/60 inch) long. They form colonies in dense webs under bamboo leaves and suck the chlorophyll from the leaf cells. This makes the leaves mottled and unsightly and a heavy infestation can kill the plant altogether. The mites live about forty days inside their web, only leaving it to defecate. Radical pruning is the safest way to get rid of them, or you could try importing one of several species of larger, predatory mite to eat them (these cost about 1p each via mail order).

Another parasite that lives uniquely on bamboo is the noxious bamboo mealybug (*Dinoderus ocellaris*). This pest turns the sap of the bamboo into sugary honeydew. This in turn grows a sooty-black mould that looks nasty but which is irresistible to ants. A practical (if fairly slow) way to control bamboo mealybugs is to eat their larvae. In Thailand bamboo borer grubs are a delicacy, often appearing on menus as 'fried little white babies'.

One animal that *doesn't* live entirely on bamboo is the Giant panda (*Ailuropoda melanoleuca*). Admittedly, up to 99 per cent of its diet *is* made up of bamboo, but pandas will happily eat small mammals, fish and carrion if they can rouse themselves to catch any.

The problem is that pandas are built like carnivores but eat like herbivores. Bamboo is available all year round, but it's so low in nutrition that, to satisfy their basic needs, pandas must spend twelve hours a day munching the equivalent of a hay bale of the stuff. This leaves little time (or energy) for hunting or gathering. Nor does it produce enough fat to hibernate in the winter. Instead, it generates a tremendous amount of waste.

Pandas defecate more than forty times a day – excreting about half the weight of what they eat – and their droppings are so fibrous that one Thai zoo uses them to make souvenir paper.

Perhaps because of the endless regime of eating and sleeping, pandas aren't very sociable. When it comes to defending their territory, they avoid energy-sapping confrontations. Instead, they keep other pandas at bay by marking their boundaries with scent. They do this in four distinct ways, the most unusual being to leave a mark while doing a handstand. The higher the pee, the more dominant the signal is rated by potential rivals. No other animal in the world does this.

As well as keeping the 2,000 surviving wild giant pandas alive, bamboo has other extraordinary qualities. It is the world's fastest-growing plant: one species in China grows a metre (about 3 feet) a day (that's nearly 8 centimetres, or 3 inches, an hour) and, when fully grown, can reach 60 metres (200 feet) tall. It also has a 'bend-factor' ten times greater than that of steel, making it ideal for construction – almost all the scaffolding in Hong Kong is made of bamboo.

Which is hairier: human or chimpanzee?

Humans may look less hairy than a chimpanzee, but we have the same number of hair follicles – about 5 million – on our bodies, of which only 100,000 (2 per cent) are on our scalps.

Our hair has evolved to be finer and more transparent than in other primates. We lost our fur, and no one knows why. One theory is that it was to reduce lice. Another is that, when our ancestors moved out of the forests on to the savannah about 1.7 million years ago, we needed to lose body hair to stop overheating. As we became less hairy, we became darker-skinned to protect our skin from the sun. But that doesn't explain why the Inuit of the Arctic have less body hair than many sub-Saharan Africans.

Nor does it explain why our scalp hair is programmed to grow for such long periods: left to its own devices, it would grow down past our waists. Other mammalian fur is more like our body hair – it grows to a set length and then is replaced. (Nor can we explain why some men sprout luxuriant hair out of their ears, noses, eyebrows and backs, even as their heads go bald.)

One theory links our loss of fur with increased brain size. A bigger brain creates more heat; in order to keep our temperature under control, we evolved to sweat heavily (sweating is hopeless if you have fur). So, the less fur we had, the more efficient our cooling system became and the bigger our brains grew. Also, as humans walked upright, the only place we still needed hair was on the head, to protect our expanding brains against the sun.

Another more extreme hypothesis suggests we evolved from 'aquatic apes'. This supposes that 8 million years ago the ancestors of modern humans lived a semi-aquatic lifestyle, foraging for food in shallow waters. As fur is not an effective insulator in water, we evolved to replace it, as other aquatic mammals have, with higher levels of body fat. Unfortunately, there isn't any fossil evidence for aquatic humans (or apes) at all.

Yet another idea is that hairlessness, once it had started to evolve, was reinforced by sexual selection – in other words it became attractive to the opposite sex. Charles Darwin went along with this (though, given that, it's odd he chose to have such an enormous beard) and it may be why women are less hairy than men and why smooth, clear skin has become a sign of good health.

Nobody's really sure, though. As leading palaeoanthropologist Ian Tattersall recently remarked: 'There are all kinds of notions as to the advantage of hair loss, but they are all just-so stories.'

What did Neanderthals look like?

A lot like us.

The latest reconstructions of Neanderthals look very similar to humans. If you gave one a haircut and a tracksuit, it wouldn't look out of place on a bus.

The first fossilised remains of humanity's closest cousins were found in 1856 near Düsseldorf in the Neander river valley, hence the word *Neanderthal* (*Tal*, then spelt *Thal*, is German for 'valley'). *Homo neanderthalensis* used tools, wore jewellery, had religious rites, buried his dead and could probably talk. Like us they had the essential hyoid bone (which holds the root of the tongue in place) and recent genetic analysis shows they had exactly the same 'language gene' (FOXP2) that humans do. Using the word Neanderthal to mean 'oafish' or 'unreconstructed' is unfair. In fact, this notion derives from a misinterpretation of the very first reconstruction of a Neanderthal skeleton.

It was the work of a French palaeontologist called Pierre Marcellin Boule (1861–1942) who in 1911 put together a specimen with a curved spine, a stoop, bent knees, and a head and hips that jutted forward. In 1957 the skeleton was re-examined and it became clear that the original owner had suffered from a grossly deforming type of osteoarthritis. Not only did this not represent the average Neanderthal, but Boule had also let his preconceptions affect his work, giving the skeleton an opposable big toe like a great ape, even though the bones didn't provide any evidence for such a conclusion.

Neanderthals had barrel-shaped chests and broad, projecting noses – traits some palaeoanthropologists believe helped them breathe better when chasing prey in cold environments. They had bigger brains than modern humans, but they couldn't run as fast and were shorter and less adept at using tools. What they lacked in height they made up for in strength: Neanderthal females had bigger biceps than the average male human does today.

Humans and Neanderthals diverged into separate species somewhere between 440,000 and 270,000 years ago. Early Neanderthals moved out of Africa into the Middle East and northern Europe much sooner than *Homo sapiens* did, and lived there for four times as long. They became extinct 30,000 years ago (the last recorded Neanderthal community was on Gibraltar), which means that humans and Neanderthals co-existed for at least 12,000 years.

No one knows why the Neanderthals died out. Were they out-competed by humans or did they (for some unknown reason) fail to adapt to the last Ice Age, when Europe became a frozen, sparsely vegetated semi-desert? The oldest known ornaments in Europe (made from shells) were the work of Neanderthals and some researchers now think that humans might have learned ritual and even culture from them during the 120 centuries we shared.

But the most startling fact to emerge from analysis of the genome of the Neanderthals is that they interbred with us. So, unless you are a pure black African, between 1 per cent and 4 per cent of you is Neanderthal.

STEPHEN *How would you spot a Neanderthal if you saw one on a bus?*

JACK DEE *He'd be the one who comes and sits next to me.*

Which part of you is evolving fastest?

It's your nose.

It was once impossible to know how our sensory organs evolved because the soft parts of our bodies don't survive in the fossil record. However, genetic analysis at Cornell University has led 'sensory psychologist' Avery Gilbert to believe that the nose is the fastest-evolving human organ.

In mammals the largest single family of genes controls the sense of smell. The study of the human genome shows that ours has altered much more rapidly than those of our closest living relatives, the great apes. This means we sniff less, but taste more, sending aromas from the back of the throat to the nose as we chew. Known as 'retronasal olfaction' or 'back-of-the-nose smelling' (as opposed to orthonasal smelling through the nostrils) this ability to savour food as we are eating is almost unique to humans. In Avery's words: 'The human nose evolved to serve the human mouth.'

Two events may have contributed to this. The first was cooking with fire, first discovered 1.8 million years ago by our ancestor *Homo erectus*, bringing with it the enticing smells of roast meat and caramelised fruit. The second was the domestication of animals around 15,000 years ago, closely followed by the invention of farming. This brought a whole new range of flavours (yogurt, milk, cheese, bread and toast) and the domestication of the dog gave us a companion species with an extremely acute sense of smell. One theory is that our ancestors delegated the practical scent-tracking function of our noses to dogs, while we concentrated on the ever more complex and delicious aromas coming from the cooking pot. Eating together around the campfire transformed human culture: our shared sense of taste helped to civilise us.

The nose may be our fastest-evolving organ, but further analysis of the human genome shows that we are also evolving elsewhere. Our hair is becoming less thick, but our hearing (perhaps as a result of developing language) is much better than that of chimpanzees. More alarmingly, the Y chromosome, the one that makes a person male (men have both an X and a Y chromosome) is shrinking. It's lost 1,393 of its original 1,438 genes over the last 300 million years. The geneticist Steve Jones points out that one consequence of this is that women are now genetically closer to chimpanzees than men are, because the two X chromosomes they possess have changed much less rapidly.

There's a widespread assumption that human beings have stopped evolving, because technological advances have insulated us from the environmental pressures that drive natural selection. However, the latest genome research suggests the rate of evolutionary change among humans is much the same as that observed in the rest of nature.

A good example of this is lactose tolerance (inability to digest milk) in adults, which has arisen in some parts of the world (but not others) as the result of a single genetic mutation that took place no more than 5,000 years ago.

What were Bronze Age tools made of?

Stone, mostly.

The Bronze Age, which in Europe is dated at 2300–600 BC, began when mankind first discovered how to make and use bronze, but this would have been a *gradual* industrial revolution. For much of the period, old technology (using stone and bone) would have been more widespread than metal. Bronze would have been rare and expensive, so most everyday tools and weapons would still have been made from flint and other familiar materials.

And, just as stone flourished in the Bronze Age, so bronze-working didn't reach its peak until well into the Iron Age (1200 BC–AD 400).

We still use all three materials today. In the twenty-first century, alongside plastic bags and silicon chips, we still continue to produce iron railings, bronze bearings and statues, gravestones and grinding stones. The last people in Britain to make a living working with flint were the flintknappers who supplied the gunflints for firearms. It was a profession that only died out in the nineteenth century, when the percussion cap replaced the flintlock.

The 'Three-Age System' – in which the Bronze Age follows the Stone Age, and is succeeded by the Iron Age – stems from the early nineteenth century. It was the brainchild of Christian Jürgensen Thomsen (1788–1865), a Danish museum curator, who was looking for a nice neat way of arranging his exhibits. It was never intended to be more than a fairly crude means of placing artefacts in a chronological relationship with each other, by classifying them according to the relative sophistication of their manufacture.

Many archaeologists believe that the Stone Age – which is itself split into three eras (the Old, Middle and New Stone ages) – was probably more of a Wood Age, but that wood's predominant role in pre-history has been hidden by the fact that wooden artefacts rot, while stone ones don't.

What was not Made in China and not made *of* china?

Glass.

Though the Chinese invented the compass, the flushing toilet, gunpowder, paper, the canal lock and the suspension bridge long before anyone else, the scientific revolution that transformed the West between the sixteenth and eighteenth centuries completely passed them by.

The reason for this is that they also invented tea.

The earliest known glass artefacts are Egyptian and date back to 1350 BC, but it was the Romans who first produced transparent glass. They liked the way it enabled them to admire the colour of their wine.

By the time the Egyptians worked out how to make glass, the Chinese had been drinking tea (traditionally they began in 2737 BC) for almost 1,400 years. Its colour was less important to them than temperature, and they found it was best served in their most famous invention of all: fine porcelain, or 'china'.

Since they had no particular use for it, early Chinese glass was thick, opaque and brittle. They mainly used it for making children's toys – and soon gave up on it altogether. For almost 500 years, from the end of the fourteenth century until the nineteenth, no glass was made in China at all.

Meanwhile, in 1291 the Republic of Venice, concerned about the fire risk to its wooden buildings, moved its glass furnaces offshore to the island of Murano. Here, inspired by migrant Islamic craftsmen, the inhabitants learned to make the finest glass in the world, giving them a monopoly that lasted for centuries

The impact of high-grade glass on Western culture cannot be overstated. The invention of spectacles towards the end of the thirteenth century added at least fifteen years to the academic and scientific careers of men whose work depended on reading. The precise reflection of glass mirrors led to the discovery of perspective in Renaissance painting. Glass beakers and test tubes transformed ancient alchemy into the modern science of chemistry.

The microscope and the telescope, invented within a few years of each other at the end of the sixteenth century, opened up two new universes: the very distant and the very small.

By the seventeenth century, European glass had become cheap enough for ordinary people to use it for windowpanes (as opposed to mere holes in the wall or the paper screens of the Orient). This protected them from the elements and flooded their houses with light, initiating a great leap forward in hygiene. Dirt and vermin became visible, and living spaces clean and disease free. As a result, plague was eliminated from most of Europe by the early eighteenth century.

In the mid-nineteenth century, transparent, easily sterilised swan-necked glass flasks allowed the French chemist Louis Pasteur to disprove the theory that germs spontaneously generated from putrefying matter. This led to a revolution in the understanding of disease and to the development of modern medicine. Not long afterwards, glass light bulbs changed both work and leisure forever.

Meanwhile, new trade links between East and West in the nineteeth century meant that a technologically backward China soon caught up. Today it is the world's third-largest industrial power and its largest exporter, with total exports in 2009 of £749 billion.

It is also the world's largest producer of glass, controlling 34 per cent of the global market.

What's the name of the chemical that's bad for you and is found in Chinese food?

Despite its reputation in the press, monosodium glutamate is much less harmful than ordinary table salt.

The list of charges against MSG is a long one. It has been accused of causing obesity, nerve damage, high blood pressure, migraine, asthma and altering hormone levels. But every concerned public body that ever investigated it has given it a clean bill of health.

For centuries, it was agreed that there were only four basic tastes – sweet, sour, bitter and salty – until in 1908 Dr Kikunae Ikeda of Tokyo University discovered a fifth one: a 'meaty' taste that he named *'umami'*. This is the taste of MSG. Like soy sauce, it just makes your food a little more delicious.

The MSG scare arose out of so-called 'Chinese Restaurant Syndrome'. Dr Robert Ho Man Kwok coined the term in 1968, when a number of his patients complained of palpitations and numbness in their neck and arms after eating a large Chinese meal. Dr Kwok blamed monosodium glutamate, and though all subsequent research has proved that to generate such symptoms would require a concentration of MSG in food that would render it completely inedible, the stigma has somehow remained.

We now know that glutamate is present in almost every natural food stuff (it is particularly high in parmesan and tomato juice) and that the protein is so vital to our functioning that our own bodies produce 40 grams of it a day. Human milk contains lots of glutamate, which it uses as an alternate enhancement to sugar – MSG and sugar are the two things that get babies drinking.

A much more dangerous substance is recklessly sprinkled on food every time we eat. Excessive salt intake increases the risk of high blood pressure, strokes, coronary artery disease, heart and kidney failure, osteoporosis, stomach cancer and kidney stones. We'd be safer replacing it in our cruets with MSG.

In the European Union, monosodium glutamate is classified as a food additive – E621.

The dreaded 'e-numbers' listed on jars and tin cans are almost all completely benign; the 'E' stands for nothing more sinister than 'European'. It is simply an international way of labelling the different substances (by no means all of them artificial) that are found in our foods. If you wanted to avoid E numbers altogether, you couldn't: 78 per cent of the air we breathe is E941 (nitrogen) and even the purest water is made entirely from E949 (hydrogen) and E948 (oxygen).

Salt, apparently, doesn't have an e-number.

JOHNNY VEGAS *This is why I don't wanna do shows like this!*

STEPHEN *Why is that, Johnny?*

JOHNNY *Well, 'cause now, I'm gonna lie awake at night, fearing that I'm lactating poison! I feel like I've already hurt people enough in my lifetime.*

STEPHEN *It's not poison; it's good. We're trying to suggest that MSG is not as bad as it's been painted. You may not like the flavour, in which case, certainly, don't have any.*

JOHNNY *Yeah, but I don't want meaty-tasting breasts!*

Does eating chocolate give you acne?

No. Nothing we eat 'causes' acne (but go easy on the breakfast cereals).

Acne affects over 96 per cent of teenagers at some time during their adolescence.

Each human hair grows in an individual pouch in the skin called a follicle (from the Latin for 'little bag'). Feeding into each follicle is a gland that secretes a waxy substance called sebum (Latin for 'grease' or 'suet'). Next to each follicle is another gland, which carries sweat up to the surface of the skin through a tiny pore (from *poros*, Greek for 'passage').

During puberty, testosterone levels increase in both boys and girls giving rise to an over-production of sebum. This spills out into the sweat pores, clogging them up with oily compost ripe for bacteria. The result is a pimple. A colony of these is called acne vulgaris ('acne' for short). Boys have higher levels of testosterone than girls, which is why they also tend to have worse acne.

So it's not chocolate, but testosterone, that 'causes' acne. But diet is a factor too, and some foods definitely make it worse.

In 1981 Professor David Jenkins, a Toronto-based nutritionist, measured the effects of carbohydrates on blood-sugar levels. He found that starchy foods (like white bread, cereals and potatoes) raised blood-sugar levels dramatically; but sugary foods had much less effect. Starchy foods have a simpler chemical structure and are easier for the digestive system to convert into glucose, the most absorbable form of sugar. Protein, fats and more complex sugars (like chocolate) are harder to absorb. From this, Jenkins devised a scale called the GI, or Glycaemic Index (from Greek *glykys*, 'sweet', and *haima*, 'blood').

Foods with a high GI score – the ones that raise blood-sugar levels most – create a surge in the production of insulin, the hormone that regulates the body's intake of glucose. Insulin is itself controlled by testosterone, and dairy products are in turn thought to stimulate testosterone. So at breakfast, it's the cereal and the milk (a double dose of hormonal stimulants) rather than the sugar that may aggravate the acne.

The English word acne was first used in 1835, but it comes from a 1,500-year-old Assyrian spelling mistake. In the sixth century, Aëtius Amidenus, a physician from the city of Amida (now in modern Turkey), accidentally coined a new word – *akne* – to describe a pimple. He had meant to write *akme* (Greek for 'point').

Munching your favourite chocolate bar produces endorphins, which help relieve pain, reduce stress and lower the risk of heart disease and cancer. But pure cacao doesn't have the same effect. Mere chemicals are not enough to satisfy the craving: we also need taste, texture and memories to set our hearts (literally) racing. In 2007 a research company, The Mind Lab, showed that, for some people – especially women – eating a piece of dark chocolate made the heart beat faster, and for longer, than a passionate kiss.

Who gets over-excited by sugary drinks?

Parents.

There isn't a shred of scientific evidence that children become 'hyperactive' when given sugary drinks, sweets or snacks.

In one test, a group of children were all given the same sugar-rich drink, but the parents of half the sample were told they'd been given a sugar-*free* drink. When questioned afterwards, the parents who thought their children *hadn't* had any sugar (even though they had) reported far less hyperactive behaviour.

In another study, some children were put on high-sugar diets and others sugar-free ones. No difference in behaviour was observed. Not even when (according to the *British Medical Journal* in 2008) the children had already been diagnosed with attention deficit hyperactivity disorder (ADHD). Because parents expect sugar to cause hyperactivity, that's what they see.

It all began in 1973, when a US allergy specialist called Benjamin Feingold (1899–1982) first showed that hyperactivity in children is linked to what they eat, and proposed a diet for preventing it. He recommended cutting out all artificial colourings and flavourings, including sweeteners such as aspartame. The Feingold Diet didn't ban sugar but, as medical opinion gradually came to accept the connection between hyperactivity and diet, sugar somehow became confused in the public mind with 'sweeteners'.

No one has ever come up with a decent theory to explain exactly *how* sugar might have this effect on youngsters. If high blood-sugar levels were the cause, they'd be more likely to go ballistic after a bowl of rice or a baked potato.

Throughout the centuries, food has been blamed for causing the behaviour that people were most worried about at the time. The sixteenth-century herbalist John Gerard warned against the herb chervil, which 'has a certain windiness, by means whereof it provoketh lust'. Buddhist monks are forbidden to eat any member of the onion family, because they, too, are thought to cause lust when cooked – and anger when raw.

In the nineteenth century, moralising Victorians attributed 'degeneracy and idleness' in the Irish to the supposed soporific effect of the potato. Englishwomen, by contrast, were warned off eating meat. Such 'stimulating' food was liable to bring on debilitating periods, nymphomania and insanity.

ALAN *Speaking as an uncle, I am often discouraged from giving them too much chocolate, because they go, in quotes, 'mental'.*

How many glasses of water should you drink every day?

Eight is too many.

You lose water every second of the day through excreting, sweating or simply breathing, so you need to take in liquid to avoid becoming dehydrated. But the advice that you should drink eight glasses of water a day is just plain wrong.

In 1945 a *British Medical Journal* report advised that adults should consume 2.5 litres of water daily but specified that 'most of this quantity is contained in prepared foods'. In the sixty years since, this important final sentence seems to have fallen by the wayside. A normal diet contains enough embedded water for us, theoretically, not to need to drink anything at all.

Drinking lots of glasses of water on top of your normal consumption of food and drink will only make you urinate more.

It's often said that drinking water is good for flushing out your system and keeping your skin blemish-free, but the evidence is patchy. Your kidneys may be helped to remove excess salt in the short term but unless you've been overdosing on crisps (or alcohol) there is no particular benefit. Chronic dehydration makes your skin drier and less elastic, but taking in extra water won't remove your wrinkles and it's unlikely to stop you from getting spots.

Treating dehydration involves more than just water. You need to replace sugar and salts as well, so try eating watermelons. They're rich in sugar, as well as calcium, magnesium, potassium and sodium. Papaya's good, too, as are coconut, cucumber and celery.

The salts and sugar are necessary because they help transport the water around the body. If you find watermelons spoil the line of your safari suit, you can buy sachets of rehydration powders from chemists and travel agents. These contain glucose and salts – but you'll still need to source your own water to dissolve them in – which is where watermelons win: they're 92 per cent water.

Too much water, on the other hand, can be lethal. 'Water intoxication' or hyponatremia (from Greek *hypo*, 'under', Latin *natrium*, 'sodium' and Greek *haima*, 'blood') is caused by over-dilution of essential body salts. Excess water is expelled from the blood into other cells, which then expand and rupture – leading to nausea, headaches, disorientation and, eventually, death.

What use is a sauna?

Saunas do many things, but 'sweating out the body's toxins' isn't one of them.

Sweat is 99 per cent water, with tiny amounts of salt and other minerals. Its function is to cool the body as the water evaporates from the skin, not to remove waste products. It's the liver and kidneys that deal with any toxins in the body, converting them into something useful, or arranging for them to be excreted.

Nor does a sauna necessarily help you get rid of a hangover. Fifteen minutes in a sauna can lead to the loss of 1.5 litres (2½ pints) of sweat. Unless you drink lots of water to compensate, sweating heavily will only make you more dehydrated. Dehydration puts your kidneys under stress, which slows down the elimination of alcohol from your system.

What a sauna *can* do well is clean your skin, by opening your pores as you sweat. A fifteen-minute session at a temperature of 70 °C and 40 per cent humidity raises the body's surface temperature by 10 °C and its internal temperature by 3 °C. This increases blood flow to the skin and makes the lungs work harder, increasing the intake of oxygen by up to 20 per cent – which is why endurance athletes often use saunas as part of their training.

A sauna followed by a cold shower generates feel-good endorphins in the brain, and can be used to treat mild depression. Research at the Thrombosis Institute in London has shown that the sauna–cold water combination also strengthens the immune system by increasing the number of white blood cells that fight disease. Saunas can also reduce the pain of arthritis and the Finns swear by them as a cure for the common cold.

Though 'sauna' is a Finnish word, the *idea* of the sauna is an ancient one. Writing in the fifth century BC, the Greek historian Herodotus described how the Scythians, a nomadic tribe from Iran, used small tents for the purpose, in which they burned cannabis on the hot stones – so they got high as well as clean. 'The Scythians', he wrote, 'enjoy it so much that they howl with pleasure.' The Apaches of North America have always used 'sweat lodges' made from willow frames covered with skins, in which up to twelve people sit naked around heated rocks. These are periodically soused with water to make steam, cleansing both body and spirit.

The sauna has a similar spiritual significance for the Finns. Traditionally it was a place for the family to gather, for women to give birth and for the dead to be washed before burial. An old Finnish saying is *unassa ollaan kuin kirkossa* – 'behave in a sauna as in a church'.

Finns who break this rule run the risk of being punished by the only permanent resident of the sauna, the *saunatonttu*, or 'sauna elf'.

The word 'sauna' is one of only two expressions in English borrowed from the Finnish language. The other is 'Molotov cocktail'.

What effect does drinking alcohol have on antibiotics?

It doesn't usually have any effect at all.

The idea that alcohol 'stops antibiotics working' was first put about in the venereal disease clinics set up after the Second World War. Penicillin, identified by Alexander Fleming in 1928, had proved particularly effective at clearing up sexually transmitted infections. It was prescribed with the strict instruction not to drink while taking it. The reason for this was psychological rather than pharmaceutical. Drunken people are more likely to jump at the chance of casual sex. By scaring their patients into not drinking, doctors and nurses were giving the drug a chance to work before the infection could be passed on.

This advice became standard medical practice, and it worked: most people still avoid alcohol when on a course of antibiotics. It's true that it's not a good idea to drink *heavily* on antibiotics, because the alcohol competes with the drug for 'processing time' in your liver. This means the drug may work a little more slowly. What it won't do is stop it working altogether.

Of over a hundred types of antibiotic available for prescription, only five are listed as having serious side effects if taken with alcohol.

Of these, the only one commonly prescribed is Metronidazole, which is used to combat some dental and gynaecological infections and for treating *Clostridium difficile*, a bacterial infection picked up in hospitals. The drug prevents the body from breaking down alcohol properly, leading to a build up in the blood of the highly toxic chemical acetaldehyde – a close relative of formaldehyde, better known as embalming fluid. The effects are similar to an extremely bad hangover: vomiting, increased heart rate and severe headaches.

In 1942 the American microbiologist Selman Waksman (1888–1973) – and his student Albert Schatz (1922–2005) – discovered streptomycin, the first drug to be effective against tuberculosis. Waksman described it as 'antibiotic' (from the Greek *anti* 'against' and *bios* 'life') because it killed living bacteria.

Antibiotics are powerless against colds or flu, which are viral infections. It's not clear what viruses are, or even if they can be said to be 'alive'. They have genes (but no cells) and can only reproduce using a host organism. Scientists tend to refer to them as 'biological entities' or 'organisms at the edge of life'.

What *does* stop antibiotics working is not alcohol but over-prescription. In farming 70 per cent of the antibiotics used are given to perfectly healthy animals. In medicine new strains of bacteria have become resistant to former 'wonder drugs' like streptomycin and the World Health Organisation estimates that a third of the world's population now carries a drug-resistant strain of TB. There are fears that as many as 35 million people may die from it before 2020.

Can you name a narcotic?

LSD, cocaine, speed?

None of the above. Medically speaking, a 'narcotic' is an opium derivative, such as morphine. A slightly looser definition might include any drug that causes unconsciousness – technically known as 'narcosis', from the Greek *narke,* meaning 'numbness' or 'torpor'.

Law enforcement agencies in the USA use the word 'narcotic' as a blanket term to mean *any* illegal drug – even though many of them are anything but narcotic in their effects, and many true narcotics, like codeine, are legal.

To avoid this confusion the medical profession now refers to opium – and its derivatives and man-made substitutes – as 'opioids'. Opium is made from *Papaver somniferum,* a type of poppy which has been grown as a medicinal herb for thousands of years.

Nowadays opioids are mostly used in pain control, a task for which they are unrivalled. Though dependence on opioid painkillers is a common result of long-term use, actual addiction is very rare. In 2001 the American Pain Society defined addiction as 'compulsive and continued use of a drug despite harm'. The most common side effect of prescribed narcotics is constipation.

In the nineteenth century, opioids were freely available over the counter. Heroin, discovered by the same man (Felix

Hoffman) in the same year (1897) as aspirin, was originally a brand name and was marketed as a cough mixture. One of its supposed virtues was that it wasn't habit-forming. At the time, the medical authorities were much more worried about green tea, which was believed to cause anaemia, convulsions, hallucinations and suffocation.

Britain is currently aiming to become self-sufficient in home-grown opium poppies to ensure a regular supply of the powerful painkiller diamorphine (otherwise known as heroin) for those suffering from cancer or recovering from surgery. In the past, the UK has depended on imports from the Far East.

Despite a 40 per cent fall in production since 2008, Afghanistan still supplies 90 per cent of the world's opium. More than half of this comes from Helmand province, the main stronghold of the Taliban insurgents. According to the UN, the Afghan government manages to intercept only 2 per cent of the opium that is produced.

In 2009 the British army sprang into action and, shortly afterwards, the Ministry of Defence announced that they had seized 1.3 tons of 'a new strain of super poppy seeds', thus denying the Taliban revenue of some £247 million. The Ministry was later forced to admit that what the army had actually got hold of was 1,100 kilos of mung beans, a staple of the Afghan diet.

What's the best way to restart a stopped heart?

Not by using a defibrillator.

If you think otherwise, you've been watching too many medical dramas on TV. Electricity is only used when the heart is beating irregularly. If it has stopped completely, attempts to re-establish a heartbeat take the form of regular intravenous injections of adrenaline and other drugs. Survival rates for such patients are fewer than one in fifty.

The two main forms of irregular heartbeat are (1) the heart beating too fast or *ventricular tachycardia* (from the Greek *tachys*, 'fast', and *kardia*, 'heart') and (2) the random quivering known as *ventricular fibrillation* (from the Latin *fibrilla*, 'fibre', because the heart is a mass of twitching fibres). Both conditions are usually the result of a heart attack, brought on by a failure in blood supply to the heart muscle. If the flow of blood to the brain becomes so irregular that the patient loses consciousness and stops breathing, the heart attack has become a 'cardiac arrest' and requires immediate medical attention. Brain damage begins four minutes after the flow of blood has stopped.

It is at this point that the electric paddles, or defibrillator, are used to stimulate the heart muscle to return to a regular rhythm. If this takes place within three to five minutes of the onset of an arrest, then there is a 74 per cent chance of a normal heartbeat being restored and a one in three chance of survival. In 2007 the UK Department of Health announced that the 681 defibrillators installed at airports, railway stations and shopping centres had saved 117 lives.

The first defibrillator used on a human was in 1947, under the supervision of Ohio surgeon Claude Beck. Sudden cardiac arrest remains the biggest cause of death in the Western world: more than 70,000 die from it each year in the UK.

Without access to a defibrillator, the chances of survival are much lower – about 1 in 25. Nevertheless, proper use of manual resuscitation techniques saves many lives by keeping the patient's blood flowing until a defibrillator can be found. This is done by pressing rhythmically on the patient's chest to pump blood through the heart (mouth-to-mouth resuscitation is now deemed less effective). A steady beat is important and, for many years, first-aiders were taught to sing the song 'Nelly the Elephant' as they pumped. Now the recommendation is for faster chest compressions, so the 103 beats per minutes of the Bee Gee's 'Stayin' Alive' is preferred.

The face of the dummy still used to teach resuscitation techniques (known as 'Rescue Annie') is that of an unidentified young suicide pulled out of the river Seine in 1900. The pathologist at the morgue was so overcome by her beauty that he made a plaster cast of her face. Her tragic story made her a fashion icon for a whole generation of writers, artists and photographers.

When Peter Safar and Asmund Laerdal designed Rescue Annie in 1958, they had no idea that she would become the most kissed woman of all time.

STEPHEN *The defibrillators: what do you use those for?*
JACK DEE *To start the heart up again when it stops.*
JIMMY CARR *Oh. I use them for making paninis . . .*

Can a living person be a successful heart donor?

Surprisingly, it is possible for a living person to donate their heart to someone else and survive the experience – provided they get another heart in exchange.

This happens when someone with severe lung disease but a healthy heart is assessed as having a better chance of survival if they receive a heart-and-lung transplant. In return, they can donate their heart to someone who needs only a heart transplant.

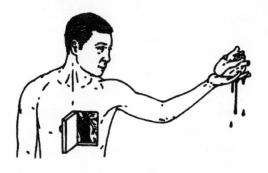

The cardiac surgeon Magdi Yacoub (now Professor Sir Magdi Yacoub) carried out the first of these so-called 'domino' transplants in the UK in 1987. We don't know the patients' names because they requested no publicity. Later that year a cystic fibrosis sufferer called Clinton House became the first US donor of a living heart. He donated his to John Couch, while he received a new heart and lungs from an unidentified car accident victim.

The first successful transplant of any kind made by a living donor took place in Boston in 1954, when one identical twin brother donated one of his kidneys to the other, both of whose kidneys had failed. In theory, everyone can survive perfectly well on one kidney, one lung, one of the two lobes of the liver and only parts of the pancreas and intestines. The liver, uniquely among such organs, has the capacity to grow back almost completely.

In 1896, the English surgeon Stephen Paget (1855–1926) wrote the standard textbook *Surgery of the Chest*, in which he predicted that it would always be too difficult and dangerous to operate on a human heart. But, later that very year, a German surgeon, Ludwig Rehn (1849–1930), successfully repaired the left chamber of a young man's heart after he had been stabbed in the chest. It was the first case of a surgeon operating on a heart and the patient surviving, and Rehn didn't dare try it again. Even in wartime, conventional surgical wisdom stated that shrapnel lodged in the heart should be left there and heart surgery for any reason was almost unheard of before the Second World War.

Things improved rapidly after the war. The South African surgeon Christiaan Barnard (1922–2001) performed the first heart transplant in Cape Town in 1967. Although his patient only lived for eighteen days, two-thirds of transplant patients now survive for more than five years. The longest recorded is Tony Huesman, a sporting goods retailer from Dayton, Ohio who lived for thirty-one years with a transplanted heart until he died of cancer, aged fifty-one, in 2009.

In the UK, these advances have led to a change in the legal definition of death. Until the 1970s, death was considered to have occurred when the heartbeat stopped. After the first heart transplants, death was redefined as the absence of brain function. This gave surgeons the chance to remove a donor heart before it stopped beating.

Which mammal has the most heartbeats in a lifetime?

Thanks to medical science, we do.

Large mammals have slow heartbeats and long lives and small ones have short lives and fast heartbeats. Because of this, no matter what size a mammal is, it has the same average number of heartbeats in a lifetime – about half a billion. This is known as 'the rate of living hypothesis' and it applies to all mammals except humans. Improvements in medicine and hygiene have extended our life expectancy so that we now get through more than five times as many heartbeats in a lifetime than all other mammals.

The world's smallest mammal is the Etruscan shrew (*Suncus etruscus*) of southern Europe, which weighs 2 grams (0.07 ounces) and is 3.5 centimetres (just over an inch) long.

Its heart hammers away at an average 835 beats per minute but it only lives for a year, just enough to allow it to reproduce before being eaten.

At the other end of the scale is the Blue whale (*Balaenoptera musculus*), which can reach 30 metres (100 feet) long and weigh 150 tons (thirty times more than an African elephant). It has a heart the size of a small car, which thumps out its stately cadence just ten times a minute for eighty years.

The beats-per-life of the two species are remarkably similar: 439 million for the shrew; 421 million for the whale. In contrast, the average human heart, at seventy-two beats per minute spread over sixty-six years, will beat 2.5 billion times.

The US astronaut Neil Armstrong was so taken by the idea of having a finite number of heartbeats that he joked that he was going to give up exercise because he didn't want to use up his allocation too quickly. But it doesn't quite work like that: though strenuous exercise makes the heart beat faster in the short term, the resultant fitness *decreases* the heart rate in general.

An even better way to slow the heart rate is to take up yoga. Research conducted over thirty days in 2004 in Bangalore, India, showed that yogic breath control and meditation led to an average reduction in the heart rate of 10.7 beats per minute. The control group, who attempted to reduce their heart rate by other means, didn't manage any lasting improvement at all.

A macabre experiment to record the effect of fear on the heart rate was conducted in 1938, when convicted murderer John Deering donated his body to science while he still was alive. Sentenced to death by firing squad in Salt Lake City, Utah, he allowed Dr Stephen Besley, the prison doctor, to wire him to an electrocardiograph. Beneath Deering's calm exterior, Besley recorded his heart rate rocketing from 72 to 120 as he was strapped down, and reaching 180 at the moment of impact. His heart stopped 15.6 seconds later.

Besley commented that, despite having 'put on a good front', the machine had confirmed what he'd expected: Deering 'was scared unto death'.

How long do mayflies live?

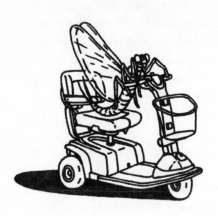

The one thing 'everybody' knows about mayflies is that they only live for a day – but their lifetimes are much longer than that.

Depending on species, the adult lives from less than a day to a week, but this is only the final stage of a much longer life-cycle. Most of the mayfly's existence is spent as an aquatic nymph, a period lasting from a few months to four years.

There are 2,500 species of mayfly, fifty-one of which live in the UK. They fly all through the summer – not just in May – and they are not actually 'flies'. True flies belong to the order *Diptera* (Greek for 'two wings'), whereas mayflies belong to the order *Ephemeroptera* (Greek for 'short-lived wings'). Mayflies are much older than true flies. They were one of the first flying insects: there are mayfly fossils that are 300 million years old. Their closest relatives are dragonflies and damselflies – neither of which are 'flies' either.

Mayflies are unique among insects, in that their final skin-shedding takes place after their wings have formed. On first emerging from the water, the immature adult, or nymph, moults and becomes a 'dun', so-called because of its small, dull-coloured wings. It flies a short distance from its pond, and rests for a while on vegetation. Then it undergoes its ultimate transformation, sloughing its final skin and emerging as the much shinier 'spinner'.

Adult mayflies never eat: their only interest is sex. Vast swarms of males take to the air simultaneously and the females fly among them to pick a partner. Mating takes place in flight, and as soon as the deed is done, the male drops to the water, dead. The female immediately lays her eggs in the water – and *then* drops dead. One species – *Dolania americana* – dies within five minutes of its final moult. In that tiny window of time, it has to dry its new wings, fly, select a partner, mate, and – if it's a female – lay its eggs. A day is a long, long time in the life of a mayfly.

In some countries, it's not only fish that benefit from these huge clouds of protein from the sky. Along the Sepik River in New Guinea, villagers skim masses of post-copulatory mayflies from the surface of the water and cook them in sago pancakes. Apparently, they taste a bit like caviar.

What comes out of a cocoon?

Not butterflies. But most moths do – and so do fleas, bees, worms and spiders.

A cocoon is a kind of silken changing room where a creature metamorphoses into a different stage of its life – such as a spider's egg into a baby spider or a caterpillar into a moth. The word comes from *kokkos*, Greek for 'berry'.

Silkworms are not worms but caterpillars. At about a month

old, they spend three days carefully winding a mile-long thread of their own saliva round their bodies that dries into a casing to keep them safe during their transformation into a silkworm moth. Unfortunately for them, it is at this stage that they are picked up by silkworm farmers and shipped off to the factory. It takes 3,000 cocoons to make a pound of silk.

Baby bees develop inside a cocoon made of royal jelly. They eat themselves out of it. Flea larvae become adults inside cocoons. They can remain in that state, buried in your carpet for months, until vibrations caused by movement nearby announce that a host animal is available for them to jump on.

After mating, an earthworm secretes mucus that hardens into a loose girdle around its body. This sheath slowly slides along the worm's length, collecting eggs and sperm from its genital openings as it goes, finally sliding off its head like a vest, where the ends seal up and it becomes a lemon-shaped cocoon. Inside the cocoon, the eggs and sperm merge into embryos. Spiders, too, place their eggs in a silken sack to hatch. They spin their thickest grade of silk for this purpose. Peasants in Romania use it as an antiseptic wound dressing.

Butterflies don't make cocoons; instead they form chrysalises (from the Greek for 'golden sheath'). A cocoon is an external structure, designed to protect the creature within, whereas the chrysalis *is* the creature. The hard exterior of the chrysalis is the final skin of the caterpillar before it becomes a butterfly.

For many centuries butterflies and moths were thought to be completely unrelated to caterpillars. Then in 1679 the German naturalist and illustrator Maria Sibylla Merian (1647–1717) published a book called *The Caterpillar: Marvelous Transformation and Strange Floral Food* which meticulously detailed the life-cycle and metamorphoses of 186 species of butterflies and moths. Because she published it in German, rather than Latin, it became one of the most talked about science books of the age.

Maria's organised approach to scientific observation and recording was far ahead of most of her contemporaries. Despite this, her discoveries were used by other scientists to justify the old theory of 'preformationism' – the idea that all life was created simultaneously at the beginning of time. They argued that, because the makings of the adult butterfly existed within its pupa form, so Adam and Eve had contained within themselves all the humans who came afterwards, already formed, like a set of smaller and smaller Russian dolls.

What does an amoeba live in?

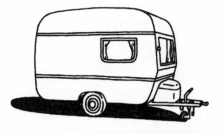

No, it's not 'soup' or 'dribble' or anything like that. It may surprise you to learn that some amoebae live in houses they design and build themselves.

Amoebae (from Greek *amoibe*, 'change') are minute single-celled organisms. No one knows how many countless thousands of different species there are: anywhere that's damp will provide a home for them – as we know to our cost. The species that causes amoebic dysentery kills over 100,000 people a year and lives in the intestines and livers of 50 million more.

Living beings don't get much simpler than an amoeba: they're just an outer membrane full of a watery fluid surrounding a nucleus containing genetic material. They have no fixed shape, but they do have a front and back, and move by squeezing bits of themselves forward in the direction of food. They eat by surrounding smaller bits of algae or bacteria and absorbing them, and they reproduce by splitting themselves in two.

Which makes it extraordinary that one branch of the amoeba family is able to build themselves portable shelters. They do it by swallowing microscopic granules of sand. Once they have enough on board, they start to glue them together by secreting a form of organic cement. As no one has ever observed this process, we have no idea how they do it.

Each species creates its own distinctive style of home. The des res of *Difflugia coronata* is a globe, with a scalloped entrance at the front, and eight points like the fins of a 1950s spaceship at the back. *Difflugia pyriform* constructs a pear-shaped urn; *Difflugia bacillefera*, a cigar-shaped tube. None of them is bigger than a full-stop.

As with so many domestic arrangements these days, inevitably the time comes to split up. The parent amoeba gets to keep the house; the offspring inherits whatever spare building material is left lying around so it can start knocking up one of its own. How is any of this possible without a brain, or even a nervous system?

In 1757 an Austrian miniature painter and naturalist called Johann Rösel von Rosenhof (1705–59) described and drew an amoeba for the first time. He called it Proteus after the Greek god who could change his shape at will. Since that time, the word 'amoeba' has become universal shorthand for something basic or unsophisticated.

Maybe it's time to revise our ideas. We have recently learnt that the genetic information packed into the single nucleus of *Amoeba proteus* is 200 times greater than our own.

They may be brainless, but you can hardly call an amoeba 'simple'.

What do Mongolians live in?

Don't call it a yurt. They hate that.

Yurt is a Turkish word meaning 'homeland'. Mongolians live in a tent called a *ger*, which means 'home' in Mongolian.

In recent years, 'yurt' has come to be used indiscriminately to refer to any of the portable, felt-covered, lattice-framed structures that are common to many cultures across the Central Asian steppe.

It's a great insult to a Mongolian to call his *ger* a 'yurt'. The English word 'yurt' comes from the Russian *yurta*, a disparaging term for the kind of jerry-built hovels you find in shanty towns. The Russians borrowed it from the Turkic languages where its original meaning was 'the imprint left on the ground by a tent'. Mongolian is a member of an entirely separate language family from Turkic and Russian, and the whole of Mongolian culture is built around the ger. To call their beloved dwelling a yurt is akin to calling a Yorkshireman's home *un chateau* or *ein Schloss* rather than his castle.

Two-thirds of Mongolians still live in gers – not out of bull-headed national pride, but because they are such practical structures. The walls are circular, made from a lattice of willow held together with leather strips, and topped with a domed roof made from slender, flexible poles. The whole thing is covered in layers of felt and they can be put up or taken down in less than an hour. Their aerodynamic shape makes them very stable in the howling winds of the steppe and their thick felt lining keeps them incredibly warm. Rural Mongolia has the widest temperature range in the world: from a sweltering 45 °C in summer to winter lows of −55 °C. Even those Mongolians who do own houses tend to move into a ger for the winter, just because they are so cosy.

There are strict rules governing layout. To minimise draughts, the door always faces south. The kitchen is to the right of the door and the traditional Buddhist altar is at the back. The beds are to the left and right of the altar. Guests sit at the top left end of the ger; the more honoured you are, the further you sit from the door. Family members sit on the right. In the middle is the wood- or dung-burning stove with its flue poking through the central roof vent. In summer the walls can be rolled up for extra ventilation.

When a Mongolian couple gets married, their families buy or build them a brand-new ger.

The earliest archaeological evidence for the ger only dates back to the twelfth century, but rock carvings, and accounts of ancient travellers like Herodotus, suggest that something similar has been in use on the steppes for at least 2,500 years.

The armies of Genghis Khan (1162–1227) were housed in similar collapsible structures, and the great Khan himself administered the whole of the Mongol empire from a huge ger known as a *gerlug*. It was permanently mounted on a cart pulled by twenty-two bulls.

STEPHEN *What do Mongolians live in?*

ROB BRYDON *They're called something like yak . . . it's like a yult or a yak.*

JO BRAND *Do you mean a yurt?*

ROB *Yes, that's the one.*

KLAXON

ROB *No, that's *not* the one. No, no.*

Can you name a tapestry?

Go to the top of the class if the medieval Apocalypse Tapestry from Angers in north-west France sprang to mind. Or the second-century BC ancient Greek tapestry found in Sampul, western China; or the four fifteenth-century Devonshire Hunting Tapestries hanging in the Victoria and Albert Museum in London.

But it's minus 10 if you said 'Bayeux Tapestry'. This isn't a tapestry at all: it's embroidery. A tapestry is a heavy textile with a design woven in as it's made on a loom, while embroidery is the business of stitching decorations on to a piece of existent fabric – in this case, coloured wool on linen.

The Bayeux *embroidery* is long and thin. It's 70 metres (230 feet) long but only 50 centimetres (20 inches) high. It's a piece of Norman propaganda and the person most likely to have commissioned it is William the Conqueror's half-brother, Odo (1037–98), Bishop of Bayeux and Earl of Kent, who features prominently in the narrative. Today it hangs in France, but the workmanship is English and it was probably made at Canterbury.

Apart from King Harold himself, it's easy to tell who's who: the English are depicted with lavish moustaches while the Normans are clean-shaven. French commentators at the time were shocked by the long-haired English 'with their combed and oiled tresses', calling them 'reluctant warriors' or 'boy-women' (*feminei iuvenes*). The French, on the other hand, look like skinheads.

The battle of Hastings didn't take place at Hastings but several miles away on Senlac Ridge, just outside the helpfully renamed village of Battle. The English king mustered his troops at a vantage point on the crest of the hill known as the 'Hoary Apple Tree' and the Saxon line held until he was lured down to his death by a faked Norman retreat.

Harold is traditionally supposed to be the figure shown with an arrow in his eye, but there are two other figures near where his name is stitched – one with a spear through his chest, and one being cut down by a horseman. He could well be both, or neither, of these people.

In August 1944 Heinrich Himmler, Hitler's second-in-command, ordered the head of the SS in France to bring the Bayeux Tapestry with him as the German Army retreated from France. Four days later, the SS tried to snatch it from the Louvre, but they were too late – the Resistance had occupied the building.

If Himmler had acted faster, the so-called 'tapestry' of Bayeux would have left France on a Nazi truck – an ordeal it might very well not have survived.

Who became king of England after the battle of Hastings?

WHO HE?

Edgar the Ætheling. **ED**

There were four kings of England in 1066, one after the other. Edward the Confessor died in January and was succeeded by Harold. When Harold was killed at Hastings in October, Edgar the Ætheling was proclaimed king. He reigned for two months before William the Conqueror was crowned on Christmas Day.

Among many things the Normans brought with them that the English didn't like was the idea that a king's eldest son automatically succeeded him. Anglo-Saxon kings were elected, not born. The duty of organising this fell to a council of religious and political leaders called the Witan (short for *Witangemot*, or 'wise-meeting').

Royal blood was only one of the factors taken into account. The king had to be able to defend the country and a dying king could nominate anyone as his heir. When Edward the Confessor died childless and without naming his successor, there was a constitutional crisis. His reign had ended thirty years of Danish rule (begun with Cnut's conquest of England in 1016) and his mother was a Norman. This gave both Cnut's great-nephew, William, Duke of Normandy, and King Harald Hardrada of Norway and (in his opinion) Denmark, claims to the English throne.

Edgar was Edward the Confessor's great-nephew. The word *Ætheling* ('prince') marked him out as a potential king, but he was only fifteen. With invasion imminent, the Witan rejected him as too inexperienced and opted instead for Harold Godwinson, Earl of Wessex and Edward the Confessor's brother-in-law.

Harold promptly marched up to Yorkshire where he defeated (and killed) Harald Hardrada at the battle of Stamford Bridge, before having to rush all the way back down again, to lose his own life near Hastings on the Sussex coast. As soon as news of Harold's death reached London, the surviving members of the Witan met to elect Edgar as king. But their heart wasn't really in it. They soon rescinded their decision and surrendered the boy to William. He hadn't even been crowned.

But Edgar, like Harold, was no milksop. Born in Hungary, son of Edward the Exile, he escaped Norman custody and became known as Edgar the Outlaw. He tried several times to recover the English throne, invaded Scotland, attempted to conquer parts of Italy and Sicily, took part in the First Crusade (in 1098) and may even have joined the Byzantine Emperor Alexios I's elite band of axe-wielding, sea-going mercenaries known as the Varangian Guard. Based in Constantinople, feared across the Mediterranean, it was mostly composed of exiled Englishmen.

When Henry I (1069–1135), William the Conqueror's fourth son, married Edgar's niece Matilda, he pardoned the former boy king. Edgar died in Scotland in 1126, at the venerable age of seventy-five. Unmarried and childless, he was buried in an unmarked grave: the last Anglo-Saxon king and the last of the male line of the House of Wessex, England's first royal family.

Who invented Gothic architecture?

Not the Goths. It was the French, if anyone.

The Renaissance artist and historian Giorgio Vasari (1511–74) invented the term 'Gothic' for the now much-admired style of architecture in 1550. He meant it as an insult. In his opinion, pointed arches and huge vaulted ceilings were 'monstrous and barbarous' horrors of bad taste that he blamed on the Goths, the Nordic invaders who had sacked Rome and defiled Italy's classical past.

Best known today for his *Lives of the Artists* – short biographies of contemporary painters, sculptors and architects such as Leonardo and Michelangelo – Giorgio Vasari was also an architect himself. He designed the Uffizi Palace in Florence for Cosimo de' Medici (1519–74). Now world-famous as a museum, it was originally an office block for lawyers (*uffizi* is Italian for 'offices').

Vasari thought the northern French medieval style that reached its peak in the great cathedrals of Chartres, Reims and Lincoln was ugly, fussy and old-fashioned, denouncing it as 'German' as well as 'Gothic'. In fact, it had no connection with either and had evolved out of Romanesque, the simpler, rounder, sturdier style known in Britain as 'Norman' architecture. If you'd asked a medieval cathedral mason what he was doing, he'd have said *opus Francigenum*: 'French work'.

But Vasari's contemptuous nickname stuck, just as the words Baroque, Cubist and Impressionist (all once terms of abuse) would later do. The 'Gothic' style soon spread all over Western Europe, but it wasn't until the late eighteenth century that it lost its negative connotations, as artists and writers looked to the Middle Ages for inspiration. In architecture the 'Gothic Revival' led to buildings like Augustus Pugin's Houses of Parliament (1835) and in literature to a new school of 'gothic' novels, full of ghostly ruins, haunted houses and fainting heroines. It was this literary sense of the word that led (in 1983) to teenagers who wore black clothes, painted their faces white and listened to gloomy music being called Goths.

The original Goths came from southern Sweden (still known today as Götaland) and the name 'Goth' simply meant 'the people' (from Old Norse *gotar*, 'men'). Over four centuries, they migrated east and south to conquer large areas of France, Spain and Italy. In AD 410, Alaric, the military commander of the western branch of Goths (known as Visigoths) attacked and looted Rome – the first time the city had fallen to a foreign power in 800 years. Although the emperor Honorius (AD 384–423) had transferred his capital to Ravenna eight years earlier, it was still a psychological shock and a key moment in the long decline of the Roman Empire.

But the Goths weren't all doom and gloom. They founded cities, converted to Christianity and established a written legal code that was still used in Spain centuries later. By the end of the sixth century, however, defeated by other Germanic tribes in the East and driven out of Spain by Islamic invaders from North Africa, the Goths gradually started to fade from history.

The last traces of the Gothic language were written down in sixteenth-century Crimea. All that survives is a list of eighty words, and a song whose meaning no one now understands.

JACK DEE *I was a Goth for a while.*

STEPHEN *Were you?*

JACK *Yeah. I was asked to leave because I was just too miserable.*

Which country do Huns come from?

Neither Hungary nor Germany. The original Huns were more of an army than a tribe, so no modern country can claim to be descended from them.

The Huns arrived in Europe from Central Asia in the fourth century AD. In just eighty years, they built an empire that stretched from the steppes of central Asia to what is now modern Germany, and from the Black Sea to the Baltic. They rode small, fast horses, and spent almost all their time on them. The Romans said that the Huns fought, ate, slept and carried out diplomacy on horseback – so much so that they became dizzy when they set foot on the ground.

We don't know exactly where they came from or what language they spoke, but most historians now believe the Huns were a multi-ethnic, multilingual army. All they had in common was their loyalty to their great leader, Attila (about 404–53), and their superlative technique as mounted archers.

After Attila the Hun died, his three sons quarrelled and his empire disintegrated almost as rapidly as it had formed. The remnants of his armies were defeated in 454 by an alliance of Goths and other German tribes at the battle of Nedao (now in western Hungary). Since there was no Hun state – no buildings, laws, culture or common language – almost nothing of them has survived except stories. This has allowed many people across Europe and Asia to claim Hun blood (the implication being, of course, that they are related to the heroic warrior-king Attila). Given the racial diversity of the Huns, this is meaningless. If the Huns can be said to live anywhere today, they live everywhere.

In nineteenth-century English, 'Hun' meant much the same as 'vandal': someone given to mindless acts of destruction. It wasn't until the very beginning of the twentieth century that 'the Huns' came to mean the Germans – and it was a German who started it. On 27 July 1900, Kaiser Wilhelm II was addressing his troops on their way to join an alliance of colonial powers putting down an anti-Western revolt in China. He urged them to show no mercy to the 'Boxer' rebels (the sarcastic Western name for the movement who called themselves 'The Righteous Fists of Harmony'). 'The Huns under the leadership of Attila', he told them, 'gained a reputation that is still remembered today. May the name of Germany become equally well known in China, so that no Chinaman will ever again dare to look askance at a German.'

When the First World War began in 1914, Allied propagandists seized on this remark. An editorial in *The Times*, headlined 'The March of the Huns', set the tone. It painted the Germans as even worse than the barbarians of old. Unlike the Kaiser, the article thundered, 'even Attila had his better side'.

By the Second World War 'Kraut' and 'Jerry' had become the popular British nicknames for the Germans, although Churchill (a keen historian) still preferred 'the Hun'. In a 1941 broadcast he described the German invasion of the Soviet Union as the 'brutish masses of the Hun soldiery, plodding on like a swarm of crawling locusts'.

STEPHEN *You'll find Alans on the Russian border in the northern Caucasus Mountains, where the Alan tribe has lived since being driven there by the Huns in the fourth century.*

ALAN *That was a bad weekend.*

STEPHEN *Yeah.*

ALAN *We still talk about that.*

STEPHEN *You, and Alan Coren, and Alan Bennett, and Alan Parsons...*

ALAN *We get together. We conference call.*

STEPHEN *Yeah.*

ALAN *And if someone mentions the Huns, quite often there's a lull in the conversation, and we have to gather ourselves.*

How did Attila the Hun die?

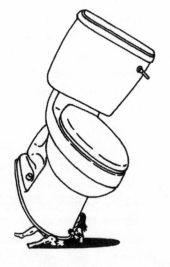

Leading his army to victory on the battlefield? Laying waste to a Roman city? Murdered by a scheming henchman? No. Attila the Hun – the greatest warrior of his age, the man the Romans called *flagellum Dei*, 'the scourge of God', died in bed. Of a nosebleed.

We know this from the Roman historian Priscus, who visited Attila's court in AD 448. According to his account, Attila was celebrating his marriage to a young Gothic woman called Ildico and retired to bed drunk. Next morning his new wife was found weeping over his corpse. The blood vessels in his nose had burst while he slept and he had drowned in his own gore. Attila was about forty-seven years old and he had led the Hunnish army for almost twenty years.

Attila owed much of his success to the devastating speed and manoeuvrability of his troops. Unlike other land armies of the time, they could fight in any weather, not just in summer. In a battle or siege Hun archers could unleash 50,000 arrows in the first ten minutes. But Attila was more than just a ruthless general: he was also a shrewd negotiator. As city after city fell, he liked to pose as a reasonable man, accepting gold in exchange for his victims' future security and building an empire on fear, like a mafia boss or a drugs baron. He didn't want land or power, just obedience and booty. Because of this pragmatic approach, even today his name means barbarism and chaos for some people, but heroic defiance for others.

To manage his set of shifting alliances, Attila had to make sure there was always a plentiful supply of gold (which meant more fighting to acquire it). From his base in Hungary he switched his military focus from the Persians to the Eastern Romans in Constantinople, and then to the Western Romans in Italy and Gaul. Finally, in AD 451, at the battle of Châlons in Gaul, the Huns clashed head-on with the Roman forces of the West. Such was the range of Attila's deal-making skills that almost every tribe in mainland Europe found themselves on one side or the other.

This battle marked the beginning of the end for both the Huns and the old Roman Empire. The Romans and their Gothic allies won, but only just: the Roman legions were decimated and never fought again. Rome was sacked once more in 455 (this time by Vandals) and the Empire relocated to Constantinople, where it stayed for the next 800 years. The complex network of allegiances Attila had built up didn't survive his death two years later and, a year after that, the much-reduced Hun army suffered their final defeat and were scattered, never to return.

Attila's personal style was modest in comparison to the gold-bedecked gangsters around him. He used wooden goblets and plates, dressed simply, and his sword carried no decoration. Not so his funeral. He was buried in a gaudy triple-walled coffin, with a layer each of gold, silver and iron, all of them stuffed full of treasure.

He died somewhere in what is now Hungary, but his grave has never been found. To ensure its location remained secret, all the men in the burial party were killed when they returned to camp.

What should you do when you get a nosebleed?

Don't tilt your head back!

This can divert the nosebleed into the throat. Swallowing blood irritates the stomach and can lead to nausea and vomiting, or if it finds its way into the lungs it can choke you – as Attila the Hun found to his cost. The best treatment is to sit down with your back straight and lean *forward*. Keeping your head above your heart lessens the bleeding. Leaning forward helps drain the blood from your nose.

According to the *British Medical Journal* you can stop the bleeding by using your thumb and index finger to squeeze the soft part of your nose for five to ten minutes. This helps the blood to clot. A cold compress or ice pack placed across the bridge of your nose also helps. If the nosebleed lasts for more than 20 minutes – or if it was caused by a bang on the head – you should go to the doctor.

The scientific term for a nosebleed is epistaxis, which is Greek for 'dripping from above'. The two most common causes of nosebleeds are being punched in the face and nose-picking. The web of blood vessels in your nose can also rupture owing to sharp changes in air pressure or temperature caused by cold weather or central heating, or if you blow your nose too hard.

Almost all nosebleeds occur in the front section of the nose, under the nose bone or septum. This is known as Kiesselbach's area, and it's vulnerable because four facial arteries connect there. Wilhelm Kiesselbach (1839–1902) was a German ear, nose and throat specialist who wrote the definitive textbook on the subject called *Nosenbluten* (German for 'nosebleeds').

High levels of the hormone oestrogen during a woman's period can lead to an increase in blood pressure causing nasal blood vessels to inflate and burst. This is no mere nosebleed. It goes by the alarming name of 'vicarious menstruation'.

STEPHEN *What are the commonest causes of nosebleeds?*
ALAN *Bouncy castles.*
STEPHEN *A classic, yeah. Another one is being punched in the face.*

What happens if you swallow your tongue?

Nothing. It's physically impossible to swallow your own tongue.

The airway of an unconscious person can sometimes briefly become blocked as the muscle of their tongue becomes limp and it collapses into the back of their throat. However, it will return to its normal position in a few seconds. The tongue is kept in place by a small piece of tissue underneath called the frenulum linguae (from Latin *frenulum*, 'little bridle', and *lingua*, 'tongue'), which stops it being swallowed.

The idea that the tongue is in danger of being swallowed dates back to the early years of first aid in the late nineteenth century. First-aiders were taught that, if someone fainted or was having a fit, they should use forceps to pull the tongue forward, or, if none were available, to grab it with their fingers, using a handkerchief. Some well-meaning (but misguided) people still do this today, inserting pieces of wood – or even their wallets – into the mouths of people who are having fits. This is not a good idea. It stops the patient from being able to breathe.

If someone faints, don't start stuffing the contents of your pockets down their throat, put them into the recovery position: lay them on one side, with their chin tilted up so they can breathe clearly.

Swallowing occurs about 2,000 times a day. Except for the initial conscious decision to do it, it is an automatic process that involves twelve separate muscle movements. Alzheimer's patients and victims of strokes sometimes lose the ability to swallow. They are helped to relearn how to do it by speech therapists. This is because speech uses exactly the same combination of muscles as swallowing.

When someone is close to death, the swallowing reflex often fails. This leads to a build up of saliva and mucus in the back of the throat, causing the so-called 'death rattle'. Before writing the patient off, however, check their airway for wallets.

Which part of your tongue tastes bitter things?

All of it.

The 'tongue map', once widely taught in schools, purported to show how each area of the tongue was solely responsible for one of 'the four basic tastes' – sweet, sour, bitter and salty. In fact, this is quite wrong. Wherever you have taste buds – all over the tongue and the roof of the mouth – you can detect all tastes more or less equally. Plus, there are more than four basic ones.

According to the tongue map, the tip of the tongue tasted sweet things and the back, bitter ones. The sides of the tongue at the front were for tasting salt while the sides at the back did sour. The map was based on German research published in 1901 but an influential Harvard psychologist with the unfortunate name of Edwin Boring (1886–1968) mistranslated it. What the original research had shown was that the human tongue has areas of *relative* sensitivity to different tastes – but Boring's translation stated that each could *only* be tasted in one zone.

What is really mysterious about the tongue map is that it was the official truth for such a long time, even though it's so easily disproved. (Just put some sugar on the part of your tongue that the map says tastes only salt.) It wasn't until 1974 that another American scientist, Dr Virginia Collings, re-examined the original theory. She showed that, though sensitivity to the four main tastes did vary around the tongue, it was only to an insignificant degree. She also demonstrated that all taste buds taste all tastes.

The other myth the tongue map perpetuated was that there are only four basic tastes. There are at least five. Umami is the taste of protein in savoury foods such as bacon, cheese, seaweed or Marmite. It was first identified by Professor Kikunae Ikeda, professor of chemistry at Tokyo

University, as long ago as 1908, but was only formally confirmed as the 'true' fifth taste in 2000 when researchers at the University of Miami discovered protein receptors on the human tongue.

'Umami' is derived from *umai*, the word for 'tasty' in Japanese. Professor Ikeda found out that its key ingredient is monosodium glutamate, now known as MSG. Ikeda was shrewd – he sold his recipe for it to the Ajinomoto Company, which still holds one third of the 1.5-million-ton global annual market for synthetic MSG.

Given the importance of protein in our diet, it makes sense for umami to stimulate the pleasure centre of our brains. A robust, mature red wine, for example, has an 'umami' taste. A bitter taste, by contrast, alerts us to the possibility of danger.

'Taste' shouldn't be confused with *flavour*, which is a broader experience involving not just taste, but also smell, sight, touch and even hearing (it's thought that the sound of crunchy food contributes to its flavour).

Lexical-gustatory synaesthesia is a rare condition whereby taste and language are confused in the brain, so that each word has a specific taste. In one experiment a woman tasted tuna whenever she thought of the word 'castanet'.

What does cracking your knuckles do?

Don't worry: it won't cause arthritis. At worst, it might leave you with a limp handshake.

We know this because of the selfless dedication of Dr Donald L. Unger, an octogenarian physician from California. Warned as a child by his mother that if he didn't stop cracking his knuckles he would end up with arthritis, he embarked on an experiment, cracking the knuckles of his left hand (but not those of his right) every day for more than sixty years. His conclusion was that knuckle-cracking had no serious effect. At the end of the experiment, he claims, he 'looked up to the heavens and said: "Mother, you were wrong, you were wrong, you were wrong."' His efforts won him the 2009 IgNobel prize for Medicine, a parody of the Nobel Prize started in 1991 and awarded annually for improbable research that 'first makes us laugh and then makes us think'.

This is not to say that knuckle-cracking is entirely harmless: it can make your joints swell and inflame your ligaments, and, over time, can reduce the strength of your grip.

Our finger joints, like most moving joints in our bodies, are called synovial joints because they contain a strange liquid called synovial fluid whose job is to cushion and lubricate the joint. But it doesn't 'flow' as most bodily fluids do: it has a thick, gel-like consistency, rather like egg white (hence the word *synovial*, from the Greek *syn-*, 'with', and Latin *ovum*, 'egg'). Between each joint is a capsule, filled with synovial fluid and sealed by a membrane. When you pull the bones apart, the membrane stretches. This reduces the pressure inside the capsule and, as the fluid moves to fill the vacuum, bubbles of carbon dioxide form. The 'pop' that we hear is the bubbles *forming* (not bursting) inside the capsule.

If you X-ray a joint just after it has been cracked, the bubbles of carbon dioxide are clearly visible. The joint can't be cracked again until they've dissolved back into the fluid, which explains why you can't crack the same knuckle repeatedly.

The cracking of knuckles (and the creaking of joints) has a scientific name: *crepitus*, from the Latin *crepare*, 'to crack'.

Arthritis comes from the Greek *arthron*, 'joint', and *-itis*, a suffix denoting 'inflammation'. It's been around as long as animals have had articulated skeletons (there is evidence that some dinosaurs' ankle joints were arthritic). The first evidence of human arthritis can be found in ancient Egyptian mummies that date back to 4500 BC.

Arthritis comes in over a hundred different forms and afflicts all ages and ethnic groups. After stress, it's responsible for more lost working days in the UK than any other medical condition, at an estimated annual cost of £5.8 billion. A quarter of all adult Britons consult their GP each year with arthritis-related complaints.

Cracked knuckles are responsible for none of them.

What are the symptoms of leprosy?

In the popular mind, lepers have rotting flesh and parts of their bodies drop off.

It doesn't work like that. Leprosy – or Hansen's disease as it's now called – is an infectious bacterial disease that affects the skin and damages nerve-endings. This means that sufferers can't feel pain and so repeatedly injure their fingers and toes. Over time these wounds become infected and leave disfiguring scars.

It is these injuries, not the disease itself, that cause the deformities leprosy is famous for. People can live into old age with the disease as it doesn't attack vital organs but, left untreated, it can cause crippling disabilities and even blindness.

Leprosy is from the Greek *lepros* ('scaly'). Ironically, it comes from the same root as the word *Lepidoptera* ('scale wings'), the scientific name for butterflies. For many centuries, the word 'leprosy' was used indiscriminately to cover a broad range of disfiguring skin diseases. A 'leper' might just as easily have been someone with a bad case of psoriasis. It wasn't until 1873, when the Norwegian physician Gerhard Armauer Hansen (1841–1912) identified *Mycobacterium leprae* as the cause of leprosy, that its accurate diagnosis was possible. Hansen's discovery was groundbreaking. It was the first time a bacterium had been proven to cause a disease in humans.

Until this point, it had been assumed that leprosy was hereditary because, despite its scary reputation, it's quite difficult to catch. About 95 per cent of people are naturally resistant to the bacterium, and even those who aren't require prolonged close contact to become infected. In 1984, to get this point across, Pope John Paul II kissed a number of lepers in a South Korean leper colony.

The good news is that Hansen's disease has been treatable with antibiotics since 1941. Over the last twenty years, 15 million patients have been cured but there are still some 250,000 new cases a year, and a million people worldwide are receiving, or are in need of, treatment. In 2009 121 countries recorded cases of leprosy. Even the USA recorded 150 and the UK twelve. More than half of all new cases are reported in India. Although 150,000 new cases a year sounds high, this is an infection rate of less than 1 in 10,000. According to World Health Organization standards, this officially qualifies leprosy for 'eliminated' status.

Europe's only remaining leper colony is in Tichilesti in Romania. In 1991 the colony was opened and residents were free to leave. Many of them had known nothing else since childhood and decided to stay on: the colony is more like a village than a hospital, with its own farm, two churches and even a vineyard,

Leprosy is a rare example of a bacterial disease that almost exclusively attacks humans: the only other animals that can catch leprosy naturally are chimpanzees, mangabey monkeys and nine-banded armadillos.

Why did lepers start carrying bells?

Leper's bells were designed to attract people, not to keep them away.

From the earliest times, lepers were forced to live separately. In Europe they were legally forbidden to marry, make a will or appear in court – and were only allowed to talk to a non-leper if they stood downwind. In the Old Testament, God himself instructs Moses to 'put out of the camp every leper'.

This was because leprosy was regarded as a punishment rather than an infectious disease: it was an outer 'uncleanness' caused by inner sin, something that God would smite you with if you harboured lustful or heretical thoughts. It was the priest, not the doctor, who declared you a leper.

In the early twelfth century two things happened to change this attitude. The first was that a number of Christian soldiers returning home from the First Crusade of 1099 were found to have picked up the disease. The second was a shift in the theological consensus concerning a key passage in the Bible. Referring to the Messiah, the prophet Isaiah wrote: 'We did esteem him stricken, smitten of God, and afflicted.' The Hebrew for 'smitten' is *nagua*. When some unknown Biblical scholar realised that everywhere else the word occurs in the Old Testament it means specifically 'smitten with leprosy', the inescapable conclusion was that Isaiah had predicted Jesus would suffer on our behalf by being treated like a leper.

The effect was to rebrand leprosy as a 'holy disease'. The

stricken Crusaders, far from being punished, were being marked out by God for special reward. St Francis of Assisi (1182–1226) overcame his revulsion to embrace a leper and made the care of lepers a central part of the monastic order he founded. Henry I's daughter, Matilda (1102–67), established a hospital for lepers at Holborn in London and publicly washed and kissed their feet. All over Europe monarchs and aristocrats competed with one another to endow leper colonies.

Lepers themselves were granted special privileges: the most important being the right to beg. In some places they were entitled to a fixed portion of all the produce sold on market day. For 200 years, although they lived separately, they mingled freely at shrines and travelled on pilgrimages. This was when the practice of lepers carrying bells and rattles started. They were used, not to warn people away, but to attract donations from them: helping a leper was a sacred act.

Attitudes hardened again after the Black Death (1348–50) – the plague was sometimes called 'a leprosy' – but, by the mid-fifteenth century, it hardly mattered: lepers had all but disappeared from Britain.

Lepers were particularly vulnerable to bubonic plague and tuberculosis (the TB bacterium is leprosy's closest bacterial relative). As waves of infectious diseases spread across Europe in the fourteenth and fifteenth centuries, the lepers' already weakened immune systems succumbed first. Their numbers declined; soon there were too few of them left to spread the disease and their bells stopped ringing for good.

STEPHEN *Why did lepers carry bells?*
ALAN *They were doing an act, you know, one of those bell-ringing acts. For 'A Leper's Got Talent'.*

Who wore horned helmets?

Not Viking warriors but Celtic priests.

None of the horned helmets discovered in Europe by archaeologists can be dated to the Viking Age (AD 700–1100). Most are Celtic and were produced during the Iron Age (800 BC–AD 100), including the famous helmet found in the Thames in the 1860s and now displayed in the British Museum. The lightness of its metal and its fine decoration strongly suggest that the Thames helmet must have been worn for ceremonial occasions rather than in battle. To a modern observer, the 'horns' are more like the cones on Madonna's famously pointy bra.

Technically speaking, the only authentic Viking helmet ever found dates from the tenth century AD (though it's in the same style as the pre-Viking Vendel period helmets). Made from iron plate, it was found inside the burial mound of a Viking chieftain and resembles a peaked cap with built in eye-protectors that look like iron-rimmed specs. But there's not even a hint of a horn. It's likely that only senior Vikings wore metal helmets, if they wore them at all. The surviving illustrations from the period show most warriors wearing simple leather skullcaps or fighting bareheaded.

The association of horned helmets with Vikings dates back no further than the nineteenth century, a period when many imperial European nations were re-inventing their mythic heritage. In Britain Druids and the Arthurian legends were all the rage; the Germans were lapping up operas about medieval Teutonic knights; and, not to be outdone, Scandinavians were dusting off their Old Norse sagas. In one of these, a republished edition of *Frithiof's Saga,* a Swedish illustrator called Gustav Malmström included small horns and dragon wings on the hero's headgear.

Frithiof's Saga (1825) became an international hit. Until

then the word 'Viking' was virtually unknown in English ('Dane' or 'Norseman' were the usual terms), so the saga literally made the Vikings' name – and their supposed horned helmets created a powerful visual image of them that has lasted to this day.

On the other hand, the tradition of adorning the head with horns for religious purposes seems to have been widespread across the Celtic world. There are several depictions of the god Cernunnos sporting enormous antlers and, in the first century BC, the Greek historian Diodorus Siculus described the Gauls as having helmets with horns, antlers or even whole animals attached. No one knows exactly what Celtic religious rituals involved, but it is likely that the ceremonial antlers were a symbol of fertility and rebirth, because they are shed and regrown each year.

The cern element in Cernunnos means 'horn' in Old Irish and is derived from an Indo-European root that also gives us unicorn, keratin (the substance horn is made from) and corn (a patch of hard, hoof-like skin).

Can you name an animal with horns?

Strictly speaking, not all the pointed projections that stick out of an animal's head are horns.

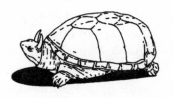

True horns have a permanent bone core surrounded by compacted strands of a protein called keratin – the same stuff that human hair and nails are made from. Animals that have them include cattle, buffalo, sheep, antelopes and horned lizards.

Animals with pointed projections that *aren't* horns include rhinos (their 'horns' are made of keratin but have no bone core); deer (they have antlers which are made of bone, but covered in velvety skin not keratin, and they drop off and are regrown each year); giraffes (they have ossicones – literally 'big bones' – covered with furry skin but not keratin); and elephants, pigs, walruses and narwhals (they all have tusks, which are overgrown teeth, made of ivory).

Keratin is a remarkable substance. In its softer alpha form, it is what ensures our skin is flexible and waterproof and, as well as producing horn, forms the hair, fur, claws, hooves and nails of mammals. In its harder beta form, it makes the shells and scales of reptiles and the feathers and beaks of birds.

Horns, tusks and antlers have a variety of functions – they can be used as tools, or weapons, or to attract a mate – but only true horns are used to cool down. The blood vessels surrounding the bone core turn the whole horn into a device similar to a car radiator, cooling the liquid by spreading its exposure to the air, in much the same way an elephant uses its large ears. Watusi cattle, a longhorn variety native to central Africa, have enormous horns for this reason. The largest true horns ever recorded belong to a Watusi bull called Lurch: they measured 92.5 centimetres (3 feet) long and weighed 45 kilograms (7 stones) each.

When the keratinous part of a true horn is slid off its bone core, it becomes a useful hollow object. Since prehistory, humans used these for drinking vessels and musical instruments and, later, to carry gunpowder in. The substance known as 'horn' was carved into buttons, handles and combs, made into book bindings or windows (it is translucent if shaved thinly) and boiled down for glue.

There are various accounts of humans growing 'horns' of the non-bony type. One of the strangest concerns Anna Schimper, 'the horned nun of Filzen'. In 1795 her nunnery in the Rhineland was occupied by French troops and the nuns evicted. The shock sent Anna mad and she was committed to an asylum. After years spent banging her head against a table, a horn started to grow from the bump on her forehead. The more it grew, the less deranged she became until she was soon sane enough to return to the nunnery, where she became abbess.

By 1834 her horn had grown to such a length that it was hard to conceal under her wimple, so she decided to have it removed. Although she was eighty-seven and the operation was both bloody and painful, she survived and lived for two more years. By the time she died her mysterious therapeutic horn had started to grow again.

How do you milk a yak?

You don't – any more than you would milk a bull.

Yaks are the males of the species *Bos grunniens* (Latin for 'grunting ox'), and they live in Tibet and Nepal. Westerners who speak of milking yaks are a staple butt of Tibetan jokes.

The female of the species is called a 'dri' or 'nak'. Their milk contains twice as much fat as that of lowland cows. Contrary to some web sources, it is not pink: on the rare occasions it is drunk, blood is sometimes added for flavour. It is golden-coloured and mainly made into yoghurt, cheese and butter. Tibetans put butter in their tea, use it for face lotion and lamp fuel and make it into ritual sculptures.

In Lhasa, fresh yak meat is for sale, draped in slabs over the branches of trees, or stacked in wheelbarrows direct from the slaughterhouse. Butchery is a hereditary trade and all butchers are Muslims. Rancid butter is piled directly on to the paving stones. The whole of Tibet smells of dri butter.

Wild yaks can be 1.95 metres (6 feet 5 inches) at the shoulder; domestic yaks are usually half that height. To operate effectively in the thin air at heights of 5,500 metres (18,000 feet) and temperatures of –40°C (or –40°F – they are the same at that value), yak blood cells are half the size and three times as numerous as those of ordinary cattle.

Yak bones are used to make jewellery and tent fastenings. The horns are carved into knife handles and musical instruments. The tails are exported to India where they are used as fly whisks. The dung is collected and burnt as fuel.

Yaks have the longest hair of any animal. It can grow to be 60 centimetres (2 feet) long on the torso and is used to make rope, clothing, bags, sacks, shoes, tents and coracles. In the seventeenth and eighteenth centuries, it was the most sought-after material (after human hair) for making gentlemen's wigs.

The fashion for wearing wigs began with Louis XIII (1601–43) – who went prematurely bald in 1624 – and ended with the French Revolution. Wigs were often as expensive as the rest of a man's clothing put together. Today, the BBC can call upon yak-hair wigs from the 10,000 false hair items available to it, and fancy-dress shops offer Santa Claus beards in 100 per cent yak hair.

Dob-dobs were monks from the Se-ra monastery in Tibet who specialised in the collection of yak dung. By the late nineteenth century they'd evolved into a combination of monastic police force and predatory gay mafia. They would occasionally venture down to the nearby city of Lhasa to pick fights and kidnap young boys. They were easily recognised because they kept the skirts of their habits kilted up higher than regular Buddhist monks. This gave them a bulky look round the thighs, which they exaggerated by swinging their buttocks as they walked.

STEPHEN *Whose job is it in Tibet to milk the yaks?*
ROGER McGOUGH *I know who cleans the hooves.*
STEPHEN *Who's that?*
ROGER *Yaksmiths.*

What do you say to get a husky to move?

Just about anything except 'Mush!' You can call 'Hike!', 'Hike on!', 'Ready!', 'Let's go!', or simply 'OK!' – but a sled driver will only shout 'Mush!' when he doesn't want to disappoint the tourists.

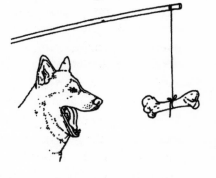

'Mush', far from being an authentic Inuit word, is a Hollywood mishearing of the command given by French Canadian sled drivers: *Marche!* It's most unlikely that any real-life husky handler ever said 'Mush!', but it's certainly not favoured today. It's too soft a sound for the dogs to hear clearly.

Stopping sled dogs is the problem, not starting them. They are born to run. If they ever get free, they'll just head for the horizon until exhaustion overtakes them and you'll never see them again. While they're in harness, though, yelling 'Whoa!' and standing on the sled's brake pad should be enough to hold them. To get them to turn right, use 'Gee!' and for left 'Haw!' (no, they're not Inuit words either). Only the lead dog needs to understand your commands; the rest just follow the leader.

Huskies, the best known of the many kinds of dog that have been used to pull sleds, were originally bred for winter transport by the Chukchi people of Siberia. In the summer, the dogs ran free, fending for themselves. This combination of tameness and independence made them perfect working dogs.

They're surprisingly small – weighing between 15 and 25 kilograms (35–55 pounds) – but those who race huskies for sport prefer dogs with outsize appetites. After marathon runs, covering as much as 160 kilometres (100 miles) in twenty-four hours, they will need to eat and drink enthusiastically to replace lost calories and prevent dehydration.

If you're thinking of getting a husky as a pet, you might want to take some advice from the Siberian Husky Club of Great Britain concerning the breed's 'bad points'. Siberian huskies have no guarding instinct: they will greet a burglar with the same sloppy kiss they give their master. They howl like wolves when happy. They're notorious killers of pets and livestock: if you take them for walks, they have to be kept on a lead. They must have company: they'll wreck your home if you leave them alone. They'll wreck your garden, in any case – and you'll need a 1.8-metre (6-foot) fence to keep them in it. Also, they moult massively – twice a year. In conclusion, the Club says, the Siberian husky isn't suitable for anyone looking for a 'civilised' dog.

The Swiss polar explorer Xavier Mertz (1883–1913) is remembered today as the first person to die of vitamin A poisoning. He was on a three-man mapping mission to the interior of Antarctica when one of the team, most of the sleds and half the dogs fell into a crevasse. On the 480 kilometre (300-mile) trek home, the two survivors were forced to eat the remaining dogs – a necessity which caused Mertz (who was a vegetarian) great anguish. Both men became ill, but Mertz died.

The polar food chain is based on marine algae that are rich in vitamin A. The further up the chain you go, the more it concentrates. Huskies – like seals and polar bears – have evolved to cope with it. Humans haven't. There is enough Vitamin A in just 100 g (3½ ounces) of husky liver to kill a grown man.

On which day should you open the first door on an Advent calendar?

Advent usually starts in November, not on 1 December.

In the Western Christian tradition, Advent begins on Advent Sunday, the fourth Sunday before Christmas, which also begins the Church's year. This can occur on any day between 27 November and 3 December, so there's only a one-in-seven chance of it falling on 1 December. As a result, Advent varies in length from twenty-two to twenty-eight days. The next time Advent Sunday falls on 1 December will be in 2013. For five of the next seven years, Advent will begin in November.

Not that anyone seems to care. Despite their name, 'Advent' calendars are now firmly established as a secular custom and the first door is opened (or the first chocolate consumed) on 1 December, a date whose main function is to remind us that there are only twenty-four shopping days to Christmas. In the UK and USA, a quarter of all personal spending for the year takes place in December.

Counting down the days to Christmas grew up among German Lutherans in the early nineteenth century. At first, they would either light a candle every day or cross off each day on a blackboard. Then, in the 1850s, German children started to draw their own home-made Advent calendars. It wasn't until 1908 that Gerhard Lang (1881–1974), of the Bavarian publishers Reichhold & Lang, devised a commercial version. It was a piece of card accompanied by a packet of twenty-four small illustrations that could be glued on for each day of the season.

Because it wasn't practical to manufacture a different number of stickers each year, this was the moment that Advent became a standard twenty-four days long and the tradition of starting the calendar on 1 December began. By 1920 Lang had introduced doors that opened, and his invention was spreading across Europe. It was known as the 'Munich Christmas Calendar'.

Lang's business failed in the 1930s – Hitler's close association with Munich can't have helped – but after the war, in 1946, another German publisher, Richard Sellmer from Stuttgart, revived the idea. He focused his efforts on the US market, setting up a charity endorsed by President Eisenhower and his family. In 1953 he acquired the US patent, and the calendar became an immediate success, with Sellmer earning the title of 'the General Secretary of Father Christmas'. His company still produces more than a million calendars a year in twenty-five countries. The first Advent calendars containing chocolate were produced by Cadbury in 1958.

Advent comes from the Latin *adventus*, meaning 'arrival', and it was meant to be a season of fasting and contemplation, in preparation for the feast of Christmas.

Despite this, it often started with the raucous celebration of St Andrew's Day on 30 November. 'Tandrew' customs included schoolchildren locking their teachers out of the classroom, organised squirrel hunts and cross-dressing. An 1851 account describes how 'women might be seen walking about in male attire, while men and boys clothed in female dress visited each other's cottages, drinking hot "eldern wine", the staple beverage of the season'.

How many days are there in Lent?

Forty-six. Or forty-four if you're a Catholic.

Lent runs from midday on Ash Wednesday to midnight on Holy Saturday, the day before Easter Sunday. For Catholics it ends two days earlier, at midnight on Maundy Thursday. The 'forty days' of Lent commemorate the forty days that Jesus (and before him, Moses) spent fasting and praying in the wilderness, but the Sundays don't count because you aren't supposed to fast on them.

The technical term for the period is *quadragesima*, Latin for 'fortieth'. In the late Middle Ages, when preachers in Britain began using English instead of Latin, they cast around for a simple but appropriate word to replace it, and fastened on 'Lent' – which then just meant 'Spring' and was related to the days 'lengthening'.

The reason why penance and fasting are suspended for the six Sundays that fall during Lent is that they are considered celebratory tasters for Easter Day, the most important feast of the Christian year.

Some may consider this weak-willed or against the spirit of the thing, but the terms of the Lenten fast have always been treated as negotiable. Even in the sixth century, when Pope Gregory the Great first came up with the idea of giving up meat, milk, cheese, butter and eggs for forty days, it was loosely interpreted. The Celtic church advised fasting during the day but having a hearty supper of bread, eggs and milk in the evening. In tenth-century England, Archbishop Aelfric went the other way and took a hard-line approach – banning sex, fighting and fish as well.

In general, though, fish have always been the saving grace of Lent. Henry VIII encouraged Lent to support the nation's fishing industry. As hungry Christians carried the Good News to distant climes, the definition of 'fish' became quite flexible.

At various times, muskrat, beaver and barnacle geese have all been officially counted as 'fish' – as has the capybara, a kind of giant South American guinea pig that can stay underwater for five minutes. In Venezuela today it forms a magnificent centrepiece for Lenten feasts: it's the world's largest rodent. Perhaps because of all these shenanigans, or perhaps because fasting implies the value of its opposite (feasting), the Puritans abolished Lent completely in 1645.

Easter is a 'moveable feast', calculated according to a complex formula that the Church took centuries to agree. It moves about because it has to fall on a Sunday but must never coincide with the Jewish Passover, which was dishonoured when the Crucifixion was held on the same day. There are thirty-five possible dates for Easter. The earliest in the year, 22 March, last fell in 1818 and won't happen again until 2285. The latest is 25 April, which last happened in 1943 and is next due in 2038. The whole sequence repeats itself once every 5.7 million years.

You might think a fixed date would be simpler. The confectionery industry certainly does – 10 per cent of the UK's annual chocolate sales take place in the run-up to Easter. As long ago as the 1920s, they successfully lobbied Parliament to fix it as the first Sunday after the second Saturday in April. The Easter Act (1928) was even passed but, despite having the support of both main churches, it was never implemented as law. No one knows why.

How did the Church of England react to Darwin's Theory of Evolution?

Rather positively, on the whole.

In 1860, the year after the publication of *On the Origin of Species*, there was a debate at Oxford University between Samuel Wilberforce, Bishop of London, and one of the theory's fiercest supporters, T. H. Huxley (known as 'Darwin's

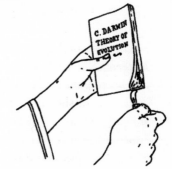

bulldog'). At one point the Bishop sarcastically asked Huxley whether he was descended from a monkey on his grandfather's or his grandmother's side. But this wasn't typical of the Church of England's reaction in general.

Much mainstream biblical scholarship in the nineteenth century viewed the Bible as a historical document backed up by archaeological evidence, rather than as the actual word of God. As a result, many senior Victorian Anglicans already thought of the Bible in the same way moderate contemporary Christians do: as a series of metaphors rather than a literal account.

In the same year as the Oxford debate, Frederick Temple, headmaster of Rugby School and later Archbishop of Canterbury, gave a sermon praising Darwin. He said that scientists could have all the laws in the universe they liked, but that 'the finger of God' would be in all of them. The influential author Rev. Charles Kingsley also congratulated Darwin. 'Even better than making the world,' Kingsley wrote to him, 'God makes the world make itself!'

By the time Darwin himself addressed the debate about human origins directly – in *The Descent of Man* (1871) – there were at least as many leading churchmen who had accepted his theory on similar grounds as those (like Wilberforce) who still opposed it. At the same time, many scientists (Huxley included) continued to support compulsory Bible study in schools.

On the Origin of Species by Means of Natural Selection, or the Preservation of Favoured Races in the Struggle for Life — as it was originally called — was the first genuinely popular work of scientific theory. Published by John Murray, the first print run sold out before it had even been printed and Darwin produced another five revised editions. Many of the initial reviews were hostile, anti-evolution organisations were formed, and Darwin was often ridiculed, but the mockery came as much from politicians and editors as from churchmen. Darwin had to get used to pictures of his head on a monkey's body in newspapers, and when he went to collect his honorary degree from Cambridge University, students dangled a stuffed monkey from the roof.

Sometimes his work was simply ignored. Just before *On the Origin of Species* came out, in 1859, the president of London's Geological Society awarded Darwin a medal of honour for his geological expeditions to the Andes and for his four-volume work on barnacles without even mentioning the book.

Darwin lost his own faith, but he hadn't intentionally set out to subvert religion. He always claimed he was an agnostic, not an atheist. And the Anglican Church certainly didn't abandon him. When he died in 1882, it awarded him its highest accolade. He was buried in Westminster Abbey, next to England's greatest scientists Michael Faraday and Isaac Newton.

Who is the only person on Earth who can never be wrong?

No, not even the Pope is 'always right'. He can still commit sins and not everything he says is 'infallible'.

The First Vatican Council introduced the Doctrine of Papal Infallibility on 18 July 1870. Under the doctrine, certain specific statements by the Pope are preserved forever from any possibility of error by the action of the Holy Spirit. This does not mean that *all* the Pope's private or public statements are beyond argument. Many of the Church's strictest laws (those against contraception, for example) are binding on all Catholics, but are not protected by the doctrine of papal in-fallibility. Nor does the doctrine imply that the Pope himself is 'impeccable', or 'incapable of sin' (*peccare* is Latin for 'to sin').

For a papal statement to be 'infallible' it has to fulfil strict conditions. The Pope must be speaking *ex cathedra* (literally, 'from his chair'), in his official capacity as pastor of all Christians, not as a private individual. He has to make it clear he is pronouncing on a doctrine of faith or morals and that this is the last word on the matter. Finally, he must confirm that the statement binds the whole Church and that everyone must agree to it, on pain of what the Catholic Church calls 'spiritual shipwreck'.

An infallible teaching by a pope can contradict previous Church teachings (as long as they were not themselves issued infallibly) but the Pope cannot use his infallibility to make other people's statements retrospectively infallible by agreeing with them. Nor is the whole of a statement made *ex cathedra* necessarily infallible: the Pope has to make clear which bit is which.

This is quite a tall order, even for a pope, so it isn't surprising that, since 1870, only one infallible papal statement has actually been issued. In 1950 Pope Pius XII stated that the Virgin Mary was bodily taken up to Heaven at the end of her life. This is known as the Assumption of the Blessed Virgin Mary, and it is celebrated on 15 August. The Pope did this because, although the Assumption had been taught and observed since the sixth century, it had no direct scriptural authority. By making it a dogma (from the Greek verb *dokein*, 'to seem good'), all doubt was removed (although theologians still can't agree whether Mary was carried up to Heaven before or after she died).

Though only one pope has ever made only one infallible statement, the Vatican has since decided that the content of Pope John Paul II's 1994 pronouncement *Ordinatio Sacerdotalis* ('Ordination to the Priesthood'), in which it was made explicit that Roman Catholic priests have to be men, *was* infallible even though the Pope had failed to say so at the time.

If the Vatican is correct, any future pope who permits female priests will instantly excommunicate himself.

What are the four main religions of India?

Hinduism, Islam, Christianity and Sikhism in that order. Not Buddhism: although Buddhism was founded in India, its spiritual home today is Tibet.

The figures from the latest available census (2001) are: Hindu 80.5 per cent, Muslim 13.4 per cent, Christian 2.3 per cent and Sikh 1.9 per cent. More than three-quarters of the population of India describe themselves as followers of Hinduism, the oldest continually practised faith in the world, and India's Muslim community, at around 145 million, is the third largest in the world, after Indonesia and Pakistan. There are about 25 million Christians in India (almost as many as the UK's 29 million) and 15 million Sikhs.

Buddhists in India account for only 0.7 per cent of the population. New Zealand has a higher percentage of people professing Buddhism (1.08 per cent) than India does. The members of the influential Indian ascetic sect known as Jainism are even fewer in number – about 0.5 per cent. The number of Indian atheists is smallest of all: only 0.1 per cent of the population are rated 'unspecified' by the census.

Buddhism was founded in India and grew rapidly there for a thousand years. But most of its adherents now live in China (notably in Tibet where, until quite recently, one in every six males was a Buddhist monk) as well as Indochina and Japan. It is also the majority religion in Sri Lanka.

Buddhism disappeared gradually from India from the sixth century AD. Though Hinduism absorbed many of its practices (such as vegetarianism) and accepted Buddha into the pantheon of gods, Buddhism was a monastic religion, based on detachment and meditation. This made it less attractive to the state rulers of India who liked to court popularity by staging lavish and colourful Hindu festivals. With the arrival of Islam in the tenth century, Buddhism was finally relegated to its present 'tiny minority' status.

This is only 'tiny' in relative terms. 0.7 per cent of the population of India is 7.5 million people, making it the ninth largest Buddhist community in the world.

There are also twice as many Buddhists as Jains in India. Mahavira (599–527 BC), whose name means 'Great Hero', founded Jainism in north-east India, in the same area and at almost the same time as the Buddha (563–483 BC), whose name means 'Awakened One'. Both men were born to high-caste families, which they both abandoned at about the age of thirty. Mahavira lived as an ascetic, much of the time naked.

Though Jainism declares that everything in the universe, including non-living things, has a soul, it is atheistic in nature and the existence of God is seen as an irrelevance. They believe the taking of any life is a sin and Orthodox Jain monks wear a net over their mouths to avoid swallowing spiders and gently sweep the street before them as they walk to avoid crushing insects.

Gandhi was greatly influenced by Jainism. The Jains' symbol is the *fylfot*, an old English word for the good luck sign better known as the swastika.

From which country did the Gypsies originate?

The Gypsies, or *Romani*, are not from Egypt, or Rome or Romania. Their ancestral home was India.

There are an estimated 10 million Romani people spread across Europe, Asia and the Americas, of which the biggest concentration are the Roma of Central and Eastern Europe. From their first arrival in Europe in the fourteenth century they have travelled under many different names: 'gypsy' and the Spanish *gitano* are just two, and both derive from the mistaken assumption that they came from Egypt. *Romani*, the name they call themselves, doesn't come from a geographic area at all, but from their word *Rom*, meaning 'man'.

Romani had survived as an oral rather than a written language and it wasn't until the mid-nineteenth century that linguists were able to solve the puzzle of its origin. Analysis of the structure and vocabulary confirmed Romani as an Indo-European language descended from Sanskrit, the ancient language of northern India – just like Hindi, Bengali, Gujarati and Punjabi. Romani also contains elements of Greek, Turkish and Iranian, which suggest that they migrated out of India, through Turkey and eventually into Europe.

A century and a half later, geneticists have come to the same conclusion. In 2003 several hundred Romani were analysed for evidence of five genetic mutations linked to certain diseases. The results confirmed that a founder group of perhaps a thousand Romani emerged from India in AD 1000 and then spread out in smaller units. This explains the complex pattern of Romani dialects that are found all across Europe.

For most of the last thousand years, the ability of the Romani to move and adapt has only been matched by the persecution they have suffered at the hands of the sedentary populations they encountered. Forced into slavery in Eastern Europe, ghettoised in Spain, marked out by head shaving and ear removal in France and England, they have been discriminated against legally and socially in every state they have travelled through.

Their painful history culminated in the Nazi regime's attempt at genocide, known as the *Porjamos* ('the devouring' in Romani). This killed an estimated 1.5 million people between 1935 and 1945. And, as recently as 2008, the Italian government blamed a rise in city crime specifically on Romani migration, describing their presence as a 'national emergency'.

The Romani have enriched European culture for centuries with music, stories and language. A surprising number of English words are borrowed from them, including pal (from *phal*, 'friend'); lollipop (from *loli phabai*, 'red apple'); gaff, in the sense of a place (from *gav*, 'town'); nark, meaning 'informant' (from *naak*, 'nose') and, most prominently in recent times, chav – which comes from the Romani *chavi* meaning 'young boy'.

What was shocking about the first cancan dancers?

It wasn't young women showing their knickers. The cancan started as a dance for both men and women – and neither was saucily dressed. The familiar line of whooping, high-kicking girls didn't come along till almost a hundred years later.

The cancan originated in the working-class dance halls of Montparnasse in the Paris of the 1830s, where it was first known as the *chahut* (meaning 'uproar'). It was for men and women, dancing in quartets, and it quickly became the rock-and-roll of its day, shocking polite society by the amount of bodily contact it allowed between the couples. A contemporary account makes it sound like a demented tango: 'They mingle, cross, part, meet again, with a swiftness and fire that must be felt to be described.' On a visit to Paris, the German poet Heinrich Heine (1797–1856) called the *chahut* a 'satanic ruction'.

Some of the earliest *chahut* stars were men, whose athletic high-kicks and mid-air splits (or *grand écart*) were copied from stage acrobats of the time. When women began to try the high-kicks, they often revealed more than just their athleticism. As the fashion for wider hoop-reinforced skirts brought with it ever-frillier layers of undergarment, the kicking, skirt-lifting and bottom-waggling began to take over. The *chahut* was a dance for everyone, but the *cancan* that evolved from it was the pole dance of the 1860s, performed on stage by semi-professional 'dancers' (often a euphemism for prostitutes).

The cancan's reputation grew increasingly sensational. An attempt to bring it to Moscow in the mid-1850s led Tsar Nicholas I to ban the dance, imprison the promoter and deport the performers under armed Cossack guard. The first 'French Cancan' was staged in England in 1861 by the impresario Charles Morton (1819–1904) in his new Oxford Street music hall. It wasn't particularly French (the cancan quartet were mostly Hungarian) but it was an immediate hit with the audience and the police threatened the theatre with closure for promoting indecency.

By the time the great Parisian cabaret clubs opened at the end of the century, female cancan dancers like Jane Avril (immortalised in Toulouse-Lautrec's famous poster) and La Goulue (who danced in expensive clothes, borrowed from her mother's laundry business) had become Paris's highest-earning celebrities. Their provocative routines at the Folies Bergère and the Moulin Rouge were incorporated into the cancan chorus lines that started in the 1920s and which still attracts the tourists to Paris today.

But high-kicks and skirt twirls weren't invented in Paris in the nineteenth century. A country dance in sixteenth-century Brittany had women doing high-kicks in billowy skirts, and there are reliefs of ancient Egyptians doing something similar at the Tomb of Mehu in Saqqara. They date back to 2400 BC.

The cancan bears out George Bernard Shaw's observation that dance is 'the vertical expression of a horizontal desire, legalized by music'. It probably gets its name from the French verb *cancaner*, which means 'to quack' — ducks are great bottom-wagglers. *Cancaner* also means 'to spread scandal'.

Where does tartan come from?

Tartan isn't particularly Scottish.

Making cloth involves inter-lacing vertical and horizontal threads called the *warp* and the *weft*. This produces an almost infinite possibility for bands and

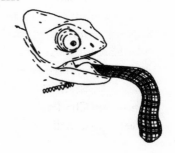

blocks of colour. Patterns similar to those we call 'tartan' have appeared in almost every culture since the invention of weaving in prehistoric times.

Nor is the word itself Scottish. First recorded in English in 1454, it probably comes from the French *tiretaine*, meaning 'strong, coarse fabric'. In medieval Scotland, 'tartan' merely meant woven (as opposed to knitted) cloth. Plaid, now used interchangeably with tartan, was originally Gaelic for blanket. By the late sixteenth century, individual weavers all over the Highlands were producing their own tartan cloths known as 'setts', much as the weavers of Harris do today with tweed. And, just as there are 4,000 registered patterns of tweed, what drove the patterns of the setts was the taste and skill of the individual weaver, the availability of coloured dyes and the quality of the local wool. It had nothing to do with any official 'clan' identity.

The original kilt was a much longer, over-the-shoulder garment, shunned by most lowland Scots and banned by the British after the defeat of the Jacobite Rebellion in 1745. The short kilt was the invention of an English industrialist, Thomas Rawlinson, who opened an ironworks in the Highlands in the mid-eighteenth century and needed something practical for his local workers to wear.

At the time English regiments stationed in Scotland were filled with lowland Scots, loyal to the Crown but keen to create an identity distinct from other British regiments. What we now call 'traditional' Scottish dress (short kilt, sporran, dirk) was the creation of these regiments and they were the first to commission regimental tartans such as the Black Watch. A growing sense of 'Scottishness' turned into a full-scale Scottish Revival led by Romantic writers like Sir Walter Scott (1771–1832). By the 1820s kilts, ballads, Highland games and retellings of Scottish legends were the height of fashion. The high point was the state visit of King George IV to Edinburgh in 1822 – the first by an English monarch for 170 years, and expertly stage-managed by Scott himself.

'Clan tartans' were a hoax from the beginning. John and Charles Allen, two brothers claiming to be Bonnie Prince Charlie's grandsons – but who were actually from Egham in Surrey – 'discovered' a late fifteenth-century manuscript called the *Vestiarium Scoticum*. Its authenticity was assured, they said, because they'd asked clan chieftains to 'check' their tartans against the book. In fact, it had happened in reverse. Clan chieftains had chosen tartans they liked and the Allens had turned it into a book. Much like the brothers, it was a complete fake. Even Sir Walter Scott was forced to conclude that the 'idea of distinguishing the clans by their tartans is but a fashion of modern date . . .'

Who wrote 'Auld Lang Syne'?

According to Robert Burns, it wasn't him.

Robert Burns (1759–96) never claimed to have written the song 'Auld Lang Syne'. 'I took it down from an old man's singing,' he wrote in 1793, in a note accompanying the lyric. He sent it to James Johnson, the editor of the *Scottish Musical Museum* (an anthology of traditional Scottish songs) stating that it was 'an olden song' that had never been written down. In fact, Burns was wrong about that – versions of it had been in print several times, including one as recently as 1770.

'Auld Lang Syne' originated in an anonymous fifteenth-century poem that went under various names in various different versions such as: 'Auld Kindries Foryett', 'Old Longsyne' and finally, in 1724, 'Auld Lang Syne'.

Pretty conclusive, you might think – but the song's

authorship remains a hot topic among Burns scholars. Only Burns's first verse and chorus bear much similarity to the song's previous incarnations. Some say he claimed the song was a traditional one to give his work extra credibility amongst antiquarians. Others argue that, whether the story of the old man was true or not, Burns had taken a traditional source, as in several other of his most famous poems (such as *My love is like a red, red rose*) and remoulded it into something stronger and more affecting than the original.

If you thought 'Rabbie Burns' wrote 'Auld Lang Syne', you'd be doubly wrong. Burns never signed his name 'Rabbie' or 'Robbie' (or, indeed, 'Bobbie' Burns, as some North Americans insist on calling him). His signatures included 'Robert', 'Robin', 'Rab' – and, on at least one occasion, 'Spunkie'.

Another piece of Burns-related pedantry you might want to bear in mind for New Year's Eve is this: the last line of the chorus isn't 'For *the sake of* Auld Lang Syne'. Since 'auld lang syne' already means 'old times' sake', this is tautologous (from Greek *tautos*, 'the same', and *logos*, 'word'). In Scots, 'for the sake of Auld Lang Syne' is the nonsensical 'for the sake of old time's sake'.

The two extra notes in the line – which is what makes people feel they need to add 'the sake of" – should be dealt with by singing two extra notes for each of 'for' and 'old'. Try singing 'For-or oh-old la-ang syne' next Hogmanay and be ready with the explanation. And say we sent you.

STEPHEN *What does it mean, Auld Lang Syne?*
DAVID TENNANT *Old long remembrance.*
BILL BAILEY *Old long signs . . .*

Which writer introduced the most words into the English language?

Not Shakespeare, but Milton.

According to Gavin Alexander of Cambridge University, who has trawled the entire *Oxford English Dictionary*, John Milton (1608–74) is responsible for introducing 630 words to the English language, beating Ben Jonson with 558 and John Donne with 342 – all of them way ahead of Shakespeare, who notches up a disappointing 229. Milton's neologisms include *pandemonium, debauchery, terrific, fragrance, lovelorn* and *healthy*.

Not that we can say for sure that these any of these authors actually 'invented' all these words; their work simply contains the first *recorded* use, and famous writers are much more likely to be read than obscure ones. If Milton or Shakespeare had filled their books with hundreds of completely new words, their readers and audiences would have struggled to understand them.

But English in the seventeenth century was in a state of creative expansion, rapidly overtaking Latin as the language of culture and science. All you had to do was find a reasonably familiar word in French or Latin and anglicise it: most educated people would quickly guess the meaning. It didn't always work, however. For example, Milton's *intervolve* ('to wind within each other') and *opiniastrous* ('opinionated') never quite caught on.

Readers who struggled with new vocabulary could turn to Robert Cawdrey's *Table Alphabeticall*. Published in 1604, it is generally considered the first English dictionary – although it isn't much more than a list of 3,000 'hard usual English wordes, borrowed from the Hebrew, Greeke, Latine, or French'.

English had to wait more than 150 years to get the dictionary it deserved. Despite being half-deaf, blind in one eye, scarred from scrofula, prone to melancholy and suffering from Tourette's syndrome, Samuel Johnson (1709–84) managed to write 42,773 definitions in nine years, assisted by six copyists. The equivalent French Dictionary took forty scholars fifty-five years.

Johnson's *Dictionary of the English Language* was published in 1755 and cost £4 10 shillings a copy (equivalent to £725 today). It didn't make him rich (it sold 6,000 copies in its first thirty years) but it did make him famous: for the next two centuries it was simply referred to as 'the Dictionary'.

Johnson's lexicographical standards remained unmatched until the *Oxford English Dictionary* appeared in the 1880s. His definitions were so thorough that 1,700 of them were carried over into the first edition of the *OED*. On the other hand, he had no words beginning with X and his etymologies were often dodgy ('May not *spider* be *spy dor*, the insect that watches the dor?').

One of the many pleasures of Johnson's *Dictionary* is discovering obsolete words ripe for revival. For example: *bibacious* (addicted to binge drinking); *feculent* (foul or grimy); *grum* (bad tempered); *keck* (to heave the stomach as if about to vomit); *lusk* (idle or worthless) and *tonguepad* (a great talker).

What were Richard III's last words?

'A horse, a horse, my kingdom for a horse' is one of the best-known lines in English literature, but the real Richard III never uttered them. His last words are among the few things about the battle of Bosworth Field in 1485 that were accurately recorded. They were 'Treason, Treason, Treason!' It was the last time an English king died in battle and it ended the Wars of the Roses in which two branches of the Plantagenet family – the Yorkists and the Lancastrians – effectively snuffed one another out, leading to the founding of a new ruling dynasty, the Tudors.

The last Lancastrian king was Henry VI. When his son Edward was killed at the battle of Tewkesbury in 1471, the Yorkists resumed power under Edward IV – followed by his son Edward V, then Edward IV's brother Richard III.

As a Lancastrian with a tenuous claim to the throne, Henry Tudor, Earl of Richmond, had spent much his life in exile. His arrival at the Welsh port of Milford Haven in August 1485 was at the urging of older exiled Lancastrians like John de Vere, Earl of Oxford, who sensed a chance of turning the tide in their favour with a new candidate for king. When Henry reached Bosworth in Leicestershire he had fewer than 1,000 Englishmen in his army. Most of his troops were French mercenaries or Welshmen. He'd never fought in a battle before, so he left the strategy to his generals.

What he was good at was marketing. After he'd won, he set about rewriting history, painting Bosworth Field as a contest between good and evil: the young idealistic moderniser versus a bitter, misshapen representative of a corrupt regime. This was so successful that definite facts about the battle are scarce. We don't even know where it was fought. In 2009 archaeological evidence suggested it was probably 2 miles south of the present official site. What we do know is that Richard became detached from his army and was surrounded by Henry's Welsh bodyguards. His supposed allies, Thomas Stanley, Earl of Derby, and his brother Sir William Stanley, chose this moment to switch sides. Hence the king's cry of: 'Treason, Treason, Treason!' as he was skewered by a Welsh poleaxe. Even Henry's official historian was impressed: 'King Richard, alone, was killed fighting manfully in the thickest press of his enemies.'

Richard, at thirty-two, was only four years older than Henry. The idea that he was a hunchback came from John Rouse's *Historia Regius Angliae* (1491), which merely said he had 'uneven shoulders'. He was certainly short but, according to contemporaries, he was good-looking with a strong, sporting physique. He wore heavy armour: an impossible feat for someone with a misshapen back.

Shakespeare was a playwright, not a historian. One of his main sources was the Tudor grandee, Sir Thomas More (1478–1535), who described Richard as 'ill featured of limbs, crook backed, hard favored of visage, malicious, wrathful, envious, from before his birth ever forward'. By no means everyone has bought into this enduring Tudor propaganda. As early as 1813 a plaque appeared at Bosworth putting the alternative version: 'Near this spot, on August 22nd 1485, King Richard III fell fighting gallantly in defence of his realm & his crown against the usurper Henry Tudor.'

When does 'i' come before 'e'?

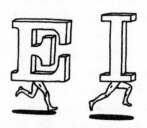

The 'i before e except after c' rule was abolished in 2009.

The old mnemonic was taught to British schoolchildren for generations, but *Support for Spelling*, a teaching aid published in 2009 as part of the British government's National Primary Strategy, now advises: 'The "i before e" rule is not worth teaching. It applies only to words in which the 'ie' or 'ei' stand for a clear 'ee' sound, so it is easier to learn the specific words.'

In fact, even with 'ee' sounds, there are still plenty of exceptions owing to the proliferation of foreign words in English. Caffeine, weird and Madeira all break the rule in one direction; species, concierge and hacienda in the other. Judging solely by the list of official Scrabble words, it turns out that the 'i before e except after c' rule is twenty-one times more likely to be wrong than right. No wonder the government dropped it.

English spelling is hellishly complicated. Many people, particularly in America, have tried to simplify it. In 1768, Benjamin Franklin published a phonetic *alfabet* containing all the familiar letters except c, j, q, w, x and y, and adding six new letters for specific sounds.

Melville Dewey (1851–1931), the inventor of the Dewey Decimal library system, changed the spelling of his Christian name to Melvil and toyed with adapting his surname to Dui. Late in life, he founded a health club in Florida where he put his spelling reforms into action. At one dinner in 1927 the menu featured *Hadok*, *Poted Beef with Noodles* and *Parsli & Masht Potato with Letis*.

George Bernard Shaw was another passionate advocate of spelling reform, leaving money in his will for a competition to create an easier system. The most extreme example of the way English doesn't always sound the way it's written (although Shaw himself never used it) is the made-up word *ghoti*.

In theory, this could be pronounced 'fish', using 'gh' as in rough, 'o' as in women, and 'ti' as in mention.

In the USA Mark Twain helped draft the Simplified Spelling Board's list of 300 recommended changes, which was accepted in principle by President Theodore Roosevelt in 1906 but rejected by Congress. Nevertheless, many of the simpler spellings did catch on, such as color, defense, mold and sulfate. Others like *profest* (professed), *mixt* (mixed) and *altho* didn't make the cut.

In the UK the Spelling Reform Bill passed its second

reading by 65 votes to 53 in 1953 but, after opposition from the House of Lords, it was withdrawn with assurances from the Minister of Education that research would be undertaken into the impacts and benefits of such a change.

The research confirmed the fundamental problem with all new language systems: that, unless they are adopted wholesale, by everyone at once, they lead to more confusion than clarity. The Spelling Reform Bill, like the 'i before e' rule, was relegated to the mists of history.

How many letters are there in Llanfairpwllgwyngyllgogerychwyrndrobwll-llantysiliogogogoch?

Admittedly, it looks like fifty-eight, but there are actually only fifty-one. Both *ll* and *ch* count as single letters in Welsh — along with *dd*, *ff*, *ng*, *ph*, *rh* and *th*. They're called digraphs: two consonants joined together to form a single sound.

Not that it matters, as only tourists (and tourist brochures) call it Llanfairpwllgwyngyllgogerychwyrndrobwll-llantysiliogogogoch. The village on the island of Anglesey, famous for having the longest officially recognised place name in the UK, is known locally as Llanfair. There are a lot of Llanfairs in Wales (it means 'church of St Mary'), so it's sometimes called Llanfairpwll or Llanfair PG, to distinguish it from the others.

Signposts opt for Llanfairpwllgwyngyll, while the Ordnance Survey map prefers Llanfair Pwllgwyngyll. Even the full name is seen with several variants of spelling, and sometimes with a hyphen between *drobwll* and *llan*. The English translation of the full name is: 'The church of St Mary in the hollow of white hazel trees near the rapid whirlpool by St Tysilio's of the red cave.'

When the first railway station on Anglesey was opened at Llanfair, local businessmen looked for a way to turn the unremarkable former fishing village into a tourist destination and came up with the idea of creating the longest station sign in Britain, made up of the existing names of the village, a nearby hamlet and a local whirlpool.

The local council adopted the imaginary place name, jokingly known as 'The Englishman's Cure for Lockjaw', in 1860. It was a hugely successful publicity stunt. A century and a half later, visitors still come to be photographed beside the station sign and to buy elongated souvenir platform-tickets. The village website also has the world's longest domain name. Llanfair PG has one other claim to immortality: it's the home of the first British branch of the Women's Institute (a Canadian invention), which opened in 1915.

Llanfair PG's full name is the longest in Europe, but the world record is held by the official name for Bangkok. This begins *Krung-Thep-Mahanakhon* . . . and stretches for 167 characters. In second place is a hill in Hawke's Bay, New Zealand, which comes in three lengths of 85, 92 and 105 characters. The most involved of these is: *Taumata-whakatangihanga-koauau-o-Tamatea-haumai-tawhiti-ure-haea-turi-pukaka-piki-maunga-horo-nuku-pokai-whenua-ki-tana-tahu*. Translated from the Maori it means, 'The hill of the flute playing by Tamatea to his beloved (he who was blown hither from afar, had a slit penis, grazed his knees climbing mountains, fell on the earth and encircled the land). Understandably, the locals just call it Taumata.

England's longest place name is only eighteen letters long. Blakehopeburnhaugh (pronounced *Black-op-bun-or*) in Northumberland combines elements of Middle English (*blake*, 'black'), Old English (*hope*, 'valley', *burn*, 'stream') and Old Norse (*haugh*, 'flat riverside land').

What's the proper name for the loo?

There isn't one.

The 'smallest room in the house' doesn't have a formal, standard, non-slang name. Whatever you choose to call it, you're using either a *euphemism* (from the Greek *euphemizein*, 'to speak nicely', *eu*, 'well' or 'good') or a *cacophemism* (from its Greek opposite *kakos*, 'bad'). In other words, you are intentionally using either a more polite or a ruder word for what you want to get across.

The John
Khazi
The Bowl
Porcelain
Throne
Dunny
The Can
The Lav
Privy

Lavatory comes from the Latin *lavatorium*, 'place for washing'. A *toilette* was originally a lady's dressing table – from *toile*, the 'cloth' laid across her shoulders when her hair was cut. By extension, the room became her *chambre de toilette*, in which she might attend to all manner of private functions.

No one knows where the word 'loo' originated, but it's probably a corruption of the French *l'eau*, 'water', or *lieu*, 'place'. Most English terms, whether coy, bawdy or comical, are euphemisms – such as restroom, washroom, bathroom, convenience, WC, comfort station, bog, chapel of ease, jakes, john, khazi, thunderbox, the necessary house, lavvy, the lavabo and 'the facilities'. In Edward Albee's play *Who's Afraid of Virginia Woolf* (1962), a dinner-party guest asks if she may powder her nose, to which the host replies, 'Martha, won't you show her where we keep the euphemism?'

This is a perfect demonstration of what linguist Stephen Pinker has called the 'euphemism treadmill', whereby one generation's polite term begins to attract the negative connotations of the object (or place) it is trying to hide, requiring a new euphemism to replace it. Toilet becomes lavatory, lavatory becomes WC, WC becomes restroom and so on.

Fashions change. Plain speaking about defecation and urination hasn't always been considered so ill-mannered. A respectable person in the first half of the eighteenth century might, without giving any offence, announce that they were going out to have a *piss* in the *shithouse*. But, unlike body parts, where we can sidestep both slang and euphemism by reverting to classical terminology – *penis, vagina, anus* – we have never had a single, universally accepted term to describe the place where we go when we ask '*to be excused*'.

This is an extraordinary achievement, given that every single one of us goes there on average 2,500 times a year.

STEPHEN *In Britain in 1994, you might be interested to know, 476 people were injured while on the lavatory. There you are. Underwear hurt eleven people.*
ALAN *How many of those people were drunk?*

How much does your handwriting tell about you?

It reveals who you are, but not what you're like.

We all find it easy to recognise the handwriting of someone we know well: the shape, size and slope of the letters are remarkably consistent. Graphology (from the Greek *graphein*, 'to write', and *logos*, 'study' from its original meaning, 'word') makes a much broader claim: that a person's character can be predicted from their handwriting.

For some reason, it's an appealing idea, but it's as inaccurate as judging a book by its cover, or a person's character from their clothes. All research studies into graphology have shown that it's much less useful in predicting a candidate's personality than, say, psychometric tests like the Meyers-Briggs Type Indicator, which uses ninety-three multiple-choice questions.

For this reason, the British Psychological Society ranks graphology alongside astrology as possessing 'zero validity'. The only reliable results handwriting tests can produce are to show whether you are male or female or have suicidal tendencies. Research published in the *International Journal of Clinical Practice* in 2010 confirmed that when graphological analysis was conducted on a group of forty people who had attempted suicide against a control group who hadn't, the graphological results clearly identified those 'at risk'.

There's a difference between using graphology to detect mental illness and employing it to see if someone has a talent for sales, or is 'trusting' or 'non-trusting'. Despite this, some 3,000 UK businesses regularly use graphology to vet potential employees. The suspicion is that this is used as a cover for illegal discrimination as regards a candidate's age, sex, race or faith. Consequently, in the US it's against the law to use graphology in job interviews. Such tests may be used to authenticate handwriting (when looking for forged signatures) but not to try to ascertain the physical or mental condition of the writer.

In its more reliable role of identifying someone, it was hand-writing analysis that sent Al Capone (1899–1947) to prison. Police accountant Frank J. Wilson (1887–1970) found three ledgers recording the business of an illegal gambling operation. The profits were recorded as going, in part, to a man named as 'A' or 'Al'. In an attempt to prove this was Al Capone, over three weeks Wilson collected handwriting samples of every one of

Capone's known associates in Chicago. Finally he found a deposit slip from a bank which matched the handwriting in the ledger. Wilson personally traced the bookkeeper who had written the ledgers (a man named Louis Shumway) to a dog track in Miami, and persuaded him to testify against Capone in return for immunity.

The highwayman Dick Turpin (1705–39) was also caught thanks to his handwriting. While in prison under the false name John Palmer he wrote to his brother-in-law asking for help. His brother-in-law refused to pay the sixpence due on the letter and it was returned to the local post office, where the postmaster – Turpin's old schoolmaster – recognised his handwriting. His identity was revealed and he was publicly hanged in York six weeks later.

How can you tell if someone's pleased to see you?

Ignore the shape of their mouth – a true smile is in the eyes.

French physician Guillaume Duchenne (1806–75) discovered the secret of the smile in 1862 by applying electric shocks to the faces of his subjects and photographing the results. He found that an artificial smile used only the large muscle on each side of the face, known as the zygomatic major, while a true smile, induced by a funny joke, involved

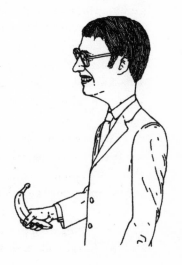

the muscles running through the eyes, or orbicularis oculi, as well. The effect is a visible wrinkling around the corners of the eyes that is outside voluntary control. In smile research circles, a genuine smile is still known as a 'Duchenne Smile', while a fake smile is a 'Pan Am Smile' – after the air hostesses in the defunct airline's adverts.

According to Duchenne, a fake smile can express mere politeness, or it can be used in more sinister ways 'as a cover for treason'. He described it as 'the smile that plays upon just the lips when our soul is sad'.

Research has borne out his thesis. In the late 1950s 141 female students at Mills College in California agreed to a long-term psychological study. Over the next fifty years they provided reports on their health, marriage, family life, careers and happiness. In 2001 two psychologists at Berkeley examined their college yearbook photos and noticed a rough fifty–fifty split between those showing a Duchenne or a Pan Am smile. On revisiting the data it was found that those with a Duchenne smile were significantly more likely to have married and stayed married and been both happier and healthier through their lives.

This was reinforced by a 2010 study of 1950s US baseball players. Those with honest grins lived an average of five years longer than players who smiled unconvincingly, and seven years longer than players who didn't smile for the camera at all.

The importance of the eyes in indicating genuine emotions is reflected in the 'emoticons' used in Japan and China. Western emoticons have a pair of fixed dots for eyes but change the mouth shape, like this:

:) meaning 'happy' and :(meaning 'sad'.

Far Eastern emoticons concentrate on changes in the eyes, but leave the mouth the same, like this:

^_^ (happy) and ;_; (sad).

This suggests that the supposedly inscrutable East is better at knowing (and telling) who's pleased to see whom than we are.

STEPHEN *What's the best way to tell if someone is lying?*
SEAN LOCK *What they've said turns out not to be true.*

What's the best way to get to sleep?

Whatever you do, don't count sheep.

In 2002 the Department of Experimental Psychology at Oxford University took a group of fifty insomniacs and got them to try different ways to fall asleep. Those using the traditional sheep-counting method took slightly *longer* than average. What worked best was imagining a tranquil scene such as a beach or a waterfall: this relaxes people and engages their imagination. Counting sheep is too boring or irritating to take your mind off whatever's keeping you awake.

The same study found that 'thought suppression' – trying to block anxious thoughts as soon as they appear – was equally ineffective. This is because of what psychologists call the 'polar bear effect'. Told not to think of polar bears, your mind can think of nothing else. Even the 'the' method many insomniacs swear by – repeating a simple word like 'the' over and over – only works if the repetitions are at irregular intervals, so that the brain is forced to concentrate. As soon you lose focus, the anxiety re-emerges.

The ancient Romans recommended that insomniacs

massaged their feet with dormouse fat, or rubbed the earwax of a dog on their teeth. Benjamin Franklin proposed that people finding themselves awake on hot nights should lift up the bedclothes with one arm and one leg and flap them twenty times. Even better, he suggested, was to have two beds, so that one was always cool.

More recently, clinical research has supported Progressive Muscle Relaxation: tensing each group of muscles in turn until they hurt, and then relaxing them. The idea is that an 'unwound' body will eventually lead to an 'unwound' mind.

TATT ('tired all the time') syndrome is one of the most common reasons for visiting a GP – one in five people in the UK report some kind of sleep disorder and a third suffer from insomnia. Sleep deprivation is linked to a quarter of all traffic accidents and to rises in obesity, diabetes, depression and heart disease.

Some sleep research seems to suggest that punctuating long working hours with brief 'power naps' of just a few minutes may actually be good for you. Or you could consider extending your working hours with new eugeroic drugs. (Eugeroic means 'well awake', from Greek *eu*, 'well', and *egeirein*, to awaken.) These are powerful stimulants that double the time people stay awake with no apparent side effects – as well as boosting concentration and memory.

They are unlikely to catch on in Japan at any time soon. The business of *inemuri* – 'to be asleep while present' – is a sign of high status, and Japanese politicians and industrial leaders will openly nod off in important meetings. Their visible need to nap in public indicates how hard they have to work.

STEPHEN *Do you know about Yan Tan Tethera? It's for counting sheep. It actually goes: Yan, Tyan, Tethera, Methera, Pimp, Sethera, Lethera, Hovera, Dovera, Dick, Yan-a-dick, Tyan-a-*

dick, Tethera-dik, Methera-dick . . . Bumfit suddenly appears, which is fifteen. And it goes all the way up to Giggot, which is twenty.

ALAN *So one in every fifteen will . . .*

STEPHEN *Will be a bumfit.*

PHILL JUPITUS *Are the last three sheep Cuthbert, Dibble and Grub?*

What happens if you eat cheese before bedtime?

Sweet dreams, it seems.

In 2005 the British Cheese Board organised a study in an attempt to nail the malicious rumour that eating cheese before sleep gives you nightmares. The results were conclusive. More than three-quarters of the 200 volunteers who took part, each of whom ate 20 grams (0.7 ounces) of cheese before retiring, reported undisturbed sleep. They didn't have nightmares (though most of them found they could remember their dreams).

Interestingly, different varieties of cheese produced different kinds of dream. Cheddar generated dreams about celebrities and Red Leicester summoned childhood memories. People who ate Lancashire dreamed about work, while Cheshire inspired no dreams at all. There also seemed to be a division between the sexes: 85 per cent of women who ate Stilton recalled bizarre dreams involving such things as talking soft toys, vegetarian crocodiles and dinner-party guests being traded for camels.

The overall conclusion was that cheese is a perfectly safe late-night snack. In addition, because it contains high levels of the serotonin-producing amino acid trytophan, it is likely to reduce stress and so encourage peaceful sleep.

It may come as a surprise to find that the British Cheese Board now lists over 700 varieties of British cheese – almost twice as many as are made in France. Having said that, 55 per cent of the £2.4 billion UK cheese market is cornered by just one variety: cheddar. Plus, the definition of 'cheese' has been stretched a bit to include such 'varieties' as Lancashire Christmas Pudding and Cheddar with Mint Choc Chips and Cherries.

The ninth most popular variety of cheese in Britain, Cornish Yarg, may sound ancient, but it only dates back to the 1960s when Allan and Jenny Gray started producing it on their farm near Bodmin Moor. 'Yarg' is 'gray' spelled backwards.

Despite the profusion of new British cheeses, the French still eat twice as much cheese per head as the British, and they sleep well on it, too. No one in France thinks that eating cheese before bed gives you nightmares.

What did ploughmen have for lunch?

Beer, bread, cheese and pickle. Yes, they really did.

The British movie *The Ploughman's Lunch* (1983), written by Ian McEwan and directed by Richard Eyre, claimed that 'the ploughman's lunch' was the spurious invention of an advertising man in the 1960s to encourage people to eat in pubs, and this has become common wisdom. It's since been alleged that the term first appeared in 1970, in *The Cheese Handbook* by one B. H. Axler. In the preface, Sir Richard Trehane, chairman of the English Country Cheese Council &

Milk Marketing Board, wrote: 'English cheese and beer have for centuries formed a perfect combination enjoyed as the Ploughman's Lunch.'

Recent research by the BBC TV show *Balderdash & Piffle* found documentary proof that the Cheese Council started using the term 'ploughman's lunch' to publicise cheese in 1960. But there is also evidence that the term ploughman's (or ploughboy's) lunch was used in the 1950s. There's also photographic evidence of ploughmen in the late nineteenth and early twentieth centuries sitting in their fields lunching on what certainly looks like bread, cheese and beer.

What seems most likely is that post-war cheese marketers were determined to remind the public of the long-standing practice of eating bread and cheese in pubs, which had been interrupted by rationing in the Second World War.

So, if ad men didn't invent the lunch, did they invent the phrase? Apparently not: there are anecdotal accounts of the name being used by pubs as early as the 1940s, and there is even a mention in an 1837 *Life of Walter Scott* of 'an extemporised sandwich, that looked like a ploughman's lunch'.

The cheese men certainly *popularised* the phrase as a marketing device, and perhaps on pub menus as well. In doing so, they helped turn a traditional, local name for bread, cheese, beer and pickles into a kind of non-copyrighted super-brand, universally recognised throughout the British Isles.

In the long term, though, only the cheese has benefited. Cheese sales have continued to grow strongly (up 2.8 per cent year on year in 2010), but Britain's last pickled-onion processor, Sheffield Foods, recently described the market as 'flat'. But not as flat as the sales of traditional beer which, despite the efforts of the Campaign for Real Ale, have declined by 40 per cent in the past thirty years.

Iconic though the ploughman's lunch may be, it hasn't

saved the institution that most relies on it. Over a hundred traditional British pubs close every month.

Where is Stilton cheese made?

It's not made in Stilton. That would be illegal.

Under European law, Stilton cheese – like Gorgonzola, Camembert and Parmesan – has Protected Designation of Origin (PDO) status. This makes it unlawful to sell it unless it's made in specified areas. In the case of Stilton, this means the counties of Derbyshire, Leicestershire or Nottinghamshire.

The village of Stilton, near Peterborough, is now in Cambridgeshire and was historically part of Huntingdonshire. In 1724, Daniel Defoe noted in his *Tour Through the Villages of England and Wales* that Stilton was 'famous for cheese' and modern cheese historians have shown that a hard cream cheese was certainly made in the village – but no one knows what it was like.

In 1743 the landlord of The Bell, a coaching inn on the Great North Road between London and Edinburgh (now the A1), started to serve an interesting blue-veined cheese. Because The Bell was in Stilton, travellers took to calling this popular new item 'Stilton cheese'. In fact, the publican, Cooper Thornhill, had discovered it on a farm at Wymondham nearly 50 kilometres (about 30 miles) away, near Melton Mowbray in Leicestershire.

So today Melton Mowbray, not Stilton, is the official capital of the Stilton industry, and has been since 1996. Oddly enough, it wasn't until 2009 that the town was granted protection for its most obvious local product: Melton Mowbray pork pies, under the slightly less stringent Protected

Geographical Indication (PGI). In the past, the local pigs that went into the pies were fed on liquid whey, separated out from the milk curd that went into making Stilton. Today, the pork meat in the pie is allowed to come from anywhere in England – but the pies have to be made *in* Melton Mowbray to a particular recipe.

Melton Mowbray pork pies are among thirty-six British regional PDO or PGI products, along with Cornish Clotted Cream, Whitstable Oysters, Jersey Royal Potatoes and twelve other British cheeses apart from Stilton. But not everybody wants one. In 2004 Newcastle Brown Ale became the first product to apply to be *de*-designated by the EU, so that it could move its brewery out of Newcastle across the river to Gateshead. In 2010 it moved out of Tyneside altogether – to the John Smith Brewery in Tadcaster, North Yorkshire. So much for tradition.

One of the British film industry's earliest hits starred a piece of Stilton. *Cheese Mites* (1903) outraged cheese manufacturers and caused screams of terrified delight among audiences. The film was considered the first-ever science documentary and it had been commissioned by its producer, Charles Urban (1867–1942) for a series of popular educational shows running at the Alhambra Theatre in London that were called 'The Unseen World'. It featured a scientist inspecting a piece of ripe Stilton under a microscope – only to discover hundreds of mites 'crawling and creeping about in all directions' (as the film catalogue put it) 'looking like great uncanny crabs, bristling with long spiny hairs and legs'.

Whether this had any effect on sales of Stilton is not recorded – but it did lead to a craze for cheap microscopes. These often came with a free packet of mites.

Where does the name Milton Keynes come from?

It isn't, as some people think, a combination of the names of the poet John Milton (1608–74) and the economist John Maynard Keynes (1883–1946). The town was built around a village whose name dates back to the thirteenth century.

The original 'Milton Keynes', with its traditional cottages, thatched pub and church, was in the centre of the area designated for development as a new town in 1967. Today it has renamed itself Middleton, after its first mention in the Domesday Book (1067), when it was Mideltone (Old English for 'middle farmstead'). By the thirteenth century this had become Mideltone Kaynes, after the village's feudal masters, the de Cahaignes. Since all Keynes's are descended from this family, you could say John Maynard Keynes is named after the place, not vice versa. John Milton has no connection with the area at all.

Only two of the twenty-one 'new towns' built in England between 1946 and 1970 take their names from people. Peterlee in County Durham was named after the miner's union leader Peter Lee (1864–1935), and Telford in

Shropshire after the Scottish engineer Thomas Telford (1757–1834). Perhaps because of this, when Milton Keynes was founded, a junior minister joked that the name 'combined the poetic with the economic' and an urban myth was born.

The supposedly boring image of Milton Keynes is the butt of many jokes from outsiders, but not from the 235,000 people who live there. The experiment to create a new town on the scale of a city has been a resounding success.

By 1983 34,000 new jobs had been created and 32,000 houses built. At that point, more than 5 per cent of all houses under construction in south-east England were in Milton Keynes. Today the local economy, driven by the rapid expansion of service industries, is one of the strongest in the country and the per capita income is 47 per cent higher than the national average.

Environmentally, the city is one of the greenest in Europe. There are 4,500 acres of parks and woodland containing more than 40 million trees – with a hundred more planted every day. The road grid and roundabout system may confuse visitors but they mean there is almost no congestion for people who live there.

MK (as residents call it) hosted the UK's first multiplex cinema, the first modern hospital to be built from scratch and Europe's first purpose-built indoor skydiving centre. It's also home to Britain's most popular theatre outside London and the Open University.

There's nothing dull about MK's past either. An archaeological survey carried out in advance of building the town uncovered the 150 million-year-old skeleton of an ichthyosaurus, the tusks of a woolly mammoth and Britain's largest collection of Bronze Age gold jewellery, the Middleton Keynes Hoard.

In other countries all this might be a cause for celebration, but not in England.

As Terry Pratchett and Neil Gaiman put it in their novel *Good Omens* (1990): 'Milton Keynes was built to be modern, efficient, healthy, and, all in all, a pleasant place to live. Many Britons find this amusing.'

BILL BAILEY *Satellite navigation, in cars ... when I was on tour ... it was useless. You get to Milton Keynes, it just goes, 'Turn left. Turn left. Turn left. Turn left. Turn left. Turn left.'*

Which kind of ball bounces highest: steel, glass or rubber?

It's the glass one. Steel balls are the next bounciest and rubber balls come last.

When a ball hits the ground, some of the energy of its downward motion is lost on impact. This energy is either absorbed by the surface of the ball as it compresses, or is released as heat. In general, the harder the ball, the less energy it loses (soft balls squash).

This assumes a hard surface. 'Bounciness' isn't just about the thing bouncing, but also about what it is bouncing off. Drop a marble, or a ball bearing, on to soft sand and neither will bounce at all. All the energy passes into the sand. Drop either of them on to a steel anvil and they will comfortably out-bounce a rubber ball dropped from the same height.

The scientific term for the bounciness of an object is its 'coefficient of restitution' or COR. This is a scale measuring the energy that a material loses on impact. It runs from 0 for all energy lost, to 1 for no energy lost. Hard rubber has a COR of 0.8, but a glass ball can have a COR of up to 0.95.

That's providing it doesn't smash on impact. Astonishingly, nobody really knows why and how glass shatters. The *Third International Workshop on the Flow and Fracture of Advanced Glasses*, a conference held in 2005 involving scores of scientists from all over the world, failed to reach agreement.

Many of the unique qualities of glass are a result of its not being a normal solid, but an amorphous (or 'shapeless') solid. Molten glass solidifies so quickly that its molecules don't have time to settle into a regular crystalline lattice. This is because glass contains small amounts of soda (sodium carbonate) and lime (calcium oxide) that interfere with the structure of the silica (silicon dioxide) atoms as they cool. Without these additions, the silica would cool more slowly. This would form chemically neat and regular – but much less useful – quartz.

Some scientists think that given enough time – maybe billions of years – glass molecules will eventually follow suit and fall into line to form a true solid.

For now, though, they're like cars in a traffic jam – they want to make orderly patterns but can't because their neighbours are blocking the route. The visible result of this underlying chaos is smooth, transparent, mysterious glass.

What's the most economical speed for driving a car?

For many years car manufacturers told motorists that the optimum driving speed for fuel efficiency was about 88.5 kilometres per hour (55 miles per hour). But it's much slower than that.

A fuel-efficiency study carried out in 2008 by *What Car?* magazine tested five cars of various sizes. It found that all of them did best at below 64 kilometres per hour (40 miles per hour), while two of the models reached optimum efficiency at speeds below 32 kilometres per hour (20 miles per hour).

On average, a car uses almost 40 per cent more fuel at 112 kilometres per hour (70 miles per hour) than it does at 80 kilometres per hour (50 miles per hour). It's a simple rule, the report concluded: 'The slower you go with the vehicle running smoothly, the less fuel you will use.'

It's not only driving fast that wastes money. Modern cars are quieter than ever. This gives the impression that the car is running smoothly when it's not, so drivers don't change gear as often as they should. Cruising at 64 kilometres per hour (40 miles per hour) in sixth gear uses 20 per cent less fuel than doing the same journey in fourth.

Air-conditioning can also cut fuel efficiency – by up to a mile a gallon or 1.6 kilometres per 4.54 litres. If you try to get round this by opening the window, you'll use more petrol battling the impaired aerodynamics. Even having the car radio on increases fuel costs.

During the recent football World Cup many England supporters drove around with flags of St George flying from their windows. In 2006 tests at the School of Mechanical, Aerospace and Civil Engineering at Manchester University found that two flags flapping from a medium-sized car travelling at an average of 48 kilometres per hour (30 miles per hour) creates enough wind-resistance to use an extra litre of fuel per hour.

In the USA almost three billion dollars' worth of fuel each year is wasted lugging overweight drivers around. Americans are pumping 938 million (US) gallons more gas a year than they were in 1960. Between 1960 and 2002 the weight of the average US citizen increased by 11 kilograms (24 pounds). Combining these figures, in 2006, researchers at the University of Illinois at Urbana-Champaign worked out that, with gasoline prices at $3 a gallon, transporting all this extra fat about by road cost the country $7.7 million a day, or $2.8 billion a year.

There are other advantages of driving at the right speed. The Energy Research Centre says that, if every UK motorist obeyed the 70 miles per hour speed limit, the saving in CO_2 pollution would be equivalent to removing 3 million Ford Focuses from the nation's roads.

What happens if you leave a tooth in a glass of Coke overnight?

It won't dissolve.

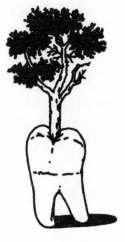

Not only do we know this is untrue, we know the person who first made the spurious claim.

In 1950 Professor Clive McCay of Cornell University told a select committee of the US House of Representatives that high levels of sugar and phosphoric acid in Coca-Cola caused tooth decay. In order to add a bit of drama to his testimony, he went further – claiming that a tooth left in a glass of Coke would begin to dissolve after two days.

It doesn't: as anyone who tries it on a lost tooth can discover for themselves. Even if McCay were correct, nobody holds Coca-Cola in their mouth for two days. The average can of soft drink contains about seven teaspoons of sugar, so it does cause tooth decay – but it does so gradually, not in a matter of hours.

Apart from sugar, the other troublesome ingredient in fizzy drinks is phosphoric acid. This stops the drinks going flat and adds a tangy flavour. It's also used in fertilisers, in detergents and in shipyards to remove rust from aircraft carriers. But it still doesn't 'rot your teeth overnight'. A 2006 study by the American Academy of General Dentistry on the effect of soft drinks on tooth enamel found that high concentrations of citric acid were much more damaging than phosphoric acid. So go easy on the orange juice.

Phosphoric acid also inhibits the digestive acids in the stomach, reducing the absorption of calcium. This means that a serious fizzy drink habit can lead to calcium deficiency, weakening teeth and bones (though not 'dissolving' them).

An occasional glass of Coke is unlikely to do anyone much harm. Coca-Cola was originally marketed as a health drink, growing out of the mid-nineteenth-century European obsession with 'tonic' wine: alcoholic beverages enhanced by herbal infusions. These often included coca, the South American plant extract better known as the source of cocaine.

In 1863 Pope Leo XIII awarded a medal to the Corsican chemist Angelo Mariani (1838–1914) for inventing Vin Mariani, the first coca-based wine. Millions of Europeans enjoyed it, including the Pope himself, Queen Victoria, Thomas Edison, Sarah Bernhardt, Jules Verne and Henrik Ibsen.

John Stith Pemberton (1831–88) of Atlanta, Georgia, soon produced an American version – Pemberton's French Wine Coca. In imitation of their European counterparts, the city's intellectual smart set took it to their hearts. But, in 1885, local prohibition laws compelled Pemberton to produce a non-alcoholic version. He pepped it up with the inclusion of caffeine-rich kola nuts from Africa and Coca-Cola was born.

Coca leaves are still used to flavour Coca-Cola – but only after they've had all the cocaine chemically extracted.

ANDY HAMILTON *My mum used to say to me, because I used to drink a lot of Coke when I was in my early teens: 'You shouldn't drink Coke because it stains the inside of your stomach.'*

HUGH DENNIS *But how do you know that's not true?*

ANDY *No, you don't, but you kind of think, well, if I ever see the inside of my stomach, it's probably going to be a bit late to worry about what colour it is.*

PHILL JUPITUS *I can't wait, Andy. I mean I don't like to talk about a friend's death, but at your post mortem: 'Look at this! Terrible stained intestines.'*

What happens if you cover a beautiful woman from head to toe in gold paint?

She won't die of suffocation.

Many people believe that we 'breathe through our skin', so that anything that blocks all our pores causes rapid asphyxiation. It's not true. We breathe only through our nose and mouth. The pores have nothing to do with it. If they did, scuba diving would be fatal.

Covering a person in gold paint might eventually kill them, if it was left on long enough. They would die from overheating, since their paint-clogged pores would be unable to sweat, which is the human body's chief means of temperature regulation. It would be a very slow and unpleasant way to go.

In the 1964 film of Ian Fleming's James Bond novel, *Goldfinger*, the actress playing the part of the woman murdered by means of body-paint was Shirley Eaton. She published her autobiography in 2000, despite the still persistent myth that she died of skin suffocation during filming. The producers of the film were as taken in by the idea of pore asphyxiation as their audience. Not only was a doctor on standby while Eaton shot her scene, but a 6-inch patch of skin was left unpainted on her stomach, to allow her skin to 'breathe'.

Human skin has about two million pores – about 700 per 6.5 square centimetres (1 square inch), each servicing a sweat gland. The skin is our largest organ, weighing an average of 2.7 kilograms (6 pounds) and covering 1.67 square metres (18 square feet). As well as the pores, a single square inch of skin contains around 4 metres (13 feet) of blood vessels, 1,300 nerve cells and 100 oil glands. Skin cells are constantly being replaced: in an average lifetime, we each get through 900 complete skins.

There is one mammal that *does* breathe through its skin. In 1998 scientists rediscovered the Julia Creek dunnart (*Sminthopsis douglasi*) – an Australian marsupial mouse 12 centi-metres (5 inches) long, named after the area in Queensland where it lives, from which it was thought to have gone extinct twenty years earlier.

Julia Creek dunnarts are unusually undeveloped at birth; their gestation period is just twelve days, and the newborn is slightly larger than a grain of rice. As a result, they can't immediately use their lungs, so they exchange oxygen and carbon dioxide through their skin instead: something previously thought impossible for a mammal. Researchers realised this after being puzzled by the fact that the newborn babies were neither breathing nor dying.

Being so tiny, the baby dunnart doesn't need much oxygen and, protected by its mother's pouch, can afford to have extremely thin, permeable skin. Indeed, its skin is *so* thin that its internal organs are visible. By the age of three weeks, however, it is getting half its oxygen from its lungs, and it

gradually switches over completely to the conventional
mammalian method of breathing.

ROB BRYDON *Do you know how he got the job, Sean Connery? He
went for the audition and then he walked away and the producers
watched him out of the window and they said he walked like a
panther. Which, when you think about it, would be on all fours,
and would make him look like a ruddy lunatic. Not the sort of man
you want botching up the schedule on an expensive film. Oh, look
at him, he's doing it again. Sean, please get up.*

What colour was Frankenstein?

Frankenstein wasn't green, nor was the monster he created.
The monster was yellow in the original book and black and
white in the film.

James Whale's movie *Frankenstein* (1931) was adapted from
the novel written by Mary Shelley in 1818. In the book, the
hero, Victor Frankenstein, isn't a doctor but an idealistic
young Swiss student, fascinated by science and alchemy. His
obsession leads him to create life from inanimate matter,
resulting in a 'creature' nearly 2½ metres (8 feet) tall made
from the body parts of corpses. In the novel, the way
Frankenstein brings him to life is barely described, but in the
movie a lightning bolt animates the monster. The spectacular
electrical effects were achieved using a Tesla coil built by the
brilliant Serbian inventor of AC current, Nikola Tesla
(1856–1943). He was then seventy-five years old.

In both the movie and the novel Frankenstein's reaction to his
creation is 'horror and disgust'. Here is Mary Shelley's version:

His yellow skin scarcely covered the work of muscles and arteries beneath; his hair was of a lustrous black, and flowing; his teeth of a pearly whiteness; but these luxuriances only formed a more horrid contrast with his watery eyes, that seemed almost of the same colour as the dun white sockets in which they were set, his shrivelled complexion and straight black lips.

It was to convey this 'corpse-like' effect that Jack Pierce, the make-up artist at Universal Studios, created the famous flat-headed, bolt-through-the-neck version of the monster, as played by Boris Karloff. Though the movie was shot in black and white, all the promotional posters showed him as green.

The film was a huge critical and commercial success, taking $53,000 (about $750,000 today) in just one New York cinema in its first week and leading to a string of sequels. When *Frankenstein* was adapted into comic book form in the early 1940s, the monster was depicted as green-skinned. This convention continued in the mid-1960s with the TV show *The Munsters*. Though the series was also made in black and white, all the publicity material shows Herman Munster (a comical parody of Boris Karloff) with lurid green skin.

Mary Shelley's creature was very different from the lumbering, inarticulate portrayal made famous by Karloff. He was agile, fast and could talk, albeit in a rather old-fashioned, ponderous way (he'd educated himself by reading Milton's *Paradise Lost*). Like a tragic parody of Adam, the first man, he refuses to eat meat and lives on 'acorns and berries'. He is driven to revenge and murder by Frankenstein's rejection of him, and by the loneliness and sense of shame he feels because of his hideous appearance. His last act is to trudge to the North Pole and burn himself on a funeral pyre to erase all traces of his existence.

Frankenstein, or The Modern Prometheus was written when Mary Shelley was only eighteen years old, and became an immediate sensation. As well as being a landmark in gothic fiction, many now consider it the first science fiction novel.

What colour were Dorothy's shoes in *The Wonderful Wizard of Oz*?

They were silver, not ruby.

L. Frank Baum's novel *The Wonderful Wizard of Oz* was the best-selling book for children in the USA for two years after its publication in 1900. Since translated into more than forty languages, it created one of the most successful publishing franchises of all time: Baum produced a series of thirteen sequels set in the land of Oz and many more were published after his death. He also wrote the script for a musical version, which ran almost continuously on Broadway between 1903 and 1904, and was the first adaptation to use the shortened title, *The Wizard of Oz*.

Under the new name, in 1939 MGM took the famous book and the famous musical and turned them into an even more famous film, directed by Victor Fleming and starring Judy Garland as Dorothy. In 2009 it was named the 'most watched' film of all time by the US Library of Congress. Although it did well at the box office, its huge budget meant it made only a small profit and it was beaten to the Best Picture Oscar by that year's other blockbuster, *Gone with the Wind*. But the immortality of *The Wizard of Oz* was assured by its annual Christmas screening on US television, which began in 1956. It's the most repeated movie on TV of all time.

Dorothy's slippers were changed to red in the film because

the producer, Mervyn LeRoy, wanted them to stand out. *The Wizard of Oz* was only the second film made in Technicolor and the new process made some colours easier to render than others. It took the art department over a week to come up with a yellow for the Yellow Brick Road that didn't look green on screen.

The new technology made the six-month shoot hazardous for the actors. The lights heated the set to a stifling 38 °C and eventually caused a fire in which Margaret Hamilton (the Wicked Witch of the West) was badly burned. The cast had to eat liquidised food through straws because their thick colour face make-up was so toxic. The original Tin Man, Buddy Ebsen, nearly died from inhaling the aluminium powder it contained and had to leave the film.

Lyman Frank Baum died in 1919, long before his book made it to the screen, although he ended his days in Hollywood as a film producer. This was the last in a long line of careers – as a breeder of fancy poultry, a newspaper editor, a theatrical impresario, the proprietor of a general store, a travelling salesman and a writer of over fifty books, many under female pseudonyms such as Edith van Dyne and Laura Metcalf. In 1900, the same year he published *The Wonderful Wizard of Oz*, he also brought out *The Art of Decorating Dry Goods Windows and Interiors*, which listed the many marketing advantages of using shop-window mannequins.

But it is *Oz* he will be remembered for and, despite all attempts at interpreting his novel as a political allegory or a feminist tract, it is best read the way he intended, as a home-grown American version of the fairy tales of the Brothers Grimm and Hans Christian Andersen that he had loved as a child.

How do you know if something's radioactive?

No, it doesn't glow in the dark.

Radioactivity isn't detectable as visible light. If it were, the whole earth would glow in the dark, as well as every plant and animal on it. Rocks, soil and living tissue all contain traces of radioactive material.

Radioactivity is not the same as radiation. Radiation is the means by which energy – radio waves, light, heat and X-rays – travels in space. These are all made of photons that spread out (or 'radiate') in waves moving at the speed of light. Though they are all made of the same stuff and travel at the same speed, their waves have different distances between the peaks and troughs, graded along a scale known as the electromagnetic spectrum. At one end are low-frequency waves (with long wavelengths) like radio waves; at the other, high-frequency waves with short wavelengths like X-rays. In the middle is 'visible light', the narrow band of electromagnetic energy that we can see.

All radiation is harmful if we're exposed to too much of it for too long. Sunshine – a mix of wavelengths from infrared (heat), through visible light, to ultraviolet – causes sunburn. At the high-frequency end of the spectrum, the energy is so intense it can knock electrons out of orbit, giving a previously neutral atom a positive electric charge. This charged atom is called an *ion* (Greek for 'going'). One ion creates another in a rapid chain reaction. This can cause terrible damage by changing the molecules in our cells, causing skin 'burns', cancerous tumours and mutations in our DNA.

Substances that do this are called 'radioactive', a term coined by the Polish chemist Marie Curie (1867–1934) in 1898. Although she invented the *word*, the French physicist Henri Becquerel (1852–1908) had accidentally discovered the actual *process* two years earlier, while working with uranium. Following in his footsteps, Marie discovered something a million times more radioactive than uranium: a new chemical element she called 'radium'.

Becquerel, Marie and her husband Pierre shared the 1903 Nobel Prize for their discovery and the 'invigorating' effects of radium salts were soon being hailed as a cure for ailments from blindness to depression and rheumatism. Radium was added to mineral water, toothpaste, face-creams and chocolate and there was a craze for 'radium cocktails'. Added radium to paint made it luminous, a novelty effect that was used to decorate clock and watch faces.

This is the origin of the radioactive 'green glow'. It wasn't the radium glowing, but its reaction with the copper and zinc in the paint, creating a phenomenon called 'radio-luminescence'. The phrase 'radium glow' stuck in the public mind. When the true consequences of exposure to radio-activity were revealed in the early 1930s, glowing and radioactivity had become inseparably linked.

Hundreds of 'radium girls', who had worked in factories applying paint containing glow-in-the-dark radium to watch-faces (and licking the brushes as they did so) were to die from painful and disfiguring facial cancers. And in 1934 Marie Curie herself died of anaemia, caused by years of handling the 'magic' substance she had discovered.

Which part of the food do microwaves cook first?

Microwave ovens don't cook food 'from the inside out'.

Microwaves are a form of electromagnetic radiation that sits on the spectrum between radio waves and infrared light. They are called 'micro' waves because they have much shorter wave-lengths than radio waves. They have a wide variety of uses: mobile phone networks, wireless connections like Bluetooth, Global Positioning Systems (GPS), radio telescopes and radar all rely on microwaves at differing frequencies. Although they carry more energy than radio waves, they're a long way from the dangerous end of the electromagnetic spectrum where X-rays and gamma rays reside.

Microwave ovens don't directly cook food; what they do is heat water. The frequency of microwaves happens to be just right for exciting water molecules. By spreading their energy evenly through food, the microwaves heat the water in it and the hot water cooks the food. Nearly all food contains water, but microwaves won't cook completely dry food like cornflakes, rice or pasta.

The molecules in the centre of your soup aren't heated any quicker than those on the outside. In fact, the opposite is true. If the food is the same consistency all the way through, the water nearest the surface will absorb most of the energy. In this regard, microwave cookery is similar to heating food in a normal oven, except that the microwaves penetrate deeper and more quickly. The reason why it sometimes appears that the middle of microwaved food has 'cooked first' is to do with the type of food. Jacket potatoes, for instance, and apple pies, are drier on the outside than the inside; so the moist centre will be hotter than the outside skin or crust.

Because microwaves work by exciting the water molecules, it also means that the food rarely gets much hotter than the 100 °C temperature at which water boils. Meat cooked in a microwave can be tender, but it is more like poaching than roasting. To break down protein and carbohydrate molecules rapidly and form a caramelised crust as in pork crackling (or to get the crisp exterior of a chip) requires temperatures of 240 °C or higher.

Microwave ovens are a by-product of the invention of radar in 1940. In 1945 Percy Spencer, a US engineer working for the defence systems company Raytheon was building a magnetron (the device at the core of radar that converts electricity to microwaves) when he noticed that a chocolate peanut bar in his pocket had completely melted. Guessing it was caused by the magnetron, he built a metal box and fed in microwave radiation. The first food he cooked in his improvised oven was popcorn; his second experiment, with a whole egg, ended in an explosion. The water in the egg had rapidly vaporised.

Raytheon was quick to introduce the first commercial microwave oven in 1947 and, by the late 1960s, smaller domestic versions had started appearing in American homes. Despite the various myths they have gathered down the years, they now occupy pride of place in 90 per cent of US kitchens.

Where did the British government plan to drop its second atomic bomb?

Yorkshire.

In 1953 British scientists seriously considered detonating a nuclear weapon next to the tiny village of Skipsea, on the East Yorkshire coast road between Bridlington and Hornsea. Home to just over 630 people, it has a medieval church and the remains of a Norman castle but not much else.

It was exactly this isolated, sleepy character – plus its convenient proximity to the RAF base at Hull – that commended the village to the scientists at the Atomic Research Establishment at Aldermaston. They were looking at various coastal sites in the UK for an above-ground atomic bomb explosion following their successful test detonation under the sea off the Monte Bello Islands, north-west of Australia, in 1952. Skipsea ticked all the boxes.

Unsurprisingly, the local community leaders were un- animously opposed to the idea, pointing out that the test site was dangerously close to bungalows and beach huts and that a public right of way ran through it. The Aldermaston team eventually relented and switched their plans back to Australia.

The results of the Maralinga tests in South Australia, in which seven above-ground atomic devices were detonated between 1956 and 1957, show just how close Skipsea – and the rest of the UK – came to total disaster. The interior of the whole Australian continent was severely contaminated, with testing stations 3,200 kilometres (2,000 miles) apart reporting a hundredfold increase in radioactivity. Significant fallout even reached Melbourne and Adelaide.

Maralinga was a site of great spiritual importance to the local Pitjantjatjara and Yankunytjatjara peoples (its name means 'Place of Thunder') and their evacuation was incompetently managed. After the detonations, there was little attempt to enforce site security and all the warnings signs were in English. As a result, many Aboriginals returned to their homeland soon afterwards.

Even more shocking, British and Australian servicemen were intentionally sent to work on the site to gauge the effect of radioactivity on active troops. It is estimated that 30 per cent of the 7,000 servicemen who worked at the location died from various cancers before they turned sixty. The effect on the Aboriginal inhabitants has been even worse – with blindness, deformity and high levels of cancer reported across the local population.

After pressure from the troops' veterans' association and aboriginal groups, the McClelland Royal Commission was set up in 1984. It concluded that all seven tests had been carried out 'under inappropriate conditions' and ordered a comprehensive clean-up of the site, which was eventually completed in 2000. In 1994 a compensation fund of $13.5 million was set up for the local people and limited payments have been made to Australian veterans.

At the time of writing, the UK government has produced no formal compensation scheme for British survivors of its nuclear testing programme.

STEPHEN *Where did Britain originally plan to test their atomic bombs?*

SANDI TOKSVIG *Was it Paris?*

Which two counties fought each other in the Wars of the Roses?

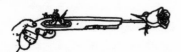 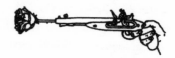

Neither the Yorkists nor the Lancastrians were based in the counties that bear their names, and neither side called the conflict 'the Wars of the Roses'.

The Houses of York and Lancaster were branches of the House of Plantagenet, which had ruled England for 300 years. They were unconnected with either Yorkshire or Lancashire. If anything, more Lancastrians than Yorkists came from Yorkshire and the remainder of the Duke of Lancaster's estates were in Cheshire, Gloucestershire and North Wales.

Most Yorkist supporters were from the Midlands, not from Yorkshire, and the Duke of York's estates were mainly concentrated along the Welsh borders and down into south Wales.

The 'Wars of the Roses' weren't wars in the traditional sense. The people involved certainly didn't think of them as such. They were really just an extended bout of infighting between two branches of the royal family. The event that provoked this rivalry was the overthrow of Richard II by Henry Bolingbroke, Duke of Lancaster, who was crowned Henry IV in 1399. There followed half a century of intrigue, treachery and murder, peppered with minor skirmishes, but it wasn't until 1455 that the first real battle was fought. And, even though the throne changed hands between the two sides three times over the period – with Edward IV (York) and Henry VI (Lancaster) getting two goes each – most of England was unaffected by the strife.

After the murder of Henry VI in 1471, there were three Yorkist kings in a row: Edward IV (again), Edward V and Richard III. Although Henry Tudor, the man who wrested the throne from Richard III to become Henry VII, was nominally a Lancastrian, his real intention was to start a new dynasty named after himself. The creation of the red-and-white Tudor rose was a brilliant bit of marketing on his part, supposedly merging the white rose of York and the red rose of Lancaster to symbolise a new united kingdom. In fact, until then, the roses had been just two of many livery signs used by either side. Most of the troops were conscripts or mercenaries who tended to sport the badge of their immediate feudal lord or employer. Even at Bosworth Field in 1485, the climactic battle that finally ended the conflict, the Lancastrian Henry fought under the red dragon of Wales, and the Yorkist Richard III under his personal symbol of a white boar.

But Henry's image manipulation was so successful that, when Shakespeare wrote *Henry VI Part I* in 1601, he included a scene where supporters of each faction pick different coloured roses. This so inspired Sir Walter Scott that – in *Ivanhoe* (1823) – he named the period 'the Wars of the Roses'. So it was 338 years after the conflict ended that the phrase was used for the very first time.

Even if they weren't really wars, or much to do with roses, and didn't involve inter-county rivalries, they were neither romantic nor trivial. The Yorkists' crushing victory at Towton in 1461 remains the largest and bloodiest battle ever fought on British soil. Some 80,000 soldiers took part (including twenty-eight lords, almost half the peerage at that time), and more than 28,000 men died – roughly 3 per cent of the entire adult male population of England.

Who led the English fleet against the Spanish Armada?

It wasn't Sir Francis Drake – he was only second-in-command. The top man was Lord Howard of Effingham, who later led the peace talks with Spain.

The defeat of the Spanish Armada in 1588 was the major engagement in the nine-year war between Protestant England and Catholic Spain that had begun in 1585. The Armada (Spanish for 'fleet' or 'navy') was the largest naval force ever assembled in Europe, with 151 ships, 8,000 sailors and 15,000 soldiers. It sailed from Lisbon in May 1588, with the intention of invading England.

Bizarrely, only thirty years before, Philip II of Spain had been King of England. He had co-ruled the country with his Catholic wife Mary I until her death in 1558. When Mary's younger Protestant sister, Elizabeth, succeeded her, Philip saw her as a heretic and unfit to rule. At first he tried to unseat her by guile, but his best hope ended when Elizabeth executed Mary, Queen of Scots (a Catholic, and the next in line to the throne) in 1587. His patience exhausted, Philip decided to resort to violence. He asked Pope Sixtus V to bless a crusade against the English so he could reclaim the benighted realm for the true faith.

Although it's often described as the greatest English victory since Agincourt, a full-blown battle never really took place. Instead, over several days there was a series of inconclusive skirmishes, in which no ship on either side was sunk by direct enemy action, although five Spanish ships ran aground in August at the minor battle of Gravelines, off what is now northern France. Drake's famous fire ships failed to ignite a single Spanish vessel – although they caused enough panic to break up the Armada's disciplined formation, allowing the smaller and nimbler English ships to get in and scatter them.

Eventually, both sides ran out of ammunition but Effingham had just enough shot left to harry the invaders northwards up the eastern coast of Britain. As the Spanish fleet, thirsty and exhausted, rounded Scotland and sailed down the west coast of Ireland going the long way home, many of their huge ships succumbed to unseasonably fierce storms. Only half of the 'invincible' Armada (and fewer than a quarter of the men) made it back. Although the English lost only a hundred men during the fighting, an estimated 6,000 English troops died in the months afterwards, from typhus and dysentery contracted while on board.

Drake may not have been commander on the day but, to the English, he was already the foremost hero of the age. In 1581, he became the first Englishman to circumnavigate the globe, returning with enough plundered Spanish gold and treasure to double the Queen's annual income. King Philip, of course, regarded him as no more than a common pirate and set a price of 20,000 ducats on his head (£4 million in today's money). The Spanish called the despised Drake by his Latin name 'Franciscus Draco' – 'Francis the Dragon'.

Did Drake really finish his leisurely game of bowls on Plymouth Hoe as the Spanish sailed into the Channel? We'll never know. The story is first mentioned in a pamphlet of 1624, which merely said that various 'commanders and captaines' had been playing; but such was Drake's mythic status that, by the 1730s, the story was told exclusively about him.

What did Cornish wreckers do?

They stole things that were washed up on beaches. There's no evidence to suggest that any Cornish wrecker ever actually caused a shipwreck.

The traditional picture of swarthy Cornish brigands on cliff tops, luring ships to their doom by waving lanterns or lighting signal fires, was invented in the mid-nineteenth century. It seems to have originated with Methodist preachers and then to have been fleshed out in graphic detail by Daphne du Maurier's romantic novel *Jamaica Inn* (1936).

During the great Methodist revival in Victorian times, clergymen used reformed 'wreckers' as living examples of the miraculous transformations that their brand of Christianity could effect; even the most debased sinners could be saved from their criminal pasts and go on to lead decent lives.

But such dramatic propaganda only worked inland. Coastal dwellers knew exactly what the ancient practice of 'wrecking' involved. It meant going down to the site of a wreck and scrounging anything you could get your hands on. It wasn't legal, but it was hardly murderous barbarism either.

Although an Act was passed in 1753 explicitly outlawing the setting out of 'any false light or lights, with intention to bring any ship or vessel into danger', no Cornishman was ever charged with the crime, and no authentic mention of the alleged practice has ever been found in contemporary Cornish documents.

The only such case ever to reach the courts involved the wreck of the *Charming Jenny* on the coast of Anglesey in 1773. Captain Chilcote, the sole survivor, claimed his ship had been lured to shore by false lights, after which three men had stripped his dead wife naked on the beach, and stolen the silver buckles from his shoes as he lay exhausted. One of the men was hanged and another condemned to death, his sentence later commuted to transportation.

The reason why this is the one known example of the crime in English history is because it doesn't make any sense for communities making a living from the sea – including working as pilots, helping ships reach shore safely – to set out to create shipwrecks. They could never be sure that vessels approaching on stormy nights were crewed by outsiders, rather than by sons or neighbours.

The belief that wreckers used false lights (sometimes allegedly tied to the tails of donkeys or cows) probably arose because smugglers used cliff-top lights to signal to their comrades offshore when it was safe to land. Luring fellow mariners to a watery end is no more authentic than the 'traditional Cornish wreckers prayer': *'Oh please Lord, let us pray for all on the sea. But if there's got to be wrecks, please send them to we.'* In fact, these words are part of an original song lyric written by London musician Andy Roberts in 2003.

Today, those who harvest the fruits of the sea in Cornish wrecker style can even avoid breaking the law entirely, provided they report their finds to the Office of the Receiver of Wrecks in Southampton.

How did the USA react to the sinking of the *Lusitania*?

Not by declaring war on Germany, as many people think. The *Lusitania* was sunk in May 1915. America didn't enter the First World War until April 1917.

From the summer of 1914 most of Europe was at war. Germany routinely attacked merchant shipping en route to Britain in an attempt to starve the country into surrender, but the US was determined to remain neutral.

At first, German submarines followed the so-called 'Cruiser Rules' laid down at the 1907 Hague Convention, by which civilian ships could only be sunk after all those aboard had been given an opportunity to evacuate. But when the British started disguising naval vessels as merchantmen and using merchant ships to transport arms, Germany adopted a 'sink on sight' policy. Winston Churchill, First Lord of the Admiralty, actually welcomed this, hoping that the Germans would sink a neutral ship, dragging America into the war. In a now infamous memo to the President of the Board of Trade, he wrote: 'We want the traffic – the more the better; and if some of it gets into trouble, better still.'

The *Lusitania* was a magnificent luxury liner, the jewel of the Cunard line. (She wasn't, as a common misconception has it, the sister ship of the *Titanic*, which was owned by the White Star Line.) As the *Lusitania* prepared to set off from New York to Liverpool, Germany placed adverts in US papers warning that passengers sailing through a war zone did so 'at their own risk'. Captain Turner of the *Lusitania* described this as 'the best joke I've heard in many days,' and reassured his passengers that with a top speed of 26 knots (nearly 50 kilometres per hour or 30 miles per hour) she was too fast for any German U-boat.

Just one torpedo was all that was needed to sink the ship, 13 kilometres (8 miles) off the coast of Ireland, on 7 May 1915. She went down in eighteen minutes with the loss of 1,198 lives – including over a hundred children, many of them babies. One survivor recalled swimming through crowds of dead children 'like lily-pads on a pond'.

On being rescued from the wreck, the hapless Captain Turner remarked, 'What bad luck – what have I done to deserve this?' Only 239 bodies were recovered, a third of whom were never identified. Among the dead were 128 Americans.

The British, and the pro-war faction in America, were delighted by the effect that this proof of Germany's 'frightfulness' had on US public opinion. The Germans, under the pressure of international outrage, promptly abandoned their 'sink on sight' strategy. (It wasn't re-adopted until January 1917, by which time Germany knew that war with the US was inevitable.)

Though President Woodrow Wilson's government refused to be swept into the war by popular anger, the military significance of the atrocity is not in doubt.

Some historians even argue that, by forcing Germany to suspend 'sink on sight' at a crucial stage of the conflict, the sinking of the *Lusitania* gave the Allies a strategic advantage that determined the outcome of the whole war.

When America did finally declare war in 1917, the US army recruited under the slogan 'Remember the *Lusitania*!'

Which radio play first made people think the world was coming to an end?

It was the BBC's *Broadcasting the Barricades* (1926). The work of an English Catholic priest, it inspired Orson Welles to adapt H. G. Wells's *The War of the Worlds* for radio in 1938.

On 16 January 1926 Father Ronald Knox interrupted his regular BBC radio show to deliver a news bulletin, complete with alarming sound effects. Revolution had broken out in London, he announced. The Savoy Hotel had been burned down and the National Gallery sacked. Mortar fire had toppled the clock tower of Big Ben and angry demonstrators were roasting the wealthy broker Sir Theophilus Gooch alive. 'The crowd has secured the person of Mr Wurtherspoon, the Minister of Traffic, who was attempting to make his escape in disguise. He has now been hanged from a lamp post in Vauxhall.'

It should have been obvious it was a spoof. For one thing, Knox was a famous satirist who had once written a scholarly essay claiming that Tennyson's *In Memoriam* was the work of Queen Victoria. Listeners who missed the BBC's announcement of the programme as a 'burlesque' should have guessed it was a joke on hearing that the leader of the uprising was a Mr Popplebury, Secretary of the National Movement for Abolishing Theatre Queues.

But this was only eight years after the Russian Revolution. Many upper- and middle-class people believed a communist takeover of Britain was imminent and took the ludicrous reports seriously. Women fainted and hundreds of people phoned police stations for details of the anarchy. The following day, as luck would have it, snow prevented newspapers reaching many rural areas, confirming the impression that civilisation had, indeed, come to an end.

The BBC rushed to offer its 'sincere apologies for any

uneasiness caused' and the press (which for commercial reasons was deeply hostile to radio) lost no time in exaggerating the depth of the 'unease' with headlines like 'Revolution Hoax by Wireless: Terror caused in villages and towns'. The BBC's Director General, Lord Reith, calmly totted up the complaints (249), compared them to messages of appreciation (2,307), and declared the show such a success that he wanted more of the same. Knox later obliged with a programme about an invention to amplify the sounds of vegetables in pain.

Ronald Knox (1888–1957) was the top classicist of his year at Oxford. Though his father and both his grandfathers had been Anglican bishops, he was inspired by G. K. Chesterton to convert to Roman Catholicism and became a respected theologian. Like Chesterton, Knox was also a prolific and successful writer of crime fiction. In 1928, he published 'The Ten Commandments for Detective Novelists'. They included: 'All supernatural or preternatural agencies are ruled out as a matter of course'; 'Not more than one secret room or passage is allowable'; 'The detective must not himself commit the crime'; and, more mysteriously, 'No Chinaman must figure in the story'.

The *New York Times* smugly reported Knox's *Broadcasting the Barricades* with the words: 'Such a thing as that could not happen in this country.' Twelve years later Orson Welles was to prove them entirely wrong.

What did US bankers do after the Wall Street Crash of 1929?

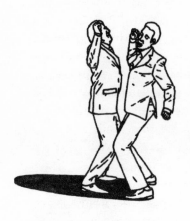

Only two people jumped to their death, and neither were bankers.

The prosperity of the 1920s encouraged millions of Americans to buy stocks and shares by using the value of the stock they were buying as collateral to borrow the money they needed to buy the stock itself. It was a classic economic bubble, and it finally burst on 'Black Thursday', 24 October 1929, when 14 billion dollars were wiped off the value of shares in a single day. Panic selling was so rapid that the New York Stock Exchange was unable to keep pace with the transactions as they were made.

Within hours, the legend had started: reporters were running around Wall Street chasing stories about ruined investors leaping out of skyscrapers. The following day's *New York Times* reported that 'wild and false' rumours were spreading across America, including the popular belief that eleven speculators had already killed themselves, and that a crowd had gathered when they mistook a man working on a Wall Street rooftop for a financier about to jump.

Comedians immediately started telling gags about the supposed jumpers, with Will Rogers tastefully noting that 'You had to stand in line to get a window to jump out of.'

None of it was true. Though there was a lot of panic and uncertainty, a fortnight after the Crash, New York's Chief Medical Examiner announced that suicides for the period were actually *down* on the previous year. John Kenneth Galbraith, the economist, corroborated this in his authoritative history, *The Great Crash* (1954), which concluded: 'The suicide wave that followed the stock market crash is also part of the legend of 1929. In fact, there was none.'

A detailed study of suicide records of the time, carried out in the 1980s, confirmed this. In New York, between 1921 and 1931, jumping from a high place was the second-most frequent method of suicide. Between Black Thursday and the end of 1929, a hundred suicide attempts, fatal or otherwise, were reported in the *New York Times*. Of these, only four were jumps linked to the crash, and only two were in Wall Street.

The two who actually did jump in Wall Street did so in November. Hulda Borowski, a fifty-one-year-old bond clerk, was said to be 'near exhaustion from overwork', while George E. Cutler, a successful wholesale greengrocer, became frustrated when told that his attorney was unavailable to see him, and leapt from the seventh floor of the lawyer's building.

In general, recessions do lead to suicide, though. A 30 per cent rise in the suicide rate was noted in the US and Britain during the Great Depression that followed the 1929 crash, and that pattern has been repeated in more recent downturns. A study of twenty-six European countries published in *The Lancet* in 2009 found a 0.8 per cent rise in the number of suicides for every 1 per cent increase in unemployment.

In the wake of the financial crash of 2008, American psychologists have even invented a term to describe the phenomenon. They call it 'econocide'.

Who was the first American to be buried in Britain?

Pocohontas. She was buried in the churchyard of St George's Church, Gravesend in 1617, aged twenty-two. She was also the first Native American to be baptised a Christian, to learn English and to marry an Englishman.

Pocahontas was born at Werowocomoco, near what is now Richmond, Virginia. The English translated her name to mean 'Bright Stream between Two Hills' but, in her native language, it seems it was a childhood nickname meaning 'Little Wanton One'. Her real name, like the other children's, was a secret known only to the tribe. Hers was Matoax, 'Little Snow Feather'.

She was the daughter of Wahunsunacawh, the Supreme Chief of the Powhatan Confederacy, an alliance of Algonquin tribes who lived around Chesapeake Bay. This was the area the English first settled when they established the new colony of Virginia in 1607. Pocohontas's father, known as 'The Powhatan', had ten daughters altogether, and he was about sixty when the English arrived.

When Pocohontas was ten, a hunting party led by the Powhatan's brother captured an English soldier and leading colonist called John Smith (1580–1631). According to his account, the little girl intervened to save his life, and he went on to become president of the Virginia colony.

At first, partly owing to Pocohontas's popularity with the settlers, relations with the Powhatans were good. But the situation deteriorated and, in 1610, the first Anglo-Powhatan war broke out. Pocahontas was kidnapped and held hostage.

Four years later, as part of the peace settlement, she was married off to an English widower, John Rolfe (1585–1622), the first man to export tobacco to England from Virginia. It was a political marriage. Rolfe wrote that he was 'motivated not by the unbridled desire of carnal affection but for the good of this plantation, for the honor of our country, for the Glory of God, for my own salvation'. The teenage bride's views are not recorded.

Baptised a Christian and renamed Rebecca, Pocahontas moved to England in 1616, living in Brentford with her husband, their son, Thomas, and a retinue of Powhatans. She appears to have been used as a kind of walking advert for the Virginia Company to show potential colonists and investors how charming the native Americans could be. For the last year of her life, she was famous. The Powhatans were a sensation at court, where Pocahontas was presented as a foreign royal, 'the Indian princess'. The diminutive King James I made so little impression on her that his status had to be explained to her afterwards.

A year later, the Rolfes boarded a ship to return to Virginia, but Pocahontas became gravely ill (possibly of smallpox), was taken ashore, and died. Her last words to her husband were: 'All must die. It is enough that the childe liveth.'

Though the Powhatan were dispossessed of most of their lands within a few years of her death, 'the childe' survived. Thomas's many descendants include Nancy Reagan and Wayne Newton, the Las Vegas entertainer, who is trying to recover Pocohontas's remains from Gravesend for reburial in Virginia.

Is there any part of Britain that is legally American soil?

Yes. It's the John F. Kennedy Memorial overlooking Runnymede, the meadow on the banks of the Thames where King John signed Magna Carta in 1215.

The acre of ground on which the memorial stands was a gift to the United States of America from the people of Britain in 1965. Formerly owned by the Crown, it is the only bit of Britain that is American territory.

Contrary to popular belief, the grounds of foreign embassies are not the sovereign territory of their state, nor are they beyond the law of the land in which they sit. The reason for the confusion is that nationals of the host country may not enter embassies without permission: refugees sometimes use them for this reason. If the authorities believe something illegal is going on inside the building, they have to wait for suspects to leave before arresting them. This doesn't apply to an ambassador or other diplomat, however, who can refuse arrest by claiming diplomatic immunity.

All diplomats in their host countries are immune in this way. The Vienna Convention on Diplomatic Relations states that they can't be arrested or criminally prosecuted by the host country for any violations of local law. The most the host country can do is to expel them, declaring them *persona non grata* (literally 'a person no longer welcome'). However, the diplomat is still covered by the laws of his home country and may be prosecuted under those laws when he returns home. The home country can also waive immunity for its own diplomats, leaving them open to prosecution by the host country.

The US Embassy is currently in Grosvenor Square in London (though it is shortly due to move to a new location in Wandsworth).

When the US government recently attempted to buy the freehold of the Grosvenor Square site from their landlord, the Duke of Westminster, he said that he would let them have it if the Americans returned to him the State of Virginia, confiscated from his ancestors during the War of Independence.

Which was the first film to star Mickey Mouse?

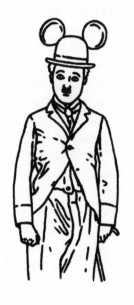

It wasn't *Steamboat Willie*, released on 18 November 1928 – even though the Walt Disney Company still celebrates this date as Mickey's official birthday.

There were two Mickey Mouse cartoons made earlier that year. The first was *Plane Crazy*. In it, Mickey tries to emulate the American aviator Charles Lindbergh (1902–74) by building a plane. He spends much of his first flight trying to force a kiss on Minnie Mouse, eventually causing the plane to crash-land. The second, *The Gallopin' Gaucho*, was a topical parody of *The Gaucho* (1927), starring matinée idol Douglas Fairbanks Junior (1909–2000). The film was set in a bar in the Argentine pampas, where Mickey smokes, drinks, dances a tango and fights the evil outlaw Black Pete to win the affections of the saucy barmaid, Minnie.

Both these films show a much raunchier Mickey than the saintly character he became. But they weren't widely distributed and didn't do well at the box office. Walt Disney (1901–66), and his friend and chief animator Ub Iwerks, had previously enjoyed great success with a series of shorts featuring their first animated character, Oswald the Lucky Rabbit. Universal Studios was the distributor for Oswald, but when Disney asked for a bigger budget, the studio demanded a 20 per cent budget cut instead and Disney walked out – without the rights to Oswald, and without his staff: only Iwerks joined him.

The two men decided to go it alone. They tried out cartoon dogs, cats, horses and cows but eventually Disney found inspiration in the pet mouse he'd once kept, growing up on a farm in Missouri. 'Mortimer Mouse' was renamed 'Mickey' at the suggestion of Disney's wife Lillian. In the first two shorts, Mickey was only slightly different (for copyright reasons) from Oswald the Lucky Rabbit, which may be why he didn't catch the public imagination.

Disney's solution was to make the kind of technical leap forward which would become a hallmark of his films. For his third Mickey Mouse short, *Steamboat Willie*, he recorded a synchronised soundtrack. Given that the first talkie, *The Jazz Singer* with Al Jolson, had been released only a year earlier, this was a remarkably bold move. *Steamboat Willie* was not only the first cartoon with a fully synchronised soundtrack: it was the first use of a soundtrack for a comedy. It was snapped up by a distributor and audiences loved it. Within a year Mickey Mouse was the most popular cartoon character in America.

Walt Disney went on to become the most awarded filmmaker of all time, winning a record twenty-six Oscars from a total of fifty-nine nominations. Mickey Mouse remained his talisman throughout and from 1929 to 1947 he voiced his most famous creation himself. As one employee put it: 'Ub designed Mickey's physical appearance, but Walt gave him his soul.'

Disney's life wasn't the wholesome, happy one he liked to portray. Addicted to sleeping pills and alcohol, he suffered from bouts of compulsive hand-washing, impotence and insomnia, which put his relationship with Lillian under great strain. He once remarked, only half-jokingly, 'I love Mickey Mouse more than any woman I've ever known.'

What was Dan Dare's original job?

He was a vicar. The legendary comic-strip hero started life as an Anglican priest: Chaplain Dan Dare of the Interplanet Patrol.

From 1950 to 1969, 'Dan Dare' was the lead strip in the *Eagle*. It sold more than 750,000 copies a week – unprecedented for a UK comic both before and since – and Dan Dare merchandise saturated the toy market in a way that wasn't matched until the advent of *Star Wars* and *Harry Potter*.

The *Eagle* was the brainchild of an Anglican priest and former RAF chaplain, Reverend Marcus Morris (1915–89), and a young graphic illustrator called Frank Hampson (1918–85). In 1949 Morris wrote a piece in the *Sunday Dispatch* attacking the importation of horror comics from America: 'Morals of little girls in plaits and boys with marbles bulging in their pockets are being corrupted by a torrent of indecent coloured magazines that are flooding bookstalls and newsagents.' What was needed, he said, was a popular children's comic where adventure is once more 'a clean and exciting business'.

Hampson and Morris's first co-creation was a strip featuring a tough East-End vicar called Lex Christian for the *Empire News*. However, the sudden death of the paper's editor meant it never ran, so Morris conceived a whole comic, which Hampson's wife christened the *Eagle*, after the shape of the traditional church lectern. The first two pages of the new magazine introduced a revised version of Lex Christian, now set in the future. Enter Chaplain Dan Dare of the Interplanet Patrol, complete with dog collar.

With Arthur C. Clarke as scientific adviser, Chad Varah (founder of the Samaritans) as script consultant and Hampson's revolutionary use of a studio of artists working from a huge library of photos, diagrams and 3-D models to create realistic blueprints for each frame, the *Eagle* idea found an enthusiastic publisher in Hulton (owners of the *Radio Times*). It was Hulton's eleventh-hour intervention that spared the children of Britain their first comic strip about a priest. The company felt that 'Dan Dare, Pilot of the Future' was a more commercial proposition and Hampson and Morris eventually agreed. Produced on the dining table of Frank Hampson's council house in Southport, the launch issue sold close to a million copies.

Hampson worked on Dan Dare until 1959, when the relentless pressure and recurring depressive illness became too much for him. He left the *Eagle* and toiled as an anonymous freelance illustrator for the next twenty-five years. In 1975 a jury of his peers voted him the best writer and artist of strip cartoons since the war. His *Eagle* had been a magnet for illustrators: it featured the first published work by David Hockney and Gerald Scarfe.

Dan Dare's Christian past was not without precedent. Superman's adopted parents were committed Methodists, although the Man of Steel never went to church in his tights – unlike Captain America, who was openly Protestant. Spiderman's Peter Parker had regular conversations with God, and The Thing in the *Fantastic Four* is Jewish. Wonder Woman, on the other hand, was explicitly conceived and drawn as an unreconstructed pagan goddess.

Why were postcards invented?

Not as tourist souvenirs – but as a speedy way of keeping in touch.

Postcards were the email of the pre-electronic age and the first medium of personal mass communication. Between 1905 and 1915, about 750 million postcards were sent in Britain each year, more than 2 million a day. The seven daily deliveries of post meant it was perfectly possible to arrange and confirm an appointment in the evening by sending a postcard in the morning.

The postcard era started in the 1870s when government postal services in Europe and the US began issuing pre-paid postal cards. By the 1890s, private printers had produced their own versions, with illustrations on the front and the words 'Post Card' moved to the back.

Between 1901 and 1907 postcard production doubled every six months. At the time, this frenetic activity was known as 'postal carditis' or 'postcard mania' and it was driven by three factors. Technological advances in printing meant that high-quality colour images could be mass-produced cheaply for the first time. Efficient postal services meant they were cheap to send (1 cent in the US; 1 penny in the UK). Finally, better public transport meant people had begun to travel much more regularly and adventurously.

This was the era of the great fairs and exhibitions. If you visited contemporary marvels like the Eiffel Tower, or the 1908 Franco-British exhibition at the White City, or the amusement arcades at Coney Island in New York, a postcard was the perfect way to prove it. On one day in 1906 200,000 of them were sent from Coney Island alone. Postcard collecting (or *deltiology* – from the Greek *deltion*, 'little writing tablet') became the world's number one pastime.

The parallels with email are striking. Advertising quickly saw the benefits and most of the nineteenth-century postcard traffic was a kind of spam, selling unsolicited goods and services. In 1906 Kodak brought out the 3A folding pocket camera that had postcard-sized negatives and a door that opened allowing a message to be scratched directly on to them. This meant that people could then have their own postcards printed – rather in the way we send attachments.

As with email, postcards had their detractors. The satirist John Walker Harrington wrote of postcard mania in *American Magazine* in March 1906: 'Unless such manifestations are checked, millions of persons of now normal lives and irreproachable habits will become victims of faddy degeneration of the brain.'

As 75 per cent of US postcards were printed in Germany, the advent of the First World War destroyed the German printing industry. This, and the arrival of the telephone, ended the golden age of the postcard.

But still they continue to thrive in the UK, especially from people at the seaside. The Royal Mail estimated that 135 million postcards were sent during the summer of 2009. The top five places they came from were, in order: Brighton, Scarborough, Bournemouth, Blackpool and Skegness.

Who made the first computer?

The key word here is *made*.

The mathematician Charles Babbage (1791–1871) is known as the 'father of modern computing', but more for his ideas than for any concrete achievement. The first full-size Babbage Engine, using his original designs, made exclusively from materials available in his day, wasn't completed until 2002. It is 3.3 metres (11 feet) long, weighs 5 tons, contains 8,000 parts and took seventeen years to build. It can be seen at the Science Museum in London.

In the nineteenth century, the British Empire ran on lists of calculations. From banking to shipping, every aspect of trade was dependent on accurate tables. Mistakes could cost money and lives and the books of tables were notoriously unreliable. It was in 1821 that Babbage decided to build a machine to replace them. Confronted by an error-strewn set of astronomical tables, he exclaimed to a colleague: 'I wish to God these calculations had been executed by steam!'

Babbage was a brilliant mathematician but found human beings difficult to deal with. His intolerance of street musicians led to an organised campaign against him: his London home in Portland Place was bombarded by noise at all hours and abusive placards were hung in local shops. He wasn't much better at handling the politicians whose support he needed to fund his work. Asked by MPs whether his machine would still produce the right answers even if wrong figures were entered, he replied, 'I am not able rightly to apprehend the kind of confusion of ideas that could provoke such a question.'

Despite patenting the cowcatcher for locomotives, and a pair of shears that made the metal tips for shoelaces, Babbage died embittered and forgotten. He had failed to find the money to build his greatest invention, a computer in the modern sense, with a memory and a printer, run by a programme that used punched cards. This first programming 'language' was the work of Ada Lovelace (1815–52), daughter of the poet Lord Byron, who understood the potential of Babbage's work even better than he did, predicting (in the 1840s) that computers would one day play chess and music.

Using Babbage's plans, two Swedish engineers, George and Edward Schuetz, completed the first prototype of what Babbage called his 'Difference Engine' in 1853. The father and son team not only built the first working computer of modern times, they sold two – one to an observatory in New York and the other to the Registrar-General's office in London. Each was the size of a piano.

But they weren't the *very* first. In 1900 a rusty artefact was discovered off the Greek island of Antikythera. We now know that the 'Antikythera mechanism' was a 2,000-year-old clock-work calculator that could predict astronomical phenomena with striking accuracy and detail.

What we now call 'computers' were originally called 'computing machines'. Until the mid-twentieth century, 'computers' were simply 'people who carried out computations'. So, strictly speaking, the correct answer to the question 'Who made the first computer?' should really be 'the computer's parents'.

What is paper money made from?

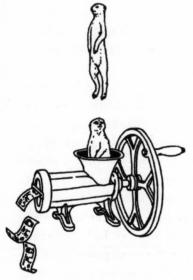

Money doesn't grow on trees. Not metaphorically and not actually.

Paper is made from pressed wood pulp. 'Paper money' is made from cotton or linen (sometimes called 'rag paper'). Cotton and linen fibres contain far fewer acids than wood pulp, so they don't discolour or wear out so easily. The cloth is then infused with gelatine to give it extra strength. This material is still used for folding money in the UK, the US and the European Union. The average lifespan of such banknotes is two years.

In 1988, after several years of research and testing by the Commonwealth Scientific and Industrial Research Organisation (CSIRO), Australia introduced a new set of banknotes made of polypropylene plastic. These last longer and are harder to counterfeit, as they make it easier to incorporate security devices such as holograms. New Zealand, Mexico, Brazil, Israel and the Northern Bank of Northern Ireland have now all switched to plastic notes. In 2005 Bulgaria introduced banknotes using the world's first cotton–polymer hybrid.

The first paper currency *was* made from wood-pulp paper. When gold and silver coins became too heavy to carry around, in the eleventh century during the Song dynasty, 'promissory notes' were issued in China. These were pieces of paper agreeing to pay over to the bearer the equivalent value in gold or silver coins if asked. The notes were made of dried, dyed mulberry bark printed with official seals and signatures. It was called 'convenient money'. It is thought that local issues of non-metal money were made as early as the Tang dynasty in Sichuan. Japanese banknotes still use paper made from mulberry bark.

This state guarantee of paper currency is the principle upon which most money is now issued. In the past, individuals and private banks were also able to issue promissory notes and this led to problems over guarantees. In 1660 Stockholms Banco in Sweden was the first bank in Europe to issue notes but four years later it ran out of coins to redeem them and collapsed.

Times of crisis have often led to emergency currency being issued on material other than cotton or paper. In 1574, when the Dutch were struggling to regain their independence from the invading Spanish, the city of Leyden produced cardboard coins minted from the covers of prayer books. During the Russian administration of Alaska in the late nineteenth century, banknotes were printed on sealskin. In Africa, during the Boer War in 1902, bits of khaki shirt were used.

Sometimes, the value of banknotes falls below the cost of producing them. The hyperinflation in Germany and Austria after the First World War meant that, by 1922, a single gold krone coin was worth 14,400 paper krone (a stack of cash that would weigh about 15 kilograms or 33 pounds). As a result, people improvised their own currency out of playing cards instead.

On a pirate's treasure map, what does X mark?

There are no documented cases of a real pirate ever drawing up a treasure map, let alone putting an 'X' on it to mark where the treasure is buried. Only one pirate, William Kidd (about 1645–1701), is ever recorded as having buried any treasure at all.

There is even some doubt as to whether Kidd was a pirate. Protected by a 'letter of marque' from King William III, he was privately employed by the British governors of New York, Massachusetts and New Hampshire to protect their coastline from genuine pirates or from the French. Legally, this meant he was not a pirate but a 'privateer' (like Sir Francis Drake). His enemies didn't agree; they vilified him as a ruthless, disrespectful and violent brigand. For example, Kidd's sailors once showed their backsides to a Royal Navy yacht instead of saluting it, and Kidd himself killed a disobedient member of his crew in cold blood. He became a political embarrassment and, when he was eventually arrested, the wealthy Englishmen who financed his voyages chose to hand him over to the authorities rather than be accused of piracy alongside him.

It is known that Kidd buried some of his wealth on Gardiners Island, off the coast of Long Island. He had hoped to use it as a bargaining tool to clear his name. However, he'd given the details to one of his backers who then dug it up and sent it on to London to be used in evidence against him. Kidd was tried and found guilty of piracy and murder. He was hanged on 23 May 1701, at 'Execution Dock' at Wapping, in London. His body was hung in a steel-hooped cage over the Thames and remained there for twenty years.

The first treasure map with an X marking the spot appears in the novel *Treasure Island* (1883) by Robert Louis Stevenson. Stevenson also introduced the Black Spot (the pirate's curse) and several piratical expressions including 'Avast', 'Yo-ho-ho' and 'matey' – though 'Shiver my timbers!' came from the pen of another Victorian novelist, Captain Frederick Marryat (1792–1848). It seems that 'walking the plank' was also a literary invention: the only recorded real-life case happened in 1829, well after most piracy had ceased.

Hardly any pirate booty was 'treasure'. The majority was food, water, alcohol, weapons, clothing, ships' fittings or whatever commodity was in the hold. The victims' ship itself might be sold or taken over if it was better than the pirates' own, and the crew and passengers were also valuable – either for ransom or to be sold as slaves. During the seventeenth century, over a million Europeans were captured and sold into slavery by Barbary pirates from Algiers.

Few pirates (or privateers) sailed in galleons. Most used galleys (with banks of oars rather than sails). Unlike the sailing ships that were their prey, these could be rowed against the wind and in any direction, even on a windless day.

Two privateers (though no pirates) are known to have had wooden legs: the sixteenth-century Frenchman François Le Clerc, known as Jambe de Bois, and Cornelis Corneliszoon Jol (1597–1641), nicknamed Houtebeen ('Pegleg').

There is no historical evidence for any pirate ever owning a pet parrot.

STEPHEN *Why would a pirate want to bury treasure?*

PHILL JUPITUS *Well, they can hardly go to the Bradford &*
Bingley, can they? 'Hello, we've got a chest full of doubloons
and booty.' 'Yes, would you like fixed term or extended
interest?'

What did early nineteenth-century whalers use to kill whales?

Not harpoons, but lances.

For the early whalers, the harpoon wasn't a killing weapon; it was used to attach a line to the whale. This was thrown by a specialist harpooner who stood up in a rowing boat with one knee jammed into a cut-out section of thwart called the 'clumsy cleat'. He hurled the harpoon into the whale from up to 6 metres (20 feet) away. The harpoon was attached to a 150-fathom (275-metre or 900-foot) rope impregnated with animal fat to help it run smoothly, coiled in a huge bucket on the deck and kept wet to prevent it catching fire from friction as it paid out.

When it reached its limit, the whalers were treated to a 'Nantucket sleigh ride'. This meant being pulled along by the whale at up to 42 kilometres per hour (26 miles per hour), the fastest speed any man had then reached on water. (Nantucket Island, off the coast of Massachusetts, was the centre of whaling in the North Atlantic in the nineteenth century.) Many hours later, the whale would eventually tire and the boat would row over to it. An officer would then change places with the harpooner to deliver the death blow with a lance (only officers could lance a whale). The cry of 'There's fire in the chimney' meant that blood was spouting from the whale's blowhole and the end was near.

The carcass was then towed alongside the mother vessel and cut up or 'flensed' from the deck using long-handled tools. Often, this exercise was a race against teeming sharks, which tore pieces of blubber from the whale while it was being butchered. Harpooning was such a dangerous profession that the Norwegians allowed only single men to do it.

Things changed in 1868 when Sven Foyn, a Norwegian engineer, invented an exploding harpoon gun. This did kill the whale and could be used from the deck of large, steam-powered vessels. It transformed whaling, allowing the hunting of faster, more powerful species, such as rorquals like the blue whale (from the Norwegian *röyrkval*, meaning 'furrowed whale', after the long pleats in their underbellies). Because rorquals sank when they died, later versions of the exploding harpoon also injected air into the carcass to keep it afloat.

The blue whale became the most profitable of all whale catches: a 27-metre (90-foot) whale yielded 15,900 litres (3,500 gallons) of oil. By the 1930s more than 30,000 blue whales were being killed annually. When the International Whaling Commission banned hunting them in 1966, the population of blue whales had dropped from an estimated 186,000 in 1880 to fewer than 5,000.

The eponymous whale in Herman Melville's *Moby-Dick* (1851) was named after a real albino sperm whale called 'Mocha Dick' who was often seen near the Chilean island of Mocha and who carried with him dozens of harpoons left embedded in his body from more than a hundred battles with whalers throughout the 1830s and 1840s.

In 2007 Alaskan whalers killed a Bowhead whale that had

the tip of a bomb harpoon dated to 1880 embedded in its blubber, which meant it was at least 130 years old when it died.

What makes the Penny Black stamp so special?

It's not their rarity, but their relative commonness that sets them apart.

A staggering 69 million Penny Blacks have been in circulation at one time or other. Many have survived intact. This is because, instead of using envelopes, Victorian letters were written on one side of a sheet of paper, which was then folded and sealed, so the address and stamp were on the reverse of the letter itself. If the letter was kept, so was the stamp.

If you have a Penny Black in your collection, you'll be lucky to get more than £100 for it. Even this is rather a lot considering how many of them there are – their value is kept artificially high by collectors sitting on hundreds of them and releasing them on to the market very slowly.

The world's most valuable stamp, the Tre Skilling Yellow, was sold at auction in Zurich in 1996 for 2.88 million Swiss Francs (about £1.8 m) and again in Geneva in May 2010 for an undisclosed price, all bidders at the auction being sworn to secrecy. If the paper that the stamp is printed on were a commodity sold by weight, it would retail at £55 billion a kilo. The best-known rare stamp is the 1856 British Guiana 1 cent Magenta, which has been kept in a vault since it last changed hands in 1980. Its owner, John du Pont, heir to the Du Pont chemicals fortune, is currently serving a life sentence for murder.

The most valuable British stamp is a Penny Red printed from plate number 77 in 1864. Plate 77 was corrupt and a few defective stamps went into circulation. There are only six known examples left. One is in the Tapling Collection at the British Library priced at £120,000.

Until Sir Rowland Hill (1795–1879), the social reformer and Secretary of the Post Office, introduced the Penny Black in 1840, it was the receiver not the sender of a letter who paid for the postage. MPs could send letters for free: they did this by stamping it with their 'frank' (a 'true' or 'frank' mark).

Sir Rowland Hill also invented postcodes. He divided London into ten districts each with a compass point and a central office. The original ten areas were EC (Eastern Central), WC (Western Central), NW, N, NE, E, SE, S, SW and W. All were contained within a circle of 12 miles' radius from central London. The present system was introduced in Croydon in 1966. It is made up of the outward code (e.g. OX7 – needed to sort from one town to another) and the inward code (e.g. 4DB – required for sorting within the town).

The first letterboxes were set up in Jersey, thanks to the novelist Anthony Trollope (1815–82). Hill sent Trollope to the Channel Islands in 1852 to see how best to collect mail on the islands, given the unpredictable sailing times of the Royal Mail packet boats. Trollope suggested using a 'letter-receiving pillar' that could be picked up whenever there was a sailing. The first box, erected in November 1852, was olive green. It worked so well that the Post Office rolled them out across the nation. By 1874 so many people had walked straight into the green boxes that red was settled on as a better choice. The Royal Mail still has a trademark on the colour 'pillar box red'.

STEPHEN *Do you know Jimmy Tarbuck? He was doing one of those Royal Command performances, and as he was going off, he looked up into the royal box and said, 'Ooh, that reminds me. I must buy a stamp.'*

When did women first show cleavage?

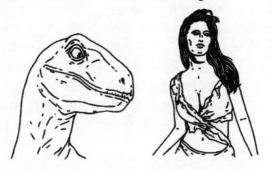

Not until 1946.

Until then cleavage was a word used exclusively by geologists to describe the way a rock or crystal splits.

In the 1940s, the British film studio Gainsborough Pictures produced a series of raunchy bodice-rippers collectively known as the 'Gainsborough Gothics'. *The Wicked Lady* (1945) was an eighteenth-century tale of a husband-murdering, society-beauty-cum-highwaywoman, starring Margaret Lockwood (then Britain's most bankable female star), James Mason and Patricia Roc. It was a huge hit in Britain, but the revealing costumes caused problems in the USA.

The Motion Picture Production Code Administration, popularly known as The Hays Code, was a voluntary system of movie censorship introduced in 1930 by Will Hays (1879–1954), the US Postmaster General. Its job was to spell out what was and wasn't acceptable to show on the screen. In 1945 it changed its name to The Motion Picture Association of America. The MPAA is still with us today: it's the body responsible for rating films as PG, PG-13, R and so forth.

When *The Wicked Lady* hit the USA, the MPAA demanded changes, but it seems they were overcome by coyness. They hid their embarrassment by using a dry geological term as a euphemism for 'the shadowed depression dividing an actress's bosom into two distinct sections'.

In 1946 *Time* magazine picked up the word when it reported:

> Low-cut Restoration costumes worn by the Misses Lockwood and Roc display too much 'cleavage'. The British, who have always considered bare legs more sexy than half-bare breasts, are resentfully re-shooting several costly scenes.

A new usage was born. Until the end of the Second World War, the partial exposure of a woman's breasts was covered by the French term *décolletage*, first recorded in English in 1894 and derived from *décolleté*, 'low-necked' (1831), from the verb *décolleter*, 'to bare the neck and shoulders'.

It's arguable that *décolletage* is still the prettiest way of putting it. In Middle English the 'cleavage' was bluntly called 'the slot' and, today, the best the International Federation of Associations of Anatomists can manage is the intermammary cleft or intermammary sulcus (*sulcus* is the Latin for 'fold' or 'furrow').

So it seems cleavage is here to stay: and the way it's used is proliferating. A lateral view of breasts is 'side cleavage'. A glimpse beneath is 'neathage' or 'Australian cleavage'. Bottom cleavage – a visible buttock cleft – has been known as 'builder's bum' since 1988. Toe cleavage, the partial exposure of toes by 'low-cut' shoes, is considered both sexy and stylish. According to shoe guru Manolo Blahnik, 'The secret of toe cleavage, a very important part of the sexuality of the shoe, is that you must only show the first two cracks.'

The back of a thong peeking over the top of a pair of jeans (which implies cleavage without revealing it) is called a 'whale-tail'. In 2005 the American Dialect Society voted it the most creative new word of the year.

What effect does testosterone have on men?

Contrary to popular belief, it's a *lack* of testosterone that makes people aggressive; if anything, surplus testosterone seems to make them friendlier.

Both men and women make testosterone, though the levels in women are, of course, significantly lower. It helps grow muscle mass, increases bone density and prevents osteoporosis.

In 2009 Ernst Fehr of the University of Zurich gave 120 women either testosterone pills or placebos, and then involved them in a role-playing situation. The mythic reputation of testosterone is so powerful that those women who *thought* they had been given it acted aggressively and selfishly (even if they'd actually received the placebo), whereas those who really *did* get testosterone behaved more fairly and were better at interacting socially, whether they believed they had received the pill or not.

Testosterone is linked to aggression in animals, so until very recently it was assumed to have a similar effect on humans. This seems not to be the case. It appears that *low* testosterone levels are more likely to cause mood disorders and aggression. Studies into testosterone have only been going on for ten years, so its function is not yet fully understood. Oddly, in the first few weeks of life, baby boys are pumped full of as much testosterone as they'll have in their teens, though this reduces to barely detectable levels by four to six months.

In 2004 Donatella Marazziti and Domenico Canale of the University of Pisa measured testosterone levels in two groups, each composed of twelve men and twelve women. The 'Love Group' consisted of people who had fallen in love in the previous six months, and the 'Control Group' were either single or in stable long-term relationships. The study found that men from the Love Group had lower levels of testosterone than men in the Control Group, while women from the Love Group had higher testosterone levels than their Control Group counterparts. The researchers theorised that, in the falling-in-love stage of a relationship, this apparent balancing act may serve to temporarily eliminate or reduce emotional differences between the sexes.

Testosterone is a hormone. Hormones (from the Greek word for 'impulse' or 'attack') are chemicals released by glands in one part of the body that use the bloodstream to transport messages to, and have an effect on, cells elsewhere.

Progesterone, a hormone associated with pregnant women, is also present in both willow trees and yams, which suggests it has a role that predates the evolution of modern animals.

Oxytocin is a hormone associated with maternal bonding, affectionately referred to by biologists as 'the cuddle chemical'. It can reduce fear, anxiety and inhibitions, and promotes social and sexual bonding as well as parenting. Neuro-economists (who combine psychology, economics and neuro-science to study how decisions are made) have experimented on subjects participating in a game called 'Investor'. They found that a squirt of oxytocin up the nose doubled levels of trust among players.

After a disaster, what's the greatest threat to the water supply?

No, we thought that as well – but it's not the dead bodies. It's the survivors.

The World Health Organization (WHO) states unequivocally:

It is important to stress that the belief that cholera epidemics are caused by dead bodies after disasters, whether natural or man-made, is false.

Cholera is an acute diarrhoeal infection, caused by the bacterium *Vibrio cholerae*. It is transmitted from infected faeces to the mouth, or by food or water that are contaminated. It kills through dehydration and kidney failure. In Europe in the nineteenth century, cholera was so common that it proved a great boon to unscrupulous heirs. People poisoned by means of small quantities of arsenic – known as 'inheritance powder' – were often assumed to have died of cholera, which has similar symptoms.

It can take mere hours to incubate – which is why it spreads so rapidly, overwhelming attempts to contain it – and can kill a healthy adult within a day. Although around 75 per cent of people infected with cholera don't develop symptoms, the germs can be present in their faeces for up to a fortnight, thus helping to spread the disease. People with damaged immune systems – through malnutrition, for instance, or HIV – are the most likely to die.

Most horribly of all, the perfect situation for cholera to spread is a refugee camp, where survivors of disasters are huddled together with inadequate supplies of clean water, and where human waste isn't safely processed. The same applies to a city where the infrastructure has been damaged by, say, an earthquake, a flood, or a 'humane intervention' with so-called 'smart bombs'.

Dead bodies don't come into it: cholera pathogens in a corpse rapidly become harmless. Yet the myth that the disease is caused by 'bodies piling up' is almost universally believed, with even the most respectable news outlets repeating it every time there's an outbreak of cholera following a disaster.

Perhaps the greatest tragedy – or disgrace, depending on

your point of view – is that cholera is far from incurable. Effective treatment – a solution of sugar and salts taken by mouth called oral rehydration – is simple and cheap. Given promptly, it saves the lives of more than 99 per cent of sufferers. And yet the WHO estimates that 120,000 people die of cholera every year.

Not that we want to alarm you, but we feel you ought to know: the seventh cholera pandemic in history began in Indonesia in 1961 – and it's still going on, having spread through Asia, Europe and Africa. In 1991 it reached Latin America – which hadn't seen cholera for more than a century. It is, by some margin, the longest of the cholera pandemics so far, probably because modern transport spreads infected people and foodstuffs with such rapid efficiency.

A pandemic is a worldwide epidemic. Pandemics generally end when there aren't enough people left to keep them going – because they've developed immunities, or been vaccinated, or (if you'll pardon the expression) died.

What positive effect did the Great Fire of London have?

It gave Sir Christopher Wren the opportunity to rebuild St Paul's Cathedral. What it didn't do was clear the city of plague.

No one knows what stopped the Great Plague of 1665–66, but despite what generations of schoolchildren have been taught, it definitely wasn't the Great Fire of September 1666.

The plague flared up in early 1665, probably carried on ships bringing cotton from Amsterdam. It was the first major outbreak in thirty years but, by the beginning of the following year, it had already begun to die out. In the last week of February 1666 there were only forty-two plague deaths reported in London, compared to more than 8,000 in each week of September 1665. The king had returned to London on 1 February 1666. Although it killed an estimated 100,000 people (20 per cent of London's population), the plague crisis was over six months before the Great Fire in September.

Also, the areas of London that burned down in the fire – the City, mainly, where 80 per cent of property was destroyed – were not the areas where the plague had been at its worst, which were the suburbs to the north, south and east.

No one really knows why the plague stopped. Perhaps it was spontaneous. That's how epidemics often end: by burning themselves out because they spread so quickly, and have such a high mortality rate, that they have nowhere left to go. It's one of the reasons the Ebola virus hasn't killed more people in Africa: a high (99 per cent) mortality rate means a quicker burn out.

Another possible reason for the disappearance of the plague in London was that the ancient method of barring the houses of known victims was policed much more aggressively. Doors were locked from the outside for twenty to twenty-eight days and guarded by watchmen. It's a fate that doesn't bear thinking about.

Even more difficult to comprehend is the story of the small hamlet of Eyam in Derbyshire. In September 1665 a bundle of infected cloth arrived from London for the local tailor. He was dead within a week. As the plague began to rage, the villagers (led by the Anglican vicar and the Puritan minister) voluntarily cut themselves off from the rest of the world so that it wouldn't spread elsewhere. When the first visitors were finally allowed to enter a year later, they found that three-quarters of the inhabitants were dead.

The disease had struck viciously, but apparently at random. Elizabeth Howe never became ill, despite the fact that she had buried her husband and their six children. Another survivor, against all probability, was the man who helped her do it – Marshall Howe, the unofficial local gravedigger.

Can anything live forever?

Yes.

Introducing the Immortal jellyfish . . .

The adult form of the species *Turritopsis nutricula* looks like any other small jellyfish. It has a transparent bell-like body, about 5 millimetres (⅕ inch) wide, fringed with eighty or so stinging tentacles. Inside is a bright red stomach, which forms the shape of a cross when seen from above.

Like most of the *Cnidaria* family (from *knide*, Greek for 'stinging nettle'), the tiny *Turritopsis* is predatory, using its tentacles to first stun plankton and then waft them up through its mouth-cum-anus. The females squeeze their eggs out through the same passage, after which the males spray them with sperm. The fertilised eggs fall to the ocean floor where each one attaches itself to a rock and starts growing into what looks like a tiny sea anemone: a stalk with tentacles called a *polyp* (from the Greek *poly* 'many' and *pous* 'foot').

Eventually these polyps form buds that break off into minute adult jellyfish – and the whole process starts all over again.

Reproduction by budding occurs in thousands of species – including sponges, hydras and starfish – and has gone on with few modifications for half a billion years. What makes *Turritopsis nutricula* so special is that it has evolved a skill unmatched, not just by other jellyfish, but by any other living organism.

Once the adult *Turritopsis* have reproduced, they don't die but transform themselves back into their juvenile polyp state. Their tentacles retract, their bodies shrink, and they sink to the ocean floor to restart the cycle. Their adult cells — even their eggs and sperm — melt into simpler forms of themselves, and the whole organism becomes 'young' again.

Newts and salamanders can grow new limbs using this cell reversal process, but no other creature enjoys an entire second childhood. Among laboratory samples, all the adult *Turritopsis* observed, both male and female, regularly undergo this change. And not just once: they can do it over and over again.

So although many *Turritopsis* succumb to predators or to disease, if left to their own devices, they never die. And, because individual specimens haven't been studied for long enough, we have no idea how old some of them may already be. What we do know is that, in recent years, they have spread out from their original home in the Caribbean to all the oceans of the world, carried in the ballast water discharged by ships.

It's an extraordinary thought. All other living things on earth are programmed to die. What does the future hold for a species that isn't?

A life-form in which each individual has the potential to found colony upon colony of fellow immortals . . .

THE USES OF INTERESTINGNESS

There are books in which the footnotes, or the comments scrawled by some reader's hand in the margin, are more interesting than the text. The world is one of those books.
GEORGE SANTAYANA (1863–1952)

We think all books, even the ones that are handsomely bound and come with an index, are still works in progress. If the pursuit of interestingness has taught us anything it is that there is no final word on any subject. For this reason we encourage you to scrawl furiously in the margins of this book or, better still, visit our website and pick up the conversation with us there. The address is www.qi.com/generalignorance. We'll happily share our sources and correct any errors we have made (and there are bound to be some) in future editions.

QI books are the product of long months of research by many people. The one you hold in your hands would not have happened without the first-class input of James Harkin, Mat Coward and Andy Murray, who researched and wrote the early drafts of many of the questions. They, in turn, relied on the work of the extended Elven family: Piers Fletcher and Justin Pollard (QI's Producer and Associate Producer respectively), Molly Oldfield, Arron Ferster, Will Bowen, Dan Kieran and the members of the QI Talkboard.

In the fourth century BC, Euripides, the great Athenian playwright, wrote that 'the language of truth is simple'. He didn't say it was easy. What success we have had in making complicated things seem simpler is due to the clear-sighted editing of Sarah Lloyd.

As for book-making, no one does it better than the team at Faber. Special thanks must go, once more, to Stephen Page, Julian Loose, Dave Watkins, Eleanor Crow, Hannah Griffiths and Paula Turner.

In a low moment the Victorian aesthete, John Ruskin, once complained: 'How long most people would look at the best book before they would give the price of a large turbot for it?' It's a good question. As we write, the wholesale price of turbot is about £9 per kilogram. We will make no further claims, except to say interestingness lasts longer and contains no bones.

The Two Johns,
Oxford

INDEX